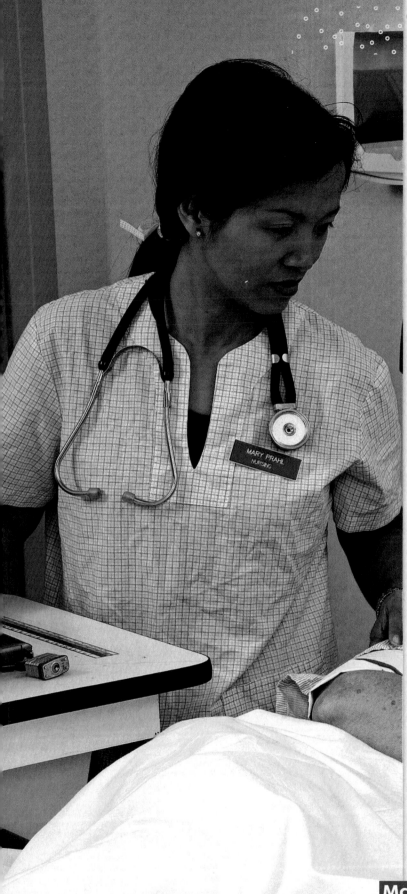

Essentials of Medical Language

2024 Release

Rachel C. Basco, MHS, RRT

Tim W. Gilmore, PhD, RRT

David M. Allan, MA, MD

Mc
Graw
Hill

ESSENTIALS OF MEDICAL LANGUAGE

Contents

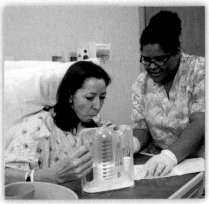
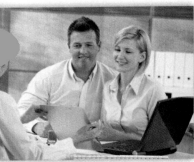

Chapter 3

The Integumentary System: *The Essentials of the Language of Dermatology* *34*

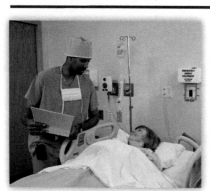

Rick Brady/McGraw Hill

Chapter 4

The Skeletal System: *The Essentials of the Language of Orthopedics* *63*

Rick Brady/McGraw Hill

Chapter 5

Muscles and Tendons: *The Essentials of the Languages of Orthopedics and Rehabilitation* **96**

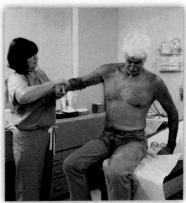

Rick Brady/McGraw Hill

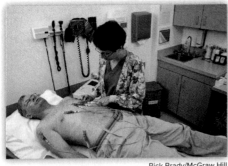

Rick Brady/McGraw Hill

Chapter 6

The Cardiovascular and Circulatory Systems: *The Essentials of the Language of Cardiology* **115**

Chapter 7

The Blood, Lymphatic, and Immune Systems: *The Essentials of the Languages of Hematology and Immunology* 144

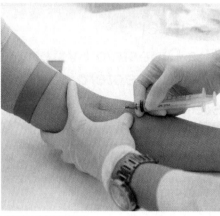

mikumistock/Shutterstock

Chapter 8

The Respiratory System: *The Essentials of the Language of Pulmonology* 183

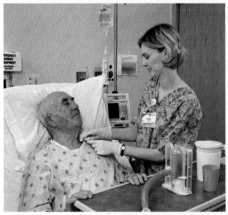

Rick Brady/McGraw Hill

Chapter 9

The Digestive System: *The Essentials of the Language of Gastroenterology* 209

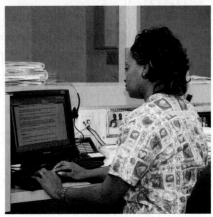

Rick Brady/McGraw-Hill Education

Chapter 10

The Nervous System and Mental Health: *The Essentials of the Languages of Neurology and Psychiatry* 248

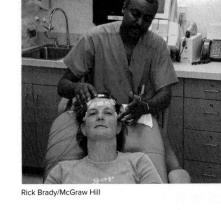
Rick Brady/McGraw Hill

Chapter 11

Special Senses of the Eye and Ear: *The Essentials of the Languages of Ophthalmology and Otology* 292

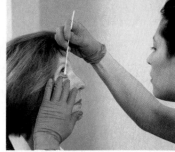

Rick Brady/McGraw Hill

Chapter 12

The Endocrine System: *The Essentials of the Language of Endocrinology* 331

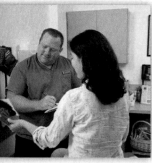

Rick Brady/McGraw Hill

Chapter 13

The Urinary System: *The Essentials of the Language of Urology* 359

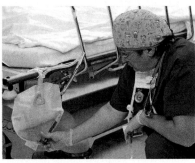

Rick Brady/McGraw Hill

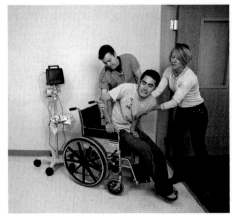

Rick Brady/McGraw-Hill Education

Chapter 14

The Male Reproductive System: *The Essentials of the Language of the Male Reproductive System* 378

Chapter 15

The Female Reproductive System: *The Essentials of the Languages of Gynecology and Obstetrics* 397

Rick Brady/McGraw-Hill Education

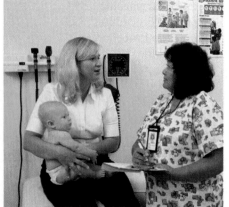

Rick Brady/McGraw-Hill Education

Chapter 16

Infancy to Old Age: *The Languages of Pediatrics and Geriatrics* 440

WHAT HELPS STUDENTS LEARN MEDICAL TERMINOLOGY

THIS TEXTBOOK INCORPORATES FEATURES DESIGNED TO ADDRESS THESE FACTORS:

Motivation to learn	→	For students to stay motivated and engaged in their learning, it's important that what they're studying feels relevant and meaningful. To make sure that each chapter of *Essentials of Medical Language* meets this standard, students are invited to imagine themselves as allied health professionals as they work through the material. By using authentic patient scenarios, the text demonstrates how medical language is applied in real-world job settings.
Retention of the material	→	When students encounter new medical terms within the context of a patient case, they are able to remember it more effectively. In addition, each chapter presents medical terms from one body system or medical specialty, which further serves to "tie it all together" to help students retain the knowledge and skills.
Opportunities for application and practice	→	Practice makes perfect. This is especially true for learning medical terminology. This textbook provides many opportunities for students to apply what they are learning. Exercises are included at the end of each chapter section, and are available in Connect for practice. Chapter review questions are also included in Connect to reinforce students' mastery of the terminology in each chapter.

Essentials of Medical Language will help you learn the terminology and language of modern health care in a way that bridges the gap between the classroom and a clinical setting.

RELEVANT MATERIALS—YOUR MOTIVATION TO LEARN!
Essentials of Medical Language provides you with terminology, exercises, images and examples you can apply to other courses and within your career. You will step into the role of a health professional in every chapter and experience medical language illustrated through authentic patient cases.

BODY SYSTEMS AND MEDICAL SPECIALTIES—REMEMBER AND APPLY THE MATERIAL!
Encountering new medical terms within the context of each patient case will help you remember them more effectively. Every chapter presents medical terms from one body system or medical specialty, which helps tie it all together!

APPLICATION AND PRACTICE—YOUR KEY TO MASTERING MEDICAL TERMINOLOGY!
Practice makes perfect, especially when you are learning medical terminology. You will have plenty of opportunity to apply what you learn through exercises at the end of every section. Additional practice opportunities and exercises are available through SmartBook and Connect.

EXERCISES

A. Build *your knowledge of the elements and terms that make up the language of the cardiovascular system. Fill in the blanks.* **LO 6.2 and 6.6**

1. A small vein leading away from a capillary network: _____ .

2. To disseminate or spread out: _____

3. State of equilibrium in the body is called _____ .

4. The two largest veins in the body are collectively called _____ .

B. Construct *the correct medical term to match the definition. If the term does not have a particular element, insert N/A. Fill in the blanks.* **LO 6.1, 6.2, and 6.7**

1. minute blood vessel between the arterial and venous systems:

_____ / _____ / _____		
P	R/CF	S

2. small terminal artery leading into the capillary network:

_____ / _____ / _____		
P	R/CF	S

3. state of equilibrium in the environment:

_____ / _____ / _____		
P	R/CF	S

4. small vein leading from the capillary network:

_____ / _____ / _____		
P	R/CF	S

To the instructor

McGraw Hill knows how much effort it takes to prepare for a new course. Through focus groups, symposia, reviews, and conversations with instructors like you, we have gathered information about what materials you need in order to facilitate successful courses. We are committed to providing you with high-quality, accurate instructor support.

New!

1. The Word Analysis and Definition (WAD) tables and review exercises have been updated, and new terms have been added.

2. Every chapter has been reorganized into sections that are consistent across all chapters.

3. Case Reports and Exercises have been grouped to the end of each section.

4. Pronunciation questions have been added to each chapter to develop effective communication.

5. PowerPoint slides are updated to reflect the change in chapter organization. Slides contain chapter images along with questions relevant to course content.

Word Analysis and Definition

S = Suffix   P = Prefix   R = Root   R/CF = Combining Form

WORD	PRONUNCIATION	ELEMENTS		DEFINITION
cardiomegaly	KAR-dee-oh-MEG-ah-lee	S/ R/CF	-megaly *enlargement* cardi/o- *heart*	Enlargement of the heart
cardiomyopathy	KAR-dee-oh-my-OP-ah-thee	S/ R/CF R/CF	-pathy *disease* cardi/o -*heart* -my/o- *muscle*	Disease of the heart muscle, the myocardium
cor pulmonale	KOR pul-moh-NAH-lee	 S/ R/	cor Latin *heart* -ale *pertaining to* pulmon- *lung*	Right-sided heart failure arising from chronic lung disease
endocarditis (**Note:** The extra "i" from the root *cardi* is dropped when joined to the suffix -*itis.*)	EN-doh-kar-DIE-tis	S/ P/ R/	-itis *inflammation* endo- *within* -cardi- *heart*	Inflammation of the lining of the heart
exudate	EKS-you-date	S/ P/ R/	-ate *pertaining to* ex- *out of* -sud- *sweat*	Fluid that has passed out of a tissue or capillaries as a result of inflammation or injury
hypertrophy (can be a noun or a verb)	high-PER-troh-fee	P/ R/	hyper- *above, excessive* -trophy *development*	Increase in size, but not in number, of an individual tissue element
incompetence (**Note:** *Same as insufficiency*)	in-KOM-peh-tense	S/ P/ R/	-ence *quality of* in- *not* -compet- *strive together*	Failure of a valve to close completely
insufficiency (**Note:** *Same as incompetence*)	in-suh-FISH-en-see	S/ P/ R/CF	-ency *quality of* in- *not* –suffic/i- *enough*	Lack of completeness of function; e.g., a heart valve that fails to close properly
myocarditis (**Note:** The extra "i" from the root *cardi* is dropped when joined to the suffix -*itis.*)	MY-oh-kar-DIE-tis	S/ R/CF R/	-itis *inflammation* my/o- *muscle* -cardi- *heart*	Inflammation of the heart muscle
pericarditis (**Note:** The extra "i" from the root *cardi* is dropped when joined to the suffix -*itis.*)	PER-ih-kar-DIE-tis	S/ P/ R/	-itis *inflammation* peri- *around* -cardi- *heart*	Inflammation of the pericardium, the covering of the heart
prolapse	pro-LAPS		Latin a *falling*	An organ slips out of its normal position
regurgitate	ree-GUR-jih-tate	S/ P/ R/	-ate *pertaining to* re- *back* -gurgit- *flood*	To flow backward; e.g., blood through a heart valve
stenosis	ste-NOH-sis	S/ R/CF	-sis *abnormal condition* sten/o- *narrow*	Narrowing of a canal or passage, e.g., of a heart valve
tamponade	tam-poh-NAID	S/ R/	-ade *a process* tampon- *plug*	Pathologic compression of an organ, such as the heart

When you use *Essentials of Medical Language,* you will be supported at every point in the program. Each chapter in the book is broken down into sections, and the Instructor's Manual provides lesson plans and additional materials for each section. Following are features of the textbook designed to address student needs.

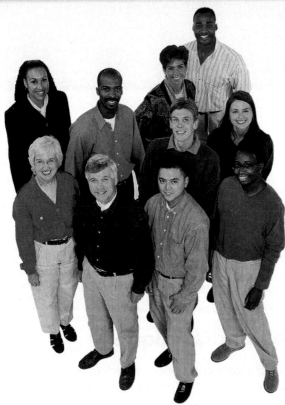

C Squared Studios/Getty Images

Chapter Organization

In this new edition, chapters have been organized for consistency and continuity to enhance student retention. For all major organ systems, the chapters will be placed in sections and will begin with an overview of the anatomy and physiology of the system. The following section will cover the common pathology associated with that organ system. The final sections will cover diagnostic and therapeutic procedures along with pharmacology. Each chapter is structured around a consistent and unique framework of learning devices including illustrations, Word Analysis and Definition (WAD) tables, and end-of-section Exercises. Regardless of the organ system being covered, the structure enables you to develop a consistent learning strategy.

Chapter Outcomes

The major learning outcomes for each chapter are presented in the beginning so you and your students can focus on what they need to know and be able to do by the end of the chapter.

Word Analysis and Definition (WAD) Tables and Case Reports

Each section contains **Word Analysis and Definition (WAD)** tables listing important medical terms and their pronunciation, elements, and definition. Prefixes, suffixes, and combining forms are color-coded. These tables provide your students with an at-a-glance view of the terms covered. The tables are excellent for reference as well as for studying and reviewing. **Case Reports** can be found within end of section exercises providing the students opportunities to apply and reinforce their knowledge of medical terms.

Exercises

In addition to the exercises at the end of each section, chapter review exercises are included in *Connect* (http://connect.mheducation.com). All these exercises are graded in their difficulty according to Bloom's Taxonomy and are tied to Chapter Learning Outcomes.

Attention is given to developing skills in spelling, forming plurals, using accepted abbreviations, writing medical language, and pronunciation. The exercises take the learner beyond memorization and teach how to think critically about the realistic application of the medical language being learned.

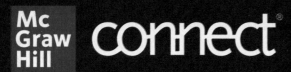

A complete course platform

Connect enables you to build deeper connections with your students through cohesive digital content and tools, creating engaging learning experiences. We are committed to providing you with the right resources and tools to support all your students along their personal learning journeys.

65%
Less Time Grading

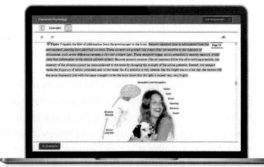

Laptop: Getty Images; Woman/dog: George Doyle/Getty Images

Every learner is unique

In Connect, instructors can assign an adaptive reading experience with SmartBook®. Rooted in advanced learning science principles, SmartBook delivers each student a personalized experience, focusing students on their learning gaps, ensuring that the time they spend studying is time well spent. **mheducation.com/highered/connect/smartbook**

Study anytime, anywhere

Encourage your students to download the free ReadAnywhere® app so they can access their online eBook, SmartBook®, or Adaptive Learning Assignments when it's convenient, even when they're offline. And since the app automatically syncs with their Connect account, all of their work is available every time they open it. Find out more at **mheducation.com/readanywhere**

"I really liked this app— it made it easy to study when you don't have your textbook in front of you."

Jordan Cunningham, a student at *Eastern Washington University*

Effective tools for efficient studying

Connect is designed to help students be more productive with simple, flexible, intuitive tools that maximize study time and meet students' individual learning needs. Get learning that works for everyone with Connect.

Education for all

McGraw Hill works directly with Accessibility Services departments and faculty to meet the learning needs of all students. Please contact your Accessibility Services Office, and ask them to email **accessibility@mheducation.com**, or visit **mheducation.com/about/accessibility** for more information.

Affordable solutions, added value

Make technology work for you with LMS integration for single sign-on access, mobile access to the digital textbook, and reports to quickly show you how each of your students is doing. And with our Inclusive Access program, you can provide all these tools at the lowest available market price to your students. Ask your McGraw Hill representative for more information.

Solutions for your challenges

A product isn't a solution. Real solutions are affordable, reliable, and come with training and ongoing support when you need it and how you want it. Visit **supportateverystep.com** for videos and resources both you and your students can use throughout the term.

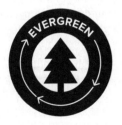

Updated and relevant content

Our new Evergreen delivery model provides the most current and relevant content for your course, hassle-free. Content, tools, and technology updates are delivered directly to your existing McGraw Hill Connect® course. Engage students and freshen up assignments with up-to-date coverage of select topics and assessments, all without having to switch editions or build a new course.

Digital Assets for Essentials of Medical Language

Application-Based Activities in McGraw Hill Connect®

Prepare students for the real world with Application-Based Activities in Connect. These highly interactive, assignable exercises boost engagement and provide a safe space to apply concepts learned to real-world, course-specific problems. Each Application-Based Activity involves the application of multiple concepts, providing the ability to synthesize information and use critical thinking skills to solve realistic scenarios.

Proctorio

Remote Proctoring & Browser-Locking Capabilities

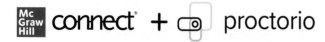

Remote proctoring and browser-locking capabilities, hosted by Proctorio within Connect, provide control of the assessment environment by enabling security options and verifying the identity of the student.

Seamlessly integrated within Connect, these services allow instructors to control the assessment experience by verifying identification, restricting browser activity, and monitoring student actions.

Instant and detailed reporting gives instructors an at-a-glance view of potential academic integrity concerns, thereby avoiding personal bias and supporting evidence-based claims.

 ## ReadAnywhere® App

Read or study when it's convenient with McGraw Hill's free ReadAnywhere® app. Available for iOS and Android smartphones or tablets, give users access to McGraw Hill tools including the eBook and SmartBook® or Adaptive Learning Assignments in McGraw Hill Connect®. Students can take notes, highlight, and complete assignments offline—all their work will sync when connected to Wi-Fi. Students log in with their Connect username and password to start learning—anytime, anywhere!

OLC-Aligned Courses

Implementing High-Quality Instruction and Assessment through Preconfigured Courseware

In consultation with the Online Learning Consortium (OLC) and our certified Faculty Consultants, McGraw Hill has created preconfigured courseware using OLC's quality scorecard to align with best practices in online course delivery. This turnkey courseware contains a combination of formative assessments, summative assessments, homework, and application activities, and can easily be customized to meet an individual instructor's needs and desired course outcomes. For more information, visit https://www.mheducation.com/highered/olc.

Evergreen

Content and technology are ever-changing, and it is important that you can keep your course up to date with the latest information and assessments. That's why we want to deliver the most current and relevant content for your course, hassle-free.

Reflecting the Diverse World Around Us

McGraw Hill believes in unlocking the potential of every learner at every stage of life. To accomplish that, we are dedicated to creating products that reflect, and are accessible to, all the diverse, global customers we serve. Within McGraw Hill, we foster a culture of belonging, and we work with partners who share our commitment to equity, inclusion, and diversity in all forms. In McGraw Hill Higher Education, this includes, but is not limited to, the following:

- Refreshing and implementing inclusive content guidelines around topics including generalizations and stereotypes, gender, abilities/disabilities, race/ethnicity, sexual orientation, diversity of names, and age.
- Enhancing best practices in assessment creation to eliminate cultural, cognitive, and affective bias.
- Maintaining and continually updating a robust photo library of diverse images that reflect our student populations.
- Including more diverse voices in the development and review of our content.
- Strengthening art guidelines to improve accessibility by ensuring meaningful text and images are distinguishable and perceivable by users with limited color vision and moderately low vision.

The Instructor Online Learning Center is available through your Connect course. Your McGraw Hill sales representative can provide you with the access you need to easily prepare for using *Essentials of Medical Language.* Our Online Learning Centers include:

- The **Instructors' Manual,** which contains valuable information that makes course prep a snap!

  - This manual includes information about student learning styles and instructor strategies; innovative learning activities; assessment techniques and strategies; classroom management tips; and answer keys.

  - **Lesson Planning Guide.** Our Lesson Planning Guide comes complete with a customizable lesson plan for each of the sections in this text. Each plan contains a step-by-step 50-minute teaching plan and master copies of handouts. Use these lessons alone or combined to accommodate different class schedules—you can even revise them to reflect your preferred topic or sequence. Each lesson plan is designed to be used with a corresponding PowerPoint® presentation that is also available on the OLC.

- **PowerPoint® Lecture Outlines.** The PowerPoint lectures with speaking notes correlate to the Lesson Plans mentioned above and include the art and photos from the text. Covering the most important parts of every section, the slides are customizable to fit your course needs.

- **Test Builder in Connect,** making creating tests easy!

  Available within McGraw Hill Connect®, Test Builder is a cloud-based tool that enables instructors to format tests that can be printed, administered within a Learning Management System, or exported as a Word document. Test Builder offers a modern, streamlined interface for easy content configuration that matches course needs, without requiring a download.

  Test Builder allows you to:

  - access all test bank content from a particular title.
  - easily pinpoint the most relevant content through robust filtering options.
  - manipulate the order of questions or scramble questions and/or answers.
  - pin questions to a specific location within a test.
  - determine your preferred treatment of algorithmic questions.
  - choose the layout and spacing.
  - add instructions and configure default settings.

  Test Builder provides a secure interface for better protection of content and allows for just-in-time updates to flow directly into assessments.

Acknowledgments

We wish to thank the talented efforts of a group of dedicated individuals at McGraw Hill Education who have made this book and its digital ancillary products come together:

Michelle Vogler, Portfolio Director; Marah Bellegarde, Portfolio Manager; Robin Reed, Director of Content Development; Krystal Faust, Lead Product Developer; Beth Baugh, Freelance Product Developer; Angela Fitzpatrick, Program Manager; Kelly Hart, Lead Content Project Manager; Paula Patel, Core Content Project Manager; Brent dela Cruz, Assessment Content Project Manager; Laura Fuller, Manufacturing Project Manager; David Hash, Designer; Lorraine Buczek, Content Licensing Specialist; and Scott Chrysler, Marketing Manager.

We also wish to recognize and express our appreciation for the contributions made by David Allan, a valued co-author of this book since its inception. David passed away in 2023.

Rachel Basco and Tim Gilmore
Authors

Rachel Curran Basco

Rachel Basco earned her BS in Cardiopulmonary Science and MS in Health Sciences from Louisiana State University Health Sciences Center, School of Allied Health Professions (SAHP). She worked as a registered respiratory therapist for ten years and then began her career in college instruction in respiratory therapy at LSU-SAHP in Shreveport, LA. She then found her interest to be in nonclinical education and began instructing biology courses at Bossier Parish Community College (BPCC) in Bossier City, LA. Ms. Basco is employed as an Associate Professor of biology, instructing courses in medical terminology along with human anatomy I and II.

Ms. Basco resides in Shreveport with her husband. While very busy with her family, work, and studies, Rachel always finds time to visit her relatives in her home state of Wisconsin.

Tim W. Gilmore

Tim Gilmore is an Associate Professor of Cardiopulmonary Science (CPS) and the CPS Program Director at Louisiana State University (LSU) Health in Shreveport, Louisiana. He earned a PhD in Health Science from Nova Southeastern University, a Masters in Health Sciences and Bachelor of Science in Cardiopulmonary Science from LSU Health Shreveport, and an Associate of Science in Respiratory Therapy from Bossier Parish Community College. Tim is a member of the Louisiana Society for Respiratory Care, American Association for Respiratory Care, and National Board for Respiratory Care. He is a Registered Respiratory Therapist with specialty credentials as a Neonatal Pediatric Specialist and Adult Critical Care Specialist, with national certifications as a Pulmonary Functions Technologist and Asthma Educator. He also serves as a peer reviewer for *Respiratory Care Journal* and an item-writer for the National Board for Respiratory Care.

David M. Allan

David Allan received his medical training at Cambridge University and Guy's Hospital in England. He was Chief Resident in Pediatrics at Bellevue Hospital in New York City before moving to San Diego, California.

Dr. Allan worked as a family physician in England, a pediatrician in San Diego, and Associate Dean at the University of California, San Diego School of Medicine. He designed, written, and produced more than 100 award-winning multimedia programs with virtual reality as their conceptual base. Dr. Allan passed away in 2023.

Learning the Essentials of Medical Language

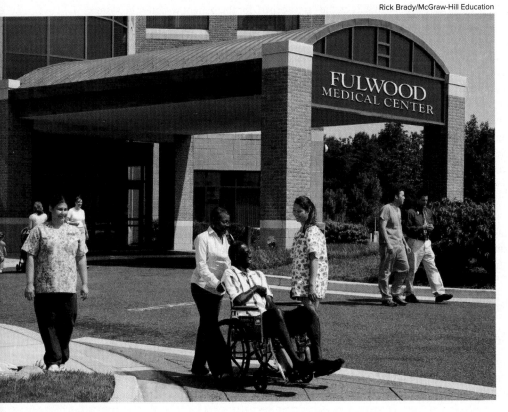

Learning Outcomes

To get the most out of your learning experiences and this textbook, you need to:

LO W.1 Establish a commitment to learn medical terminology.

LO W.2 Recognize the knowledge and skills you will need to be an active learner.

LO W.3 Understand how the contextual approach of this book promotes active learning.

LO W.4 Use the pedagogical devices in each chapter and lesson.

LO W.5 Use the vivid illustrations, photos, and tables in the book to enhance understanding of the concepts being taught.

LO W.6 Solve the exercises in each lesson and at the end of each chapter to demonstrate understanding of the material.

LO W.7 Implement the effective organizational strategies and study habits described in this chapter of the book.

LO W.8 Understand how a commitment to lifelong learning will enhance your professionalism.

LO W.9 Differentiate the roles of the various members of a health care team in different medical specialties and settings.

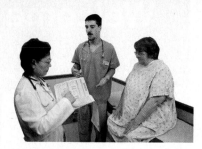

▲ **FIGURE W.1**
Direct Communication with Doctor and Patient.

Rick Brady/McGraw-Hill Education

The Health Care Team (LO W.9)

The team leader is a medical doctor, or physician, who can be an **MD** (doctor of medicine) or a **DO** (doctor of osteopathy) with other ordering providers such as Physician Assistants or Nurse Practitioners working under the supervision of a licensed physician. Most **managed care systems** require the patient to have a **primary care physician.** This physician can be a **family practitioner, internist,** or **pediatrician** (for children) and is responsible for the continuing overall care of the patient. In managed care, the primary care physician acts as the "gatekeeper" for the patient to enter the system, supervising all care the patient receives.

If needed medical care is beyond the expertise of the primary care physician, the patient is referred to a medical specialist whose expertise is based on a specific body system or even a part of a body system. For example, a **cardiologist** has expertise in diseases of the heart and vascular system, whereas a **dermatologist** specializes in diseases of the skin and an **orthopedist** in problems with the musculoskeletal system. A **gastroenterologist** is an expert in diseases of the whole digestive system, whereas a **colorectal surgeon** specializes only in diseases of the lower gastrointestinal tract. Some specialists are considered sub-specialists with additional, very specific training and specialization and may be consulted to further contribute to a patient's diagnosis and treatment.

Other health professionals work under the supervision of the physician and provide direct care *(Figure W.1)* to the patient. These can include a **registered nurse, respiratory therapist, medical assistant** and, in specialty areas, various therapists, technologists, and technicians with expertise in the use of specific therapeutic and diagnostic tools.

Still other health professionals on the team provide indirect patient care *(Figure W.2)*. These include **administrative medical assistants, transcriptionists, health information technicians, medical insurance billers,** and **coders,** all of whom are essential to providing high-quality patient care.

"Why Do I Need to Learn Medical Terminology?"

Communication Needs

Throughout your career as a health professional, you will need to communicate with other health professionals. This need is present whether you are providing direct patient care—for example, as a CMA like Luis Guitterez—or whether you are providing indirect patient care—for example, as a medical transcriptionist, biller, or

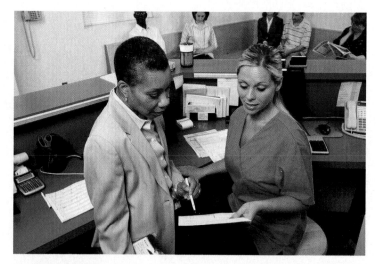

▲ **FIGURE W.2**
Administrative Medical Assistants.
Administrative medical assistances are among the health professions who provide indirect care to patients.

Rick Brady/McGraw-Hill Education

coder. In this book, you will find all the medical terms necessary to equip yourself with the essential medical vocabulary needed for work and further study in any of the allied health professional careers.

Health professionals use specific terms and a different language to describe to each other situations they encounter each day. You need to be able to understand, spell, and pronounce the terms they use.

Modern medical terminology is an artificial language constructed over centuries using words and elements from Greek and Latin origins (where healing professions began). Some 15,000 or more words are formed from 1,200 Greek and Latin roots. New words are being added continually as new medical discoveries are made. Medical terminology enables health professionals from different fields, different specialties, and different countries to communicate clearly and precisely with each other. Every profession has its own language *(Figure W.3)*.

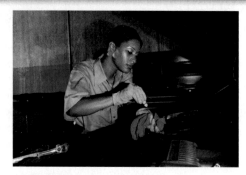

▲ **FIGURE W.3** Every Profession Has Its Own Language.
You may have difficulty understanding your auto mechanic when she tells you that the expansion valve, evaporator core, and orifice tubes in your air-conditioning system need to be replaced.

Jupiterimages/Stockbyte/Getty Images

Listening, Speaking, Reading, Writing, and Critical Thinking

Daily in your practice as a health professional you will:

Listen to information from physicians about patient care, and carry out their instructions.

Listen to patients describing their symptoms, and translate their descriptions into medical terms.

Speak to physicians and other health professionals to report information and ask questions.

Speak to patients to translate and clarify information given to them by physicians and other health professionals.

Read physicians' comments and treatment plans in patient medical records and insurance reports.

Read the results of physical examinations, procedures, and laboratory and diagnostic tests.

Write to document actions taken by yourself and other members of the health care team *(Figure W.4)*.

Write to precisely record verbal orders, test results given over the phone, and other phone messages.

Think critically to evaluate medical documentation for accuracy.

Think critically to analyze and discover the meaning of unfamiliar medical terms using the strategies outlined in *Chapter 1* of this book.

IF YOU CANNOT SPEAK AND UNDERSTAND THE LANGUAGE, YOU CANNOT JOIN THE CLUB.

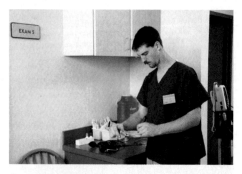

▲ **FIGURE W.4**
Accurate Documentation of Care Is Critical.

Rick Brady/McGraw-Hill Education

"What Is Lifelong, Active Learning?"

Lifelong Learning

Your current training in medical terminology is necessary for you to be able to continue your education in your health care profession. But it is important to recognize that school is only one of the many places where you acquire knowledge.

You also acquire knowledge:

• Each time you ask a question about a patient or a report and receive an answer.

• Each time you analyze an unfamiliar medical term and discover its meaning.

• Each time you interact with a patient and see how that patient is coping with his or her problems *(Figure W.5)*.

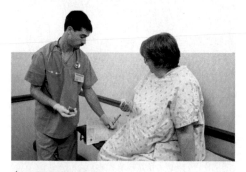

▲ **FIGURE W.5**
Every Patient Interaction Is an Opportunity for Learning.

Rick Brady/McGraw-Hill Education

All these are opportunities for learning to discover *your own* answers to *your own* problems or lack of knowledge.

This type of knowledge—discovered through your own experience and driven by your own needs and goals—is genuine, real, and trustworthy for you. It is not like what you learn in school, which is determined by some distant authority.

The authentic knowledge you gain from solving your own problems, whether by yourself or with the help of other people or resources, motivates you to acquire still more knowledge and helps you grow as a person and as a professional.

Throughout your working life, additional classroom training will be needed to keep your skills and professional knowledge up to date with new developments in medicine. You will also continue to learn through your own experience. Everything you do in life can result in learning.

Your own experience and judgment become your most valuable resources for making your life vibrant, strong, creative, and what *you* want *it* to be.

Your own experience and judgment maximize your professional and personal success.

Your own learning never ends.

Actively Experiencing Medical Language

Medical terms were created to provide health care professionals a way to communicate with each other and document the care they provide. To provide effective patient care, all health care professionals must be fluent in medical language. One misused or misspelled medical term on a patient record can cause errors that can result in injury or death to patients, incorrect coding or billing of medical claims, and possible fraud charges.

When medical terms are separated from their intended context, as they are in other medical terminology textbooks, it is easy to lose sight of how important it is to use them accurately and precisely. Learning medical terminology in the context of the medical setting reinforces the importance of correct usage and precision in communication.

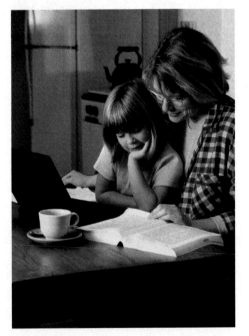

▲ **FIGURE W.6**
Preview The Book Before Class.
Identify your own personal preferences for learning, and seek out the resources that will best help you with your studies. Recognize your weaknesses, and try to compensate for or work to improve them.

Scott T. Baxter/Photodisc/Getty Images

Active Learning

It is not acceptable to sit back and expect someone else to pour knowledge into your head. You have to **actively work at learning** *(Figure W.6)*.

Get the Most Out of Lectures

- *Prepare* for your classroom experiences. Preview the book chapter before class *(Figure W.6)*, and the material will be much easier to understand.

- *Listen actively.* You cannot do this if you are looking at your phone, daydreaming, or worrying about what you have to get for dinner.

- *Ask* a question if you do not comprehend something the instructor is saying.

- *Write* good notes. Focus on the main points, and capture key ideas; review and edit your notes within 24 hours of the class.

Get the Most Out of Reading

- *Concentrate* on what you are reading. Review the titles, objectives, headings, and visuals for each lesson to identify what the lesson is all about.

- *Read* actively using the SQ3R method (see the Study Hint) to help you.

- *Write* down any questions you have.

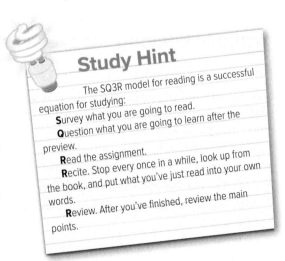

Study Hint

The SQ3R model for reading is a successful equation for studying:
Survey what you are going to read.
Question what you are going to learn after the preview.
Read the assignment.
Recite. Stop every once in a while, look up from the book, and put what you've just read into your own words.
Review. After you've finished, review the main points.

Study with a Partner or Group

- *Find* a study partner. Schedule study dates, compare notes, talk through concepts and questions, and quiz each other.
- *Establish* a small study group, including your study partner. Again, compare notes and quiz each other.

Perform Well on Tests

- *Read* the directions carefully, and scan the entire test so that you know how long it is and what types of activities it contains.
- *Answer* the easy questions or sections first so that you finish as much as possible before doing the difficult questions, which might slow you down.
- *Use* any extra time, after you have finished the test, to check that you have answered all the questions and then to confirm your answers.

Know and Motivate Yourself

- What type of learner are you? **Visual**—who responds best by **seeing** information. **Auditory**—who works best by listening. **Tactile**—who prefers hands-on applications. Recognize your type and motivate yourself by emphasizing your best method of learning to help achieve your goals.

A few months of committed study now is a small price to pay for a lifetime of professionalism.

"How Can I Help Myself Learn Better?"

You have a lot of time and money invested in your education. To succeed, you need to be able to focus and manage your time and your studies.

- *Recognize* the stresses in your life at different times.
- *Prioritize* mentally, and handle each task in the order of importance. In this case, eat a healthy meal with your kids, enjoy putting them to bed, pay the bills, and then relax (or meditate) for 10 minutes. When you are relaxed, settle down to review the text, and go to bed at a reasonable hour. Picking up around the house will have to wait because study and sleep are a higher priority. Sounds too easy? What other choices do you have to be able to study in an effective way?
- *Actively develop a support group.* Enlist the support of your spouse, parents, siblings, friends—any people you can trust and rely on. If you have a test every Thursday, get one of them to come over Wednesday night and put the kids to bed while you go over to his or her house or the library to study.
- *Find your own space.* Create a place where you keep everything for your courses at your fingertips, clutter-free.
- *Study when you are most productive.* Are you a night owl or an early bird? Set a daily study time for yourself.
- *Balance your life.* While studying should be a main focus, plan time for family, friends, leisure, exercise, and sleep.
- *Resist distractions.* Avoid the temptation to surf the Web, send instant messages, and make phone calls. Stick to your schedule.
- *Be realistic* when planning—know your limits and priorities.
- *Be prepared* for the unexpected (child's illness, your illness, inclement weather) that can turn your schedule into shambles.
- *Reprioritize* daily on the basis of schedule disruptions and other conflicts.
- *Identify* clear goals for what you need to get done today, this week, this month, before the end of the semester, and so on.

EXERCISES

Write out *all of your activities for a typical week. On average, how many hours each week do you spend sleeping, grooming, eating, working, running errands, studying, attending your children's activities, and on social media? Add all the hours up. There are 168 hours in the week. How many hours do you have left for studying? A sample time budget is shown below.*

Activity	Number of Hours per Day	Number of Days per Week	Number of Hours per Week
Sleeping	8	7	56
Grooming	1	7	7
Meals: preparation, eating, cleanup	1	7	7
Cleaning, laundry	1	3	3
Commuting to and from school	1	5	5
In class	4	5	20
Doing errands	1	3	3
Family time	3	7	21
Church, workout, hobbies			5
Job			30
Friends, going out, TV, entertainment			6
TOTAL			163
TOTAL HOURS IN A WEEK			168
Hours remaining for study			5

- ARE 5 HOURS ENOUGH FOR STUDY?
- WHEN ARE THEY AVAILABLE?
- WHAT CAN YOU DO TO INCREASE THEM?

STUDY HOURS SHOULD BE SPENT IN A SETTING THAT ALLOWS YOU TO CONCENTRATE ON YOUR WORK AND NOT BE DISTRACTED. TURN OFF YOUR CELL PHONE AND TV. THE BIGGEST QUESTION TO ASK YOURSELF IS, "AM I INVESTING MY TIME WISELY?" IF NOT, HOW CAN YOU BUDGET YOUR TIME DIFFERENTLY SO THAT MORE TIME IS SPENT ON HIGHER-PRIORITY ACTIVITIES?

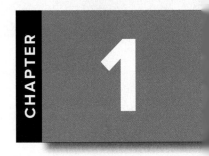

CHAPTER 1

The Anatomy of Medical Terms

The Essential Elements of the Language of Medicine

Rick Brady/McGraw Hill

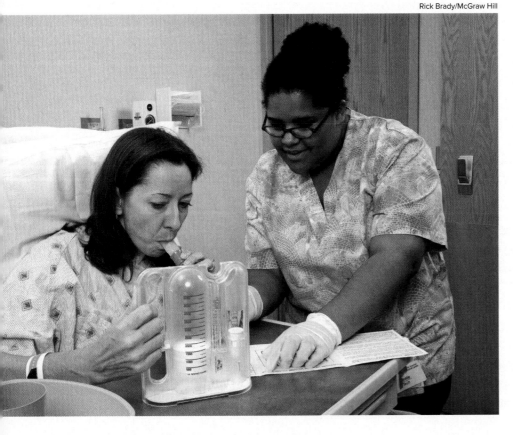

Learning Outcomes

The technical language of medicine has been developed logically from Latin and Greek roots. In fact, it was in Latin and Greek cultures that the concept of treating patients began. Medical terms are built from their individual parts, or **elements,** which form the **anatomy** of the word. The information in this chapter will enable you to:

LO 1.1 Select the roots, combining vowels, **and combining forms** of medical terms.

LO 1.2 Demonstrate the importance of suffixes and prefixes in forming medical terms.

LO 1.3 Construct (build) medical terms from separate elements.

LO 1.4 Deconstruct (break down) medical terms into their elements.

LO 1.5 Use correctly the plurals of medical terms.

LO 1.6 Articulate the correct pronunciations of medical terms.

LO 1.7 Demonstrate precision and accuracy in documentation and other written and verbal communication of medical terms.

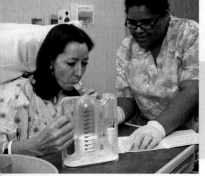

Section 1.1

The Construction of Medical Words

Your confidence in using and understanding the medical terms in this book will increase as you become familiar with the logic of how these terms are constructed.

Roots

- A **root** is the constant foundation and core of a medical term.
- **Roots** are usually of Greek or Latin origin.
- All medical terms have *one or more* **roots**.
- A **root** can appear anywhere in the term.
- More than one **root** can have the same meaning.

Combining Forms

- A **root** plus a **combining vowel** creates a **combining form**.
- Can be attached to another **root** or **combining form**.
- Can precede another word element called a **suffix**.
- Can follow a **prefix**.

Keynotes

- Throughout this book, look for the following patterns:

  Roots, combining forms, and **combining vowels** will be colored **red**.

  Prefixes will be colored **green**.

  Suffixes will be colored **blue**.

- Different **roots** can have the same meaning. *Pulmon-* and *pneumon-* both mean *lung, air*.

Roots (LO 1.1)

Every medical term has a **root**—the element that provides the core meaning of the word.

- The word *pneumonia* has the **root** *pneumon-*, taken from the Greek word meaning *lung* or *air*. The Greek **root** *pneum-* also means *lung* or *air*. Pneumonia is an infection of the lung tissue.

- A *pulmonologist* will likely be involved in diagnosing patients with pneumonia. The **root** *pulmon-* is taken from the Latin word meaning *lung*. A *pulmonologist* is a specialist of the **respiratory** system who treats lung diseases.

Combining Forms (LO 1.1)

Roots are often joined to other elements in a medical term by adding a **combining vowel,** such as the letter "o," to the end of the **root,** like *pneum-,* to form **pneum/o-.**

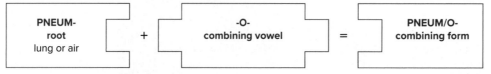

| PNEUM-
root
lung or air | + | -O-
combining vowel | = | PNEUM/O-
combining form |

Throughout this book, whenever a term is presented, a **slash (/)** will be used to separate the combining vowel from the **root.** Other examples of this approach are as follows:

- Adding the **combining vowel "o"** to the Latin **root** *pulmon-* makes the **combining form** *pulmon/o-.*

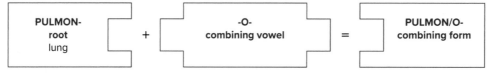

| PULMON-
root
lung | + | -O-
combining vowel | = | PULMON/O-
combining form |

Any vowel, "a," "e," "i," "o," or "u," can be used as a **combining vowel.**

- The **root** *respir-* means *to breathe.* Adding the **combining vowel "a"** makes the **combining form** *respir/a-.*

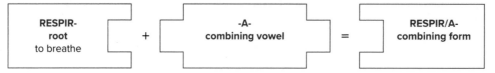

| RESPIR-
root
to breathe | + | -A-
combining vowel | = | RESPIR/A-
combining form |

- The **root** *bronch-* is derived from the Greek word for *windpipe* and is one of the two subdivisions of the trachea that carry air to and from the lungs. Adding the **combining vowel "o"** to the **root** *bronch-* makes the **combining form** *bronch/o-.*

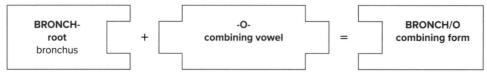

| BRONCH-
root
bronchus | + | -O-
combining vowel | = | BRONCH/O
combining form |

Many medical terms contain more than one **root;** when two roots occur together, they are always joined by a **combining vowel,** as in the following example:

- The word **hemopneumothorax** has the root *hem-,* from the Greek word meaning *blood,* the root *pneum-,* from the Greek word meaning *air* or *lung,* and the **root** *-thorax,* from the Greek word meaning *chest.* The **combining vowel "o"** joins these two roots together to make the **combining form,** *pneum/o-.* A **hemopneumothorax** is the presence of air and blood in the space that surrounds the lungs in the chest. As blood and air fill the pleural cavity, the lungs cannot expand and **respiration** is not possible, often compressing the affected lung and causing it to collapse.

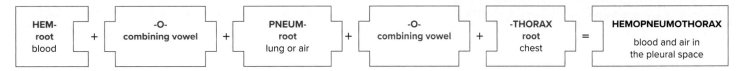

Suffixes (LO 1.2)

A **suffix** is an element added to the end of a **root** or **combining form** to give it a new meaning. You can add different **suffixes** to the same **root** to build new words, all with different meanings. For example:

- Add the **suffix** *-ary* to the **root** *pulmon-* to create the term **pulmonary.** The **suffix** *-ary* means *pertaining to* or *relating to.* The adjective **pulmonary** means *pertaining to the lung.* **Pulmonary circulation** means the *passage of blood through the lungs.*

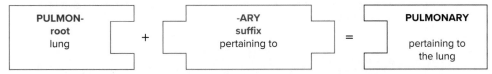

- Add the **suffix** *-logy* to the **combining form** *pulmon/o-* to make the term **pulmonology.** The **suffix** *logy* means *study of.* **Pulmonology** is the study of the structure, functions, and diseases of the lungs.

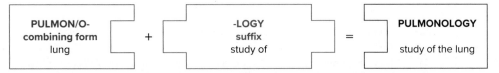

- Add the **suffix** *-ia* to the **root** *pneumon-* to make the term **pneumonia.** The **suffix** *-ia* means *a condition of.* **Pneumonia** is a condition of the lungs that involves an infection of the lung tissue.

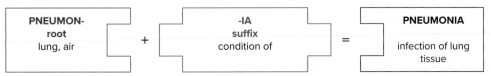

- Add the **suffix** *-ation* to the **root** *respir-* to make the term **respiration.** The **suffix** *-ation* means *a process.* **Respiration** is the process of breathing in and out.

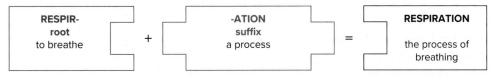

- Add the **suffix** *-itis* to the **root** *bronch-* to make the term **bronchitis.** The **suffix** *-itis* means *inflammation.* **Bronchitis** is an inflammation of the bronchial tubes.

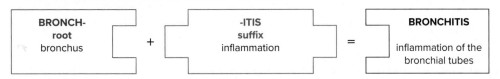

Suffixes

- A **suffix** is a group of letters attached to the end of a **root** or **combining form.**
- A **suffix** changes the meaning of the word.
- If the **suffix** begins with a consonant, it must follow a **combining vowel.**
- If the **suffix** begins with a vowel, no **combining vowel** is needed.
- A few medical terms can have two **suffixes.**
- A **suffix** always appears at the end of a term.
- **Suffixes** that are different can have the same meaning.

Keynotes

Adjectival **suffixes** meaning *pertaining to:*

-ac, -al, -ale, -alis, -ar, -aris, -ary, -atic, -ative, -eal, -ent, -etic, -ial, -ic, -ica, -ical, -ine, -ior, -iosum, -ious, -istic, -ius, -nic, -ous, -tic, -tiz, -tous, -us.

There are times when two medical terms have the same meaning. Add the **suffix** *-itis* to the **root** *pneumon-* to make the term **pneumonitis. Pneumonitis** is an inflammation of the lung **parenchyma** (tissue). It is a synonym, or means the same as, the medical term pneumonia. Although most **roots** are specific to body systems and medical specialties, **suffixes** are universal and can be applied to all body systems and specialties.

Review all the terms in the Word Analysis and Definition (WAD) table before you start any exercise.

Word Analysis and Definition

S = Suffix   P = Prefix   R = Root   R/CF = Combining Form

WORD	PRONUNCIATION		ELEMENTS	DEFINITION
bronchitis	brong-**KI**-tis	S/ R/	-itis *inflammation* bronch- *bronchus*	Inflammation of the bronchi
bronchoscopy	brong-**KOS**-koh-pee	S/ R/CF	-scopy *to examine, view* bronch/o *bronchus*	Examination of the interior of the tracheobronchial tree with an endoscope
bronchoscope	**BRONG**-koh-skope	S/	-scope *instrument for viewing*	Endoscope used for bronchoscopy
hemopneumothorax	**HEE**-moh-**NEW**-moh-**THOR**-ax	R/CF R/CF R/	hem/o- *blood* pneum/o- *air, lung* -thorax *chest*	Blood and air in the pleural cavity
parenchyma	pah-**REN**-ki-mah		Greek *to pour in*	The specific functional cells of a gland or organ (e.g., the lung) that are supported by the connective tissue framework
pneumonia	new-**MOH**-nee-ah	S/ R/	-ia *condition* pneumon- *lung, air*	Inflammation of the lung parenchyma (tissue)
pneumonitis (same as *pneumonia*)	**NEW**-moh-**NI**-tis	S/	-itis *inflammation*	
pneumothorax	new-moh-**THOR**-ax	R/CF R/	pneum/o- *air, lung* -thorax *chest*	Air in the pleural cavity
pulmonary (adj)	**PULL**-moh-**NAR**-ee	S/ R/	-ary *pertaining to* pulmon- *lung*	Pertaining to the lungs
pulmonology	**PULL**-moh-**NOL**-oh-jee	S/ R/CF	-logy *study of* pulmon/o- *lung*	Study of the lungs, or the medical specialty of disorders of the lungs
pulmonologist	**PULL**-moh-**NOL**-oh-jist	S/	-logist *one who studies, specialist*	Specialist in treating disorders of the lungs
respiration	**RES**-pih-**RAY**-shun	S/ R/	-ation *process* respir- *to breathe*	Process of breathing; fundamental process of life used to exchange oxygen and carbon dioxide
respiratory (adj)	**RES**-pih-rah-tor-ee	S/	-atory *pertaining to*	Pertaining to respiration

Prefixes (LO 1.2)

Prefixes

- A **prefix** always appears at the beginning of a term.
- A **prefix** precedes a **root** to change its meaning.
- **Prefixes** can have more than one meaning.
- **Prefixes** never require a **combining vowel.**
- An occasional medical term can have two **prefixes.**
- Not every term has a **prefix.**

A **prefix** is an element added to the beginning of a **root** or **combining form** to further expand the meaning of a medical term. Prefixes usually indicate time, number, size, or location.

Examples of **prefixes** defining time are as follows:

- The term **mature** can refer to an infant born after a normal length of pregnancy, between 37 and 42 weeks.

- An infant born before 37 weeks is called **premature.** The **prefix** *pre-* means *before.* **Premature** means that the infant was born *before 37 weeks.*

- An infant born after 42 weeks is called **postmature.** The **prefix** *post-* means *after.* **Postmature** means that the *infant was born after 42 weeks.*

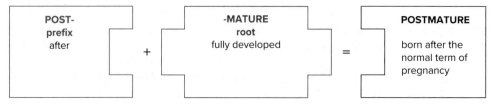

| POST-
prefix
after | + | -MATURE
root
fully developed | = | POSTMATURE
born after the
normal term of
pregnancy |

- The term **natal** contains the **root** *nat-* (*birth* or *born*) and the **suffix** *-al* (*pertaining to*); it means *pertaining to birth.*

- Add the **prefix** *pre- (before)* to form **prenatal**, which means *pertaining to the time before birth.*
- Add the **prefix** *post- (after)* to form **postnatal**, which means *pertaining to the time after birth.*
- Add the **prefix** *peri- (around)* to form **perinatal**, which means *pertaining to around the time of birth.* This includes the time immediately *before, during,* and *after birth.*

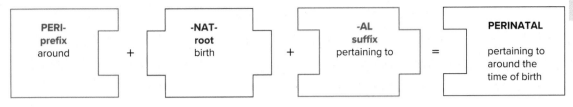

Examples of **prefixes** indicating number are as follows:

- The term **lateral** contains the **root** *later- (side)* and the **suffix** *-al (pertaining to).* **Lateral** means *pertaining to a side of the body.*
- Add the **prefix** *uni- (one)* to form **unilateral**, which means *pertaining to one side of the body only.*
- Add the **prefix** *bi- (two)* to form **bilateral**, which means *pertaining to both sides of the body.*

Examples of prefixes indicating location are as follows:

- The term **gastric** contains the **root** *gastr- (stomach)* and the **suffix** *-ic (pertaining to).* **Gastric** means *pertaining to the stomach.*
- Add the **prefix** *epi- (above)* to form **epigastric**, which means *pertaining to above the stomach.*
- Add the **prefix** *hypo- (below)* to form **hypogastric**, which means *pertaining to below the stomach.*

Examples of **prefixes** indicating size are as follows:

- The **root** *-cyte* means *cell.*
- Add the **prefix** *macro- (large)* to form **macrocyte**, which means *a large cell.*
- Add the **prefix** *micro- (small)* to form **microcyte**, which means *a small cell.*

Word Analysis and Definition

S = Suffix   P = Prefix   R = Root   R/CF = Combining Form

WORD	PRONUNCIATION	ELEMENTS		DEFINITION
gastric	GAS-trik	S/	-ic *pertaining to*	Pertaining to the stomach
		R/	gastr- *stomach*	
epigastric	ep-ih-GAS-trik	P/	epi- *above*	Abdominal region above the stomach
hypogastric	high-poh-GAS-trik	P/	hypo- *below*	Abdominal region below the stomach
hypotensive (adj)	HIGH-po-TEN-siv	S/	-ive *pertaining to*	Pertaining to or suffering from low blood pressure
		P/	hypo- *low*	
		R/	-tens- *pressure*	
lateral	LAT-er-al	S/	-al *pertaining to*	Pertaining to one side of the body
		R/	later- *side*	
bilateral	by-LAT-er-al	P/	bi- *two*	Pertaining to both sides of the body
unilateral	you-nih-LAT-er-al	P/	uni- *one*	Pertaining to one side of the body only
macrocyte	MACK-roh-site	P/	macro- *large*	Large cell
		R/	-cyte *cell*	
macrocytic (adj) (Note: *The "e" in cyte is deleted to allow the word to flow.*)	mack-roh-SIT-ik	S/	-ic *pertaining to*	Pertaining to a macrocyte
mature	mah-TYUR		Latin *ready*	Fully developed
postmature	post-mah-TYUR	P/	post- *after*	Infant born after 42 weeks of gestation
		R/	-mature *fully developed*	
premature	pree-mah-TYUR	P/	pre- *before*	Occurring before the expected time; e.g., an infant born before 37 weeks of gestation.
microcyte	MY-kroh-site	P/	micro- *small*	Small cell
		R/	-cyte *cell*	
microcytic (adj) (Note: *The "e" in cyte is deleted to allow the word to flow.*)	my-kroh-SIT-ik	S/	-ic *pertaining to*	Pertaining to a small cell
natal	NAY-tal	S/	-al *pertaining to*	Pertaining to birth
		R/	nat- *birth, born*	
perinatal	per-ih-NAY-tal	P/	peri- *around*	Pertaining to around the time of birth
postnatal	post-NAY-tal	P/	post- *after*	Pertaining to after the birth
prenatal	pree-NAY-tal	P/	pre- *before*	Pertaining to before the birth

EXERCISES

Case Report 1.1

You are

. . . a **respiratory therapist** working with Tavis Senko, MD, a pulmonologist at Fulwood Medical Center.

You are communicating with. . .

. . . Mrs. Sandra Omotoye, a 43-year-old woman referred to Dr. Senko by her primary care physician, Dr. Andrew McDonald, an **internist**. Mrs. Omotoye has a persistent abnormality on her chest **X-ray.** You have been asked to determine her **pulmonary** function prior to a scheduled **bronchoscopy**.

From Mrs. Omotoye's medical records, you can see that 2 months ago she developed a right upper lobe (**RUL**) **pneumonia**. After treatment with an **antibiotic**, a follow-up chest **X-ray (CXR)** showed some residual collapse in the RUL and a small right **pneumothorax**. Mrs. Omotoye has smoked a pack a day since she was a teenager. Dr. Senko would like to further evaluate for potential lung cancer and has scheduled her for a **bronchoscopy**.

This summary of a Case Report illustrates the use of some simple medical terms. Modern health care and medicine have their own language. The medical terms all have precise meanings, which enable you, as a health professional, to communicate clearly and accurately with other health professionals involved in the care of a patient. This communication is critical for patient safety and the delivery of high-quality patient care.

A. Read Case Report 1.1 *and review the content from Section 1.1 to correctly answer the questions.* **LO 1.1, 1.2, and 1.7**

1. Mrs. Omotoye's lung condition seen on the X-ray is:

   A. blood surrounding the lung   **C.** air in the pleural cavity

   B. infection in the RLL   **D.** cancer in the RUL

2. The task that Dr. Senko has asked you to do is:

   A. determine how well her lungs are working   **C.** schedule her for an MRI

   B. insert a tube into her lungs   **D.** insert a needle into her pleural space

3. **Correct use of terms is required when communicating** *on paper, with other members of the health care team, and with patients and their families. Use the words provided below to correctly complete each sentence.*

   antibiotic   bronchoscope   bronchoscopy   pneumonia   pneumothorax

   1. The patient with a _____ has air in the RUL.

   2. Dr. Senko asked you to get the _____ so he could perform the _____ on Mrs. Omotoye.

   3. The internist prescribed a(n) _____ to treat her _____.

B. Review *what you have just learned about roots and combining forms. Select the correct answer to the statement.* **LO 1.1**

   root   combining form   combining vowel   suffix   prefix

1. Roots and combining forms can go before a _____.

2. This element does not have a meaning; it serves to make the word easier to pronounce: _____.

3. A _____ can go before a root, but never after.

4. The _____ is the root plus a combining vowel.

C. Identify *the word parts of a medical term. Use the provided medical term to correctly answer the questions.* **LO 1.1**

1. In the word **pneumonia**, the root is:

   a. pneum-   **b.** pneumon-   **c.** -ia   **d.** -nia

2. In the medical term **pulmonologist**, the root is:

   a. pulm-   **b.** pulmon-   **c.** -logist   **d.** -gist

3. The combining vowel in the medical term **respiratory** is:

   a. -a-   **b.** -o-   **c.** -i-   **d.** -e-

Elements: *It is important for you to recognize the identity of an element. Is it a root, combining form, or suffix? This will help you to determine its place in the term when you are building terms.*

D. Build the appropriate medical term *to match the definitions given. The placement of the elements is noted for you under the line; each different element is separated on the line. Insert the correct elements on the line. The first one is done for you.* **LO 1.1 and 1.2**

1. Study of the lungs: _____ pulmon/o _____/_____ logy _____
                              R/CF   S

2. Pertaining to the lung: _____/_____
                              R/CF   S

3. The process of breathing: _____/_____
                              R/CF   S

4. Condition of the lung: _____/_____
                              R/CF   S

E. Suffixes *can provide clues to the meanings of terms. Answer the following questions using terms related to the respiratory system. Fill in the blanks.* **LO 1.1 and 1.2**

1. What is another term with the same meaning as pneumonia? _____

2. Which term is a body process? _____

3. Which suffix can be applied to a specialist? _____

Prefixes: *Solid knowledge of prefixes will quickly help increase your medical vocabulary.*

F. Answer the first question, *and then build the correct term on the line next to the definitions in 2 through 4.* **LO 1.1, 1.2, and 1.4**

natal	prenatal	postnatal	perinatal

1. The term *natal* means: _____

2. Pertaining to around the time of birth: _____ / _____ / _____

                                       P   R/CF   S

3. Pertaining to after the birth: _____ / _____ / _____

                                       P   R/CF   S

4. Pertaining to before the birth: _____ / _____ / _____

                                       P   R/CF   S

G. Prefixes usually indicate time, number, size, or location. *Given the prefix, select the correct category of meaning.* **LO 1.2**

1. hypo

    a. time   **b.** number   **c.** size   **d.** location

2. uni

    a. time   **b.** number   **c.** size   **d.** location

Section 1.2

Word Deconstruction, Plurals, Pronunciation, and Precision

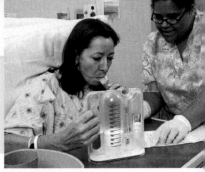

Rick Brady/McGraw Hilly

When you see an unfamiliar medical term, you can learn its meaning by **deconstructing** it—reducing it to its basic elements.

Word Deconstruction (LO 1.1, 1.2, and 1.4)

When you see an unfamiliar medical term, the first step toward deconstructing the term is to break it down into its components, or parts. For words you need to define, first identify the **suffix**. Take the term **cardiologist**. Here, the **suffix** at the end of the word is *-logist,* which means *one who studies and is a specialist in*. This leaves the element *cardi/o-,* which is the **combining form** for *heart*. The term **cardiologist** means *a specialist in the heart and its diseases.* It has a **combining form** and a **suffix**.

In the term **myocardial**, the **suffix** at the end of the word is **-al,** which means *pertaining to,* as you learned earlier in this chapter. The **combining form** *my/o-,* which means *muscle,* is at the beginning of the word. The **root** *-cardi-,* which means *heart,* is in the middle of the word. So, the term **myocardial** means *pertaining to the heart muscle.* It has a **combining form,** a **root,** and a **suffix**.

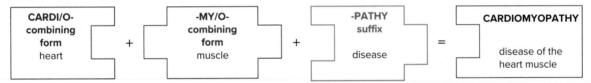

MY/O- combining form		**-CARDI-** root		**-AL** suffix		**MYOCARDIAL**
muscle	+	heart	+	pertaining to	=	pertaining to heart muscle

Changing the **suffix** to *-um,* meaning *a structure,* results in the term **myocardium,** *the structure called the heart muscle.*

The term **cardiomyopathy** contains the **suffix -pathy,** meaning *a disease,* the **combining form** *cardi/o-,* meaning the *heart,* and the **combining form** *my/o-,* meaning *muscle.* When you put this all together, the term **cardiomyopathy** means *a disease of the heart muscle.*

CARDI/O- combining form		**-MY/O-** combining form		**-PATHY** suffix		**CARDIOMYOPATHY**
heart	+	muscle	+	disease	=	disease of the heart muscle

The term **ischemia** has the **suffix** *-emia,* which means *a blood condition.* The **root** *isch-* means *to block.* **Ischemia** means *a blockage of blood flow.* The term **myocardial ischemia** means *a blockage of blood flow to the heart muscle.*

A **diagnosis** is made based on the symptoms of the patient and the results of one or more procedures that confirm the signs of a disease or disorder. The term **diagnosis** does not have a suffix; therefore, start at the beginning of the term with the **prefix** *dia-,* which means complete, and finish with the **root** *-gnosis,* which means *knowledge of an abnormal condition.* The meaning of the term is *complete knowledge of an abnormal condition.* A term used with a diagnosis is a **prognosis. Prognosis** begins with the **prefix** *pro-,* which means *before,* or project forward. A **prognosis** means *a forecast of the probable course and outcome of a disease.*

A **therapeutic** procedure is a treatment for a disorder or diseases. The term **therapeutic** is the adjectival form of therapy, which means *a treatment.*

Diagnostic and **therapeutic** procedures often include a root element of the organ or structure being diagnosed or treated. In the term *electrocardiogram,* the **suffix** (at the end of the term) **-gram** means record, the **combining form** *electr/o-* means *electricity*, and the **combining form** *cardi/o-* means *heart*. Putting this together you get a *record of the electrical signals of the heart.*

Changing the **suffix** *-emia* to *-emic,* which means *pertaining to a condition of the blood,* creates a new term, **ischemic,** which is an adjective. It means *pertaining to a blockage of blood flow.* It has a **root** and a **suffix**.

Keynotes

- Always begin deconstructing a medical term by identifying its suffix.

- Abbreviations are listed in Abbreviations Boxes throughout the book.

WORD	PRONUNCIATION	ELEMENTS		DEFINITION
cardiologist	kar-dee-**OL**-oh-jist	S/	**-logist** *one who studies and is a specialist in*	A medical specialist in the diagnosis and treatment of disorders of the heart
		R/CF	**cardi/o-** *heart*	
cardiology	kar-dee-**OL**-oh-jee	S/	**-logy** *study of*	Medical specialty of diseases of the heart
cardiomyopathy	**KAR**-dee-oh-my-**OP**-ah-thee	S/	**-pathy** *disease*	Disease of the heart muscle, the myocardium
		R/CF	**cardi/o-** *heart*	
		R/CF	**-my/o-** *muscle*	
diagnosis (noun)	die-ag-**NO**-sis	P/	**dia-** *complete*	The determination of the cause of a disease
		R/	**-gnosis** *knowledge of an abnormal condition*	
diagnoses (pl)	die-ag-**NO**-seez			
diagnostic (adj)	die-ag-**NOS**-tik	S/	**-tic** *pertaining to*	Pertaining to or establishing a diagnosis
(**Note:** *The "is" in -gnosis is deleted to allow the word to flow.*)				
diagnose (verb)	die-ag-**NOSE**	R/	**-gnose** *recognize an abnormal condition*	To make a diagnosis
electrocardiogram	ee-lek-troh-**KAR**-dee-oh-gram	S/	**-gram** *record*	Record of the heart's electrical signals
		R/CF	**electr/o-** *electricity*	
		R/CF	**-cardi/o-** *heart*	
infarct	in-**FARKT**	P/	**in-** *in*	
		R/	**-farct** *area of dead tissue*	An area of cell death resulting from blockage of its blood supply
infarction	in-**FARK**-shun	S/	**-ion** *action, condition*	Sudden blockage of an artery
ischemia	is-**KEY**-me-ah	S/	**-emia** *a blood condition*	Lack of blood supply to tissue
		R/	**isch-** *to block*	
ischemic (adj)	is-**KEY**-mik	S/	**-emic** *pertaining to a condition of the blood*	Pertaining to the lack of blood supply to tissue
myocardial (adj)	**MY**-oh-**KAR**-dee-al	S/	**-al** *pertaining to*	Pertaining to heart muscle
		R/CF	**my/o-** *muscle*	
		R/	**-cardi-** *heart*	
myocardium	**MY**-oh-**KAR**-dee-um	S/	**-um** *structure*	All the heart muscle
prognosis (noun)	prog-**NO**-sis	P/	**pro-** *before, project forward*	A forecast of the probable course and outcome of a disease
		R/	**-gnosis** *knowledge of an abnormal condition*	

Plurals (LO 1.5)

Many words in the English language allow you to change them from singular to plural by adding an "s." For medical terms, this rarely happens, as these plurals are formed in ways that were once logical to Greeks and Romans but now have to be learned by memory in English. Examples of medical terms with Greek and Latin plurals are shown in *Table 1.1.*

Table 1.1 Singular and Plural Forms

Singular Ending	Plural Ending	Examples
-a	-ae	axilla axillae
-ax	-aces	thorax thoraces
-en	-ina	lumen lumina
-ex	-ices	cortex cortices
-is	-es	diagnosis diagnoses
-is	-ides	epididymis epididymides
-ix	-ices	appendix appendices
-ma	-mata	carcinoma carcinomata
-on	-a	ganglion ganglia
-um	-a	septum septa
-us	-era	viscus viscera
-us	-i	villus villi
-us	-ora	corpus corpora
-x	-ges	phalanx phalanges
-y	-ies	ovary ovaries
-yx	-ices	calyx calices

Throughout this book, the Greek and Latin plurals of medical terms appear in the Word Analysis and Definition box with the singular medical term.

Pronunciation (LO 1.6)

Being able to pronounce words correctly is essential to effective communication. In the medical world, this concept is especially important. As a health professional, you will routinely use medical terms, and your colleagues must be able to understand what you are saying. Correct pronunciation is crucial to patient safety and your ability to provide high-quality patient care.

Throughout this book, the pronunciation of medical terms is spelled out phonetically using modern English forms to show you exactly how the terms are pronounced. The word part to be emphasized is shown in bold, uppercase letters.

For example, **pulmonary** is phonetically written **PUL**-moh-nar-ee, and **pulmonology** is written **PUL**-moh-**NOL**-oh-jee. This illustrates that words derived from the same **root** can have their emphasis placed on different parts of the word and that the emphasized part can be from different elements. The emphasized syllable **NOL** comes partly from the **combining form** *pulmon/o-* and partly from the **suffix** *-logy.* You can hear glossary terms pronounced correctly by visiting the audio glossary in Connect® (connect.mheducation.com).

Communication

Some medical terms are pronounced the same but spelled differently. For example:

- Both *ilium* and *ileum* are pronounced **ILL**-ee-um. *Ilium* is a bone in the pelvis; *ileum* is a segment of the small intestine.
- Both *mucus* and *mucous* are pronounced **MYU**-kus. *Mucus* is a noun and is the name of a fluid secreted by *mucous* (adjective) membranes that line body cavities.

A medical term may relate to more than one anatomical structure.

- The term *cervical* means relating to a neck in any sense.
- It can pertain to the neck that joins the head to the trunk with the cervical vertebrae.
- It can also pertain to the cervix of the uterus, with its cervical canal.

Some words, when incorrectly pronounced, sound the same. For example:

- The term *prostate,* pronounced **PROS**-tate, refers to the gland at the base of the male bladder. The term *prostrate* means to be physically weak or exhausted, or to lie flat on the ground.
- Train your ear to hear the differences—*reflex* is not *reflux.*

Many medical terms form a verb, a noun, a plural, and an adjective, and you have to know them all, as in diagnose, diagnosis, diagnoses, and diagnostic (see the WAD on the previous spread).

Word Analysis and Definition

S = Suffix   P = Prefix   R = Root   R/CF = Combining Form

WORD	PRONUNCIATION		ELEMENTS	DEFINITION
axilla axillae (pl) axillary (adj)	AK-sill-ah AK-sill-ee AK-sill-air-ee	 S/ R/	Latin *armpit* -ary *pertaining to* axill- *armpit*	Medical term for the armpit Pertaining to the armpit
cervical (adj) cervix	SER-vih-kal SER-viks	S/ R/	-al *pertaining to* cervic- *neck* Latin *neck*	Pertaining to the cervix or to the neck region Lower part of the uterus
ganglion ganglia (pl)	GANG-lee-on GANG-lee-ah		Greek *a swelling or knot*	A fluid-filled cyst or a collection of nerve cells outside the brain and spinal cord
ileum ilium ilia (pl)	ILL-ee-um ILL-ee-um ILL-ee-ah		Latin *to twist or roll up* Latin *groin*	Third portion of the small intestine. Large wing-shaped bone at the upper and posterior part of the pelvis
mucus (noun) mucous (adj) mucosa	MYU-kus MYU-kus myu-KOH-sah	 S/ R/ S/	Greek *slime* -ous *pertaining to* muc- *mucus* -osa *full of; like*	Sticky secretion of cells in mucous membranes Pertaining to mucus or the mucosa Lining of a tubular structure that secretes mucus
prostate	PROS-tate		Greek *one who stands before*	Organ surrounding the urethra at the base of the male urinary bladder
prostrate prostration (noun)	pros-TRAYT pros-TRAY-shun		Latin *to stretch out*	To lay flat or to be overcome by physical weakness and exhaustion
reflex reflux	REE-fleks REE-fluks		Latin *bend back* Latin *backward flow*	An involuntary response to a stimulus Backward flow
septum septa (pl)	SEP-tum SEP-tah		Latin *a partition*	A thin wall separating two cavities or two tissue masses
uterus	YOU-ter-us		Latin *womb*	Organ in which an egg develops into a fetus
vertebra vertebrae (pl)	VER-teh-brah VER-teh-brae		Latin *bone in the spine*	One of the bones of the spinal column

Keynotes

- Many words, when they are written or pronounced, have an element that if misspelled or mispronounced gives the intended word an entirely different meaning. A treatment response to the different meaning could cause a medical error or even the death of a patient.
- Precision in written and verbal communication is essential to prevent errors in patient care.
- The medical record in which you document a patient's care and your actions is a legal document. It can be used in court as evidence in professional medical liability cases.

Keynotes

- Communicate verbally and in writing with attention to detail, accuracy, and precision.
- When you understand the individual word elements that make up a medical term, you are better able to understand clearly the medical terms you are using.

Precision in Communication (LO 1.7)

It is important for you to note that being accurate and precise in both your written and verbal communication with your health care team can save someone's life. Each year in the United States, more than 400,000 people die because of drug reactions and medical errors, many of which are the result of poor communication. On the next page, you will find some specific examples of how certain medical terms could be seriously miscommunicated and misinterpreted.

If **hypotensive** (suffering from **low** blood pressure) were confused with **hypertensive** (suffering from **high** blood pressure), incorrect and dangerous treatments could be prescribed.

- In the word **hypotensive**, the **suffix** *-ive* means *pertaining to*. The **prefix** *hypo-* means *below or less than normal.* The **root** *-tens-* means *pressure.* The term **hypotensive** means *pertaining to or suffering from a below normal or low blood pressure.*

- In the word **hypertensive**, the **prefix** *hyper-* means *above or higher than normal.* The term **hypertensive** means *pertaining to or suffering from an above normal or high blood pressure.*

To deconstruct the term **hypotensive,** start with the **suffix** *-ive,* which means *pertaining to* or *suffering from.* Next, the **prefix** *hypo-* means *below or less than normal.* Then the **root** *-tens-* means *pressure.* Now, place the pieces together to form a word meaning *suffering from a below-normal pressure* or *low blood pressure.*

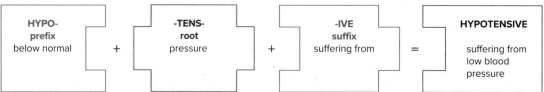

| HYPO-
prefix
below normal | + | -TENS-
root
pressure | + | -IVE
suffix
suffering from | = | HYPOTENSIVE
suffering from low blood pressure |

The term **neurology**, the specialty of the nervous system *(see Chapter 10),* can sound very similar to **urology**, the study of the urinary system *(see Chapter 13).* In the urinary system, if a patient's **ureter** (the tube from the kidney to the bladder) were confused with the **urethra** (the tube from the bladder to the outside), the consequences could be serious.

As you can see from the above examples, your ability to correctly identify, spell, and pronounce different medical terms is essential. Being a health care professional requires the utmost attention to detail, as a patient's life could be in your hands. Incorrect spelling and poor pronunciation not only reflect badly on you and your health care team—it could also be a matter of life and death.

Word Analysis and Definition

S = Suffix   P = Prefix   R = Root   R/CF = Combining Form

WORD	PRONUNCIATION	ELEMENTS		DEFINITION
hypertension	HIGH-per-TEN-shun	S/ P/ R/	-ion *condition, action* hyper- *above normal* -tens- *pressure*	Persistent high arterial blood pressure
hypertensive (adj) hypotension hypotensive (adj)	HIGH-per-TEN-siv HIGH-poh-TEN-shun HIGH-poh-TEN-siv	S/ P/	-ive *pertaining to* hypo- *below normal*	Pertaining to or suffering from high blood pressure Persistent low arterial blood pressure Pertaining to or suffering from low blood pressure
neurology	nyu-ROL-oh-jee	S/ R/CF	-logy *study of* neur/o- *nerve*	Medical specialty of disorders of the nervous system
neurologist	nyu-ROL-oh-jist	S/	-logist *one who studies and is a specialist in*	Medical specialist in disorders of the nervous system
ureter	you-REE-ter		Greek *urinary canal* Greek *passage for urine*	Tube that connects a kidney to the urinary bladder Canal leading from the bladder to the outside
urethra	you-REE-thrah			
urology	you-ROL-oh-jee	S/ R/CF	-logy *study of* ur/o- *urine*	Medical specialty of disorders of the urinary system

EXERCISES

 ### CASE REPORT 1.2

You are . . .

. . . a medical assistant working in the office of Lokesh Bannerjee, MD, a cardiologist in Fulwood Medical Center.

You are communicating with. . .

. . . the 70-year-old spouse and the 45-year-old son of James Donovan, a 75-year-old man who will be admitted to the hospital's acute care **cardiology** unit.

Dr. Bannerjee has **diagnosed** Mr. Donovan with an acute myocardial infarction **(AMI),** confirmed by changes in his **electrocardiogram (ECG/EKG)**. One of your tasks is to explain Mr. Donovan's **diagnosis** and reasons for admission to the hospital to Mrs. Donovan and her son. While Mr. Donovan is waiting to be admitted, he is receiving oxygen through nasal cannula. He is **hypotensive**, and an intravenous **(IV)** infusion of normal saline has been started. His medical record indicates that he is also being seen in the neurology clinic for early dementia.

The bold terms in the Case Report are used as examples in the text and/or are deconstructed in the Word Analysis and Definition box that immediately follows a group of text.

Mr. Donovan is waiting to be admitted to the hospital and is receiving oxygen through nasal cannula. He is **hypotensive,** and an **intravenous (IV) infusion** of normal saline has been started. According to his medical record, he is also being seen in the **neurology** clinic for early dementia.

A. Read Case Report 1.2 and review the content from Section 1.2 to correctly answer the questions. **LO 1.5, 1.6, and 1.7**

1. From which branch of specialty medicine is the provider who is caring for Mr. Donovan? _____

2. Which medical term refers to the specific heart muscle that was damaged? _____

3. From the description of Mr. Donovan's condition while awaiting hospital admission, he is experiencing:

    a. high blood pressure   **b.** low blood pressure   **c.** pain   **d.** nausea

4. Which test, read by Dr. Bannerjee, allowed an appreciation of the changes in the electrical signals of Mr. Donovan's heart?

Precision in communication: *In addition to using the precise medical terms and speaking and spelling them correctly, you must use the appropriate form of the term as well.*

B. There are several forms for the term diagnosis. *Note that there are singular and plural forms of the term, as well as the noun, adjective, and verb forms. Insert the correct form of the term in the documentation below.* **LO 1.1, 1.2, and 1.7**

    Note: A noun is a person, place, or thing.   Singular: One

            A verb denotes action.   Plural: More than one

            An adjective usually describes something.

1. The primary _____ for this patient is myocardial ischemia.

2. Dr. Bannerjee is unable to _____ this patient until he receives the lab results.

3. The _____ tests have been ordered for this patient first thing in the morning.

4. It is possible for this patient to have multiple _____ if there is more than one condition present.

C. **Identify the form of the term diagnosis.** *Fill in the blanks.* **LO 1.4 and 1.7**

1. The verb form: _____

2. Plural form: _____

3. Singular noun: _____

4. Adjective form: _____

D. **Medical language:** *Many terms in medicine sound and/or look very similar. The difference of only one letter can create a new term. Train your eye and ear to recognize the difference. Select the correct choice of terms in the following documentation.* **LO 1.6 and 1.7**

1. The patient's nasal (mucus/mucous) membrane is severely inflamed.

2. Schedule this patient for a (prostrate/prostate) exam at his next annual physical.

3. The doctor checked the (reflex/reflux) in the patient's knee.

4. The patient's (ilium/ileum) was severely fractured in the motor vehicle accident.

E. **Plurals:** *Select the correct form of the plural in the following sentences.* **LO 1.5**

1. Because of additional medical problems needing treatment, this patient's insurance claim form will include multiple (diagnoses/diagnosis).

2. Check both (axilla/axillae) for any evidence of enlarged lymph nodes.

3. Several (septa/septum) exist in the body—e.g., in the heart and in the nose.

4. A cluster of (ganglia/ganglion) has formed on her left wrist.

F. **Terminology challenge:** *Use your knowledge of the new medical terms you have learned in this chapter and choose the correct answer.* **LO 1.7**

1. The term *cervical* can apply to two different places in the body. Where are they?
   a. neck of the body and neck of the femur
   b. neck of the uterus and neck of the humerus
   c. neck of the femur and neck of the humerus
   d. neck of the body and neck of the uterus

2. The terms *ileum* and *ilium* are pronounced the same but are in two different body systems. Where are they?
   a. muscular and nervous systems
   b. digestive and skeletal systems
   c. circulatory and integumentary systems
   d. endocrine and respiratory systems

G. **Patient documentation:** *Read the following excerpts from patient charts and insert the medical term that correctly completes each sentence.* **LO 1.7**

1. This patient has several badly fractured _____ in his spinal column.

2. This patient has nerve damage. Refer him to the department of _____ .

3. Schedule this patient for an _____ of chemotherapy drugs today.

4. This patient has low blood pressure—he is _____ and anemic.

5. I am ordering an immediate _____ of 2 units of whole blood for this patient.

6. Send this patient for _____ X-rays of his neck immediately.

H. **Brain teaser:** *Challenge yourself to analyze the question and insert the correct answers.* **LO 1.1, 1.2, and 1.7**

1. If a medical specialist in the study of disorders of the nervous system is a neurologist, what is a medical specialist in the study of disorders of the urinary system called?
   (Hint: Use your knowledge of suffixes and roots to help you.)

2. What element is the difference between high blood pressure and low blood pressure? _____

3. What is the tube that connects a kidney to the bladder? _____

4. What substance goes through a transfusion but not through an infusion? _____

Additional exercises available in **connect** | **Chapter Review exercises, along with additional practice items, are available in Connect!**

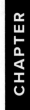
The Body as a Whole, Cells, and Genes

The Essentials of the Languages of Anatomy and Genetics

Classic Collection/Shotshop GmbH/Alamy Images

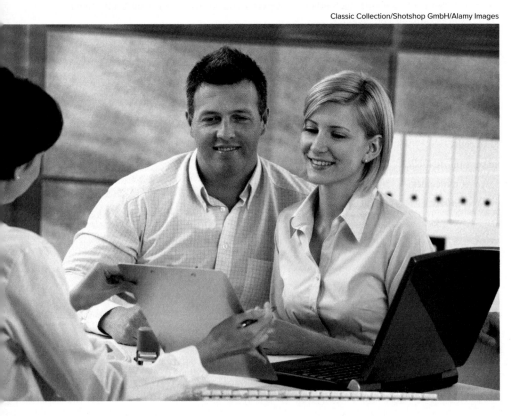

Learning Outcomes

Effective medical treatment recognizes that each organ, tissue, and cell in your body, no matter where it is located, connects to and functions in harmony with every other organ, tissue, and cell. To understand these concepts, you need to be able to:

LO 2.1 Use **roots, combining forms, suffixes, and prefixes** to construct and analyze (deconstruct) medical terms related to the anatomy and physiology of the body as a whole.

LO 2.2 Spell and pronounce correctly medical terms related to the body as a whole in order to communicate with accuracy and precision in any health care setting.

LO 2.3 Discuss the medical terms associated with cells and tissues.

LO 2.4 Explain the terms genes, genetics, and gene therapy.

LO 2.5 Describe the primary tissue groups and their functions.

LO 2.6 Relate individual organs and organ systems to the organization and function of the body as a whole.

LO 2.7 Integrate the medical terms of the different anatomic positions, planes, and directions of the body into everyday medical language.

LO 2.8 Describe the nine regions of the abdomen.

LO 2.9 Map the body cavities.

LO 2.10 Apply your knowledge of the medical terms of the body as a whole to documentation, medical records, and medical reports.

LO 2.11 Translate the medical terms of the body as a whole into everyday language to communicate clearly with patients and their families.

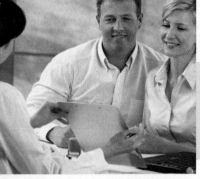

Section 2.1

Composition of Body and Cells

All the different elements of your body interact with each other to support constant change as your body reacts to your environment and to the nourishment you give it.

Abbreviation

IVF   in vitro fertilization

Keynotes

- **In vitro fertilization (IVF)** combines eggs and sperm in a laboratory dish.

- After fertilization occurs, the embryos are placed into the woman's uterus.

Composition of the Body (LO 2.1 and 2.2)

- The whole body or organism is composed of **organ systems** *(Figure 2.1)*.
- Organ systems are composed of **organs.**
- Organs are composed of **tissues.**
- Tissues are composed of **cells.**
- Cells are composed in part of **organelles.**
- Organelles are composed of **molecules.**
- Molecules are composed of **atoms.**

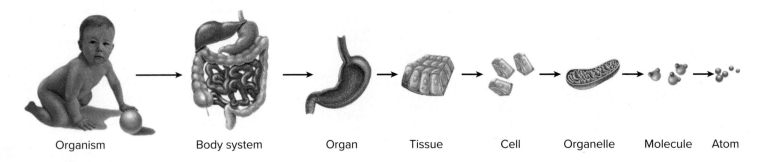

Organism   Body system   Organ   Tissue   Cell   Organelle   Molecule   Atom

▲ **FIGURE 2.1**
Composition of the Body.

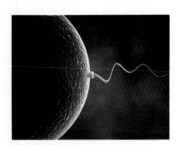

The Cell (LO 2.3)

The result of the **fertilization** of an egg by a sperm is a single fertilized cell called a **zygote** *(Figure 2.2)*. This process is also called **conception**. This zygote is the origin of every cell in your body. It divides and multiplies into trillions of cells, which become the basic unit of every tissue and organ. These cells are responsible for the structure and all the functions of your tissues and organs.

    Cytology is the study of cell structure and function, and this forms the basis of the knowledge of the anatomy and physiology of every tissue and organ.

▲ **FIGURE 2.2**
Fertilization of Egg by Single Sperm.

WORD	PRONUNCIATION		ELEMENTS	DEFINITION
atom	**AT**-om		Greek *indivisible*	A small unit of matter
cell	**SELL**		Latin a *storeroom*	The smallest unit of the body capable of independent existence
conception	kon-**SEP**-shun		Latin *something received*	Fertilization of the egg by sperm to form a zygote
cytology	sigh-**TOL**-oh-jee	S/ R/CF	-**logy** *study of* **cyt/o-** *cell*	Study of the cell
cytologist	**SIGH**-tol-oh-jist	S/	-**logist** *one who studies, a specialist*	Specialist in the structure, chemistry, and pathology of the cell
fertilization (noun)	**FER**-til-eye-**ZAY**-shun	S/ R/	-**ation** *process* **fertiliz-** *to make fruitful*	Union of a male sperm and a female egg
fertilize (verb) in vitro	**FER**-til-izeen-**VEE**-troh IN **VEE**-troh		Greek *to bear* Latin *glass*	Penetration of the egg by sperm In vitro fertilization is the process of combining sperm and eggs in a laboratory dish and placing resulting embryos inside a uterus
molecule	**MOLL**-eh-kyul\	S/ R/	-**ule** *small* **molec-** *mass*	Very small particle consisting of two or more atoms held tightly together
molecular (adj) (*Note:* The two suffixes are joined by two vowels: therefore, the *e* in *ule* is not used.)	mo-**LEK**-you-lar	S/	-**ar** *pertaining to*	Pertaining to a molecule.
organ	**OR**-gan		Latin *instrument, tool*	Structure with specific functions in a body system
organelle	**OR**-gah-nell	S/ R/	-**elle** *small* **organ-** *organ*	Part of a cell having specialized function(s)
organism	**OR**-gan-izm	S/	-**ism** *condition, process*	Any whole living, individual plant or animal
tissue	**TISH**-you		Latin *to weave*	Collection of similar cells
zygote	**ZYE**-goat		Greek *yolk*	Cell resulting from the union of sperm and egg

Structure and Function of Cells (LO 2.3)

As the zygote divides, every cell it creates becomes a complex little factory that carries out these basic life functions:

- **Manufacture** of **proteins** and **lipids;**
- **Production** and use of energy;
- **Communication** with other cells;
- **Replication** of **deoxyribonucleic acid (DNA)**; and
- **Reproduction** of itself.

All cells contain a fluid called **cytoplasm** (intracellular fluid) surrounded by a cell **membrane** *(Figure 2.3)*. Your cell membrane—made of **proteins** and **lipids**—allows water, oxygen, glucose, **electrolytes**, **steroids**, and alcohol to pass through it. On the outside of the cell membrane, you have receptors that bind to chemical messengers like **hormones** sent by other cells. These are the chemical signals by which your cells communicate with each other.

Organelles (LO 2.3)

Organelles are small structures in the cytoplasm of the cell that carry out special **metabolic** tasks (the chemical processes that occur in the cell).

The **nucleus** is the largest organelle *(Figure 2.3)*. It is surrounded by its own membrane and directs all the cell's activities. The 46 molecules of DNA in the nucleus form 46 **chromosomes**.

A **nucleolus** is a small, dense body composed of **ribonucleic acid (RNA)** and protein found in the nucleus. It is involved in the manufacture of proteins from simple materials—a process called **anabolism**.

Mitochondria are the cell's powerhouses. They produce energy by breaking down compounds like glucose and fat in a process called **catabolism**.

- **Metabolism** is the sum of the constructive processes of anabolism and the destructive processes of catabolism within a cell (**intracellular**).

The **endoplasmic reticulum** manufactures steroids, cholesterol and other lipids, and proteins. It also detoxifies alcohol and other drugs.

Keynote

- The cytoplasm is a clear, gelatinous substance containing different organelles.

Abbreviations

DNA   deoxyribonucleic acid
RNA   ribonucleic acid

▼ **FIGURE 2.3**
Structure of a Representative Cell.

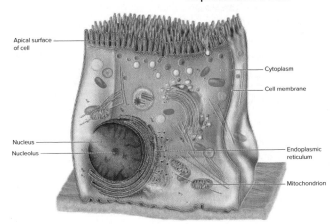

Apical surface of cell
Cytoplasm
Cell membrane
Nucleus
Nucleolus
Endoplasmic reticulum
Mitochondrion

WORD	PRONUNCIATION	ELEMENTS		DEFINITION
anabolism	an-**AB**-oh-lizm	S/ R/	-ism *process, condition* anabol- *build up*	The buildup of complex substances in the cell from simpler ones as a part of metabolism
catabolism	kah-**TAB**-oh-lizm	S/ R/	-ism *process, condition* catabol- *break down*	The breakdown of complex substances into simpler ones as a part of metabolism
chromosome	**KROH**-moh-sohm	S/ R/CF	-some *body* chrom/o- *color*	Body in the nucleus that contains DNA and genes
cytoplasm	**SIGH**-toh-plazm	S/ R/CF	-plasm *something formed* cyt/o- *cell*	Clear, gelatinous substance that forms the substance of a cell, except for the nucleus
deoxyribonucleic acid (DNA)	dee-**OCK**-see-rye-boh-nyu-**KLEE**-ik **ASS**-id		deoxyribose *a sugar* nucleic acid *a protein*	Source of hereditary characteristics found in chromosomes
electrolyte	ee-**LEK**-troh-lite	S/ R/CF	-lyte *soluble* electr/o- *electricity*	Substance that, when dissolved in a suitable medium, forms electrically charged particles
endoplasmic reticulum	**EN**-doh-**PLAZ**-mik reh-**TIC**-you-lum ribonucleic acid	S/ P/ R/ S/ R/	-ic *pertaining to* endo- *inside, within* -plasm- *something formed* -um *structure* -reticul- *fine net, network*	Structure inside a cell that synthesizes steroids, detoxifies drugs, and manufactures cell membranes
hormone hormonal (adj)	**HOR**-mohn hor-**MOHN**-al	 S/ R/	Greek *set in motion* -al *pertaining to* hormon- *hormone*	Chemical formed in one tissue or organ and carried by the blood to stimulate or inhibit a function of another tissue or organ Pertaining to a hormone
intracellular (adj)	in-trah-**SELL**-you-lar	S/ P/ R/	-ar *pertaining to* intra- *within* -cellul- *small cell*	Within the cell
lipid	**LIP**-id		Greek *fat*	General term for all types of fatty compounds; for example, cholesterol, triglycerides, and fatty acids
membrane membranous (adj)	**MEM**-brain **MEM**-brah-nus	 S/ R/	Latin *parchment* -ous *pertaining to* membran- *cover, skin*	Thin layer of tissue covering a structure or cavity Pertaining to a membrane
metabolism metabolic (adj)	meh-**TAB**-oh-lizm met-ah-**BOL**-ik	S/ R/ S/	-ism *condition, process* metabol- *change* -ic *pertaining to*	The constantly changing physical and chemical processes occurring in the cell that are the sum of anabolism and catabolism Pertaining to metabolism
mitochondria (pl) mitochondrion (singular)	my-toe-**KON**-dree-ah my-toe-**KON**-dree-on	S/ R/CF R/ S/	-ia *condition* mit/o- *thread* -chondr- *granule* -ion *condition*	Organelles that generate, store, and release energy for cell activities
nucleolus	nyu-**KLEE**-oh-lus	S/ R/CF	-lus *small* nucle/o- *nucleus*	Small mass within the nucleus
nucleus nuclear (adj)	**NYU**-klee-us **NYU**-klee-ar	 S/ R/	Latin *command center* -ar *pertaining to* nucle- *nucleus*	Functional center of a cell or structure Pertaining to a nucleus
protein	**PRO**-teen		Greek *protein*	Class of food substances based on amino acids
ribonucleic acid (RNA)	**RYE**-boh-nyu-**KLEE**-ik **ASS**-id	S/ P/ R/	-ic *pertaining to* ribo- *from ribose, a sugar* -nucle- *nucleus*	The information carrier from DNA in the nucleus to an organelle to produce protein molecules
steroid	**STAIR**-oyd	S/ R/	-oid *resembling* ster- *solid*	Large family of chemical substances found in many drugs, hormones, and body components

EXERCISES

 Case Report 2.1

You are . . .

. . . a certified medical assistant (**CMA**) employed as an in vitro fertilization coordinator in the Assisted Reproduction Clinic at Fulwood Medical Center.

You are communicating with . . .

. . . Mrs. Mary Arnold, a 35-year-old woman who has been unable to **conceive. In vitro fertilization (IVF)** was recommended. After **hormone** therapy, several healthy and mature eggs were recovered from her **ovary**. The eggs were combined with her husband's **sperm** in a laboratory dish where **fertilization** occurred to form a single cell, called a **zygote**. The cells were allowed to divide for five days to become **blastocysts**, and then four blastocysts were implanted in her uterus.

Your role is to guide, counsel, and support Mrs. Arnold and her husband through the implementation and follow-up for the IVF process.

Mrs. Arnold achieved pregnancy and delivered a healthy girl at term.

A. Read Case Report 2.1 and answer the following questions. **LO 2.10**

1. The procedure of in vitro fertilization can be abbreviated. Provide the abbreviation here: _____

2. There is a term in Case Report 2.1 that can be replaced with oocytes. Insert the term here (make sure it is in plural form): _____

3. Which test would indicate that successful implantation has taken place?

    a. genomic evaluation   **b.** pregnancy test   **c.** phenotyping   **d.** prenatal therapy

B. Read *the terms related to the composition of the body and the cell. Pay careful attention to word elements and meanings. Fill in the blanks.* **LO 2.1 and 2.3**

1. Put the following terms in ascending order of their size (smallest to largest):

organism	**cells**	**molecules**	**organs**
organ systems	**organelles**	**atoms**	**tissues**

    a. _____

    b. _____

    c. _____

    d. _____

    e. _____

    f. _____

    g. _____

    h. _____

C. Use the terms *and their elements related to the cell to answer the questions.* **LO 2.1 and 2.2**

1. The suffix _____ means *study of.* The suffix that means *specialist (in the study of)* is. _____

2. What part of *cyt/o-* makes it a combining form rather than a root? _____

3. What is the medical term for *union of a sperm and an egg?* _____

4. What suffix related to the composition of the body and the cell describes the size of something? _____

5. What does a cytologist study? _____

D. Knowledge *of elements is your best clue to determining the meaning of medical terminology. Deconstruct the elements in these questions to find your answers. Select the BEST ANSWER to the question.* **LO 2.3**

1. Which term relates to electrically charged particles?

    a. protein   **b.** hormonal   **c.** electrolyte

2. Which term relates to change?

    a. steroid   **b.** metabolic   **c.** lipid

3. Which term has an element meaning "condition"?

    a. metabolism   **b.** cytoplasm   **c.** hormone

4. What is a thin layer of tissue that covers a structure or cavity?

    a. lipid   **b.** membrane   **c.** hormone

Section 2.2

Genes and Genetics

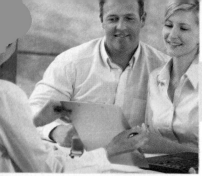

Abbreviations

A	adenosine
C	cytosine
G	guanine
T	thymine
DNA	deoxyribonucleic acid

Keynotes

- Deoxyribonucleic acid (DNA) is the hereditary material in humans.
- DNA molecules are packaged into chromosomes.
- Genes are the basic functional and physical unit of **heredity** and are made up of DNA.
- Genes regulate the division and replication of cells.
- Cancer can result when cell division and replication are abnormal.
- Chemical compounds can be added to a gene and can lead to abnormal **genetic** (epigenetic) activity producing cancers and degenerative and metabolic diseases.

DNA and Genes (LO 2.4)

Inside the cell nucleus are packed 46 molecules of **deoxyribonucleic acid (DNA)** as thin strands called **chromatin.** When cells divide, the chromatin condenses with **histone** proteins to form 23 pairs (46 total) of densely coiled bodies called **chromosomes**. Twenty-two of these pairs look the same in both males and females. In the 23rd pair, females have two copies of the X chromosome; males have one X and one Y. The picture of the human chromosomes lined up in pairs is called a **karyotype** *(Figure 2.4).*

The information in DNA is stored as a code of four chemical bases: adenine (A), guanine (G), cytosine (C), and thymine (T). The total human DNA contains about 3 billion bases, and more than 99% of those bases are the same in all people. The sequence of these bases determines the building and maintaining of the organism's cells, similar to the way in which letters of the alphabet appear in order to form words and sentences.

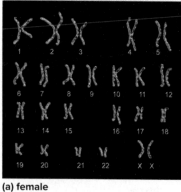
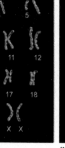
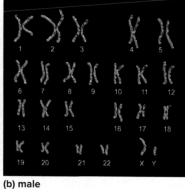

(a) female   (b) male

◀ **FIGURE 2.4** Human Karyotype.

Kateryna Kon/Shutterstock

The **chromosomal** DNA bases pair with each other—A with T and C with G—and are attached to a sugar molecule and a phosphate molecule. A base, sugar, and phosphate form a **nucleotide.** Nucleotides are arranged in two long strands to form a spiral called a double **helix.**

The nuclear DNA in the chromosomes is the **hereditary** material, each unit of which is called a **gene.** The genes act as instructions to make molecules of different proteins. Each person has two copies of each gene, one inherited from each parent. Most genes are the same in all people; only less than 1% is slightly different between people. These small differences contribute to each person's unique physical features. Humans are thought to have between 20,000 and 25,000 genes. This total is called the **genome.**

Mitosis

The critical property of DNA is that it can **replicate,** make copies of itself, so that when cells divide, each new cell has an exact copy of the DNA present in the old cell. This cell division is called **mitosis**, in which a cell duplicates all of its contents, including its chromosomes, to form two identical daughter cells. When mitosis is not performed correctly, abnormal cells, such as cancer cells, can result.

Mutations and Epigenetic Changes

A permanent alteration of the nucleotide sequence of the genome of an organism is called a **mutation**. Mutations may or may not produce visible changes in the observable characteristics (**phenotype**) of an organism. Mutations play a part in both normal and abnormal biological processes including evolution, cancer, and the development of the immune system.

Chemical compounds that become added to single genes can regulate their activity to produce modifications known as **epigenetic** changes. These changes can remain as cells divide and can be inherited through generations. Environmental influences from pollution, drugs, pharmaceuticals, aging, and diets can also produce epigenetic modifications, such as cancers, mental disorders, and degenerative and metabolic disorders.

Word Analysis and Definition

WORD	PRONUNCIATION	ELEMENTS		DEFINITION
chromatin	KROH-ma-tin	S/ R/CF	-tin *pertaining to* chrom/a- *color*	DNA that forms chromosomes during cell division
chromosome	KROH-moh-sohm	R/CF R/	chrom/o- *color* -some *body*	The body in the cell nucleus that carries the genes
chromosomal (adj)	KROH-moh-SO-mal	S/	-al *pertaining to*	Pertaining to a chromosome
deoxyribonucleic acid (DNA)	dee-OCK-see-RYE-boh-noo-KLEE-ik ASS-id	S/ P/ P/ R/ R/ R/	-ic *pertaining to* de- *without* -oxy- *oxygen* -ribo- *ribose* -nucle- *nucleus* acid *acid, low pH*	The chemical repository of hereditary characteristics
epigenetics	EP-ih-jeh-NET-iks	S/ P/ R/	-etics *pertaining to* epi- *above, over* -gen- *to create*	The study of disorders produced by the effects of chemical compounds (e.g., pollutants) or environmental influences (such as diet) on genes
gene genetic (adj)	JEEN jeh-NET-ik	S/ R/ R/	Greek *birth* -etic *pertaining to* gen- *to create* -ome *body*	The functional unit of heredity on a chromosome Pertaining to genetics
genome	JEE-nome			A complete set of chromosomes
helix	HEE-liks		Greek *a coil*	A spiral of nucleotides in the structure of DNA
heredity	heh-RED-ih-tee		Latin *an heir*	The transmission of characteristics from parent to offspring
hereditary (adj)	her-ED-ih-TAIR-ee	S/ R/	-ary *pertaining to* heredit- *inherited through genes*	Transmissible from parent to offspring
histone	HIS-tone	S/ R/	-one *chemical* hist- *tissue*	A simple protein found in the cell nucleus
karyotype	KAIR-ee-oh-type	S/ R/CF	-type *model* kary/o- *nucleus*	The chromosome characteristics of an individual cell
mitosis	my-TOE-sis		Greek *thread*	Cell division to create two identical cells, each with 46 chromosomes
mutation	myu-TAY-shun		Latin *to change*	A permanent alteration in the nucleotide sequence of the genome
nucleotide	NYU-klee-oh-tide	R/CF R/	nucle/o- *nucleus* -tide *time*	Combination of a DNA base, a sugar molecule, and a phosphate molecule
phenotype	FEE-noh-type	S/ R/CF	-type *model* phen/o- *appearance*	Manifestation of a genome
replicate (verb)	REP-lih-kate		Latin *a reply*	To produce an exact copy

EXERCISES

A. Use your knowledge of medical terminology related to genetics. Insert the correct term in the appropriate statement. **LO 2.4**

gene   genome   mitosis   chromosomes   chromatin

1. When the cell is maintaining normal function, DNA and proteins are contained within thin strands of _____.

2. When the cell is dividing, DNA wraps around the proteins and is contained within densely coiled bodies called _____.

3. The unit of nuclear DNA in the chromosomes is called a _____.

4. A _____ is a complete set of chromosomes.

5. The process of _____ occurs when a cell creates an exact copy of itself and divides into two identical cells.

Genetic Medicine

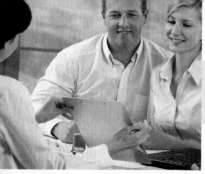

Classic Collection/Shotshop GmbH/Alamy Images

Genetic Medicine (LO 2.4)

Medical genetics is the application of genetics to medical care. Genetic medicine is the newer term for medical genetics and incorporates areas such as gene therapy, personalized (precise) medicine, and predictive medicine.

Every person has a unique variation of the human genome and an individual's health stems from this genetic variation interacting with behaviors (drinking, smoking, etc.) and influences from the environment (chemical pollution in some form). Knowing the genetic makeup will enable more accurate diagnoses to be made, the source of the disease to be understood, and earlier and more accurate treatments for the prevention of progression of the disease provided. This concept is called *personalized medicine.*

One way that the biological variant is seen is responsiveness to drugs. Attention deficit hyperactivity disorder (ADHD) medications only work for one out of ten preschoolers, cancer drugs are effective for only one out of four patients, and depression drugs work for six out of ten patients. The drug Tamoxifen used to be prescribed to women with a form of breast cancer (BRCA), but 65% developed resistance to it. These women were found to have a mutation in their CYP2D6 gene that made Tamoxifen an ineffective treatment.

Personalized medicine can assist with preventive care. Women are already being genotyped for mutations in the BRCA1 (BReast CAncer gene 1) and BRCA2 (BReast CAncer gene 2) genes if they have a family history of breast or ovarian cancer. Women who test positive for both mutations can consider preventive treatment that is specific to genetic mutations.

Cytogenetics is the study of chromosome abnormalities to determine a cause for developmental delay, intellectual disability, birth defects, and **dysmorphic** features. Chromosomal abnormalities are often detected in cancer cells.

Gene therapy is an experimental technique to replace a mutated gene that causes disease with a healthy copy, inactivate a mutated gene that is functioning improperly, or introduce a new gene into the body to prevent or help cure a disease. The **therapeutic** genes are introduced into body cells, and some 600 clinical trials using this form of therapy are underway in the United States.

Predictive medicine looks at the probability of a disease and allows preventive measures to be taken. Examples are newborn screening to identify genetic disorders that can be treated early in life, and **prenatal** testing to look for diseases and conditions in an **embryo** or **fetus** whose parents have an increased risk of having a baby with a genetic or chromosomal disorder.

Word Analysis and Definition

S = Suffix   P = Prefix   R = Root   R/CF = Combining Form

WORD	PRONUNCIATION	ELEMENTS		DEFINITION
cytogenetics	SIGH-toh-jeh-NET-iks	S/ R/CF R/	-etics *pertaining to* cyto- *cell* -gen- *create*	Study of chromosomal abnormalities in a cell
dysmorphology	dis-mor-FOLL-oh-jee	S/ P/ R/CF	-logy *study of* dys- *difficult, bad* -morph/o- *form*	Study of developmental structural defects
dysmorphic (adj)	dis-MOR-fik	S/	-ic *pertaining to*	Possessing a developmental structural defect
embryo	EM-bree-oh		Greek *a young one*	Developing organism from conception until the end of the eighth week
fetus	FEE-tus		Latin *offspring*	Human organism from the end of the eighth week to birth
predictive (adj)	pree-DIK-tiv	S/ P/ R/	-ive *quality of* pre- *before* -dict- *consent*	The likelihood of a disease or disorder being present or occurring in the future
prenatal (adj)	pree-NAY-tal	S/ P/ R/	-al *pertaining to* pre- *before* -nat- *born*	Pertaining to before birth Pertaining to before birth
therapy	THAIR-ah-pee		Greek *medical treatment*	Systematic treatment of a disease, dysfunction, or disorder
therapeutic (adj)	THAIR-ah-PYU-tik	S/ R/	-ic *pertaining to* therapeut- *treatment*	Relating to the treatment of a disease or disorder
therapist	THAIR-ah-pist	S/ R/	-ist *specialist* therap- *treatment*	Professional trained in the practice of a particular therapy

EXERCISES

 Case Report 2.2

You are

. . . a physician's assistant (**PA**) in the Genetic Counseling Clinic at Fulwood Medical Center.

Your patient is

. . . Mrs. Patricia Bennet, a 52-year-old office manager with two daughters, aged 30 and 25. Mrs. Bennett's sister, aged 55, recently had a mastectomy for breast cancer and is now receiving chemotherapy. Their mother died of ovarian cancer in her late fifties. Mrs. Bennet wants to know her risk for breast or ovarian cancer, what she can do to prevent it, and what her daughters' risks are.

A. After reading Case Report 2.2, select the correct answer to each question. **LO 2.3 and 2.11**

1. The purpose of Mrs. Bennett's visit with you today is to determine her:

   a. gene therapy   **c.** personalized medicine

   b. predictive medicine   **d.** cytogenetics

2. Mrs. Bennett wants to determine if the cause of her mother's and sister's cancer is:

   a. genetic   **c.** causative

   b. dysmorphic   **d.** therapeutic

3. The types of cancer that affected Mrs. Bennett's sister and mother were of which system?

   a. digestive   **c.** endocrine

   b. urinary   **d.** reproductive

B. Discuss *the applications of medical genetics. Choose the correct answer to complete the following statements.* **LO 2.4**

1. The replacement of a mutated gene with a healthy copy is termed:

   a. predictive medicine   **c.** gene therapy

   b. cytogenetics   **d.** personalized medicine

2. The study of chromosome abnormalities in a cell is:

   a. cytogenetics   **c.** prenatal therapy

   b. dysmorphology   **d.** precise medicine

3. _____ medicine uses genetics to determine accurate treatments for an existing condition.

   a. Personalized   **c.** Cytogenetic

   b. Preventive   **d.** Predictive

C. Not all terms can be deconstructed. *It is sometimes necessary to memorize the medical terms of Greek and Latin origin. Given the definition, provide the term that is being described. Fill in the blanks.* **LO 2.2 and 2.4**

1. Systematic treatment of a disease, dysfunction, or disorder. _____

2. Human organism from conception to the end of the eighth week. _____

3. Human organism from the end of the eighth week to birth. _____

4. Curing or capable of curing a disorder or disease. _____

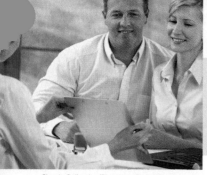

Section 2.4

Tissues, Organs, and Organ Systems

Your tissues, organs, and organ systems must continually adapt and adjust in order to work in sync with each other.

Tissues (LO 2.5)

Tissues have many functions, including storage, transport, and support of the framework for the body. Each tissue is different but made of similar cells with unique materials around them manufactured by the cells. The many tissues of your body have different structures that enable them to perform specialized functions. **Histology** is the study of the structure and function of tissues. The four primary tissue types are outlined in *Table 2.1.*

Table 2.1 The Four Primary Tissue Groups (LO 2.5)

Type	Function	Location
Connective	Bind, support, protect, fill spaces, store fat	Widely distributed throughout the body, e.g., in blood, bone, cartilage, and fat
Epithelial	Protect, secrete, absorb, excrete	Cover body surface, cover and line internal organs, compose glands
Muscle	Movement	Attached to bones; found in the walls of hollow tubes, organs, and the heart
Nervous	Transmit impulses for coordination, sensory reception, motor actions	Brain, spinal cord, nerves

Adapted from David Shier, Jackie L. Butler, and Ricki Lewis, *Hole's Human Anatomy and Physiology,* 10th ed.

Connective Tissues (LO 2.5)

The relation of structure to function in your body tissues is key. To help you understand this important connection, this lesson uses the knee joint to illustrate the structures and functions of the different tissues found in this joint.

Connective Tissues in the Knee Joint (LO 2.5)

The **connective** tissues in your knee joint make it possible for you to enjoy your daily life—from standing, sitting, walking, bending, and running. These tissues and their roles are listed below:

- The **bones** of the knee joint are the **femur**, **tibia**, and **patella** *(see Chapter 4).* Bone is the hardest connective tissue in your body because it contains calcium mineral salts (mainly calcium phosphate). Bones have a good blood supply so they can heal well after a fracture. Bones in general are covered with a thick fibrous tissue called the **periosteum**.

- **Cartilage** has a flexible, rubbery **matrix** (in the knee as a **meniscus**) that allows it to function as a shock absorber and a gliding surface where two bones meet to form a joint. Cartilage has very few blood vessels and therefore heals poorly—sometimes not at all. When it is injured or torn, surgery is often needed. Cartilage also forms the shape of your ear, the tip of your nose, and your larynx.

- **Ligaments** are strips or bands of fibrous, connective tissue made of **collagen** fibers. Hold the knee joint together. The knee joint has four major ligaments that hold it together. Two ligaments outside the joint cavity on each side of the joint are the **medial collateral ligament (MCL)** and the **lateral collateral ligament (LCL)** *(Figure 2.5).* Two other ligaments located inside the joint cavity are called the **anterior cruciate ligament (ACL)** and the **posterior cruciate ligament**; they cross over each other to form an "X". *(Figure 2.5a).* The blood supply to these ligaments is poor, so they do not heal well without surgery.

Keynotes

- Certain tissues are made of specialized cells that manufacture unique fluids. The epithelial layer of the synovial membrane is an example, as it produces synovial fluid.

- Each connective tissue has distinct functions that enable a structure or organ to function correctly.

- There are four major ligaments of the knee joint:

  1. anterior cruciate ligament (ACL)
  2. posterior cruciate ligament (PCL)
  3. medial collateral ligament (MCL)
  4. lateral collateral ligament (LCL)

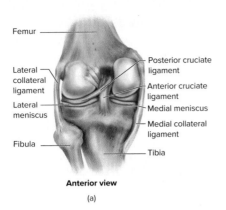

Femur
Lateral collateral ligament
Lateral meniscus
Fibula
Posterior cruciate ligament
Anterior cruciate ligament
Medial meniscus
Medial collateral ligament
Tibia

Anterior view

(a)

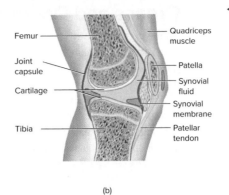

Femur
Joint capsule
Cartilage
Tibia
Quadriceps muscle
Patella
Synovial fluid
Synovial membrane
Patellar tendon

(b)

◀ **FIGURE 2.5** Ligaments of Knee Joint, with the Patellar Tendon Removed.

- **Tendons** are thick, strong ligaments that attach muscles to bone. Tendons can become inflamed and sometime even torn, thereby allowing muscles to detach from the bone.

- The **joint capsule** *(Figure 2.5b)* of the knee joint encloses the joint cavity. It's made of thin, fibrous connective tissue and strengthened by fibers that extend over it from the surrounding ligaments and muscles. These features are common to most joints.

- The **synovial membrane** *(Figure 2.5b)* lines many joint capsules and secretes **synovial fluid**—a slippery lubricant stored in the joint cavity. This fluid makes joint movement almost friction-free. It distributes **nutrients** to the cartilage on the joint surfaces of bone.

- **Muscle tissue** stabilizes the joint. Extensions of the large muscle tendons in the front and the rear of the thigh are major stabilizers of the knee joint. The muscles alone extend and flex the knee joint *(see Chapter 4)*.

- **Nervous tissue** carries messages between the brain and the knee structures. The knee structures are packed with nerves, which is why a knee injury is excruciatingly painful.

Word Analysis and Definition

S = Suffix   P = Prefix   R = Root   R/CF = Combining Form

WORD	PRONUNCIATION		ELEMENTS	DEFINITION
capsule	KAP-syul	S/	Latin *little box*	Fibrous tissue layer surrounding a joint or other structure
capsular (adj)	KAP-syu-lar	R/	-ar *pertaining to* capsul- *box*	Pertaining to a capsule
cartilage	KAR-tih-lij		Latin *gristle*	Nonvascular, firm connective tissue found mostly in joints
collagen	KOLL-ah-jen	S/ R/CF	-gen *produce, form* coll/a- *glue*	Major protein of connective tissue, cartilage, and bone
connective tissue	koh-NECK-tiv TISH-you	S/ R/	-ive *pertaining to* connect- *join together* tissue Latin *to weave*	The supporting tissue of the body
cruciate (adj)	KRU-she-ate		Latin *cross*	Shaped like a cross
histology	his-TOL-oh-jee	S/ R/CF	-logy *study of* hist/o- *tissue*	Study of the structure and function of cells, tissues, and organs
histologist	his-TOL-oh-jist	S/	-logist *one who studies, specialist*	Specialist in histology
ligament	LIG-ah-ment		Latin *band*	Band of fibrous tissue connecting two structures
matrix	MAY-triks		Latin mater *mother*	Substance that surrounds and protects cells, is manufactured by the cells, and holds them together
meniscus	meh-NISS-kuss		Greek *crescent*	Disc of cartilage between the bones of a joint
muscle	MUSS-el		Latin *muscle*	A tissue consisting of contractile cells
nutrient	NYU-tree-ent	S/ R/	-ent *end result* nutri- *nourish*	A substance in food required for normal physiologic function
periosteum	PAIR-ee-OSS-tee-um	S/ P/ R/	-um *tissue* peri- *around* -oste- *bone*	Fibrous membrane covering a bone
synovial (adj)	si-NOH-vee-al	S/ P/ R/CF	-al *pertaining to* syn- *together* -ov/i- *egg*	Pertaining to the synovial membrane or fluid
tendon	TEN-dun		Latin *sinew*	Fibrous band that connects muscle to bone

Organs and Organ Systems (LO 2.6)

An **organ** is a structure composed of several tissues that work together to carry out specific functions. For example, your skin is an organ that contains different tissues, such as epithelial cells, hair, nails, and glands *(see Chapter 3)*.

An **organ system** is a group of organs with a specific collective function, like digestion, circulation, or respiration. For example, your nose, pharynx, larynx, trachea, bronchi, and lungs all work together to achieve the total function of respiration *(see Chapter 8)*.

The different organs in an organ system are usually interconnected. For example, in the **urinary** organ system *(Figure 2.6)*, the organs are the kidneys, ureters, bladder, and urethra, and they are all connected *(see Chapter 13)*.

All your organ systems work together to ensure that your body's internal environment remains relatively constant. This process is called **homeostasis**. It ensures that cells receive adequate nutrients and oxygen and that cell waste products are removed so your cells can function normally. Disease affecting an organ or organ system disrupts the achievement and maintenance of homeostasis.

Your body has 11 organ systems, as shown in *Table 2.2*. Muscular and **skeletal** are considered one organ system called the musculoskeletal system *(see Chapters 4 and 5)*. Each body system has a chapter in this book where the associated terms are defined.

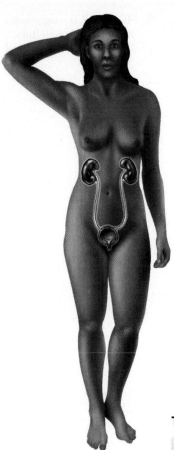

▲ **FIGURE 2.6**
The Urinary System.

Table 2.2 Organ Systems (LO 2.6)

Organ System	Major Organs	Major Functions
Integumentary	Skin, hair, nails, sweat glands, sebaceous glands	Protect tissues, regulate body temperature, support sensory receptors
Skeletal	Bones, ligaments, cartilage	Provide framework, protect soft tissues, provide attachments for muscles, produce blood cells, store inorganic salts
Muscular	Muscles	Cause movements, maintain posture, produce body heat
Nervous	Brain, spinal cord, nerves, sense organs	Receive and interpret sensory information and, in response, stimulate muscles, glands, and other organ systems
Endocrine	Glands that secrete hormones: pituitary, thyroid, parathyroid, adrenal, pancreas, ovaries, testes, pineal, thymus	Control metabolic activities of organs
Cardiovascular	Heart, blood vessels	Move blood and transport substances throughout body
Lymphatic	Lymph vessels and nodes, thymus, spleen	Defend body against infection, return tissue fluid to blood, carry certain absorbed food molecules
Digestive	Mouth, tongue, teeth, salivary glands, pharynx, esophagus, stomach, liver, gallbladder, pancreas, small and large intestines	Receive, break down, and absorb food; eliminate unabsorbed material
Respiratory	Nasal cavity, pharynx, larynx, trachea, bronchi, lungs	Intake and output air, exchange gases between air and blood
Urinary	Kidneys, ureters, urinary bladder, urethra	Remove wastes from blood, maintain water and electrolyte balance, store and transport urine
Reproductive	Male: scrotum, testes, epididymides, vasa deferentia, seminal vesicles, prostate, bulbourethral glands, urethra, penis	Produce and maintain sperm cells, transfer sperm cells into female reproductive tract
	Female: ovaries, fallopian tubes, uterus, vagina, vulva	Produce and maintain egg cells, receive sperm cells, support development of an embryo, function in birth process

Adapted from David Shier, Jackie L. Butler, and Ricki Lewis, *Hole's Human Anatomy and Physiology, 10th ed.*

WORD	PRONUNCIATION	ELEMENTS		DEFINITION
cardiovascular (adj)	KAR-dee-oh-VAS-kyu-lar	S/ R/CF R/	-ar *pertaining to* cardi/o- *heart* -vascul- *blood vessel*	Pertaining to the heart and blood vessels
digestion digestive (adj)	die-JEST-shun die-JEST-iv	S/ R/ S/	-ion *action* digest- *break down food* -ive *pertaining to*	Breakdown of food into elements suitable for cell metabolism Pertaining to digestion
endocrine (adj)	EN-doh-krin	P/ R/	endo- *within* -crine *to secrete*	Gland that produces an internal or hormonal substance
homeostasis (Note: *Hemostasis is the arrest of bleeding.*)	hoh-mee-oh-STAY-sis	S/ R/CF	-stasis *standstill, control* home/o- *the same*	Maintaining the stability of a system or the body's internal environment
integument integumentary (adj)	in-TEG-you-ment in-TEG-you-MENT-ah-ree	 S/ R/	Latin *a covering* -ary *pertaining to* integument- *covering of the body*	Organ system that covers the body, the skin being the main organ within the system Pertaining to the covering of the body
lymph lymphatic (adj)	LIMF lim-FAT-ic	 S/ R/	Latin *clear spring water* -atic *pertaining to* lymph- *lymph, lymphatic system*	Clear fluid collected from body tissues and transported by lymph vessels to the venous circulation Pertaining to lymph or the lymphatic system
nervous (adj) nervous system	NER-vus NER-vus SIS-tem	S/ R/	-ous *pertaining to* nerv- *nerve* system Greek *an organized whole*	Pertaining to a nerve or the nervous system; or easily excited or agitated The whole, integrated nerve apparatus
respiration respiratory (adj)	RES-pih-RAY-shun RES-pih-rah-tor-ee	S/ R/ S/	-ation *process* respir- *to breathe* -atory *pertaining to*	Process of breathing; fundamental process of life used to exchange oxygen and carbon dioxide Pertaining to respiration
skeleton skeletal (adj)	SKEL-eh-ton SKEL-eh-tal	 S/ R/	Greek *skeleton or mummy* -al *pertaining to* skelet- *skeleton*	The bony framework of the body Pertaining to the skeleton
urinary (adj)	YUR-ih-nair-ee	S/ R/	-ary *pertaining to* urin- *urine*	Pertaining to urine

EXERCISES

 ## Case Report 2.3

You are . . .

. . . a physical therapy assistant employed in the Rehabilitation Unit in Fulwood Medical Center.

You are communicating with . . .

. . . Mr. Richard Josen, a 22-year-old man who injured tissues in his left knee while playing football. Using **arthroscopy**, the orthopedic surgeon removed his torn **anterior cruciate ligament (ACL)** and replaced it with a **graft** from his **patellar tendon**. The torn medial collateral ligament was **sutured** together. The tear in his medial **meniscus** was repaired. Rehabilitation is focused on strengthening the **muscles** around his knee joint and regaining joint mobility and stability.

A. After reading Case Report 2.3, provide or select the correct answer to each question. **LO 2.5, LO 2.6, and 2.11**

1. The injured structures are on the _____ and _____ of the knee. Choose the two answers that correctly fill in the blanks.

   a. middle   c. front
   b. outside   d. back

2. The patellar ligament gets its name from the:

   a. muscle-to-muscle attachment   c. length of the tissue
   b. organ it originates from   d. bone it attaches to

3. Which level of structural organization do ligaments fit into?

   a. organ system   c. tissue
   b. organ   d. cell

4. Your job would be to focus on two areas. Select these two areas:

   a. joint mobility   c. bone density
   b. cartilage healing   d. muscle strength

B. Read Use your knowledge of medical terminology related to tissues, organs, and organ systems to answer the following questions. *Fill in the blanks.*
   LO 2.2, 2.5, and 2.10

1. Which therapeutic procedure is performed to examine the inside of a joint? _____

2. When a physician describes a cartilage tear to the disc of the knee joint, which structure is being described? _____

3. What type of surgeon would perform the procedures? _____

4. Which of the structures repaired is a type of cartilage? _____

5. Which structure was repaired by suturing? _____

C. Dictionary exercise: *When you are working in the medical field, you will be exposed to medical terms you may not recognize. Learn to use the glossary or a good medical dictionary, or practice going online to find the definitions you need.*

   Insert the correct term in the appropriate statement. **LO 2.2 and 2.10**

   orthopedic   **collateral**   **sutured**

1. Placing stitches to bind the wound edges together to close an incision or laceration of a body part _____ .

2. Accessory or secondary _____ .

3. Medical specialty that diagnosis and treats diseases and conditions of bones _____ .

D. Construct the appropriate medical term *to match the definitions given. The placement of the elements is noted for you under the line; each different element is separated on the line. Write the correct elements on the line. If a term does not have a particular element, leave it blank.* **LO 2.5**

1. Fibrous membrane covering a bone: _____ / _____ / _____
                                  P   R/CF   S

2. Major protein of connective tissue: _____ / _____ / _____
                                  P   R/CF   S

3. Pertaining to the synovial membrane _____ / _____ / _____
                                  P   R/CF   S

4. Substance in food that nourishes _____ / _____ / _____
                                  P   R/CF   S

E. Match *each connective tissue term to its correct description.* **LO 2.5**

1. Term that contains a word element meaning bone

2. Term that contains a word element meaning glue

3. Term that contains a word element meaning egg

4. Term that is Latin and means gristle

5. Term that is Latin and means sinew

a. cartilage

b. tendon

c. periosteum

d. synovial

e. collagen

F. Construct *the correct medical terms by working with the literal meaning of the elements. Enter the correct elements on each line to complete the term.* **LO 2.6**

1. _____ / _____
   lymph   pertaining to

2. _____ / _____
   heart and blood vessels   pertaining to

3. _____ / _____
   skeleton   pertaining to

4. _____ / _____
   covering of the body   pertaining to

5. _____ / _____
   break down food   pertaining to

G. Continue *working with the medical terms related to the organs and organ systems.* **LO 2.2 and 2.6**

1. When referring to a body system, add a suffix that means: _____

2. Which element type is different between the terms *homeostasis* and *hemostasis?* _____

3. What is the main organ in the integumentary system? _____

4. What is the bony framework of the body called? _____

5. What term refers to clear fluid? _____

Anatomical Positions, Planes, and Directions

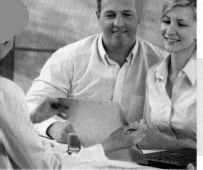

Classic Collection/Shotshop GmbH/Alamy Images

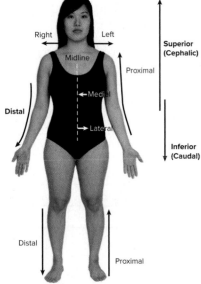

▲ **FIGURE 2.7**
Anatomical Position, with Directional Terms.

Aaron Roeth Photography

Medical terms have been developed over many centuries to help you describe clearly the location of different anatomical structures and lesions and their relation to each other in the human body.

Fundamental Anatomical Position (LO 2.7)

When all anatomical descriptions are used, it is assumed that the body is in the "anatomical position" *(Figure 2.7)*. Here is how this position looks if you are standing in front of a full-length mirror: your body is standing erect, your feet are flat on the floor, your face and eyes are facing forward, and your arms are at your sides with your palms facing forward.

When you lie down flat on your back with your palms upward, you are **supine**. When you lie down flat on your belly with your palms facing the floor, you are **prone**.

Anatomical Directional Terms (LO 2.7)

Directional terms describe the position of one body structure or part relative to another body structure or part. These directional terms are shown in *Figures 2.7* and *2.8*.

Anatomical Planes (LO 2.7)

Different views of your body are based on imaginary "slices," which produce flat surfaces called **planes** that pass through your body *(Figure 2.9)*. The **three major anatomical planes** are the following:

• **Transverse or horizontal:** a plane passing across the body parallel to the floor and perpendicular to the body's long axis. It divides the body into an upper/superior portion and a lower/inferior portion.

• **Sagittal:** a vertical plane that divides the body into right and left portions. A mid-sagittal plane divides right and left sides equally.

• **Frontal (coronal):** a vertical plane that divides the body into front (**anterior**) and back (**posterior**) portions.

▶ **FIGURE 2.8**
Other Directional Terms.

Aaron Roeth Photography

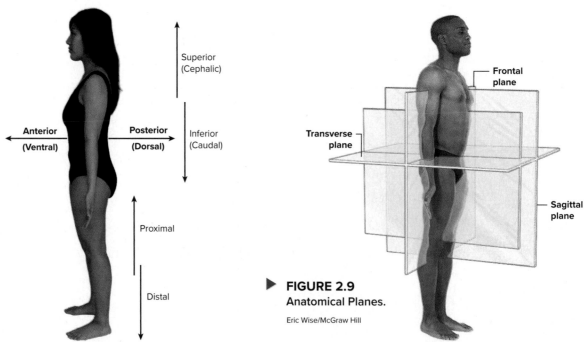

▶ **FIGURE 2.9**
Anatomical Planes.

Eric Wise/McGraw Hill

WORD	PRONUNCIATION	ELEMENTS		DEFINITION
anatomy	ah-**NAT**-oh-mee	S/ R/	-tomy *process of separating* ana- *apart from*	Study of the structures of the human body
anatomical (adj)	an-ah-**TOM**-ik-al	S/	-ical *pertaining to*	Pertaining to anatomy
anterior *(opposite of posterior)* (adj)	an-**TEER**-ee-or	S/ R/	-ior *pertaining to* anter- *before, front part*	The front surface of the body; situated in front
caudal *(opposite of cephalic, same as inferior)* (adj)	**KAW**-dal	S/ R/	-al *pertaining to* caud- *tail*	Pertaining to or nearer to the tailbone
cephalic *(opposite of caudal, same as superior)* (adj)	seh-**FAL**-ik	S/ R/	-ic *pertaining to* cephal- *head*	Pertaining to or nearer to the head
coronal *(same as frontal)* (adj)	**KOR**-oh-nal	S/ R/	-al *pertaining to* coron- *crown*	Pertaining to the vertical plane dividing the body into anterior and posterior portions
distal *(opposite of proximal)* (adj)	**DISS**-tal	S/ R/	-al *pertaining to* dist- *away from the center*	Situated away from the center of the body
dorsal *(same as posterior)* (adj)	**DOOR**-sal	S/ R/	-al *pertaining to* dors- *back*	Pertaining to the back or situated behind
frontal *(same as coronal)* (adj)	**FRON**-tal	S/ R/	-al *pertaining to* front- *front*	In front; relating to the anterior part of the body
inferior *(opposite of superior)* (adj)	in-**FEER**-ee-or	S/ R/	-ior *pertaining to* infer- *below*	Situated below
lateral *(opposite of medial)* (adj)	**LAT**-er-al	S/ R/	-al *pertaining to* later- *side*	Situated at the side of a structure
medial *(opposite of lateral)* (adj)	**ME**-dee-al	S/ R/	-al *pertaining to* medi- *middle*	Nearer to the middle of the body
posterior *(opposite of anterior)* (adj)	pohs-**TEER**-ee-or	S/ R/	-ior *pertaining to* poster- *back part*	Pertaining to the back surface of the body; situated behind
prone *(opposite of supine)* (adj)	**PROHN**		Latin *bending forward*	Lying face down, flat on your belly
proximal *(opposite of distal)* (adj)	**PROK**-sih-mal	S/ R/	-al *pertaining to* proxim- *nearest to the center*	Situated nearest to the center of the body
sagittal	**SAJ**-ih-tal	S/ R/	-al *pertaining to* sagitt- *arrow*	Vertical plane through the body dividing it into right and left portions
superior *(opposite of inferior)* (adj)	soo-**PEER**-ee-or	S/ R/	-ior *pertaining to* super- *above*	Situated above
supine *(opposite of prone)* (adj)	soo-**PINE**		Latin *lying on the back*	Lying face up, flat on your spine
transverse	trans-**VERS**		Latin *crosswise*	Horizontal plane dividing the body into upper and lower portions
ventral *(same as anterior)* (adj)	**VEN**-tral	S/ R/	-al *pertaining to* ventr- *belly*	Pertaining to the belly or situated nearer the surface of the belly

Abdominal Quadrants (LO 2.8)

To simplify your job of locating and identifying abdominal structures and sites of abdominal pain and other abnormalities, you can mentally divide the abdomen into **quadrants**, as shown in *Figure 2.10a*. This approach allows you to separate these locations into manageable parts. These divisions are known as the right upper quadrant **(RUQ),** left upper quadrant **(LUQ),** right lower quadrant **(RLQ),** and left lower quadrant **(LLQ).**

In addition, there are three main regions of your abdomen—the epigastric, umbilical, and hypogastric regions, as shown in *Figure 2.10b*.

Abbreviations

LLQ	left lower quadrant
LUQ	left upper quadrant
RLQ	right lower quadrant
RUQ	right upper quadrant

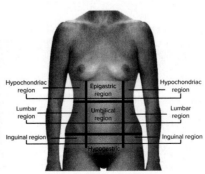

(a) Abdominal quadrants

(b) Abdominal regions

◀ **FIGURE 2.10**
Regional Anatomy.

Body Cavities (LO 2.9)

Your body contains many **cavities** or hollow spaces. Some, like the nasal cavity, open to the outside of your body. Five cavities that do not open to the outside are shown in *Figure 2.11* and listed below.

1. The **cranial cavity** contains the brain within the skull.
2. The **thoracic cavity** contains the heart, lungs, thymus gland, trachea and esophagus, and numerous blood vessels and nerves.
3. The **abdominal cavity**, separated from the thoracic cavity by the **diaphragm**, contains the stomach, intestines, liver, spleen, pancreas, and kidneys. There are nine regions in the abdomen, as shown in *Figure 2.10b*.
4. The **pelvic cavity**, surrounded by the pelvic bones, contains the urinary bladder, part of the large intestine, the rectum and anus, and the internal reproductive organs.
5. The **spinal cavity** contains the spinal cord.

The abdominal cavity and pelvic cavity can be combined as the **abdominopelvic cavity**.

▶ **FIGURE 2.11**
Major Body Cavities.

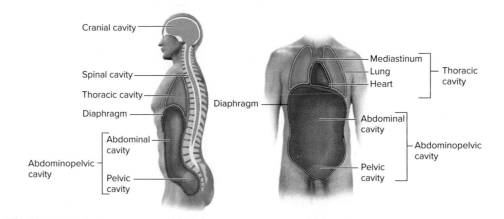

Word Analysis and Definition

S = Suffix   P = Prefix   R = Root   R/CF = Combining Form

WORD	PRONUNCIATION		ELEMENTS	DEFINITION
abdomen	AB-doh-men		Latin *abdomen*	Part of the trunk between the thorax and the pelvis
abdominal (adj)	ab-**DOM**-in-al	S/	-al *pertaining to*	Pertaining to the abdomen
		R/	abdomin- *abdomen*	
abdominopelvic (adj)	ab-**DOM**-ih-no-**PEL**-vik	S/	-ic *pertaining to*	Pertaining to the abdomen and pelvis
		R/CF	abdomin/o- *abdomen*	
		R/	-pelv- *pelvis*	
cavity	**KAV**-ih-tee	S/	-ity *state, condition*	A hollow space or body compartment
cavities (pl)	**KAV**-ih-teez	R/	cav- *hollow space*	
cranial (adj)	**KRAY**-nee-al	S/	-al *pertaining to*	Pertaining to the cranium
		R/	crani- *skull*	
cranium	**KRAY**-nee-um	S/	-um *structure*	The skull
diaphragm	**DIE**-ah-fram		Greek *diaphragm, fence*	Muscular sheet separating the abdominal and thoracic cavities
diaphragmatic (adj)	**DIE**-ah-frag-**MAT**-ik	S/	-ic *pertaining to*	Pertaining to the diaphragm
		R/	diaphragmat- *diaphragm*	
quadrant	**KWAD**-rant		Latin *one quarter*	One quarter of a circle; one of four regions of the surface of the abdomen
spine	**SPYN**		Latin *spine*	The vertebral column or a short bony projection
spinal (adj)	**SPY**-nal	S/	-al *pertaining to*	Pertaining to the spine
		R/	spin- *spine*	
thoracic (adj)	thor-**ASS**-ik	S/	-ic *pertaining to*	Pertaining to the chest (thorax)
		R/	thorac- *chest*	
thorax	**THOR**-acks		Greek *chest*	The part of the trunk between the abdomen and the neck
umbilical (adj)	um-**BILL**-ih-kal	S/	-al *pertaining to*	Pertaining to the umbilicus or the center of the abdomen
		R/	umbilic- *navel (belly button)*	
umbilicus	um-**BILL**-ih-kuss		Latin *navel (belly button)*	Pit in the abdomen where the umbilical cord entered the fetus

EXERCISES

A. Use **directional terms** to correctly answer each question. Fill in the blanks. **LO 2.2 and 2.7**

1. To examine a patient's abdomen, in which position would you place them? _____

2. To examine a patient's spine, in which position would you place them? _____

3. A patient's spine is _____ to their abdomen.

B. **Identify** *the following pairs of terms as either opposites or synonyms.* **LO 2.7**

1. anterior/posterior _____

2. ventral/anterior _____

3. prone/supine _____

4. coronal/frontal _____

5. cephalic/caudal _____

6. cephalic/superior _____

Study Hint

Help your memory with little tricks of association for medical terms. Example: The medical term *supine* has the word up in it. The meaning of *supine* is lying with the face and the anterior part of the body UP. Associate UP with sUPine and you will have no trouble remembering its definition. Then associate the opposite term and you will know the meaning of *prone* as well.

C. **Deconstruct the following terms** *into their basic elements. Note that not every type of element will appear in every term. The only element every term needs is a root or a combining form.* Fill in the blanks. **LO 2.1 and 2.9**

1. diaphragmatic _____ / _____
                 R/CF   S

2. abdominopelvic _____ / _____ / _____
               R/CF   R/CF   S

3. umbilical _____ / _____
               R/CF   S

4. cranial _____ / _____
               R/CF   S

5. thoracic _____ / _____
               R/CF   S

6. cavity _____ / _____
               R/CF   S

D. **Select** *the correct answer to answer each question or complete the statement.* **LO 2.8 and 2.9**

1. Which term contains a root and a combining form?
   a. abdominopelvic   **b.** diaphragmatic   **c.** thoracic   **d.** spinal

2. Which term is a muscle that separates body cavities?
   a. abdominopelvic   **b.** diaphragm   **c.** thoracic   **d.** spinal

3. The term "quadrant" represents what number?
   a. two   **b.** four   **c.** six   **d.** eight

4. The term "spine" also refers to:
   a. diaphragm   **b.** skull   **c.** chest   **d.** vertebral column

5. Which of the following terms is a dentist likely to use?
   a. cavity   **b.** abdomen   **c.** spinal   **d.** thoracic

Additional exercises available in **connect**

Chapter Review exercises, along with additional practice items, are available in Connect!

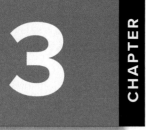
3

The Integumentary System

The Essentials of the Language of Dermatology

Rick Brady/McGraw Hill

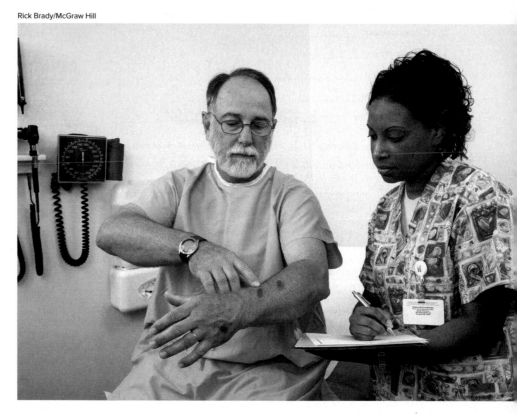

Learning Outcomes

In addition to anticipating needs for equipment to **biopsy**, diagnose, and treat skin lesions, you also have to be able to communicate clearly in medical terms and understand the language as health care providers communicate with you about the **etiology** (cause) and structure of the lesions. You will then need to document the medical history and treatment and communicate clearly with the patient about the treatment of the lesions and their **prognosis**.

To perform these tasks, you must be able to:

LO 3.1 Use roots, combining forms, suffixes, and prefixes to construct and analyze medical terms related to the integumentary system.

LO 3.2 Spell and pronounce correctly medical terms and their plurals related to the integumentary system to communicate them with accuracy and precision in any health care setting.

LO 3.3 Define accepted abbreviations related to the integumentary system.

LO 3.4 Relate the anatomical structures of the integumentary system and their locations to their functions.

LO 3.5 Describe common disorders of and injuries to the skin and its accessory glands.

LO 3.6 Identify diagnostic and therapeutic procedures and pharmacology used to treat disorders of the integumentary system.

LO 3.7 Apply your knowledge of medical terms relating to the integumentary system to documentation, medical records, and medical reports.

LO 3.8 Translate the medical terms relating to the integumentary system into everyday language to communicate clearly with patients and their families.

The health professionals involved in the diagnosis and treatment of problems with the integumentary system include the following:

- **Dermatologists** are medical doctors who are specialists in skin disorders.
- **Dermatology technicians** are medical assistants who have an additional year of training in dermatology.

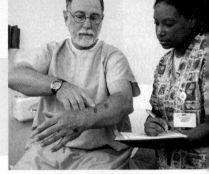

Section 3.1

Functions and Structure of the Skin

Rick Brady/McGraw Hill

Your skin is your largest organ–it covers your entire body. The outer layer of the skin is called the epidermis. Hair follicles, sebaceous glands, sweat glands, and nails are accessory organs located in your skin. Each of these skin organs has specific anatomical and physiological characteristics. This lesson looks at the structure and function of the skin, as well as of the accessory skin organs.

Your skin's nerves allow you to feel heat, cold, pain, and comfort. Your skin wards off infections and protects your body from harmful environmental elements. Your skin is constantly shedding old cells in order to make room for new skin growth.

The **integumentary system** consists of your skin and its associated organs. **Dermatology** is the study and treatment of the integumentary system. A **dermatologist** is a medical specialist in the disorders of the skin.

Functions of the Skin (LO 3.1, 3.2, and 3.4)

Your skin functions in several ways to keep you healthy and safe. These important functions include the following:

- **Protection:** Your skin is a physical barrier against injury, chemicals, **ultraviolet (UV)** rays, microbes, and toxins and is not easily breached *(Figure 3.1)*. Certain bacteria and other pathogens, called normal **flora**, populate your skin's surface.

- **Water resistance:** You do not swell up every time you take a bath because your skin is water resistant. It also prevents water from leaking out of body tissues.

- **Temperature regulation:** A network of capillaries in your skin opens up or dilates (**vasodilation**) when your body is too hot. When your body is cold, this capillary network narrows (**vasoconstriction**), blood flow decreases, and your body retains heat.

  The structure of the skin to enable these functions is detailed in the next section.

- **Vitamin D synthesis:** As little as 15 to 30 minutes of sunlight each day allows your skin cells to initiate the metabolism of vitamin D, which is essential for bone growth and maintenance.

- **Sensation:** Nerve endings that detect touch, pressure, heat, cold, pain, vibration, and tissue injury are particularly numerous in the skin of your face, fingers, palms, soles, nipples, and genitals.

- **Excretion and secretion:** Water and small amounts of waste products from cell metabolism are lost through your skin by **excretion** and **secretion** from your sweat glands.

- **Social functions:** The skin reflects your emotions: it blushes when you are self-conscious, goes pale when you are frightened, and wrinkles when you register disgust.

Structure of the Skin (LO 3.1, 3.2, 3.3, and 3.4)

Epidermis (LO 3.1, 3.2, 3.3, and 3.4)

The most **superficial** layer of the skin is the **epidermis**.

The epidermis is made of four to five layers of squamous cells called **keratinocytes.** Keratinocytes are formed at the deepest layer of the epidermis. When new keratinocytes are formed they cause the layers above them to move upward. As the keratinocytes move upward they move away from their source of oxygen and nutrients, causing them to die. The outer layer of your epidermis *(Figure 3.2)* is a keratin-packed cover of compact, dead cells that you continually shed. **Keratin**–a tough, scaly protein that is also the basis for your hair and nails–shields your body from harmful elements like chemicals and bacteria.

In the lower layers of your epidermis, cells are filled with a protein that becomes keratin. Other cells produce a brown/black pigment called **melanin**, which determines the color of your skin and protects it from ultraviolet light damage.

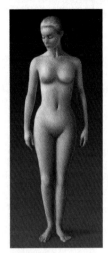

▲ **FIGURE 3.1**
Integumentary System.
The skin provides protection, contains sensory organs, and helps control body temperature.

Abbreviations

UV   ultraviolet

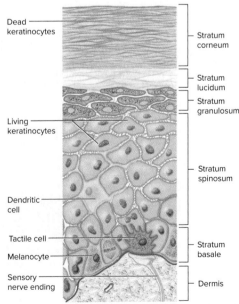

Labels: Dead keratinocytes; Living keratinocytes; Dendritic cell; Tactile cell; Melanocyte; Sensory nerve ending; Stratum corneum; Stratum lucidum; Stratum granulosum; Stratum spinosum; Stratum basale; Dermis

◀ **FIGURE 3.2**   Epidermis.

WORD	PRONUNCIATION		ELEMENTS	DEFINITION
cutaneous	kyu-**TAY**-nee-us	S/ R/CF	**-ous** *pertaining to* **cutan/e-** *skin*	Pertaining to the skin
dermatology	der-mah-**TOL**-oh-jee	S/ R/CF	**-logy** *study of* **dermat/o-** *skin*	Medical specialty concerned with disorders of the skin
dermatologist dermatologic (adj)	der-mah-**TOL**-oh-jist der-mah-toh-**LOJ**-ik	S/ S/	**-logist** *one who studies, specialist* **-ic** *pertaining to*	Medical specialist in diseases of the skin Pertaining to the skin and dermatology
excrete (verb)	eks-**KREET**	P/ R	**ex-** *out of, away from* **-crete** *separate*	To pass waste products of metabolism out of the body
excretion (noun)	eks-**KREE**-shun	S/	**-ion** *action*	Removal of waste products of metabolism out of the body
flora	**FLO**-rah		Latin *flower*	The population of microorganisms covering the exterior and interior surfaces of healthy animals
integument	in-**TEG**-you-ment		Latin *a covering*	Organ system that covers the body, the skin being the main organ within the system
integumentary (adj)	in-**TEG**-you-**MENT**-ah-ree	S/ R/	**-ary** *pertaining to* **integument-** *covering of the body*	Pertaining to the covering of the body
prognosis	prog-**NO**-sis	P/ R/	**pro-** *projecting forward* **-gnosis** *knowledge*	Forecast of the probable future course and outcome of a disease
secrete (verb)	seh-**KREET**	R/	**secret-** *produce*	To produce a chemical substance in a cell and release it from the cell
secretion (noun)	seh-**KREE**-shun	S/	**-ion** *action*	Production by a cell(s) of a physiologically active substance and its movement out of the cell.
synthesis	**SIN**-the-sis	P/ R/	**syn-** *together* **-thesis** *to organize, arrange*	The process of building a compound from different elements
synthetic (adj)	sin-**THET**-ik	S/ R/	**-ic** *pertaining to* **-thet-** *arrange, organize*	Built up or put together from simpler compounds
ultraviolet	ul-trah-**VIE**-oh-let	P/ R/	**ultra-** *beyond* **-violet** *violet, bluish purple*	Light rays at a higher frequency than the violet end of the spectrum
vasoconstriction	**VAY**-soh-con-**STRIK**-shun	S/ R/CF R/	**-ion** *action* **vas/o-** *blood vessel* **-constrict-** *narrow*	Reduction in diameter of a blood vessel
vasodilation	**VAY**-soh-die-**LAY**-shun	R/	**-dilat-** *widen, open up*	Increase in diameter of a blood vessel

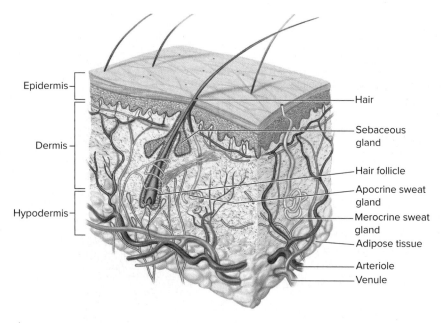

▲ FIGURE 3.3
Dermis and Its Organs.

Labels: Epidermis, Dermis, Hypodermis, Hair, Sebaceous gland, Hair follicle, Apocrine sweat gland, Merocrine sweat gland, Adipose tissue, Arteriole, Venule

Dermis (LO 3.1, 3.2, and 3.4)

Figure 3.3 shows that the **dermis** is a much thicker connective tissue layer than the epidermis. Your dermis is the middle layer of your skin between your epidermis and **hypodermis**. It contains an abundance of collagen fibers and is well supplied with blood vessels and nerves. It contains your other skin organs: sweat glands, sebaceous glands, hair **follicles**, and nail roots.

Hypodermis or Subcutaneous Tissue Layer (LO 3.1, 3.2, and 3.4)

This layer beneath your dermis is the site of **subcutaneous** fat (**adipose** tissue), nerves, and larger blood vessels. Also called the subcutaneous tissue layer, it regulates your body's temperature and helps protect your vital organs. When this layer becomes thinner or deteriorates, as with the aging process, your skin begins to sag.

Clinical Applications (LO 3.1, 3.2, 3.3, 3.4, and 3.6)

Injections are given into the three areas of the skin using the following approaches:

- **Intradermal**, in which a short, thin needle is introduced into the epidermis, raising a small **wheal** on the skin. This site is used for allergy testing or a tuberculosis (TB) test.

- **Subcutaneous (SC)**, in which a longer needle pierces the epidermis and dermis to reach the hypodermis (subcutaneous) layer. This site is used for insulin injections and immunizations.

- **Intramuscular (IM)**, in which a long needle penetrates the epidermis, dermis, and hypodermis to reach into the muscles underneath. Some antibiotics and immunizations are given this way.

In addition, there are **transdermal** applications. Here, medications are administered through the skin by an adhesive transdermal patch applied to the skin. The medication diffuses across the epidermis and enters the blood vessels in the dermis. Contraceptive hormones, analgesics, and antinausea/antiseasickness medications are examples of transdermal applications.

Abbreviations

IM	intramuscular
SC	subcutaneous

Word Analysis and Definition

S = Suffix   P = Prefix   R = Root   R/CF = Combining Form

WORD	PRONUNCIATION	ELEMENTS		DEFINITION
adipose	ADD-ih-pose	S/ R/	-ose *full of* adip- *fat*	Containing fat
cutaneous	kyu-**TAY**-nee-us	S/ R/CF	-ous *pertaining to* cutan/e- *skin*	Pertaining to the skin
dermis dermal (adj)	**DER**-miss **DER**-mal	S/ R/	Greek *skin* -al *pertaining to* derm- *skin*	Connective tissue layer of the skin beneath the epidermis Pertaining to the skin
epidermis epidermal (adj)	ep-ih-**DER**-miss ep-ih-**DER**-mal	P/ R/ S/ R/	epi- *above, upon* -dermis *skin* -al *pertaining to* -derm- *skin*	Top layer of the skin Pertaining to the epidermis
hypodermis hypodermic (adj) *(same as subcutaneous)*	high-poh-**DER**-miss high-poh-**DER**-mik	P/ R/ S/ R/	hypo- *below* -dermis *skin* -ic *pertaining to* -derm- *skin*	Loose connective tissue layer of skin below the dermis Pertaining to the hypodermis
intradermal	in-trah-**DER**-mal	S/ P/ R/	-al *pertaining to* intra- *within* -derm- *skin*	Within the epidermis
intramuscular	in-trah-**MUSS**-kew-lar	S/ P/ R/	-ar *pertaining to* intra- *within* -muscul- *muscle*	Within the muscle
keratin	**KAIR**-ah-tin	S/ R/	-in *substance* kerat- *hard protein*	Protein present in skin, hair, and nails
melanin	**MEL**-ah-nin	S/ R/	-in *substance* melan- *black pigment*	Black pigment found in skin, hair, and the retina
squamous cell	**SKWAY**-mus **SELL**		squamous Latin *scaly*	Flat, scale-like epithelial cell
subcutaneous *(same as hypodermic)*	sub-kew-**TAY**-nee-us	S/ P/ R/CF	-ous *pertaining to* sub- *below* -cutan/e- *skin*	Below the skin
superficial	soo-per-**FISH**-al		Latin *surface*	Situated near the surface
transdermal	trans-**DER**-mal	S/ P/ R/	-al *pertaining to* trans- *across, through* -derm- *skin*	Going across or through the skin
wheal *(same as hives)*	**WHEEL**		Old English *wheal*	Small, itchy swelling of the skin (wheals raised by an injection do not itch)

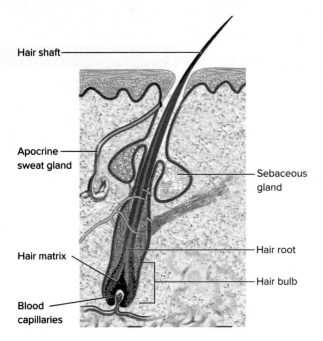

Hair shaft

Apocrine
sweat gland

Hair matrix

Blood
capillaries

Sebaceous
gland

Hair root

Hair bulb

▲ **FIGURE 3.4**
Hair Follicle and Sebaceous Gland.

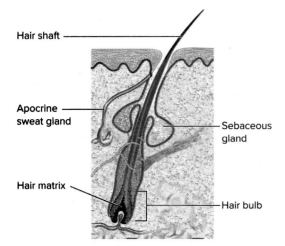

Hair shaft

Apocrine
sweat gland

Hair matrix

Sebaceous
gland

Hair bulb

▲ **FIGURE 3.5**
Hair Follicle.

Hair Follicles and Sebaceous Glands (LO 3.4)

Each hair **follicle** on your face has a **sebaceous gland** opening into it *(Figure 3.4)*. This gland secretes into the follicle oily, acidic **sebum,** which mixes with broken-down keratin cells from the base of the follicle. Sebum rises up along the hair shaft and onto the skin. The functions of sebum are to lubricate the hair and skin, water-proof the skin, and protect the skin from bacterial and fungal infections.

Hair (LO 3.4)

Every hair on your body or scalp originates from epidermal cells at the base (**matrix**) of a hair **follicle.** As these cells divide and grow, they push older cells upward, away from the source of nutrition in the hair papilla *(Figure 3.5)*. The older cells become keratinized and die.

Sweat Glands (LO 3.4)

You have 3 million to 4 million sweat glands scattered all over your skin, with clusters on your palms, soles, and forehead *(Figure 3.6)*. Their main function is to produce the watery perspiration (sweat) that cools your body. Some sweat glands open directly onto the surface of your skin. Others open into your hair follicles *(Figure 3.6)*.

In the dermis, the sweat gland is a coiled tube lined with epithelial, sweat-secreting cells. In your armpits (axillae), around your nipples, in your groin, and around your anus, different sweat glands produce a thick, cloudy secretion. This interacts with your normal skin bacteria to produce a distinct, noticeable smell. The ducts of these glands lead directly into your hair follicles *(see Figure 3.5)*.

Nails (LO 3.4)

Your nails consist of closely packed, thin, dead skin cells that are filled with parallel fibers of hard keratin. On the average, your fingernails grow about 1 millimeter (mm) per week. New cells are added by cell division in the nail matrix, which is protected by the nail fold of skin and the **cuticle** at the base of your nail *(Figure 3.7)*.

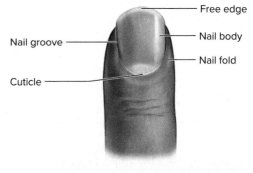

Free edge

Nail body

Nail groove

Nail fold

Cuticle

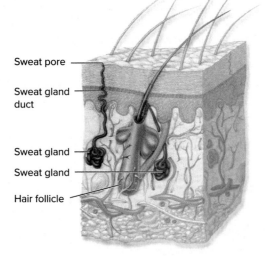

Sweat pore

Sweat gland
duct

Sweat gland

Sweat gland

Hair follicle

▲ **FIGURE 3.6**
Sweat Glands.

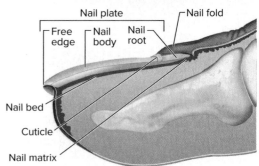

Nail plate

Free
edge

Nail
body

Nail
root

Nail fold

Nail bed

Cuticle

Nail matrix

▲ **FIGURE 3.7**
Anatomy of a Fingernail.

Word Analysis and Definition

S = Suffix   P = Prefix   R = Root   R/CF = Combining Form

WORD	PRONUNCIATION		ELEMENTS	DEFINITION
cuticle	**KEW**-tih-kull		Diminutive of cutis *skin*	Nonliving epidermis at base of fingernails and toenails
follicle	**FOLL**-ih-kull		Latin *small sac*	Spherical mass of cells containing a cavity or a small cul-de-sac, such as a hair follicle
matrix	**MAY**-tricks		Latin *mother*	The formative portion of a hair, nail, or tooth
sebaceous glands	seh-**BAY**-shus **GLANZ**	S/ R/CF	**-ous** *pertaining to* **sebac/e-** *wax*	Glands in the dermis that open into hair follicles and secrete a waxy fluid called sebum
sebum	**SEE**-bum		Latin *tallow*	Waxy secretion of the sebaceous glands

EXERCISES

 CASE REPORT 3.1

You are . . .

. . . a **dermatology technician** working with dermatologist Dr. Laura Echols, MD, a member of the Fulwood Medical Group.

You are communicating with . . .

. . . Mr. Rod Andrews, a 60-year-old man, who shows you three skin lesions—two on his left forearm and one on the back of his left hand. You learn that he has been living in Arizona for the past 10 years but has recently returned to this area to live near his daughter and young grandchildren. You find no other skin lesions on his body.

When Dr. Echols examined Mr. Andrews, she determined that two of his lesions were basal cell **carcinomas** and treated them with **cryosurgery**, an approach that involves freezing cancerous tissue. She believed that the third lesion was a **squamous cell** carcinoma and performed a biopsy removal of the **cutaneous** (skin) lesion. You sent this to the laboratory with a request for a pathologic diagnosis and determination of whether the lesion had been completely removed.

A. Read *Case Report 3.1 to select the correct answer the following questions.* **LO 3.2 and 3.8**

1. Which two types of skin lesions did Dr. Echols remove from Mr. Andrews?
   a. squamous cell carcinoma and cryosurgery
   b. basal cell carcinoma and squamous cell carcinoma
   c. cutaneous and integumentary
   d. cryosurgery and excisional biopsy

2. What different types of treatment did Dr. Echols use to remove these lesions?
   a. squamous cell carcinoma and cryosurgery
   b. basal cell carcinoma and squamous cell carcinoma
   c. cutaneous and integumentary
   d. cryosurgery and excisional biopsy

3. What two questions did Dr. Echols need the pathologist to answer?
   a. What kind of cancer is present and has the lesion been completely removed?
   b. What are the results of the biopsy and what type of flora is present?
   c. What is Mr. Andrews' prognosis and has the lesion been completely removed?
   d. What is Mr. Andrews' prognosis and should he see a dermatologist?

4. What treatment approach involves freezing cancerous tissue?
   a. excretion
   b. vasoconstriction
   c. excisional biopsy
   d. cryosurgery

5. Cutaneous means:
   a. pertaining to the skin
   b. action of the skin
   c. pertaining to icy cold
   d. process of covering the body

B. Read *Case Report 3.1 to answer the following questions.* **LO 3.5 and 3.6**

1. What type of physician is Dr. Echols? _____

2. What treatments were given for Mr. Andrews' skin cancer? _____

3. What future precautions should Mr. Andrews take? _____

C. Practice *using your medical terminology in the following exercise. When possible, be sure to deconstruct the term using the slashes provided. Fill in the blanks.*
LO 3.1, 3.4, and 3.5

1. This pigment is responsible for skin color: _____ / _____

                                                                R/CF   S

2. Skin needs protection from this type of light: _____ / _____

                                                     P   R/CF

Section 3.2

Disorders of the Skin and Accessory Organs

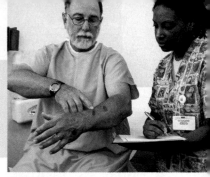

Rick Brady/McGraw Hill

Your skin provides your body's first line of defense against injury, disease, **allergens**, and pollutants. Because your skin is continually exposed to the elements, it is susceptible to various problems and disorders. The skin shows the same types of disease as most organs—infections, tumors, cancers—but because of its protective covering, it is the first responder to many irritant and **allergenic** agents.

Dermatitis (LO 3.5)

Dermatitis is an inflammatory condition that often presents as a swollen red **rash** with **pruritus** with a potential to form **vesicles** *(Figure 3.8)*.

The different types of dermatitis and their related causes are as follows:

- **Eczema** is a general term used for inflamed and **pruritic** (itchy) skin conditions. When the itchy skin is scratched, it becomes **excoriated** and produces the dry, red, scaly patches characteristic of eczema. The terms eczema and atopic dermatitis are often used interchangeably. The difference between contact and atopic dermatitis is the way the body reacts to the substance.

- **Atopic** or **allergic dermatitis** is due to allergens that include nickel in jewelry, perfume, cosmetics, poison ivy, and latex.

- **Contact dermatitis** results from direct contact with irritants or **allergens**, including soaps, detergents, cleaning products, and solvents.

- **Stasis dermatitis** occurs in the lower leg when varicose veins slow the return of blood and the accumulation of fluid interferes with the nourishment of the skin.

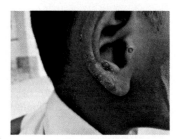

▲ **FIGURE 3.8** Dermatitis of the Ear.

Paosun Rt/Shutterstock

Word Analysis and Definition

S = Suffix P = Prefix R = Root R/CF = Combining Form

WORD	PRONUNCIATION		ELEMENTS	DEFINITION
allergen (**Note:** *The duplicate "g" is deleted to better form the word.*)	**AL**-er-jen	S/ R/ R/	-gen- *produce* all- *strange, other* -erg- *work, activity*	Substance producing a hypersensitivity (allergic) reaction
allergenic (adj)	al-er-**JEN**-ik	S/	-ic *pertaining to*	Pertaining to the capacity to produce an allergic reaction
allergy	**AL**-er-jee	S/	-ergy *process of working*	Hypersensitivity to an allergen
allergic (adj)	ah-**LER**-jik	S/	-ic *pertaining to*	Pertaining to being hypersensitive
atopy	**AT**-oh-pee		Greek *strangeness*	State of hypersensitivity to an allergen; allergic
atopic (adj)	ay-**TOP**-ik			Pertaining to an allergy.
dermatitis	der-mah-**TYE**-tis	S/ R/	-itis *inflammation* dermat- *skin*	Inflammation of the skin
eczema	**EK**-zeh-mah		Greek *to boil* or *ferment*	Inflammatory skin disease, often with a serous discharge
eczematous (adj)	ek-**ZEM**-ah-tus	S/ R/CF	-tous *pertaining to* eczem/a- *eczema*	Pertaining to or marked by eczema
excoriate (verb)	eks-**KOR**-ee-ate	S/ P/ R/	-ate *pertaining to* ex- *away from* -cori- *skin*	To scratch
excoriation (noun)	eks-**KOR**-ee-**AY**-shun	S/	-ation *process*	Scratch mark
pruritus	proo-**RYE**-tus		Latin *to itch*	Itching
pruritic (adj)	proo-**RIT**-ik	S/ R/	-ic *pertaining to* prurit- *itch*	Itchy
rash	**RASH**		French *skin eruption*	Skin eruption
stasis	**STAY**-sis		Greek *staying in one place*	Stagnation in the flow of any body fluid
vesicle	**VES**-ih-kull		Latin *blister*	Small sac containing liquid; e.g., a blister

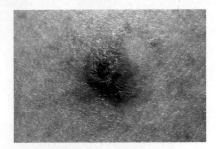

▲ **FIGURE 3.9** Basal Cell Carcinoma.

jax10289/Shutterstock

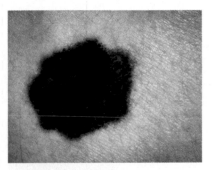

▲ **FIGURE 3.10** Malignant Melanoma.

Australis Photography/Shutterstock

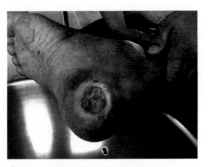

▲ **FIGURE 3.11** Decubitus (Pressure) Ulcer on the Heel.

Duangnapa Kanchanasakun/Shutterstock

Skin Cancers (LO 3.5)

Basal cell **carcinomas** *(Figure 3.9)* arise from the basal (bottom) layer of the epidermis. This is the most common and the least dangerous form of skin cancer because it does not **metastasize** (spread to elsewhere in the body).

Squamous cell carcinoma arises from cells in the middle layers of the epidermis. This skin cancer responds well to surgical removal but can metastasize to lymph glands if neglected.

Malignant melanoma *(Figure 3.10)* is the least common but most dangerous skin cancer. It arises in melanin-producing cells in the basal layer of the epidermis and metastasizes quickly. If neglected, this cancer is fatal.

Excess sunlight can also be an irritant to the skin. Too much sun can burn the skin and may lead to cancer.

Pressure Ulcers (LO 3.5)

When a patient lies in one position for a long period, the pressure between the bed and the body's bony projections, such as the lower spine or heel, cuts off the blood supply to the skin. Under these circumstances, **pressure** or **decubitus ulcers** can appear *(Figure 3.11)*. When this happens, the skin's protective function is compromised, making it easy for germs to enter the body. The elderly are often at risk for pressure ulcers because their skin is usually thin and dry. In addition, poor nutritional status can deplete the fatty protective layer in the hypodermis under the skin, making the body more susceptible to pressure ulcers. Bed-bound patients or those with limited movement ability are also at high risk for pressure ulcers.

Congenital Lesions (LO 3.5)

A birthmark caused by abnormal pigmentation or proliferation of blood vessels is called a **nevus**. Vascular nevi produce the port-wine stain or stork bite on the back of the neck and face; they resolve spontaneously in the first few years of life. The blue-gray, benign, flat Mongolian spot on the lower back of Black persons, Native Americans, and Latin Americans usually fades by two years of age.

Infections of the Skin (LO 3.5)

The skin can be susceptible to many different types of **infections**, including viral, fungal, parasitic, and bacterial.

Viral Infections (LO 3.5)

Warts (**verrucae**) are skin growths caused by the human **papillomavirus** invading the epidermis *(Figure 3.12)*.

Varicella-zoster virus causes chickenpox in unvaccinated people. Here, **macules** (small, flat spots different in color from the surrounding skin), **papules** (small, solid elevations), and vesicles (small sacs containing fluid) form. The virus can then remain dormant in the peripheral nerves (near the skin's surface) for decades before erupting as the painful vesicles of **herpes zoster**, also called **shingles** *(Figure 3.13)*.

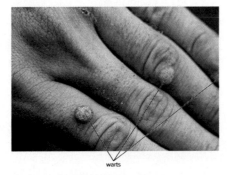

warts

▲ **FIGURE 3.12** Warts on Fingers.

Marcel Jancovic/Shutterstock

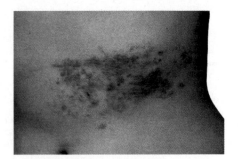

▲ **FIGURE 3.13** Shingles.

Franciscodiazpagador/iStock/Getty Images

WORD	PRONUNCIATION	ELEMENTS		DEFINITION
carcinoma	kar-sih-**NOH**-mah	S/ R/	-oma *tumor, mass* carcin- *cancer*	A malignant and invasive epithelial tumor
congenital	con-**JEN**-ih-tal	S/ P/ R/	-al *pertaining to* con- *with* -genit- *bring forth*	Present at birth
decubitus ulcer (pressure ulcer)	deh-**KYU**-bit-us **UL**-ser	P/ R/ R/	de- *from* -cubitus *lying down* ulcer *sore*	Sore caused by lying down for long periods of time
herpes zoster (shingles)	**HER**-peez **ZOS**-ter		herpes Greek *to creep or spread* zoster Greek *belt, girdle*	Painful eruption of vesicles that follows a nerve root on one side of the body
macule	**MACK**-yul		Latin *spot*	Small, flat spot or patch on the skin
malignant (adj)	mah-**LIG**-nant	S/ R/	-ant *forming, pertaining to* malign- *harmful, bad*	Tumor that invades surrounding tissues and metastasizes to distant organs
malignancy	mah-**LIG**-nan-see	S/	-ancy *state of*	State of being malignant
melanoma	**MEL**-ah-**NO**-mah	S/ R/	-oma *tumor, mass* melan- *black pigment*	Malignant neoplasm formed from cells that produce melanin
metastasis (noun)	meh-**TAS**-tah-sis	P/ R/	meta- *beyond, subsequent to* -stasis *stagnate, stay in one place*	Spread of a disease from one part of the body to another
metastasize (verb)	meh-**TAS**-tah-size	S/ R/	-ize *affect in a specific way* -stat- *stationary*	To spread to distant parts
metastatic (adj)	meh-tah-**STAT**-ik	S/	-ic *pertaining to*	Pertaining to the character of cells that can metastasize
nevus nevi (pl)	**NEE**-vus **NEE**-veye		Latin *mole, birthmark*	Congenital lesion of the skin
papillomavirus	pap-ih-**LOH**-mah-vi-rus	S/ R/CF	-oma *mass, tumor* papill/o- *papilla, pimple* virus Latin *poison*	Virus that causes warts and is associated with cancer
papule	**PAP**-yul		Latin *pimple*	Small, circumscribed elevation on the skin
verruca verrucae (pl)	ver-**ROO**-cah ver-**ROO**-kee		Latin *wart*	Wart caused by a virus

Fungal Infections (LO 3.5)

Tinea is a general term for a group of related skin infections caused by different species of **fungi.**

Tinea pedis, or athlete's foot, causes itching, redness, and peeling of the skin of the foot, particularly between the toes *(Figure 3.14)*. **Tinea capitis** describes an infection of the scalp (ringworm). **Tinea corporis** refers to ringworm infections of the body's skin and hands. **Tinea cruris,** or jock itch, is the name for infections of the groin. The fungus spreads from animals, from the soil, and by direct contact with infected individuals.

A yeastlike fungus, *Candida albicans,* can produce recurrent infections of the skin, nails, and mucous membranes. The first sign can be a frequent diaper rash or oral **thrush** in infants. Older children can show repeated or persistent lesions on the scalp. In adults, chronic **mucocutaneous candidiasis** can affect the mouth (thrush) *(Figure 3.15)*, vagina, and skin. It can also occur with diseases of the immune system *(see Chapter 7),* as those with a compromised immune system are more susceptible to chronic infections, including fungal infections.

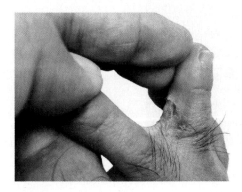

◀ **FIGURE 3.14** Tinea Pedis between the Toes.

Thiti Sukapan/Shutterstock

▶ **FIGURE 3.15** Thrush.

Timonina/Shutterstock

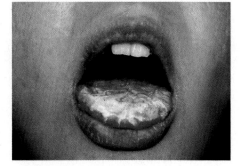

Parasitic Infestations (LO 3.5)

A **parasite** is an organism that lives in contact with and feeds off another organism or host. This process is called an **infestation** and is different from an **infection**.

Lice *(Figure 3.16)* are small, wingless, blood-sucking parasites that produce the disease **pediculosis** by attaching their nits (eggs) to hair and clothing.

Itch mites *(Figure 3.17)* produce an intense, itching rash called **scabies**, which generally occurs in the genital area or near the waist, breasts, and armpits. These mites lay eggs under the skin. Scabies is **contagious** and is typically spread when others come into physical contact with an infested person or when using shared items, such as clothing, sheets, or towels.

Bacterial Infections (LO 3.5)

Staphylococcus aureus (commonly called "staph") is the most common bacterium to invade the skin. Staph causes pimples, boils, **carbuncles**, and **impetigo** *(Figure 3.18)*. It can also produce a **cellulitis** of the epidermis and dermis. *Group A Streptococcus* (strep) can also cause cellulitis.

Occasionally, some strains of both staph and strep can be extremely **toxic**, especially when their enzymes digest the connective tissues and spread into the muscle layers. This condition is called **necrotizing fasciitis** and requires highly aggressive surgical and antibiotic treatment.

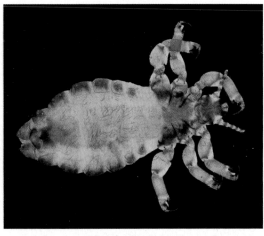

▲ **FIGURE 3.16**   Body Louse.

STEVE GSCHMEISSNER/Getty Images

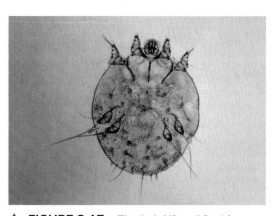

▲ **FIGURE 3.17**   The Itch Mite of Scabies.

Aliaksei Marozau/Shutterstock

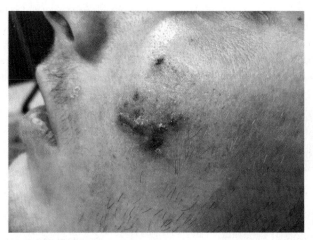

▲ **FIGURE 3.18**   Impetigo.

TisforThan/Shutterstock

Word Analysis and Definition

S = Suffix   P = Prefix   R = Root   R/CF = Combining Form

WORD	PRONUNCIATION		ELEMENTS	DEFINITION
Candida candidiasis	**KAN**-did-ah kan-dih-**DIE**-ah-sis	S/ R/	Latin *dazzling white* -iasis *state of, condition* candid- *Candida*	A yeastlike fungus Infection with the yeastlike fungus
Candida albicans thrush	**KAN**-did-ah **AL**-bih-kanz **THRUSH**		albicans Latin *white*	The most common form of *Candida* Another name for infection with *Candida*
carbuncle	**KAR**-bunk-ul		Latin *carbuncle*	Infection of many hair follicles in a small area, often on the back of the neck
cellulitis	sell-you-**LIE**-tis	S/ R/	-itis *inflammation* cellul- *cell*	Infection of subcutaneous connective tissue
contagious	kon-**TAY**-jus		Latin *touch closely*	Can be transmitted from person to person or from a person to a surface to a person
fungus fungi (pl)	**FUN**-gus **FUN**-jee or **FUN**-gee		Latin *mushroom*	General term used to describe yeasts and molds
impetigo	im-peh-**TIE**-go		Latin *scabby eruption*	Infection of the skin producing thick, yellow crusts
infection infectious (adj)	in-**FECK**-shun in-**FECK**-shus	S/ R/ S/	-ion *action* infect- *internal invasion, infection* -ious *pertaining to*	Invasion of the body by disease-producing microorganisms Capable of being transmitted, or a disease caused by the action of a microorganism
infestation	in-fes-**TAY**-shun	S/ R/	-ation *process* infest- *invade*	Act of being invaded on the skin by a trouble- some other species, such as a parasite
louse lice (pl)	**LOWSE** **LISE**		Old English *louse*	Parasitic insect
mucocutaneous	**MYU**-koh-kyu-**TAY**-nee-us	S/ R/CF R/CF	-ous *pertaining to* muc/o- *mucous membrane* -cutan/e- *skin*	Junction of skin and mucous membrane; e.g., the lips
necrotizing fasciitis *(Note the spelling.)*	**NEH**-kroh-**TIZE**-ing fash-eh-**EYE**-tis	S/ S/ R/CF S/ R/CF	-ing *quality of* -tiz- *pertaining to* necr/o- *death* -itis *inflammation* fasc/i- *fascia*	Inflammation of fascia producing death of the tissue
parasite parasitic (adj)	**PAIR**-ah-site pair-ah-**SIT**-ik	 S/ R/	Greek *guest* -ic *pertaining to* parasit- *parasite*	An organism that attaches itself to, lives on or in, and derives its nutrition from another species Pertaining to a parasite
pediculosis	peh-dick-you-**LOH**-sis	S/ R/	-osis *condition* pedicul- *louse*	An infestation with lice
scabies	**SKAY**-beez		Latin *to scratch*	Skin disease produced by mites
tinea tinea capitis tinea corporis tinea cruris tinea pedis tinea versicolor	**TIN**-ee-ah **TIN**-ee-ah **CAP**-it-us **TIN**-ee-ah **KOR**-por-is **TIN**-ee-ah **KROO**-ris **TIN**-ee-ah **PED**-is **TIN**-ee-ah **VERSE**-ih-col-or	 S/ R/ S/ R/ S/ R/ R/ R/CF R/	Latin *worm* -is *pertaining to* capit- *head* -is *pertaining to* corpor- *body* -is *pertaining to* crur- *leg* ped- *foot* vers/i- *to turn* -color *color*	General term for a group of related skin infections caused by different species of fungi Fungal infection of the scalp Fungal infection of the body Fungal infection of the groin Fungal infection of the foot Fungal infection of the trunk in which the skin loses pigmentation
toxin toxic (adj) toxicity **(Note:** *Contains two* *suffixes)*	**TOK**-sin **TOK**-sick tok-**SIS**-ih-tee	 S/ R/ S/	Greek *poison* -ic *pertaining to* tox- *poison* -ity *state, condition*	Poisonous substance formed by a cell or organism Pertaining to a toxin The state of being poisonous

Abbreviations

HIV   human immunodeficiency virus

SLE   systemic lupus erythematosus

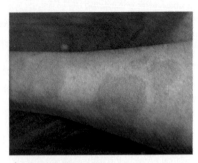

▲ FIGURE 3.19
Systemic Lupus Erythematosus.

korn ratchaneekorn/Shutterstock

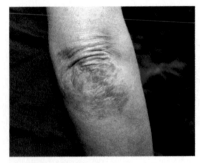

▲ FIGURE 3.20
Psoriasis Patch on the Elbow.

Dave Bolton/Getty Images

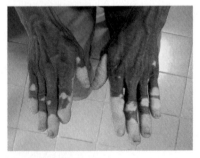

▲ FIGURE 3.21
Vitiligo.

Numstocker/Shutterstock

Collagen Diseases (LO 3.5)

Collagen, a fibrous protein, comprises 30% of your total body protein. Because your body contains so much of this protein, collagen diseases can have a dramatic effect throughout the body and in the skin.

Systemic lupus erythematosus (SLE) is an **autoimmune** disease that occurs most commonly in women. It produces characteristic skin lesions like a butterfly-shaped, red rash on both cheeks that is joined across the bridge of the nose *(Figure 3.19)*. This disease also affects multiple organs, including the kidneys, brain, heart, lungs, and joints.

Rosacea, a skin condition in which the cause is not well understood, produces a similar facial rash to that of SLE, but there are no systemic complications.

Scleroderma is a chronic, persistent autoimmune disease that also occurs more often in women. It's characterized by a hardening and shrinking of the skin that makes it feel leathery. Joints show swelling, pain, and stiffness. Internal organs, including the heart, lungs, kidneys, and digestive tract, are involved in a similar process. The **etiology** is unknown, and there is no effective treatment.

Breast cancer can often occur in a patient with scleroderma.

Other Skin Diseases (LO 3.5)

Psoriasis *(Figure 3.20)* is marked by itchy, flaky, red patches of skin of various sizes covered with white or silvery scales. It appears most commonly on the scalp, elbows, and knees, and its cause is unknown.

Vitiligo *(Figure 3.21)* produces pale, irregular patches of skin. It is thought to have an autoimmune etiology.

Skin Manifestations of Internal Disease (LO 3.1, 3.2, 3.3 and 3.5)

The presence of cancer inside the body is often shown by skin lesions visible on the body's surface, even before the cancer or other disease has produced **symptoms** or been diagnosed. **Dermatomyositis** *(Figure 3.22)* is often associated with ovarian cancer, which can appear within 4 to 5 years after the skin disease is diagnosed. This skin disease presents with a reddish-purple rash around the eyes. Muscle weakness commonly follows weeks or months after the appearance of the rash.

Kaposi sarcoma is caused by infection with herpesvirus 8 and mostly develops in association with **HIV** infection. Raised red or brown blotches or bumps in tissues occur below the skin's surface and eventually spread throughout the body.

Herpes zoster, referred to earlier in this chapter, is common in immunocompromised patients, including the elderly, individuals with HIV, and patients on chemotherapy *(see Chapter 7)*.

Acne (LO 3.5)

Around puberty, **androgens**, male sex hormones, are thought to trigger an excessive production of sebum from the sebaceous glands. Sebum brings with it excessive numbers of broken-down keratin cells. This blocks the hair follicle, forming a **comedo** (whitehead or blackhead). Comedones can stay closed, leading to papules, or can rupture, allowing bacteria to get in and produce **pustules**. These are the classic signs of **acne**. Acne affects about 85% of people between the ages of 12 and 25 years *(Figure 3.23)*. Severe forms of acne can result in the formation of fluid-filled **cysts** that leave **scars**.

A different skin problem involving the sebaceous glands is **seborrheic dermatitis**. The glands are thought to be inflamed and to produce a different sebum. The skin around the face and scalp is reddened and covered with yellow, greasy scales. In infants, this condition is called cradle cap. Seborrheic dermatitis of the scalp produces dandruff. **Dandruff** is clumps of these keratinocytes stuck together with sebum.

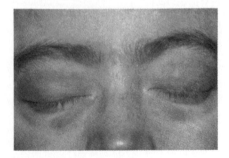

◀ FIGURE 3.22
Periorbital Rash of Dermatomyositis.

Mediscan/Alamy Images

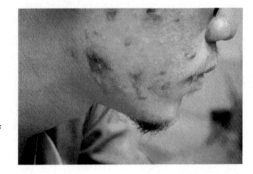

◀ FIGURE 3.23
Acne—showing pustules and papules.

NikomMaelao Production/Shutterstock

WORD	PRONUNCIATION		ELEMENTS	DEFINITION
acne	**AK**-nee		Greek *point*	Inflammatory disease of sebaceous glands and hair follicles
androgen	**AN**-droh-jen	S/ R/CF	-gen *to produce, create* andr/o- *male*	Hormone that promotes masculine characteristics
autoimmune (adj)	awe-toe-im-**YUNE**	P/ R/	auto- *self* -immune *protected from*	Diseases in which the body makes antibodies directed against its own tissues
comedo *(whitehead or blackhead)* comedones (pl)	**KOM**-ee-doh kom-ee-**DOH**-nz		Latin *eat up*	Too much sebum and too many keratin cells block the hair follicle to produce the comedo
cyst cystic (adj)	**SIST** **SIS**-tik	S/	Greek *sac, bladder* -ic *pertaining to*	Abnormal fluid-filled sac surrounded by a membrane Pertaining to a cyst
dandruff	**DAN**-druff		Source unknown	Scales in hair from shedding of the epidermis
dermatomyositis	**DER**-mah-toe-**MY**-oh-site-is	S/ R/CF R/	-itis *inflammation* dermat/o- *skin* -myos- *muscle*	Inflammation of the skin and muscles
etiology	ee-tee-**OL**-oh-jee	S/ R/CF	-logy *study of* eti/o- *cause*	The study of the causes of a disease
Kaposi sarcoma	kah-**POH**-see sar-**KOH**-mah		Moritz Kaposi, Hungarian dermatologist, 1837–1902	A form of skin cancer seen in patients with HIV
pustule	**PUS**-tyul		Latin *pustule*	Small protuberance on the skin containing pus
psoriasis	so-**RYE**-ah-sis		Greek *the itch*	Rash characterized by reddish, silver-scaled patches
rosacea	roh-**ZAY**-she-ah		Latin *rosy*	Persistent erythematous rash of the central face
scar	**SKAR**		Greek *scab*	Fibrotic seam that forms when a wound heals
scleroderma	sklair-oh-**DERM**-ah	S/ R/CF	-derma *skin* scler/o- *hard*	Thickening and hardening of the skin due to new collagen formation
seborrhea seborrheic (adj) *(The "a" is deleted to enable the word to flow.)*	seb-oh-**REE**-ah seb-oh-**REE**-ik	S/ R/CF S/	-rrhea *flow* seb/o- *sebum* -ic *pertaining to*	Excessive amount of sebum Pertaining to seborrhea
symptom *(subjective)* symptomatic (adj) sign *(objective)*	**SIMP**-tum simp-toe-**MAT**-ik **SINE**	S/ R/	Greek *event or feeling that has happened to someone* -atic *pertaining to* symptom- *symptoms* Latin *mark*	Departure from normal health experienced by the patient Pertaining to the symptoms of a disease Physical evidence of a disease process
systemic lupus erythematosus	sis-**TEM**-ik **LOO**-pus er-ih-**THEE**-mah-**TOE**-sus	S/ R/ S/ R/	-ic *pertaining to* system- *the body as a whole* lupus Latin *wolf* -osus *condition* erythemat- *redness*	Inflammatory connective tissue disease affecting the whole body
vitiligo	vit-ill-**EYE**-go		Latin *skin blemish*	Nonpigmented white patches on otherwise normal skin

Hair Follicles and Sebaceous Glands (LO 3.5)

Diseases of Hair (LO 3.5)

In most people, aging causes various degrees of **alopecia**, thinning of the hair, and baldness as the follicles shrink and produce thin, wispy hairs.

Sweat Glands (LO 3.5)

Hyperhidrosis is an uncontrollable overproduction of sweat usually experienced in the armpits, palms, and soles of the feet. Primary hyperhidrosis is caused by the hypothalamus, an area of the brain responsible for regulating body temperature, overstimulating the eccrine glands. Secondary hyperhidrosis is caused by overstimulation of the eccrine glands by anything other than the hypothalamus, such as drugs, obesity, and menopause.

Diseases of Nails (LO 3.5)

Fifty percent of all nail disorders are caused by fungal infections and are called **onychomycosis** *(Figure 3.24)*. With these infections, the fungus grows under the nail and leads to yellow, brittle, cracked nails that separate from the underlying nail bed.

    Paronychia *(Figure 3.25)* is a bacterial infection, usually staphylococcal, of the nail base. The nail fold and cuticle become swollen, red, and painful, and pus forms under the nail.

    With an **ingrown toenail,** the nail grows into the skin at the side of the nail, particularly if pressured by tight, narrow shoes. An infection can then form underneath this ingrown toenail.

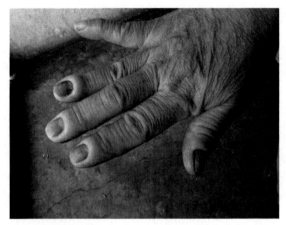

▲ **FIGURE 3.24**
Onychomycosis (Fungal Infection).

jeeraphon/Shutterstock

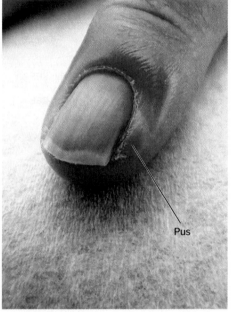

Pus

▲ **FIGURE 3.25**
Paronychia.

Robert Kirk/iStock/Getty Images

Word Analysis and Definition

S = Suffix   P = Prefix   R = Root   R/CF = Combining Form

WORD	PRONUNCIATION		ELEMENTS	DEFINITION
alopecia	al-oh-**PEE**-shah		Greek *mange*	Partial or complete loss of hair, naturally or from medication
hyperhidrosis	HIGH-per-high-DROH-sis	S/ P/ R/	-osis *abnormal condition* hyper- *excessive* -hidr- *production of sweat*	Excessive production of sweat
onychomycosis	oh-nih-koh-my-**KOH**-sis	S/ R/CF R/	-osis *condition* onych/o- *nail* -myc- *fungus*	Condition of a fungus infection in a nail
paronychia (**Note:** *The vowel "a" at the end of para is dropped to make the composite word flow more easily.*)	pair-oh-**NICK**-ee-ah	S/ P/ R/	-ia *condition* para- *alongside* -onych- *nail*	Infection alongside the nail

EXERCISES

 ### CASE REPORT 3.2

You are . . .

. . . a medical assistant working with dermatologist Dr. Echols in Fulwood Medical Center.

You are communicating with . . .

. . . Ms. Cheryl Fox, a 37-year-old nursing assistant working in a surgical unit in Fulwood Medical Center.

Recently, Ms. Fox's fingers have become red and itchy, with occasional **vesicles**. She has also noticed irritation and swelling of her earlobes and **pruritus**. Over the weekends, both the itching and the **rash** on her hands worsen. A patch test by Dr. Echols showed that Ms. Fox is **allergic** to nickel, which is present in the rings she wears on both hands and in her earrings. She only wears this jewelry on the weekends, not during her workdays.

For Ms. Fox, the **allergy** is not just a local reaction to an irritant. Her form of **atopic** or allergic **dermatitis** develops when the whole body becomes sensitive to an allergen. This whole-body involvement is shown by her systemic symptoms of **pruritus** distant from the local irritant site. Ms. Fox has stopped wearing rings and earrings that contain nickel. Her dermatitis was treated with topical steroids.

A. Read *Case Report 3.2 to answer the following questions.* **LO 3.4 and 3.5**

1. Which two parts of Ms. Fox's body were exhibiting symptoms? _____

2. Does Ms. Fox experience itching on her earlobes? _____

3. What test did Dr. Echols use to determine the cause of the symptoms? _____

4. What is Ms. Fox allergic to? _____

5. Which of the symptoms means blisters? _____

 ### CASE REPORT 3.3

You are . . .

. . . a pharmacist working in the pharmacy at Fulwood Medical Center.

You are communicating with . . .

. . . Mr. Wayne Winter, an 18-year-old man who will be starting college in a few months.

Mr. Winter has had acne since the age of 15. He has tried several over-the-counter products, all of which have been unsuccessful in treating his acne. He has even tried retinoic acid. He has numerous **comedones**, papules, **pustules**, and **scars** on his face and forehead and has severe **cystic** lesions and scars on his back. He avoids social settings, and his peers frequently tease him. He is seeking treatment prior to his upcoming attendance at college.

Your role is to explain to him how to use the medications Dr. Echols, a dermatologist, has prescribed, what their effects will be, and what possible complications may occur.

B. Read *Case Report 3.3 to answer the following questions. Fill in the blanks.* **LO 3.4, 3.5, and 3.6**

1. Does Mr. Winter have blackheads, whiteheads, or both? _____

2. Which hormone is likely triggering Mr. Winter's acne? _____

3. Evidence of previous pustules and cystic lesions are noted as: _____

4. What type of specialist did Mr. Winter consult? _____

C. Medical documentation *should always be neat, legible, and spelled correctly for patient safety. Also remember that the patient record is a legal document. After you finish this exercise, you can hear terms pronounced correctly by visiting the audio glossary contained in your Connect® course (http://connect.mheducation. com) and practice them yourself. Below, insert the correct spelling of the term on the line.* **LO 3.5, 3.6, and 3.7**

1. Medication has been prescribed for this patient's case of _____ dermatitis.

   seborheic   **seborrheic**

2. The _____ rash on the patient's face is slowly clearing after she tried the new medication.

   eczematous   exzematous

3. Ms. Fox's _____ is an allergic reaction to her jewelry, which contains nickel.

   purritis   **pruritus**

D. Identify *the italicized element in the first column of the chart, define it, and use it to determine the meaning of the medical term.* **LO 3.1 and 3.5**

Medical Term	Identity of Element (P, S, R, or CF)	Meaning of Element	Meaning of Medical Term
meta*stasis*	1.	2.	3.
*malign*ant	4.	5.	6.
melan*oma*	7.	8.	9.
decubitus	10.	11.	12.

E. Demonstrate *that you are able to spell medical terms related to disorders of the skin. Fill in the blank with the correct term from the list below. Not all terms will be used.* **LO 3.2 and 3.5**

   congenital   **herpes zoster**   **macule**   **nevi**   **nevus**   **papillomavirus**

1. The medical term that means the same as *mole* is _____.

2. Shingles is caused by the _____ virus.

3. The plural form of the term *nevus* is _____.

4. A birthmark is a _____ accumulation of pigment on the skin.

F. Demonstrate *that you are able to spell medical terms related to disorders of the skin. Fill in the blanks.* **LO 3.2 and 3.5**

1. A condition caused by lice infestation: _____

2. Inflammation of subcutaneous connective tissue: _____

3. What are lice eggs called? _____

4. A skin disease caused by mites: _____

5. An infection of the fascia that results in the death of the tissue: _____

G. Document *using the language of dermatology by inserting the correct term in the space provided. Fill in the blanks.* **LO 3.2, 3.5, and 3.7**

1. According to the patient's symptoms, the physician diagnosed a/an (body attacks its own tissues) _____ disease.

2. What we thought was originally a localized problem has now spread, and the patient's final diagnosis is (inflammatory connective tissue disease affecting the whole body) _____.

3. In consideration of this patient's past history of HIV, his new skin lesions have been diagnosed by the pathologist as (a form of skin cancer commonly seen in patients with HIV) _____.

4. Patients with (rash with reddish, silver-scaled patches) _____ often wear long sleeves to hide their elbows.

H. Building medical terms and taking them apart *force you to focus on the elements they contain. Understanding elements is the key to increasing your medical vocabulary. Deconstruct the following terms to increase your knowledge of their elements.* **LO 3.1 and 3.5**

1. In the term **erythematosus,** the root means:

   a. condition of   **b.** blemish   **c.** red   **d.** inflammation

2. In the term **symptomatic**, the suffix means:

   a. pertaining to   **b.** inflammation   **c.** painful   **d.** condition of

3. In the term **dermatomyositis**, the word element that means skin is a:

   a. root/combining form   **b.** prefix   **c.** suffix

4. In the term **autoimmune**, the word element that means self is a:

   a. root/combining form   **b.** prefix   **c.** suffix

I. Indicate if the statement is true or false. LO 3.4 and 3.5

   1. A pustule is filled with pus.   True False

   2. Acne is a degenerative disease of the skin.   True False

   3. A cystic lesion is filled with hard, packed cells.   True False

   4. A comedo can be either a whitehead or a blackhead.   True False

J. List *the plural term of the following:* **LO 3.2, 3.3, and 3.5**

1. scar: _____

2. cyst: _____

3. comedo: _____

K. Elements *are clues to the meaning of a medical term. Identify each given element in the following chart and list its meaning.* **LO 3.1 and 3.3**

Element	Identity of Element (P, R, CF, or S)	Meaning of Element
para-	1.	2.
-ia	3.	4.
myc-	5.	6.
onycho	7.	8.
-osis	9.	10.
onych	11.	12.

L. Answer the following questions. Select the correct answer that completes each statement. LO 3.4 and 3.5

1. The structure that protects the nail matrix:

   a. nail root   **b.** free edge   **c.** cuticle   **d.** dermis

2. Fungal infection of the nail:

   a. paronychia   **b.** alopecia   **c.** ingrown toenail   **d.** onychomycosis

3. Sweat glands open:

   a. into hair follicles only   **b.** onto the surface of the skin only   **c.** into the hair follicles and onto the surface of the skin

4. Alopecia is defined as a(n):

   a. infection of a hair follicle

   b. partial or complete hair loss

   c. infection alongside the nail

   d. fluid-filled sac

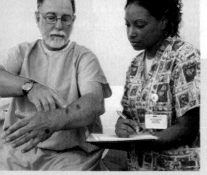

Section 3.3

Diagnostic and Therapeutic Procedures and Pharmacology for Disorders

Diagnostic Procedures (LO 3.6)

The most important procedures in making a diagnosis of a skin lesion are taking a careful medical history of the etiology and progression of the lesion and a careful visual examination to define the clinical appearance of the lesion.

Diascopy, in which a finger or a microscope slide is pressed against a lesion to see if it blanches (loses color), helps define a vascular lesion, which blanches, from a hemorrhagic (bleeding) lesion which does not blanch but rather displays petechia purpura spots.

Microscopic examination of skin scrapings helps diagnose fungal infections and scabies. Tzanck testing by scraping the base of vesicles and staining them with a Giemsa stain shows multinucleated giant cells of herpes simplex or zoster under microscopy.

Cultures using swabs taken from lesions and implanted in the appropriate growth medium are utilized to diagnose some viruses (e.g., herpes simplex) and certain bacteria.

Biopsy (Bx) of a skin lesion using a punch biopsy, excision of a whole lesion, or shaving of the lesion for microscopic examination is valuable in diagnosing malignancies, fungal diseases, and immune diseases.

Wood's light (black light) is used to define the borders of pigmented lesions before excision, show the presence of *Pseudomonas* infection (**fluoresces** green), and distinguish the **hypopigmentation** of vitiligo, which fluoresces a deep ivory white.

Therapeutic Procedures (LO 3.6)

Photodynamic therapy (**PDT**) in a series of sessions exposes the skin in acne to a high-intensity blue light and creates a toxic environment in which bacteria in the sebaceous glands cannot live. In addition to treating acne, PDT can be used to treat precancerous lesions called **actinic keratoses,** which have the potential to develop into squamous cell carcinomas.

Laser therapy is used for the management of birthmarks, vascular lesions, warts, and skin disorders like vitiligo.

Chemical peels are performed on the face, neck, or hands. An acid solution such as glycolic acid, salicylic acid, or carbolic acid (phenol) is applied to small areas of skin to reduce fine facial lines and wrinkles, treat sun damage, and reduce age spots and dark patches (**melasma**).

Cryotherapy, also referred to as **cryosurgery,** is used frequently to treat acne, scars, sebaceous plaques, and some skin cancers. Liquid nitrogen is sprayed onto the affected area of skin to cause peeling or scabbing.

Used purely for **cosmetic** procedures, Botox is a prescription medicine that blocks signals from nerves to muscles. When injected into superficial muscles, the injected muscle can no longer contract, causing facial muscles to temporarily relax, which in turn cause wrinkles and lines to soften.

Dermal fillers such as Restylane and Juvederm help to diminish facial lines and wrinkles by restoring subcutaneous volume and fullness to the face as subcutaneous fat is lost in the natural aging process.

Abbreviations

Bx	biopsy
PDT	Photodynamic therapy

WORD	PRONUNCIATION	ELEMENTS		DEFINITION
actinic	ak-**TIN**-ik	S/ R/	-ic *pertaining to* actin- *ray*	Pertaining to the sun
biopsy	**BI**-op-see	S/ R/	-opsy *to view* bi- *life*	Removing tissue from a living person for laboratory examination
cosmetic	koz-**MET**-ik		Greek *an adornment*	A concern for appearance
cryosurgery	cry-oh-**SUR**-jer-ee **CRY**-oh-**THAIR**-ah pee	S/ R/CF R/	-ery *process of* cry/o- *icy cold* -surg- *operate*	Use of liquid nitrogen or argon gas in a probe to freeze and kill abnormal tissue
cryotherapy (syn)		R/	-therapy *medical treatment*	Use of cold in the treatment of disease
culture	**KUL**-chur		Latin *tillage*	The growth of microorganisms on or in media
diascopy	di-**AS**-koh-pee	P/ R/	dia- *through* -scopy *to examine, to view*	Examination of superficial skin lesions with pressure
fluoresce	flor-**ESS**		Greek *bright color*	Emit a bright-colored light when irradiated with ultraviolet or violet-blue rays
keratosis keratoses (pl)	ker-ah-**TOH**-sis ker-ah-**TOH**-seez	S/ R/	-osis *condition* kerat- *horny*	Epidermal lesion of circumscribed overgrowth of the horny layer
melasma	meh-**LAZ**-mah		Greek *black spot*	Patchy pigmentation of the skin
pigment hypopigmentation	**PIG**-ment **HIGH**-poh-pig-men-**TAY**-shun	S/ P/ R/	Latin *paint* -ation *process* hypo- *below normal* -pigment- *color*	A coloring matter or stain Below normal melanin relative to the surrounding skin
phototherapy	foh-toe-**THAIR**-ah-pee	R/CF	phot/o	

Dermatologic Pharmacology (LO 3.6)

A wide range of **topical pharmacologic** agents of different types can be used in the treatment of skin lesions either to relieve symptoms or to cure the disease.

- **Anesthetics**: topical agents that relieve pain or itching on the skin's surface. Benzocaine is used for this purpose as a numbing **cream.** It is used prior to injections, for oral ulcers, for hemorrhoids, and for infant teething.

- **Antibacterials:** topical agents that eliminate bacteria that cause skin lesions. Mupirocin **ointment** is commonly used. Certain antibiotics taken by mouth, such as doxycycline or azithromycin, are also used to treat acne.

- **Antifungals:** topical agents that eliminate or inhibit the growth of fungi. Nystatin (*Mycostatin, Nilstat*) is used as a cream or ointment. Terbinafine (*Lamisil*) is used as a cream or ointment. Clotrimazole (*Canesten, Clomazol*) and ketoconazole (*Ketopine, Daktagold*) are *imidazoles* available in creams, sprays, **lotions,** and **shampoos.** Mycamine (*Micafungin*) is used in IV therapy for systemic fungal infections.

- **Antipruritics:** topical lotions, ointments, creams, or sprays that relieve itching. **Corticosteroids** such as hydrocortisone are most frequently used, although for systemic pruritus, certain neurological medications can also be effective.

- **Keratolytics:** topical agents that peel away the skin's stratum corneum from the other epidermal layers.
  Salicylic acid is used for this purpose in the treatment of acne, psoriasis, ichthyoses, and dandruff. It is available in the form of wipes, creams, **lotions, gels,** ointments, and **shampoos** in strengths varying from 3% to 20%.

- **Parasiticides:** topical agents that kill parasites living on the skin. Permethrin (1%) is used in lotion or shampoo form to kill lice and is also a treatment for scabies.

- **Retinoids:** derivatives of retinoic acid (vitamin A) used under the strict supervision of a physician in the treatment of acne, sun spots, and psoriasis. Tretinoin (*Retin-A*) is used topically for acne; isotretinoin (*Accutane*) is taken orally for severe acne; etretinate (*Tegison*) is taken orally to treat severe psoriasis; and adapalene (*Differin*) is used topically for psoriasis.

Classes of Topical Medications

Solutions are usually a powder dissolved in water or alcohol.

Lotions are usually a powder mixed with oil and water to be thicker than a solution.

Gels are a semisolid **emulsion** in an alcohol base.

Creams are an emulsion of oil and water that is thicker than a lotion and holds its shape when removed from its container. These penetrate the outer stratum corneum layer of skin.

Ointments are a homogenous semisolid preparation, 80% a thick oil and 20% water, that lies on the skin. They can also be used on the mucous membranes of the eye, vulva, anus, and nose, and are emulsifiable with the mucous membrane secretions.

Transdermal patches are a precise, time-released method to deliver a drug. Release of the drug can be controlled by **diffusion** through the adhesive that covers the whole patch or through a membrane with adhesive only on the patch rim.

Word Analysis and Definition

S = Suffix   P = Prefix   R = Root   R/CF = Combining Form

WORD	PRONUNCIATION	ELEMENTS		DEFINITION
anesthetic	an-es-**THET**-ik	S/ P/ R/	-ic *pertaining to* an- *without* -esthet- *sensation, perception*	Substance that takes away feeling and pain.
antibacterial	AN-tee-bak-**TEER**-ee-al	S/ P/ R/CF	-al *pertaining to* anti- *against* -bacter/i- *bacteria*	Destroying or preventing the growth of bacteria
antifungal antipruritic	AN-tee-**FUN**-gul AN-tee-pru-**RIT**-ik	R/ S/ P/ R/	fung- *fungus* -ic *pertaining to* anti- *against* -prurit- *itch*	Destroying or preventing the growth of a fungus Medication against itching
cream	**KREEM**		Latin *thick juice*	A semisolid emulsion
diffusion	dih-**FYU**-zhun	S/ R/	-ion *process* diffus- *movement*	The process by which small particles move between tissues
emulsion	ee-**MUL**-shun	S/ R/	-ion *process* emuls- *suspension in a liquid*	Very small particles suspended in a solution
keratolytic	**KAIR**-ah-toh-**LIT**-ik	S/ R/CF R/	-ic *pertaining to* kerat/o- *horn* -lyt- *loosening*	Causing separation or loosening of the horny layer (stratum cor-neum) of the skin
parasiticide	pair-ah-**SIT**-ih-side	S/ R/CF	-cide *to kill* parasit/i- *parasite*	Agent that destroys parasites
retinoid	**RET**-ih-noyd		Derived from retinoic acid	A cream that is a derivative of vitamin A used to treat acne and wrinkles
topical	**TOP**-ih-kal	S/ R/	-al *pertaining to* topic- *local*	Medication applied to the skin to obtain a local effect

EXERCISES

A. Identify *the proper diagnostic procedure or treatment for each condition. Use the words from the provided word bank to complete the sentences. Fill in the blanks.* **LO 3.6**

diascopy   Juvederm   cryotherapy   Botox   fluoresce

1. Injecting _____ into the skin will fill areas to reduce the appearance of aging.

2. Acne can be treated with _____ to freeze the cells of the affected area.

3. Pigmented or hypopigmented areas can be better seen when they _____ with Wood's light.

4. Pressing on an area of skin to see if it blanches is termed _____.

5. The injection of _____ can reduce the appearance of wrinkles by paralyzing the affected muscles.

B. Defining the meaning of word elements can help you to quickly decipher the meaning of medical terms. *Choose the correct answer to each question.* **LO 3.1**

1. The word element that means *cold*:

   a. *dia-*   b. *-therapy*   c. *cry/o-*   d. *hypo-*

2. The word element *dia-* means:

   a. to view   b. through   c. light   d. two

3. The word element *-scopy* means:

   a. to view   b. scrape   c. suture   d. inject

4. The suffix that means *condition of* is:

   a. *-osis*   b. *-ic*   c. *-itis*   d. *-al*

C. Practice *your language of pharmacology by correctly filling in the blanks of each sentence.* LO 3.6 and 3.7

Mrs. Robison brought in her 8-year-old daughter to the doctor because the child had a red ring-like rash on her abdomen. Dr. Palmer examined the child and diagnosed her with tinea corporis. She prescribed Terbinafine cream to be applied to the site twice daily for 6 weeks.

1. Dr. Palmer prescribed an _____ cream to cure the patient's tinea corporis.

2. She prefers to provide _____ application of the medication because it stays local to the site of the infection.

D. Define *the classes of topical medications. Topical medications come in a variety of forms to best deliver medication to the skin. Match the description of the form of the medication to its term.* LO 3.3 and 3.7

Term	Meaning
_____ 1. gel	a. adhesive membrane attached to the surface of the skin
_____ 2. lotion	b. semisolid emulsion in an alcohol base
_____ 3. ointment	c. powder dissolved in alcohol or water
_____ 4. transdermal patch	d. powder mixed with oil and water; thicker than a solution
_____ 5. solution	e. Semisolid preparation of oil and water

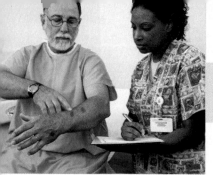

Section 3.4

Burns and Injuries to the Skin

Burns (LO 3.4 and 3.5)

In burns, the immediate threats to life are from fluid loss, infection, and the systemic effects of burned dead tissue. Burn injury to the lungs through damage from heat or smoke inhalation is responsible for 60% or more of burn-related fatalities.

Burns are classified according to the depth of burnt tissue involved *(Figure 3.26):*

First-degree (superficial) burns involve only the epidermis and produce superficial **inflammation,** with redness, pain, and slight edema. Healing takes 3 to 5 days without scarring, although skin **desquamation** (peeling) often occurs.

Second-degree (partial-thickness) burns involve the epidermis and dermis but leave some of the dermis intact. They produce redness, blisters, and more severe pain. Healing takes 2 to 3 weeks, with minimal scarring.

Third-degree (full-thickness) burns involve the epidermis, dermis, and subcutaneous tissues, which are often completely destroyed. Healing takes a long time and involves skin **grafts.**

Fourth-degree burns destroy all layers of the skin and involve underlying tendons, muscles, and, sometimes, bones. In full-thickness burns, because there is no dermal tissue left for **regeneration**, skin grafts are necessary.

The ideal graft is an **autograft**, taken from another location on the patient's body, because it is not rejected by the immune system.

If the patient's burns are too extensive, **allografts**—grafts from another person—are used. **Homograft** is another name for allograft. These grafts are provided by skin banks, which acquire them from deceased donors (**cadavers**). A **xenograft** or **heterograft** is a graft from another species, such as a pig for heart valves.

In addition, artificial skin is being developed commercially and can stimulate the growth of new connective tissues from the patient's underlying tissue.

Eschar describes the presence of dead tissue and dried secretions found at the site of a partial or full-thickness burn. Typically, the eschar will be removed by a process of debridement to avoid infection and encourage healing at the burn region. Debridement is one of the most common treatments for burns of various degrees and involves the removal of the damaged or dead tissue to accelerate healing and the regrowth of healthy tissue. Although several types of debridement exist, surgical debridement is most common in treating partial- or full-thickness burns. In surgical debridement, the burn region is thoroughly cleansed, and all dead (necrotic) tissue is removed in addition to any other foreign matter. This allows for the application of a proper dressing for protection, avoiding infection, and encouraging proper healing.

Keynotes

- Sunburn usually causes a first-degree burn.
- **Scalds** can cause second-degree burns.
- House fires with prolonged flame contact can cause third-degree burns.
- High-voltage electrical injury can cause fourth-degree burns.

Keynote

- In third- and fourth-degree burns, there is no dermal tissue left for regeneration, and skin grafts are necessary.

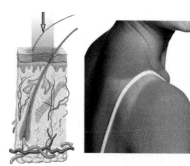
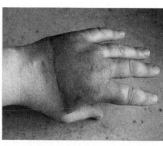
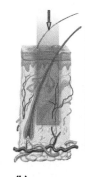
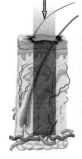
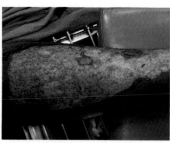

(a)   (b)   (c)

▲ **FIGURE 3.26**   Partial- and Full-Thickness Burns.
(a) First degree (superficial thickness). (b) Second degree (partial thickness). (c) Third degree (full thickness).

Rule of Nines (LO 3.4, 3.5, and 3.6)

The treatment and prognosis for a burn patient also depend on how much of the body surface is affected. This is estimated by subdividing the skin's surface into regions, each one of which is a fraction of or multiple of 9% of the total surface area (*Figure 3.27*). To give you a clearer idea of how these numbers come into play, the body's surface areas are assigned the following percentages:

- Head and neck = 9% (4½% anterior and 4½% posterior).
- Each arm = 9% (4½% anterior and 4½% posterior).
- Each leg = 18% (9% anterior and 9% posterior).
- The anterior trunk = 18%.
- The posterior trunk = 18%.
- Genitalia = 1%.

Aging of the Skin (LO 3.4 and 3.5)

With aging, the epidermis thins and the number of melanocytes decreases, but the remaining melanocytes increase in size. Aging skin, therefore, appears thinner, paler, and more translucent, and large pigmented spots (**lentigines**) appear in sun-exposed areas. The blood vessels of the dermis become fragile, leading to bruising and bleeding under the skin. Sebaceous glands produce less oil, leading to dryness and itching. Sweat glands produce less sweat, making it harder to keep cool. The subcutaneous fat layer thins, connective tissue becomes less elastic, and the skin wrinkles and tears easily. Aging skin repairs slowly and wound healing takes up to 4 times longer. Most of these skin changes are hastened and increased by sun exposure.

Wounds and Tissue Repair (LO 3.5 and 3.6)

If you cut yourself when shaving and produce a superficial **laceration** in the epidermis, the epithelial (surface tissue) cells along the laceration's edges will split rapidly and fill in the gap to heal it.

If you cut yourself more deeply, creating a **wound** in the dermis or hypodermis, blood vessels in the dermis break and blood escapes into the wound (*Figure 3.28a*). The same happens when a surgeon makes an **incision**. On the other hand, a surgeon would perform an **excision** if he or she removed a lesion from the skin or any other tissue.

Escaped blood from a wound or surgical procedure forms a **clot** in the wound. The clot consists of the protein fibrin together with platelets, blood cells, and dried tissue fluids trapped in the fibers. Cells that digest and clean up the tissue debris enter the wound (*see Chapter 7*). The surface of the clot dries and hardens in the air to form a **scab**. The scab seals and protects the wound from becoming infected (*Figure 3.28b*).

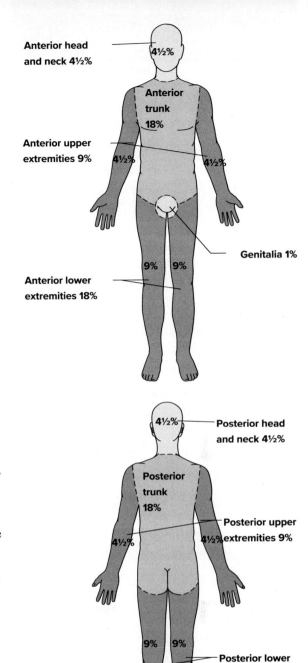

▲ **FIGURE 3.27** Rule of Nines.

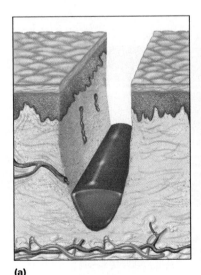

(a)

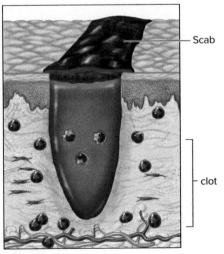

(b)

◀ **FIGURE 3.28**
Wound Healing.
(a) Bleeding into the wound. (b) Scab formation.

WORD	PRONUNCIATION	ELEMENTS		DEFINITION
allograft	**AL**-oh-graft	P/ R/	allo- *other* -**graft** *transplant*	Skin graft from another person or a cadaver
autograft	**AWE**-toe-graft	P/ R/	auto- *self, same* -**graft** *transplant*	A graft removed from the patient's own skin
cadaver	kah-**DAV**-er		Latin *dead body*	A dead body or corpse
cryotheraphy (syn)	**CRY**-oh-**THAIR**-ah pee	R/	-**therapy** *medical treatment*	The use of cold in the treatment of disease
debridement	day-**BREED**-mon (French pronunciation of -ment)	S/ P/ R/	-**ment** *resulting state* de- *take away* -**bride-** *rubbish*	The removal of injured or necrotic tissue
desquamation	des-kwa-**MAY**-shun	S/ P/ R/	-**action** *action, condition* de- *away from* -**squam-** *squamous*	The peeling of outer layer of skin; Shedding of epidermis
eschar	**ESS**-kar		Greek *scab of a burn*	The burnt, dead tissue lying on top of third-degree burns
heterograft *(same as xenograft)*	**HET**-er-oh-graft	P/ R/	hetero- *different* -**graft** *transplant*	A graft from another species (not human)
homograft *(same as allograft)*	**HOH**-moh-graft	P/ R/	homo- *same, alike* -**graft** *transplant*	Skin graft from another person or a cadaver
inflammation inflammatory (adj)	in-flah-**MAY**-shun in-**FLAM**-ah-tor-ee	S/ P/ R/ S/	-**ion** *action, condition* in- *in* -**flammat-** *flame* -**ory** *having the function of*	A complex of cell and chemical reactions occurring in response to an injury or chemical or biologic agent Causing or affected by inflammation
lentigo lentigines (pl)	len-**TIE**-go len-**TIJ**-ih-neez		Greek *lentil*	Age spot; small, flat, brown-black spot in the skin of older people
regenerate (verb) regeneration (noun)	ree-**JEN**-eh-rate ree-**JEN**-eh-**RAY**-shun	S/ P/ R/ S/	-**ate** *composed of* re- *again* -**gener-** *produce* -**ation** *process*	Reconstitution of a lost part The process of reconstitution
scald	**SKAWLD**		Latin *wash in hot water*	Burn from contact with hot liquid or steam
shock	**SHOCK**		German *to clash*	Sudden physical or mental collapse or circulatory collapse
xenograft *(same as heterograft)*	**ZEN**-oh-graft	P/ R/	xeno- *foreign* -**graft** *transplant*	A graft from another species (not human)

New capillaries from the surrounding dermis then invade the clot. Three or four days after the injury, other cells migrate into the wound. These cells form new collagen fibers that pull the wound together. This soft tissue in the wound is called **granulation** tissue *(Figure 3.29)*, which is later replaced by a scar *(Figure 3.30)*.

Suturing brings together the edges of the wound to enhance tissue healing.

▶ **FIGURE 3.29**
Formation of Granulation Tissue.

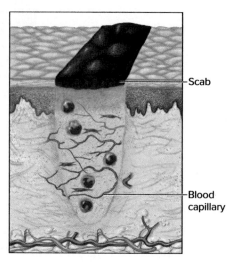

Scab

Blood capillary

▶ **FIGURE 3.30**
Scar Formation.

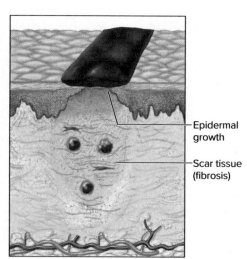

Epidermal growth

Scar tissue (fibrosis)

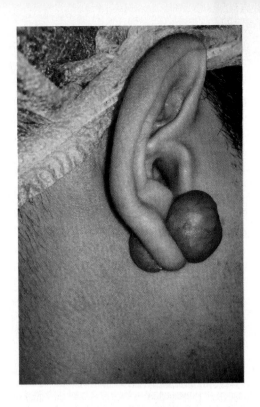

▶ **FIGURE 3.31**
Keloid of the Earlobe—resulting from piercing of the earlobe.

Karan Bunjean/Shutterstock

In some patients, there are excessive fibrosis and scar tissue, producing raised, irregular, lumpy, shiny scars called **keloids** *(Figure 3.31)*. Keloids, most commonly found on the upper body and earlobes, can extend beyond the edges of the original wound and often return even if they are surgically removed.

A superficial scraping of the skin, a mucous membrane, or the cornea of the eye *(Chapter 11)* is called an **abrasion**.

Surgery on the skin is now being performed using focused light beams called lasers. These lasers remove lesions like birthmarks and tattoos and create a fresh surface over which new skin can grow.

Cosmetic Procedures (LO 3.1, 3.2, 3.4, 3.5, 3.6, and 3.8)

Surgical procedures that cosmetically alter or improve the appearance of your face or body are becoming more and more common. These cosmetic procedures include:

Abdominoplasty: a "tummy tuck."
Blepharoplasty: the correction of defects, usually droopiness, in the eyelids.
Dermabrasion: the removal of upper layers of skin using a high-powered rotating brush.
Lipectomy: the surgical removal of fatty tissue by excision.
Liposuction: the surgical removal of fatty tissue using suction.
Mammoplasty: the surgical procedure to alter the size or shape of the breasts.
Rhinoplasty: the surgical procedure to alter the size or shape of the nose.

WORD	PRONUNCIATION	ELEMENTS		DEFINITION
abdominoplasty (tummy tuck)	ab-**DOM**-ih-noh-plas-tee	S/ R/CF	-plasty *surgical repair* abdomin/o- *abdomen*	Surgical removal of excess subcutaneous fat from abdominal wall
abrasion	ah-**BRAY**-zhun		Latin *to scrape*	Area of skin or mucous membrane that has been scraped off
blepharoplasty	**BLEF**-ah-roh-plas-tee	S/ R/CF	-plasty *surgical repair* blephar/o- *eyelid*	Surgical repair of an eyelid
clot	**KLOT**		German *to block*	The mass of fibrin and cells that is produced in a wound
dermabrasion	der-mah-**BRAY**-zhun	S/ R/ R/	-ion *action* derm- *skin* -abras- *scrape off*	Removal of upper layers of skin by rotary brush
granulation	gran-you-**LAY**-shun	S/ R/	-ation *process* granul- *small grain*	New fibrous tissue formed during wound healing
incision	in-**SIZH**-un	S/ R/	-ion *action, condition* incis- *cut into*	A cut or surgical wound
excision	ek-**SIZH**-un	R/	excis- *cut out*	Surgical removal of part or all of a structure
keloid	**KEY**-loyd		Greek *stain*	Raised, irregular, lumpy scar due to excess collagen fiber production during healing of a wound
laceration	lass-eh-**RAY**-shun	S/ R/	-ation *process* lacer- *to tear*	A tear or jagged wound of the skin caused by blunt trauma; not a cut
lipectomy	lip-**ECK**-toe-me	S/ R/	-ectomy *surgical excision* lip- *lipid, fat*	Surgical removal of adipose tissue
liposuction	**LIP**-oh-suck-shun	S/ R/CF R/	-ion *action* lip/o- *fat* -suct- *suck*	Surgical removal of adipose tissue using suction
mammoplasty	**MAM**-oh-plas-tee	S/ R/CF	-plasty *surgical repair* mamm/o- *breast*	Surgical procedure to change the size or shape of the breast
rhinoplasty	**RYE**-no-plas-tee	S/ R/CF	-plasty *surgical repair* rhin/o- *nose*	Surgical procedure to change the size or shape of the nose
scab	**SKAB**		Old English *crust*	Crust that forms over a wound or sore during healing
suture (noun) suture (verb)	**SOO**-chur		Latin *seam*	Stitch to hold the edges of a wound together To stitch the edges of a wound together
wound	**WOOND**		Old English *wound*	Any injury that interrupts the continuity of skin or a mucous membrane

EXERCISES

 CASE REPORT 3.4

You are . . .

. . . a burn technician employed in the Burn Unit at Fulwood Medical Center.

You are communicating with . . .

. . . the son and daughter of Mr. Steven Hapgood, a 52-year-old man.

Mr. Hapgood has been admitted to the Fulwood Burn Unit with severe burns over his face, chest, and abdomen. After an evening of drinking, he began smoking in bed and fell asleep. His next-door neighbors smelled smoke and called 911. In the Burn Unit, his initial treatment included large volumes of intravenous fluids to prevent shock.

Mr. Hapgood's burns were mostly third-degree. The burned, dead tissue formed an **eschar** that can have toxic effects on the digestive, respiratory, and cardiovascular systems. The eschar was surgically removed by **debridement**.

A. **Read** *Case Report 3.4 to answer the following.* **LO 3.5 and 3.7**

1. What areas of his body have the most severe burns? _____

2. How did Mr. Hapgood sustain these burns? _____

3. How do intravenous fluids get into the body? _____

4. What area of the body would also likely be burned even though flames did not directly contact?

    a. heart   **b.** lungs   **c.** kidneys   **d.** brain

B. **Read** *Case Report 3.4 to answer the following questions.* **LO 3.2, 3.5, and 3.7**

1. What degree of burns did Mr. Hapgood suffer? _____

2. The burned, dead tissue is referred to as: _____.

3. What is the surgical procedure called that removes burned, dead tissue? _____

C. **Knowledge application.** *Complete this exercise on burns. Employ your knowledge of medical terms from the integumentary system. Fill in the blanks.* **LO 3.2, 3.5, and 3.7**

1. High-voltage electrocution typically causes:

    Degree of burn: _____

    Signs: _____

    Layers of skin involved: _____

2. Scalding typically causes:

    Degree of burn: _____

    Signs: _____

    Layers of skin involved: _____

3. Prolonged flame contact in a house fire typically causes:

    Degree of burn: _____

    Signs: _____

    Layers of skin involved: _____

    What specific surgical procedure is used to promote healing for this type of burn? _____

4. Sunburn typically causes:

    Degree of burn: _____

    Signs: _____

    Layers of skin involved: _____

D. **Compare and contrast** *the meanings of word elements that describe the types of skin grafts. Fill in each blank with the correct term that completes each sentence.* **LO 3.4, 3.5, and 3.6**

1. A graft from another species is a **xenograft**, also known as a _____.

2. A graft from another person is an **allograft**, also known as a _____.

3. A graft taken from one part of a person's body and placed elsewhere on the same body: _____

E. **Remembering** *the meaning of the word element can help you easily identify the type of skin grafts. Match the prefix to its meaning.* **LO 3.3, 3.4, and 3.5**

1. hetero-	**a.** other
2. allo-	**b.** same, alike
3. xeno-	**c.** self
4. homo-	**d.** different
5. auto-	**e.** foreign

F. Wounds: *Use your knowledge of the meaning of the following medical terms to put them in the correct order of their appearance and give a brief description of each term. Fill in the chart.* **LO 3.2, 3.3, and 3.5**

keloid   scab   clot   laceration   wound   granulation

Medical Term	Brief Description
1.	2.
3.	4.
5.	6.
7.	8.
9.	10.
11.	12.

G. Construct *medical terms related to therapeutic procedures of the skin.* **LO 3.1 and 3.3**

1. Surgical repair of the nose: _____/_____
                          R/CF   S

2. Surgical removal of adipose tissue: _____/_____
                          R/CF   S

3. Surgical repair of an eyelid: _____/_____
                          R/CF   S

4. Surgical repair of the breast: _____/_____
                          R/CF   S

H. Pronunciation is important whether you are saying the word or listening to a word from a coworker. Identify the proper pronunciation of the following medical terms. **LO 3.2**

1. The correct pronunciation for a benign, localized area of melanin is:

   a. kar-sih-**NOH**-mah

   b. **KAH**-sin-oh-MAH

   c. mel-ahn-**OM**-ah

   d. **MEL**-ah-NO-mah

   Correctly spell the term: _____

2. The correct pronunciation for the protein found in the dead outer layer of skin is:

   a. **KAIR**-ah-tin

   b. **KE**-rah-TEN

   c. **MEL**-ah-nin

   d. **MEL**-a-nine

   Correctly spell the term: _____

3. The correct pronunciation for seborrheic scales from the scalp is:

   a. **DA**-nd-ryuf

   b. **DAN**-druff

   c. **SEE**-bum

   d. **SAY**-byum

   Correctly spell the term: _____

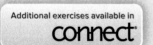

Additional exercises available in

Chapter Review exercises, along with additional practice items, are available in Connect!

CHAPTER 4

The Skeletal System

The Essentials of the Language of Orthopedics

Rick Brady/McGraw Hill

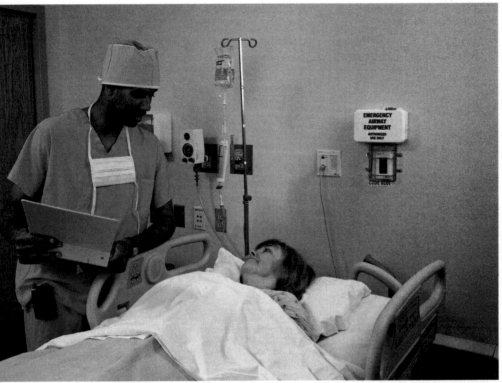

Many health professionals are involved in the diagnosis and treatment of problems in the skeletal system. You may work directly and/or indirectly with one or more of the following:

- **Orthopedic surgeons (orthopedists)** are medical doctors **(MDs)** or doctors of osteopathic medicine (DOs) who deal with the prevention and correction of injuries of the skeletal system and associated **muscles**, joints, and ligaments.
- **Osteopathic physicians** have earned a doctor of osteopathy **(DO)** degree and receive additional training in the **musculoskeletal system** and how it affects the whole body.
- **Chiropractors (DC)** focus on the manual adjustment of joints—particularly the spine—to maintain and restore health.
- **Physical therapists** evaluate and treat pain, disease, or injury by physical therapeutic measures, as opposed to medical or surgical measures.
- **Physical therapist assistants** work under the direction of a physical therapist to assist patients with their physical therapy.
- **Orthopedic technologists** and **technicians** assist orthopedic surgeons in treating patients.
- **Podiatrists** are practitioners in the diagnosis and treatment of disorders and injuries of the foot.

Learning Outcomes

In order for you to work with orthopedists to give optimal care to patients with a bone disorder or injury, you will need to be able to use correct medical terminology to:

LO 4.1 Use roots, combining forms, suffixes, and prefixes to construct and analyze (deconstruct) medical terms related to the skeletal system.

LO 4.2 Spell and pronounce correctly medical terms related to the skeletal system to communicate them with accuracy and precision in any health care setting.

LO 4.3 Define accepted abbreviations related to the skeletal system.

LO 4.4 Relate the different types of bones and their structures to their functions.

LO 4.5 Identify, list, and describe the bones and structures of the axial skeletal system.

LO 4.6 Identify, list, and describe the bones and structures of the appendicular skeletal system.

LO 4.7 Identify and describe injuries, disorders, and pathological conditions related to the skeletal system.

LO 4.8 Describe diagnostic procedures used for injuries and disorders of the skeletal system.

LO 4.9 Describe therapeutic procedures and pharmacologic agents used for injuries and disorders of the skeletal system.

LO 4.10 Identify health professionals involved in the care of patients with skeletal injuries and disorders.

LO 4.11 Apply your knowledge of the medical terms of the skeletal system to documentation, medical records medical reports, and communication.

LO 4.12 Translate the medical terms of the skeletal system into everyday language to communicate clearly with patients and their families.

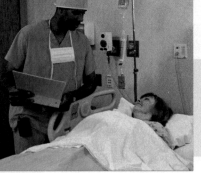

Section 4.1

Bones of the Skeletal System

Abbreviations

DO	Doctor of Osteopathy
MD	Doctor of Medicine
DC	Doctor of Chiropractic
PT	Physical Therapist

Without your bones, you would be shapeless—unable to sit, stand, walk, or move your fingers and toes. Your skeleton supports and protects your organ systems, and is the foundation for much of the medical terminology you will learn in this book. For example, the radial artery (used for checking a pulse) is so named because it travels beside the radial bone of the forearm.

Understanding the surface anatomy of bones and their markings will enable you to describe and document the sites of symptoms, signs, and diagnostic and therapeutic procedures.

Tissues and Functions of the Skeletal System (LO 4.4)

There are four components of the skeletal system *(Figure 4.1)*:

1. **bones**
2. **cartilage**
3. **tendons**
4. **ligaments**

Each plays an important role in the way your tissues and skeletal system function. Your skeletal system provides:

- **Support:** The bones of your vertebral column, pelvis, and legs hold up your body. The jawbone supports your teeth.

- **Protection:** The skull protects your brain. The vertebral column protects your spinal cord. The rib cage protects your heart and lungs.

- **Blood formation:** The marrow in many bones is the major producer of blood cells, including most of those in your immune system *(see Chapter 7)*.

- **Mineral storage and balance:** The skeletal system stores calcium and phosphorus and releases each when your body needs them for other purposes.

- **Detoxification**: Bones remove metals like lead and radium from your blood, store them, and slowly release them for excretion.

- **Movement:** Muscles cannot function without their attachments to skeletal bones, and muscles are responsible for your movements *(see Chapter 5)*.

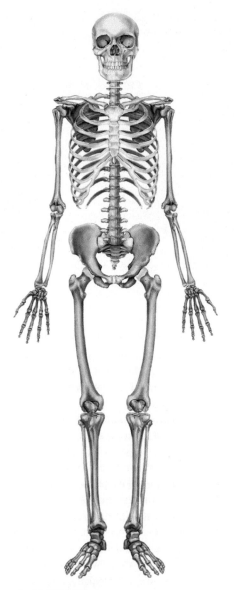

▲ **FIGURE 4.1**
Adult Skeletal System, Anterior View.

WORD	PRONUNCIATION	ELEMENTS		DEFINITION
cartilage	**KAR**-tih-laj		Latin *gristle*	Nonvascular, firm connective tissue found mostly in joints
chiropractic	kye-roh-**PRAK**-tik	S/ R/CF	-ic *pertaining to* chir/o- *hand*	Diagnosis, treatment, and prevention of mechanical disorders of the musculoskeletal system
chiropractor	kye-roh-**PRAK**-tor	R/ S/	-pract- *efficient, practical* -or *a doer*	Practitioner of chiropractic
detoxification (**Note:** *Same as* detoxication)	dee-**TOKS**-ih-fih-**KAY**-shun	S/ P/ R/	-fication *remove* de- *from, out of* -toxi- *poison*	Removing poison from a tissue or substance
ligament	**LIG**-ah-ment		Latin *band, sheet*	Band of fibrous tissue connecting two structures
muscle musculoskeletal	**MUSS**-el **MUSS**-kyu-loh-**SKEL**-eh-tal	S/ R/CF R/	Latin *muscle* -al *pertaining to* muscul/o- *muscle* -skelet- *skeleton*	A tissue consisting of cells that can contract Pertaining to the muscles and the bony skeleton
orthopedic	or-tho-**PEE**-dik	S/ R/CF R/	-ic *pertaining to* orth/o- *straight* -ped- *child*	Pertaining to the correction and cure of deformities and diseases of the musculoskeletal system; originally, most of the deformities treated were in children
orthopedist	or-tho-**PEE**-dist	S/	-ist *specialist*	Specialist in orthopedics
osteopath	**OSS**-tee-oh-path	S/ R/CF	-path *disease* oste/o- *bone*	Practitioner of osteopathy Medical practice based on maintaining the balance of the body
osteopathy	**OSS**-tee-**OP**-ah-thee	S/	-pathy *disease*	
tendon	**TEN**-dun		Latin *sinew*	Fibrous band that connects muscle to bone

Bones (LO 4.4)

Classification of Bones (LO 4.2 and 4.4)

The bones of your skeletal system are classified by their shape.
Each falls into one of the following four shape categories:

- **Long** (considerably longer than they are wide), like the main bones of the limbs, palms, soles, fingers, and toes;
- **Short** (nearly as long as they are wide), like the patella (kneecap) and the bones of the wrists and ankles;
- **Flat,** like the bones of the skull and the ribs; or
- **Irregular,** like the vertebrae.

Structure of Long Bones (LO 4.4)

Think about how long your arms and legs are, and then consider how few bones make up all that length. In that context, it is likely no surprise that long bones are the most common bones in your body (*Figure 4.2a, 4.2b*). The shaft (**diaphysis**) of a long bone contains compact bone (also called **cortical** bone), while each end of the bone (the **epiphysis**) is composed of spongy bone. Sandwiched between the diaphysis and epiphysis are thin layers of cartilage cells in the **epiphysial plate** or **line** that allow your bones to grow longer.

A tough, connective tissue sheath called **periosteum** covers the outer surface of all bones; it protects the bone and anchors blood vessels and nerves to the bone's surface. Strong collagen fibers attach the periosteum to the **cortical** (compact) bone.

Inside the diaphysis is a hollow cylinder called the **medulla** (*Figure 4.2b*), which contains bone **marrow**, a fatty tissue in adults. Red bone marrow with blood cells in varying stages of development can be found in the epiphyseal ends of the bone and in the flat bones of the skull, the sternum, and the hip bones. Because red bone marrow is normally concentrated here, the medulla of the sternum and hip bone is the ideal source for bone marrow aspiration, a procedure where a needle is inserted into the bone to withdraw a sample of bone marrow fluid and cells to be checked for abnormalities. A bone marrow transplant follows a similar process.

Most bones have a strong blood supply (*Figure 4.3*) because of the blood vessels that travel through them in a system of small central (Haversian) **canals**. The normal good supply of blood through your bones promotes healing.

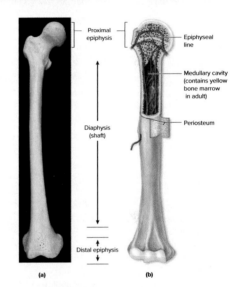

▲ **FIGURE 4.2**
Femur: Long Bone of the Thigh. (a) Anterior view. (b) Interior view.

Christine Eckel/McGraw Hill

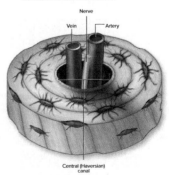

▲ **FIGURE 4.3**
Blood Supply to Bone.

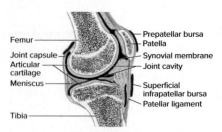

Femur —
Joint capsule —
Articular cartilage —
Meniscus —

— Prepatellar bursa
— Patella
— Synovial membrane
— Joint cavity

— Superficial infrapatellar bursa
— Patellar ligament

Tibia —

▲ **FIGURE 4.5** Synovial Joint.

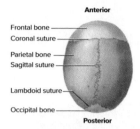

Anterior

Frontal bone —
Coronal suture —
Parietal bone —
Sagittal suture —
Lambdoid suture —
Occipital bone —

Posterior

▲ **FIGURE 4.4**
Sutures of the Skull: Superior View.

Joints (LO 4.4)

Classes of Joints (LO 4.4)

Although joints allow you to move, movable parts that rub together can wear out. Damage or disease in a joint can make movement very difficult and painful. The structure of any joint, or articulation, is directly related to its mobility and function. Joints are classified structurally into three types:

1. **Fibrous** joints are two bones tightly bound together by bands of fibrous tissue with no joint space.

   Examples include sutures occurring between the bones of the skull *(Figure 4.4),* the joining of two bones such as the tibia and fibula, and the joints between the teeth in their sockets.

2. **Cartilaginous** joints join two bones with cartilage.

   Examples include the joining of ribs to cartilage and the joining of the two pubic bones in the front of the pelvis.

3. **Synovial** joints contain synovial fluid as a lubricant and allow considerable movement *(Figure 4.5).* Most joints in the legs and arms are synovial joints. The ends of the bones are covered with **hyaline articular** cartilage. In some joints, an additional plate of fibrocartilage is located between the two bones. In the knee, this plate is incomplete and is called a **meniscus**.

A **bursa** is an extension of the synovial joint that forms a cushion between structures that otherwise would rub against each other; for example, in the knee joint between the patellar tendon and the patellar and tibial bones *(Figure 4.5).*

Word Analysis and Definition

S = Suffix   P = Prefix   R = Root   R/CF = Combining Form

WORD	PRONUNCIATION		ELEMENTS	DEFINITION
articulate	ar-**TIK**-you-late	S/ R/	-ate *composed of* articul-*joint*	Two separate bones have formed a joint
articulation	ar-tik-you-**LAY**-shun	S/	-ation *process*	A joint
bursa bursae (pl)	**BURR**-sah **BURR**-see		Latin *purse*	A closed sac containing synovial fluid
central canals (also called **Haversian canals**)	**SEN**-tra ka-**NALS** hah-**VER**-shan ka-NALS		Latin *pertaining to a center*	Vertically running canals found in cortical bones. Contain blood vessels and nerve fibers.
cortex cortical (adj)	**KOR**-teks **KOR**-tih-cal	S/ R/	-al *pertaining to* cortic- *cortex*	Latin *bark* — Outer portion of an organ, such as bone Pertaining to a cortex
diaphysis	die-**AF**-ih-sis		Greek *growing between*	The shaft of a long bone
epiphysis	eh-**PIF**-ih-sis	P/ R/	epi- *upon, above* -physis *growth*	Expanded area at the proximal and distal ends of a long bone to provide increased surface area for attachment of ligaments and tendons
epiphysial (adj) (**Note:** also spelled epiphyseal)	ep-ih-**FIZ**-ee-al	S/	-ial *pertaining to*	Pertaining to an epiphysis
epiphysial plate	ep-Pih-**FIZ**-ee-al PLATE		plate Greek *broad, flat*	Layer of cartilage between epiphysis and metaphysis where bone growth occurs
hyaline	**HIGH**-ah-line		Greek *glass*	Cartilage that looks like frosted glass and contains fine collagen fibers
marrow	**MAH**-roe		Old English *marrow*	Fatty, blood-forming tissue in the cavities of long bones
medulla medullary (adj)	meh-**DULL**-ah meh-**DULL**-ah-ree	S/ R/	-ary *pertaining to* medulla- *medulla*	Central portion of a structure surrounded by cortex Pertaining to a medulla
meniscus menisci (pl)	meh-**NISS**-kuss meh-**NISS**-key		Greek *crescent*	Disc of cartilage between the bones of a joint, in this case, the knee joint
periosteum periosteal (adj)	**PER**-ee-**OSS**-tee-um **PER**-ee-**OSS**-tee-al	S/ P/ R/ S/	-um *structure* peri- *around* -oste- *bone* -al *pertaining to*	Strong membrane surrounding a bone Pertaining to the periosteum
suture sutures (pl)	**SOO**-chur **SOO**-churs		Latin *a seam*	Place where two bones are joined together by a fibrous band continuous with their periosteum, as in the skull Also means to unite two surfaces by sewing; the material used in the sewing together; and the seam formed by the sewing together
synovial	sih-**NOH**-vee-al	S/ P/ R/CF	-al *pertaining to* syn- *together* -ov/i- *egg*	Pertaining to synovial fluid and synovial membrane

EXERCISES

A. Identify *the components of the skeletal system and the functions of the bones. Select the correct organ or tissue being described.* **LO 4.4**

1. Band of strong tissue that connects two structures (such as bone to bone).

   a. muscle   **b.** ligament   **c.** tendon   **d.** cartilage

2. Tissue containing contractile cells.

   a. muscle   **b.** ligament   **c.** tendon   **d.** cartilage

3. Firm connective tissue found mostly in joints.

   a. muscle   **b.** ligament   **c.** tendon   **d.** cartilage

4. Fibrous band that connects muscle to bone.

   a. muscle   **b.** ligament   **c.** tendon   **d.** cartilage

B. Elements *remain your best clue for understanding a medical term. In this exercise, the meaning of each element is given below the line—this is your clue to constructing the term. Insert the correct element on the line above its meaning. After you have constructed the term, give its definition in the space provided.*
LO 4.1 and 4.4

1. _____ / _____

        cortex   pertaining to

   The term is _____ .

2. _____ / _____ / _____

        around   bone   structure

   The term is _____ .

3. _____ / _____ / _____

        upon, above   growth   pertaining to

   The term is _____ .

4. _____ / _____

        medulla   pertaining to

   The term is _____ .

C. Use this exercise *to review what you've learned about bones. Select the correct answer for each question.* **LO 4.4**

1. Bones of the skeletal system are classified by their:

   a. shape   **b.** function   **c.** weight   **d.** color

2. What are the most common types of bones in the body?

   a. flat   **b.** short   **c.** long   **d.** irregular

3. What is another name for "compact" bone?

   a. cortical   **b.** diaphysis   **c.** long   **d.** spongy

4. Where can you find bone marrow? (select all that apply)

   a. between two bones   **c.** epiphysis of a long bone

   b. inside a hollow space of the diaphysis   **d.** large flat bones, such as the skull

5. The strong blood supply in bones is provided by the:

   a. red bone marrow   **b.** yellow bone marrow   **c.** blood vessels in the periosteum   **d.** blood vessels of the central (Haversian) canals

6. What is the purpose of synovial fluid?

   a. balance   **d.** weight bearing

   b. alignment   **e.** mobility

   c. lubrication

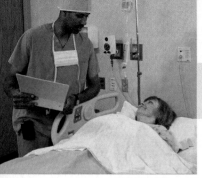

Section 4.2

Axial and Appendicular Skeleton

In order to best evaluate, treat, and educate patients, understanding the medical terminology for the structures and functions of the vertebral column, its joints, and its ligaments is a must. The vertebral column is part of the axial skeleton.

Cervical
region
(curved
anteriorly)

Thoracic
region
(curved
posteriorly)

Intervertebral
disc

Intervertebral
foramina

First lumbar
vertebra

Lumbar
region
(curved
anteriorly)

Fifth lumbar
vertebra

Sacral
promontory

Sacral and
coccygeal
regions
(curved
posteriorly)

Sacrum

Coccyx

▲ **FIGURE 4.6** Vertebral
Column, Lateral View.

Structure of the Axial Skeleton (LO 4.5)

Your axial skeleton, the upright axis of your body, includes the:

1. **vertebral column,**
2. **skull, and**
3. **rib cage.**

The axial skeleton protects the brain, **spinal** cord, heart, and lungs—most of the major centers of human physiology.

Within the vertebral column, there are 26 bones divided into the following five regions *(Figure 4.6)*:

- **Cervical** region, with 7 **vertebrae,** labeled C1 to C7 and curved anteriorly;
- **Thoracic** region, with 12 vertebrae, labeled T1 to T12 and curved posteriorly;
- **Lumbar** region, with 5 vertebrae, labeled L1 to L5 and curved anteriorly;
- **Sacral** region, with 5 bones that in early childhood fuse into 1 bone curved posteriorly; and
- **Coccyx** (tailbone), with 4 small bones fused together into 1 bone curved posteriorly.

The spinal cord lies protected in the vertebral canal of the vertebral column. Spinal nerves travel from the spinal cord to other parts of the body through the intervertebral **foramina.**

Intervertebral discs consisting of fibrocartilage (a form of cartilage) are also found in the axial skeleton. These discs inhabit the intervertebral space between the bodies of adjacent vertebrae and provide extra support and cushioning (acting as shock absorbers) for the vertebral column.

Abbreviations

C5	the fifth cervical vertebra
C5-C6	the intervertebral space between the fifth and sixth cervical vertebrae
C6	the sixth cervical vertebra

Word Analysis and Definition

S = Suffix   P = Prefix   R = Root   R/CF = Combining Form

WORD	PRONUNCIATION		ELEMENTS	DEFINITION
cervical	**SER**-vih-kal	S/ R/	-al *pertaining to* cervic- *neck*	Pertaining to the neck region
coccyx	**KOK**-sicks		Greek coccyx	Small tailbone at the lowest end of the vertebral column
disc	DISK		Latin or Greek *disk*	Flattened, round structure. In the skeletal system, a flattened round fibrocartilaginous structure between bones
foramen foramina (pl)	foh -**RAY**-men foh-**RAM**-in-ah		Latin *an opening*	An opening through a structure
intervertebral	**IN**-ter-**VER**-teh-bral	S/ P/ R/	-al *pertaining to* inter- *between* -vertebr- *vertebra*	Located between two vertebrae
lumbar	**LUM**-bar		Latin *loin*	The region of the back and sides between the ribs and pelvis
sacrum sacral (adj)	**SAY**-crum **SAY**-kral	S/ R/	Latin *sacred* -al *pertaining to* sacr- *sacrum*	Segment of the vertebral column that forms part of the pelvis Pertaining to or in the region of the sacrum
spine spinal (adj)	SPINE **SPY**-nal	S/ R/	Latin *spine* -al *pertaining to* spin- *spine*	Vertebral column or a short projection from a bone Pertaining to the spine
thoracic (adj)	thor-**ASS**-ik	S/ R/	-ic *pertaining to* thorac- *chest*	Pertaining to the chest (thorax)
vertebra vertebrae (pl) vertebral (adj)	**VER**-teh-brah **VER**-teh-brae **VER**-teh-bral	 S/ R/	Latin *spinal joint* -al *pertaining to* vertebr- *vertebra*	One of the bones of the spinal column Pertaining to a vertebra

Skull and Face (LO 4.5)

The Skull (LO 4.5)

When you glance at your face in the mirror, chances are you are not thinking about what is behind your brown eyes or your slightly crooked smile. You see one image—not its layers, pieces, or parts. However, the human skull *(Figure 4.7)* is made up of 22 separate bones. Your **cranium**, the upper part of the skull that encloses the **cranial** cavity and protects the brain, contains 8 of these 22 bones; your facial skeleton contains the remaining 14.

The bones of the cranium are joined together by sutures (joints that appear as seams), which are covered on the inside and outside by a thin layer of connective tissue. These bones have the following functions:

1. The **frontal** bone forms the forehead, roofs of the (eye) orbits, and part of the floor of the cranium and contains a pair of right and left frontal sinuses above the orbits.
2. **Parietal** bones form the bulging sides and roof of the cranium.
3. The **occipital** bone forms the back of and part of the base of the cranium.
4. **Temporal** bones form the sides of and part of the base of the cranium.
5. The **sphenoid** bone forms part of the base of the cranium and the orbits.
6. The **ethmoid** bone is hollow and forms part of the nose, the orbits, and the ethmoid sinuses.

These bones of the skull provide protection for the brain and the organs of vision, taste, hearing, equilibrium, and smell.

The lower part of the skull houses the bones of the facial skeleton *(Figure 4.8)*. These bones do the following:

1. **Maxillary** bones form the upper jaw (**maxilla**), hold the upper teeth, and are hollow, forming the maxillary sinuses.
2. **Palatine** bones are located behind the maxilla and cannot be seen on a lateral view of the skull.
3. **Zygomatic** bones are the prominences of the cheeks (cheekbones) below the eyes.
4. **Lacrimal** bones form the medial wall of each eye orbit.
5. **Nasal** bones form the sides and bridge of the nose.
6. The **mandible** is the lower jawbone, which holds the lower teeth. The mandible articulates (joins) with the temporal bone to form the **temporomandibular joint (TMJ)**.

The bones of the facial skeleton provide a frame on which the muscles and other tissues of the face facilitate eating, facial expressions, breathing, and speech.

The third component of the axial skeleton, the rib cage, is discussed in Chapter 8, "Respiratory System."

Abbreviation

TMJ   temporomandibular joint

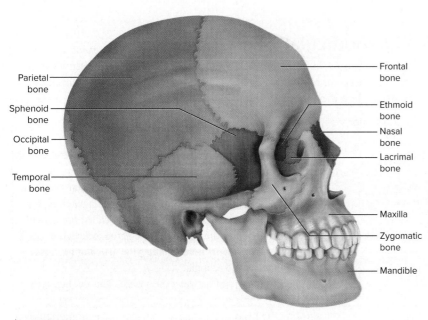

▲ **FIGURE 4.7**
Skull, Right Lateral View.

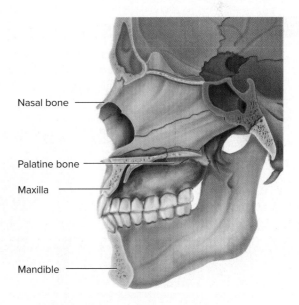

▲ **FIGURE 4.8**
Facial Bones.

WORD	PRONUNCIATION		ELEMENTS	DEFINITION
cranium cranial (adj)	KRAY-nee-um KRAY-nee-al	S/ R/	Greek *skull* -al *pertaining to* crani- *skull*	The upper part of the skull that encloses and protects the brain Pertaining to the skull
ethmoid	ETH-moyd	S/ R/	-oid *resembling* ethm- *sieve*	Bone that forms the back of the nose and encloses numerous air cells
frontal	FRUNT-al	S/ R/	-al *pertaining to* front- *front of*	Pertaining to the front
lacrimal	LAK-rim-al	S/ R/	-al *pertaining to* lacrim- *tears*	Lacrimal bone forms part of the medial wall of the orbit, *or* pertaining to tears
mandible mandibular (adj)	MAN-di-bel man-DIB-you-lar	S/ R/	Latin *jaw* -ar *pertaining to* mandibul- *mandible*	Lower jaw bone Pertaining to the mandible
maxilla maxillary (adj)	mak-SILL-ah mak-SILL-ah-ree	S/ R/	Latin *jawbone* -ary *pertaining to* maxilla- *maxilla*	Upper jawbone, containing right and left maxillary sinuses Pertaining to the maxilla
nasal	NAY-zal	S/ R/	-al *pertaining to* nas- *nose*	Pertaining to the nose
occipital	ock-SIP-it-al	S/ R/	-al *pertaining to* occipit- *back of the head*	The back of the skull
palatine	PAL-ah-tine	S/ R/	-ine *pertaining to* palat- *palate*	Bone that forms the hard palate and parts of the nose and orbits
parietal	pah-RYE-eh-tal	S/ R/	-al *pertaining to* pariet- *wall*	The two bones forming the sidewalls and roof of the cranium
sphenoid	SFEE-noyd	S/ R/	-oid *resemble* sphen- *wedge*	Wedge-shaped bone at the base of the skull
temporal temporomandibular joint (TMJ)	TEM-pore-al TEM-pore-oh-man-DIB-you-lar JOYNT	S/ R/ S/ R/CF R/	-al *pertaining to* tempor- *time, temple* -ar *pertaining to* tempor/o- *temple* -mandibul- *mandible*	Bone that forms part of the base and sides of the skull The joint between the temporal bone and the mandible
zygoma zygomatic (adj)	zye-GO-mah zye-go-MAT-ik	S/ R/	French *yoke* -ic *pertaining to* zygomat- *cheekbone*	Bone that forms the prominence of the cheek Pertaining to the cheekbone

Abbreviation

AC	acromioclavicular

Structure of the Appendicular Skeleton (LO 4.6)

Your shoulders, arms, hands, and fingers are used nearly every time you move your body, no matter where you are—at work, home, or the gym, or in the car, or relaxing on the beach. Because these bones and joints get so much use, it is necessary to understand how they work and how to care for them.

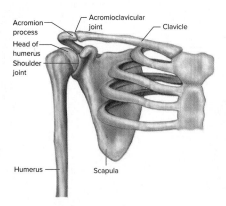

Acromion process
Acromioclavicular joint
Clavicle
Head of humerus
Shoulder joint
Humerus
Scapula

▲ FIGURE 4.9
Pectoral Girdle and Humerus.

Pectoral Girdle (LO 4.6)

The bones and joints of your **pectoral** (shoulder) **girdle** connect your axial skeleton to your upper limbs.

The bones of the shoulder girdle are the **scapulae** (shoulder blades) and **clavicles** (collarbones). The scapula extends over the top of the shoulder joint to form a roof called the **acromion**, which is attached to the clavicle at the **acromioclavicular (AC)** joint. Several ligaments hold together the **articulating** surfaces of the humerus and scapula.

The shoulder joint between the scapula and the **humerus** bone of the upper arm *(Figure 4.9)* is a ball-and-socket joint, allowing the head of the humerus greater range of motion than any other joint in the body.

Upper Arm and Elbow Joint (4.6)

Your upper arm extends from your shoulder to your elbow and contains only one bone, the humerus *(Figure 4.10)*.

The smooth surface of the hemispherical head that articulates with the socket of the scapula is covered with articular cartilage. At the lower end of the humerus, the **trochlea** articulates with the **ulna** bone of the forearm and the **capitulum** articulates with the **radius** *(Figure 4.11)*. The **olecranon** *(Figure 4.12)* is a bony projection on the posterior side of the proximal end of the ulna. This projection is the area of the ulna that is commonly referred to as the elbow.

Elbow Joint (4.6)

The elbow joint has two articulations:

1. A hinge joint between the humerus and the ulna bone of the forearm, which allows flexion and extension of the elbow; and

2. A gliding joint between the humerus and the radius bone of the forearm, which allows **pronation** and **supination** of the forearm and hand.

Forearm, Wrist, and Hand (LO 4.2 and 4.7)

The Wrist (4.6)

In your forearm, the radius bone on the thumb side and the larger ulna bone on the little-finger side articulate at your wrist joint with the small **carpal** bones *(Figure 4.12)*.

The Hand (4.6)

The five fingers of your single hand have 14 bones called **phalanges.** The thumb has two phalanges, and each of the remaining four fingers has three *(Figure 4.12)*. In your palm, the five bones closest to the fingers are **metacarpals**; these connect to the phalanges at the **metacarpophalangeal** joints. The metacarpals connect at the wrist to eight small carpal bones, which then connect the hand to the bones of the forearm. All of these bones require numerous joints with ligaments to connect and stabilize them.

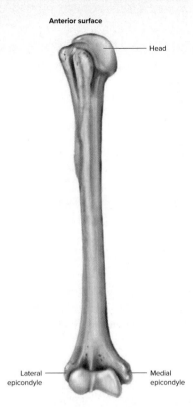

Anterior surface

▲ **FIGURE 4.10**
Humerus.

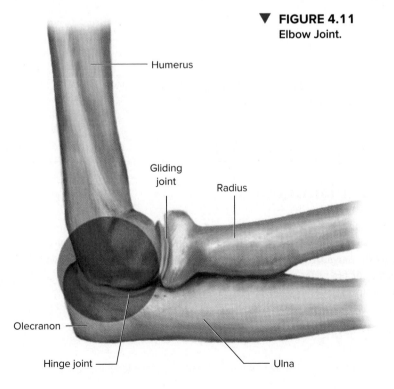

▼ **FIGURE 4.11**
Elbow Joint.

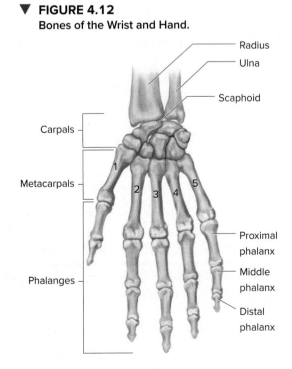

▼ **FIGURE 4.12**
Bones of the Wrist and Hand.

WORD	PRONUNCIATION	ELEMENTS		DEFINITION
acromion	ah-**CROW**-mee-on		Greek *tip of the shoulder*	Lateral end of the scapula, extending over the shoulder joint
acromioclavicular	ah-**CROW**-mee-oh-klah- **VICK**-you-lar	S/ R/CF	-**ar** *pertaining to* **acromi/o-** *acromion*	The joint between the acromion and the clavicle
clavicle	**KLAV**-ih-kul		Latin *collarbone*	Curved bone that forms the anterior part of the pectoral girdle
clavicular (adj)	klah-**VICK**-you-lar	S/ R/	-**ar** *pertaining to* **clavicul-** *clavicle*	Pertaining to the clavicle
carpus	**KAR**-pus		Greek *wrist*	The eight carpal bones of the wrist
carpal (adj)	**KAR**-pal	S/ R/	-**al** *pertaining to* **carp-** *wrist bones*	Pertaining to the wrist
metacarpal	**MET**-ah-**KAR**-pal	P/	**meta-** *after, subsequent to*	The five bones between the carpus and the fingers
capitulum	kah-**PIT**-you-lum	S/ R/CF	-**lum** *small structure* **capit/u-** *small head*	A small head or rounded extremity of a bone
eponym	**EH**-po-nim		Greek *epŏnymos, meaning eponymous*	A procedure or a diagnosis with a name derived from the name of the person who discovered it (if it is a disease or condition) or originated it (if it is a procedure)
humerus	**HYU**-mer-us		Latin *shoulder*	Single bone of the upper arm
olecranon	oh-**LECK**-rah-non		Greek *point of elbow*	Prominent, proximal extremity of ulna
metacarpophalangeal	**MET**-ah-**KAR**-poh-fay-**LAN**-jee-al	S/ P/ R/CF R/CF	-**al** *pertaining to* **meta-** *after, subsequent to* -**carp/o-** *bones of the wrist* -**phalang/e-** *phalanx, finger or toe*	The joints between the metacarpal bones and the phalanges
pectoral	**PEK**-tor-al	S/	-**al** *pertaining to*	Pertaining to the chest
pectoral girdle	**PEK**-tor-al **GIR**-del	R/	**pector-** *chest* girdle, Old English *encircle*	Incomplete bony ring that attaches the upper limb to the axial skeleton
phalanx	**FAY**-lanks		Latin *bone of finger* or *toe*	One of the bones of the digits (fingers or toes)
phalanges (pl)	fay-**LAN**-jeez			
pronation	pro-**NAY**-shun	S/	-**ion** *action, condition*	Process of lying face down or of turning a hand or foot with the volar (palm or sole) surface down
pronate (verb)	**PRO**-nate	R/	**pronat-** *bend down*	
prone	**PRONE**		Latin, *lying down*	Lying face down, flat on your belly
radius	**RAY**-dee-us		Latin *spoke of a wheel*	The forearm bone on the thumb side
radial (adj)	**RAY**-dee-al	S/ R/	-**al** *pertaining to* **radi-** *radius*	Pertaining to the radius or to any of the structures (artery, vein, nerve) named after it
supination	soo-pih-**NAY**-shun	S/ R/	-**ion** *action, condition* **supinat-** *bend backward*	Process of lying face upward or of turning a hand or foot so that the palm or sole is facing up
supine	soo-**PINE**		Latin *bend backward*	Lying face up, flat on your spine
scapula	**SKAP**-you-lah		Latin *shoulder blade*	Shoulder blade
scapulae (pl)	**SKAP**-you-lee			
scapular (adj)	**SKAP**-you-lar	S/ R/	-**ar** *pertaining to* **scapul-** *scapula*	Pertaining to the shoulder blade
trochlea	**TROHK**-lee-ah		Latin *pulley*	Smooth articular surface of bone on which another glides
trochlear	**TROHK**-lee-ar	S/ R/	-**ar** *pertaining to* **trochle-** *pulley*	Pertaining to a trochlea
ulna	**UL**-nah		Latin *elbow, arm*	The medial and larger bone of the forearm
ulnar (adj)	**UL**-nar	S/ R/	-**ar** *pertaining to* **uln-** *ulna*	Pertaining to the ulna or to any of the structures (artery, vein, nerve) named after it

Pelvic Girdle and Lower Limb (LO 4.6)

Pelvic Girdle (LO 4.6)

Your pelvic girdle consists of your two hip bones that articulate anteriorly with each other at the **symphysis pubis** and posteriorly with the sacrum (a triangular-shaped bone in your lower back). This forms the bowl-shaped **pelvis**. The two joints between your hip bones and the sacrum are called **sacroiliac joints**.

The pelvic girdle has these functions:

1. Supports the axial skeleton;
2. Transmits the upper body's weight to the lower limbs;
3. Provides attachments for the lower limbs; and
4. Protects the internal reproductive organs, urinary bladder, and distal segment of the large intestine.

Each of your hip bones is actually a fusion of three bones: the **ilium**, **ischium**, and **pubis** *(Figure 4.13a)*. This fusion occurs in the region of the **acetabulum**, a cup-shaped cavity on the lateral (outer) surface of the hip bone that receives the head of the **femur**, or thigh bone *(Figure 4.13b)*.

The lower part of the pelvis is formed by the lower ilium, ischium, and pubic bones that surround a short canal-like pelvic cavity, through which the rectum, vagina, and urethra pass. During childbirth, the infant passes down this canal.

Bones and Joints of the Hip and Thigh (LO 4.6)

Your hip joint is a ball-and-socket mechanism formed by the head of your femur (thigh bone) and the acetabulum (cup-shaped hip socket) of your hip bone *(Figure 4.14)*. The **labrum** is the articular cartilage that forms a rim around the hip joint socket, cushioning the joint and helping to keep your femoral head in place in the socket. Finally, the hip joint is secured by a thick joint capsule reinforced by strong ligaments that connect the neck of the femur to the rim of the hip socket.

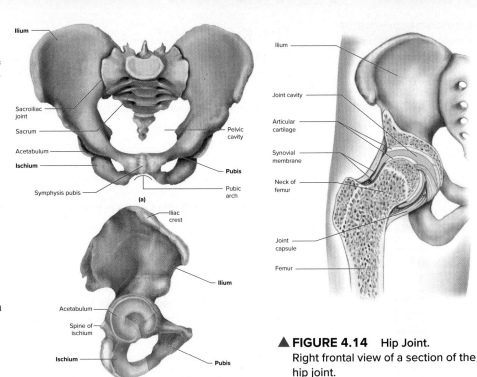

▲ **Figure 4.13** Pelvic Girdle. (a) Front view. (b) Side view.

▲ **FIGURE 4.14** Hip Joint. Right frontal view of a section of the hip joint.

Word Analysis and Definition

S = Suffix   P = Prefix   R = Root   R/CF = Combining Form

WORD	PRONUNCIATION		ELEMENTS	DEFINITION
acetabulum	ass-eh-**TAB**-you-lum		Latin *vinegar cup*	The cup-shaped cavity of the hip bone that receives the head of the femur to form the hip joint
femur femoral (adj)	**FEE**-mur **FEM**-oh-ral	S/ R/	Latin *thigh* -al *pertaining to* femor- *femur*	The thigh bone Pertaining to the femur
ilium	**ILL**-ee-um		Latin *groin*	Large wing-shaped bone at the upper and posterior part of the pelvis
ischium ischia (pl) ischial (adj)	**IS**-kee-um **IS**-kee-ah **IS**-kee-al	S/ R/	Greek *hip* -al *pertaining to* ischi- *ischium, hip bone*	Lower and posterior part of the hip bone Pertaining to the ischium
labrum	**LAY**-brum		Latin *lip-shaped*	Cartilage that forms a rim around the socket of the hip joint
pelvis pelvic (adj)	**PEL**-viss **PEL**-vik	S/ R/	Latin *basin* -ic *pertaining to* pelv- *pelvis*	Basin-shaped ring of bones, ligaments, and muscles at the base of the spine. Also, any basin-shaped cavity, like the pelvis of the kidney Pertaining to the pelvis
pubis pubic (adj)	**PYU**-bis **PYU**-bik	S/ R/	Latin *pubis* -ic *pertaining to* pub- *pubis*	Alternative name for the pubic bone Pertaining to the pubic bone
sacroiliac joint	say-kroh-**ILL**-ih-ak **JOINT**	S/ R/CF R	-ac *pertaining to* sacr/o- *sacrum* -ili- *ilium*	The joint between the sacrum and the ilium
symphysis symphyses (pl)	**SIM**-feh-sis **SIM**-feh-seez		Greek *grow together*	Two bones joined by fibrocartilage; in this case, the two pubic bones

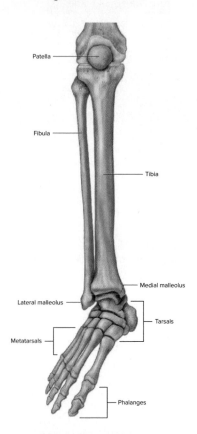

▲ **FIGURE 4.16**
Bones of the Lower Leg and Foot.

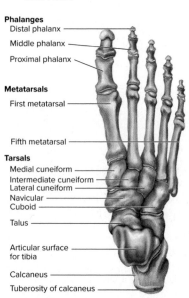

▲ **FIGURE 4.17**
Twenty-Six Bones and 33 Joints of Right Foot.

The Knee Joint (LO 4.2 and 4.9)

Your knees do plenty of bending, whether you are climbing the stairs, exercising, sitting cross-legged, or squatting down to collect something from the floor. Each knee is a hinged joint formed with these four bones:

1. Lower end of the **femur**, shaped like a horseshoe;

2. Flat upper end of the **tibia**;

3. Flat triangular **patella** (kneecap), embedded in the **patellar** tendon and articulating with the femur *(Figure 4.15a)*; and

4. **Fibula**, which forms a separate joint–the **tibiofibular** joint *(Figure 4.15b)*–by articulating with the tibia.

Mechanically, the patella's role is to provide a strength increase in the extension of the knee joint.

Within the knee joint, two crescent-shaped pads of cartilage–the **medial** and **lateral menisci**–lie on top of the tibia and articulate with the femur. This cartilage helps to distribute weight more evenly across the joint surface to minimize wear and tear.

The knee joint has a fibrous capsule, lined with synovial membrane that secretes synovial fluid to lubricate the joint. Four ligaments hold the knee joint together: the **medial** and **lateral collateral ligaments** located outside the joint and the **anterior cruciate ligament** (ACL) and **posterior cruciate ligament** (PCL) located inside the joint cavity, crossing over each other to form an "X" *(Figure 4.15b)*.

The thigh muscles that move the knee joint are described in Section 5.1 of the next chapter.

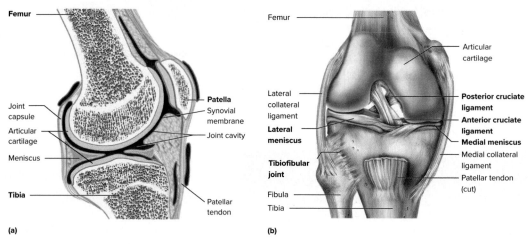

(a)

(b)

▲ **FIGURE 4.15**   Knee Joint.
(a) Section of knee joint. (b) Right knee joint, anterior view.

Bones and Joints of the Lower Leg, Ankle, and Foot (LO 4.2 and 4.9)

Your lower leg has two differently sized bones: the large medial tibia and the thin lateral fibula. The lower end of your tibia on its medial border forms a prominent process called the medial malleolus. The lower end of your fibula forms the lateral malleolus *(Figure 4.16)*. You can palpate (feel) both these prominences at your own ankle, which has two joints:

• Joint between the lateral malleolus of the fibula and the talus; and

• Joint between the medial malleolus of the tibia and the talus.

The **talus** is the most superior of the seven **tarsal** bones of the ankle *(Figure 4.16)*, and its upper surface articulates with the tibia. The heel bone is called the **calcaneus**. The tarsal bones help the ankle bear the body's weight. Strong ligaments on both sides of the ankle joint hold the joint together.

Attached to the tarsal bones are the five parallel **metatarsal** bones *(Figure 4.17)*. These bones form the instep and the ball of the foot, where they bear weight. Each toe has three phalanges, except for the big toe, which has only two. This configuration is identical to the thumb and its relation to the hand.

WORD	PRONUNCIATION	ELEMENTS		DEFINITION
calcaneus calcaneal (adj)	kal-**KAY**-knee-us kal-**KAY**-knee-al	 S/ R/	Latin *heel* -eal *pertaining to* calcan- *calcaneus*	Bone of the tarsus that forms the heel Pertaining to the calcaneus
collateral (**Note:** *An extra "l" has been inserted.*)	koh-**LAT**-er-al	S/ P/ R/	-al *pertaining to* co- *together* -later- *side*	Situated at the side, often to bypass an obstruction
cruciate	**KRU**-she-ate		Latin *cross*	Shaped like a cross. In this case, the two internal ligaments of the knee joint cross over each other to form an "X"
fibula fibular (adj)	**FIB**-you-lah **FIB**-you-lar	 S/ R/	Latin *clasp or buckle* -ar *pertaining to* fibul- *fibula*	The smaller of the two bones of the lower leg Pertaining to the fibula
metatarsus metatarsal (adj)	**MET**-ah-**TAR**-sus **MET**-ah-**TAR**-sal	S/ P/ R/ S/	-us *pertaining to* meta- *after, subsequent to* -tars- *ankle* -al *pertaining to*	The five parallel bones of the foot between the tarsus and the phalanges Pertaining to the metatarsus
patella (kneecap) patellae (pl) patellar (adj)	pah-**TELL**-ah pah-**TELL**-ee pah-**TELL**-ar	 S/ R/	Latin *small plate* -ar *pertaining to* patell- *patella*	Thin, circular bone in front of the knee joint, embedded in the patellar tendon Pertaining to the patella bone or the tendon
prepatellar	pree-pah-**TELL**-ar	S/ P/ R/	-ar *pertaining to* pre- *before, in front of* -patell- *patella*	In front of the patella
talus	**TAY**-luss		Latin *heel bone*	The tarsal bone that articulates with the tibia to form the ankle joint
tarsus tarsal (adj)	**TAR**-sus **TAR**-sal	 S/ R/	Latin *ankle* -al *pertaining to* tars- *ankle*	The collection of seven bones in the foot that form the ankle and instep Pertaining to the tarsus
tibia tibial (adj)	**TIB**-ee-ah **TIB**-ee-al	 S/ R/	Latin *large shinbone* -al *pertaining to* tibi- *tibia*	The larger bone of the lower leg Pertaining to the tibia

EXERCISES

 ## Case Report 4.1

You are . . .

. . . an orthopedic technologist working in the orthopedic department of Fulwood Medical Center with Dr. Kenneth Stannard.

You are communicating with . . .

. . . Ms. Nancy Cardenas, a 27-year-old jeweler whose car was rear-ended by another car at a traffic light 3 days ago. Ms. Cardenas suffers from severe neck pain radiating down her left arm, as well as dizziness and headaches. She is unable to go to work. Dr. Stannard has examined her and diagnosed her condition as a **whiplash** injury. An MRI shows herniation (rupture) of intervertebral discs between C5-C6 and C6-C7. Your role is to assist Dr. Stannard and document the care Ms. Cardenas receives to relieve her symptoms. Ms. Cardenas' whiplash injury caused protrusion of two cervical intervertebral discs. The centers of the discs bulge into the vertebral canal and pinch the nerves in such a way that the pain radiates to her left arm.

A. Read *Case Report 4.1 to select the correct answer to the following questions.*   **LO 4.2, 4.7, and 4.8**

1. The abbreviation MRI stands for:

    a. multiple reading interpretations   c. maximal recording indices

    b. magnetic radiographic imaging   d. magnetic resonance imaging

2. Describe herniation of a disc:
   a. lateral displacement of cartilage in the knee
   b. rupture of a disc into surrounding tissue
   c. displacement of a vertebra into the spinal canal
   d. fracture of a bone of the spine

3. The term *intervertebral* means:
   a. condition around the spine
   b. pertaining to within the backbones
   c. pertaining to between the backbones
   d. condition between the spine

4. The "C" in "C5-C6" means:
   a. cavity
   b. cervical
   c. central
   d. cartilage

B. **Apply** *the correct form of the bolded similar terms appropriately in the following documentation, and you will meet a chapter objective!*
   Fill in the blanks. **LO 4.2, 4.5, and 4.11**

   vertebra   **vertebral**   **vertebrae**

1. The patient's C5 _____ was fractured in the accident.

2. A part of the axial skeleton is the _____ column.

3. The patient's C5 and C6 _____ were fractured in the accident.

   Now supply the missing terms to complete the following sentence.

4. The designations C5-C6 and C6-C7 are for locations of _____.

C. **Construct medical terms related to the bones of the skull.** *Given the definition, complete the medical term with the correct word element.*
   Fill in the blanks. **LO 4.1 and 4.5**

1. Wedge-shaped bone at the base of the skull: _____ /oid

2. Bone that forms part of the base and sides of the skull: _____ /al

3. Bone that forms the back of the nose and encloses numerous air cells: _____ /oid

4. The two bones forming the sidewalls and roof of the cranium: _____ /al

D. **Apply** *the language of orthopedics and select the correct answer.* **LO 4.5**

1. The mandible is the:
   a. lower jawbone   b. base of the cranium   c. upper jawbone

2. Which of these bones is a bone of the cranium?
   a. lacrimal   b. frontal   c. patella

3. How many bones are in the cranium?
   a. 8   b. 14   c. 22

4. What does *articulate* mean?
   a. stretches   b. fractures   c. joins

5. What is a *suture*?
   a. seam   b. bend   c. sharp point

E. **Build medical terms** *using the language of orthopedics to complete this exercise. Each term is defined and partially complete. Add the rest of the elements to complete the term. The first one is done for you. Fill in the blanks.* **LO 4.1, 4.2, and 4.6**

1. five bones of the foot between the tarsus and phalanges _____meta_____ / _____tars_____ / _____us_____
                                                         P   R   S

2. joint between the acromion and clavicle _____ / _____ / _____ar_____
                           R/CF   R   S

3. a joint _____ / _____ / _____ation_____
             P   R   S

4. pertaining to the shoulder blade _____ / _____ / _____ar_____
                  P   R   S

F. Translate the layman's terms that describe bones to the language of medicine.

Fill in the blanks. **LO 4.2, 4.6, and 4.11**

1. The bones of the hand are called: _____

2. The bones of the wrist are called: _____

3. A finger bone is called a: _____

G. Meet *the chapter learning outcomes by answering these questions using the language of orthopedics. Select the correct answer to complete each statement.*

LO 4.6

1. The two types of joints found in the elbow are:

   a. hinge and cruciate   **b.** ball-and-socket and gliding   **c.** hinge and gliding   **d.** gliding and pivot

2. The upper arm consists of the bone(s):

   a. humerus   **b.** humerus and scapula   **c.** radius   **d.** radius and ulna

3. The lower arm consists of the bone(s):

   a. humerus   **b.** humerus and scapula   **c.** radius   **d.** radius and ulna

4. The bony projection that means *pulley*:

   a. capitulum   **b.** ulna   **c.** trochlea   **d.** olecranon

H. The statement *is either true or false. Select T if the statement is true. Select F if the statement is false.* **LO 4.6**

1. The opposite of pronation is supination.   T   F

2. The capitulum articulates with the scapula.   T   F

3. The metacarpophalangeal joint is between the wrist and the hand bones.   T   F

4. The radius is on the thumb side of the hand.   T   F

5. A hinge joint allows pronation of the hand and forearm.   T   F

I. Demonstrate your knowledge *of the precise medical term to answer the following questions. Fill in the blanks with the term that is:* **LO 4.2, 4.5, and 4.11**

1. another name for the thigh bone _____

2. a basin-shaped ring of bones _____

3. the joint between the sacrum and the ilium _____

4. the lower posterior part of the hip bone _____

5. the wing-shaped bone in the pelvis _____

J. Meet learning outcomes *and select the correct medical term based on the statement.* **LO 4.5**

1. The hip bone is a fusion of three bones: the ilium, the ischium, and the:

   a. femur   **b.** pubis   **c.** acetabulum

2. The pelvis is shaped like a:

   a. bowl   **b.** box   **c.** basket

3. One function of the pelvic girdle is to:

   a. support the cranium   **b.** attach lower limbs   **c.** transport waste products

4. What organs does the pelvic girdle protect?

   a. lungs   **b.** pancreas and gallbladder   **c.** bladder, intestines, reproductive

5. A triangular-shaped bone in the lower back is the:

   a. scapula   **b.** sacrum   **c.** symphysis

6. The cartilage that forms a ring around the hip joint:

   a. labrum   **b.** pubis   **c.** acetabulum   **d.** symphysis

7. The head of the femur fits into the _____ of the pelvis.

   a. sacrum   **b.** acetabulum   **c.** labrum   **d.** foramen

K. Spelling *medical terms is a skill that is necessary for communicating in written documentation. Given the definition, correctly spell the medical term it is defining. Fill in the blanks.* **LO 4.2, 4.6**

1. The lateral bone of the lower leg: _____

2. The medical term for the kneecap: _____

3. Situated to the side: _____

4. Disc of cartilage between the bones of a joint: _____

5. Shaped like a cross: _____

L. Challenge your knowledge *of the language of orthopedics. Fill in the blanks with the correct medical terms.* **LO 4.2, 4.7**

1. On which bone does a Pott fracture occur? _____

2. Metacarpal bones appear in the hand; what are the similar bones called in the foot? _____

3. Another name for a bunion is _____.

4. What is another name for the heel bone? _____

5. The big toe is similar in construction to the _____ of the hand.

6. What is the prominent process called at the lower end of the tibia on its medial border? _____.

7. A medical specialist that treats disorders of the foot: _____

8. How many bones form the instep? _____ Are these bones classified as tarsals, metatarsals, or phalanges? _____

M. Demonstrate *your knowledge of elements that construct medical terms. Select the correct answer that completes each statement.* **LO 4.1, 4.2, 4.6, and 4.10**

1. The suffix in the term *podiatry* means:

   a. pertaining to

   b. specialist

   c. structure

   d. treatment

2. The prefix in the term *metatarsus* means:

   a. ankle

   b. after

   c. foot

   d. bone

3. The root in the term *tarsal* means:

   a. ankle

   b. foot

   c. bump

   d. big toe

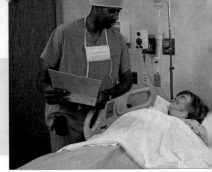

Rick Brady/McGraw Hill

Section 4.3

Disorders and Injuries of the Skeleton System

Diseases of Bone (LO 4.7)

One of the major bone diseases is **osteoporosis**, which results from a loss of bone density *(Figure 4.18)*. More common in women than in men, the incidence of osteoporosis increases with age. In the United States alone, 10 million people are living with osteoporosis and millions more have low bone density (**osteopenia**). Osteopenia puts people at risk for developing osteoporosis.

In women, production of the hormone estrogen decreases after menopause, weakening the body's protection against bone loss and potentially resulting in fragile, brittle bones. In men, lower levels of testosterone have a similar but less noticeable effect.

Other bone diseases that may not be as prevalent or publicized as osteoporosis are the following:

Osteomyelitis: an inflammation of bone and bone marrow caused by a bacterial infection, such as staphylococcus.

Osteomalacia: a disease (known as **rickets** in children) caused by vitamin D deficiency where the calcium-lacking bones become soft and flexible, lose their ability to bear weight, and become bowed.

Achondroplasia: a very rare condition where the long bones stop growing in childhood, but the axial skeleton bones are not affected *(Figure 4.19)*. People with this condition are short in stature, with the average adult measuring about 4 feet tall. Although intelligence and life span are normal, the disease is caused by a spontaneous gene mutation that then becomes a dominant gene for succeeding generations.

Osteogenesis imperfecta (OI): a rare genetic disorder producing very brittle bones that are easily fractured or broken, often **in utero** (while inside the uterus).

Primary bone cancer is found in three forms:

1. **Osteogenic sarcoma** occurs most often in bone cells around the knee in adolescents.

2. **Ewing sarcoma** occurs most often in children and adolescents.

3. **Chondrosarcoma** arises in cartilage cells, often in the pelvises of older people.

Keynote

- Osteomalacia occurs in some developing nations and occasionally in this country when children drink soft drinks instead of milk fortified with vitamin D.

Abbreviation

OI   osteogenesis imperfecta

Normal bone   Osteoporotic bone

LM 5×

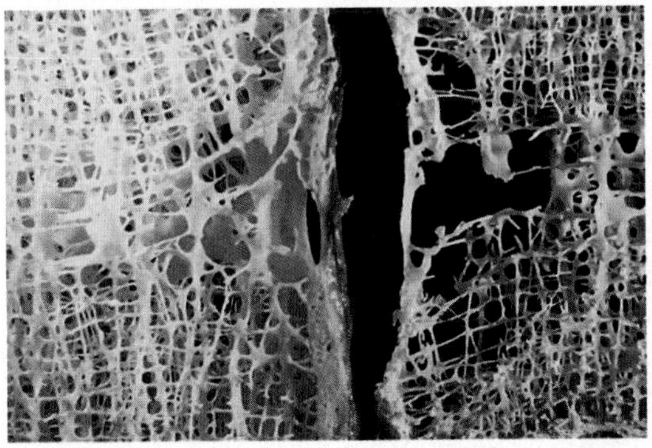

▲ **FIGURE 4.18**
Normal Bone and Osteoporotic Bone.

Michael Klein/Photolibrary/Getty Images

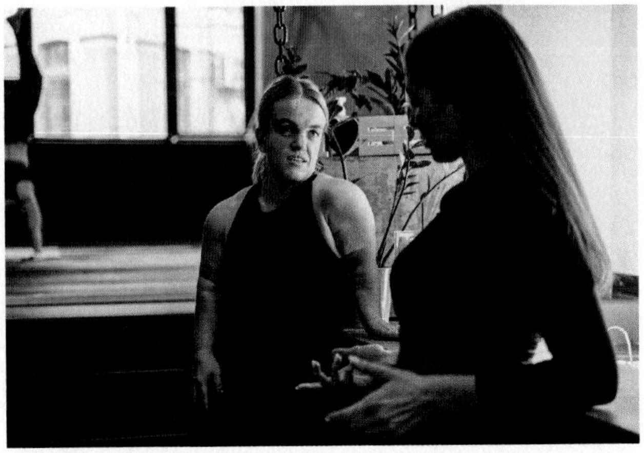

▲ **FIGURE 4.19**
Young Person with Dwarfism (Achondroplasia) Beside Her Female Trainer at Gym.

Olena Yakobchuk/Shutterstock

S = Suffix   P = Prefix   R = Root   R/CF = Combining Form

WORD	PRONUNCIATION	ELEMENTS		DEFINITION
achondroplasia	a-kon-droh-**PLAY**-zee-ah	S/ P/ R/CF	-plasia *formation* a- *without* -chondr/o- *cartilage*	Condition with abnormal, early conversion of cartilage into bone, leading to dwarfism
osteogenesis imperfecta	**OSS**-tee-oh-**JEN**-eh-sis im-per-**FEK**-tah	S/ R/CF	-genesis *creation, formation* oste/o- *bone* imperfecta, Latin *unfinished*	Inherited condition in which bone formation is incomplete, leading to fragile, easily broken bones
osteomalacia	**OSS**-tee-oh-mah-**LAY**-she-ah	S/ R/CF	-malacia *abnormal softness* oste/o- *bone*	Soft, flexible bones lacking in calcium (rickets)
osteomyelitis	**OSS**-tee-oh-my-eh-**LIE**-tis	S/ R/CF R/	-itis *inflammation* oste/o- *bone* -myel- *bone marrow*	Inflammation of bone and bone marrow
osteopenia	**OSS**-tee-oh-**PEE**-nee-ah	S/ R/CF	-penia *deficient* oste/o- *bone*	Decreased calcification of bone
osteoporosis	**OSS**-tee-oh-poh-**ROE**-sis	S/ R/CF R/CF	-sis *condition* oste/o- *bone* -por/o- *opening*	Condition in which the bones become more porous, brittle, and fragile and more likely to fracture
rickets	**RICK**-ets		Old English *to twist*	Disease due to vitamin D deficiency, producing soft, flexible bones
sarcoma	sar-**KOH**-mah	S/ R/ R/CF	-oma *tumor, mass* sarc- *flesh* chondr/o- *cartilage*	Malignant tumor originating in connective tissue Malignant tumor originating in cartilage cells
chondrosarcoma	**CHON**-droh-sar-**KOH**-mah			Malignant neoplasm in bones of the extremities before the age of 20 years
Ewing sarcoma	**YOU**-ing sar-**KOH**-mah		Dr. James Ewing, pathologist at Cornell, named in 1921	
osteogenic sarcoma	**OSS**-tee-oh-**JEN**-ik sar-**KOH**-mah	S/ R/CF R/	-ic *pertaining to* oste/o- *bone* -gen- *creation*	Malignant tumor originating in bone-producing cells

Fx   fracture

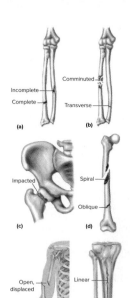

▲ **FIGURE 4.20**
Bone Fractures.

Bone Fracture (Fx) Types (LO 4.7)

Some bone fracture types can overlap in category, such as when a closed fracture is also a greenstick type or such as when an open fracture is also a displaced type.

Table 4.1 Classification and Definition of Bone Fractures

Name	Description	Reference
Closed (also called **simple** fracture)	A bone is broken, but the skin is not broken.	*Figure 4.20g*
Open (also called **compound** fracture)	A fragment of the fractured bone breaks the skin, or a wound extends to the site of the fracture.	*Figure 4.20e*
Displaced	The fractured bone parts are out of line.	*Figure 4.20e*
Complete	A bone is broken into at least two fragments.	*Figure 4.20a*
Incomplete	The fracture does not extend completely across the bone. It can be hairline, as in a stress fracture in the foot, when there is no separation of the two fragments.	*Figure 4.20a*
Comminuted	The bone breaks into several pieces, usually two major pieces and several smaller fragments.	*Figure 4.20b*
Transverse	The fracture is at right angles to the long axis of the bone.	*Figure 4.20b*
Impacted	The fracture consists of one bone fragment driven into another, resulting in shortening of a limb.	*Figure 4.20c*
Spiral	The fracture spirals around the long axis of the bone.	*Figure 4.20d*
Oblique	The fracture runs diagonally across the long axis of the bone.	*Figure 4.20d*
Linear	The fracture runs parallel to the long axis of the bone.	*Figure 4.20f*
Greenstick	This is a partial fracture. One side breaks, and the other bends.	*Figure 4.20g*
Pathologic	The fracture occurs in an area of bone weakened by disease, such as cancer.	—
Compression	The fracture occurs in a vertebra from trauma or pathology, leading to the vertebra being crushed.	—
Stress	This is a fatigue fracture caused by repetitive, local stress on a bone, as occurs in marching or running.	—

Healing of Fractures (LO 4.7)

When a bone is fractured, blood vessels bleed into the fracture site, forming a **hematoma** *(Figure 4.22a)*. After a few days, bone-forming cells called **osteoblasts** move in and start producing new bone cells (**osteocytes**), which form a **callus** *(Figure 4.22b)*. Osteoblasts continue to produce bone cells, which form **cancellous** (spongy) bone to replace the callus *(Figure 4.22c)*. As more bone cells form, the spongy bone structure is replaced by compact bone, which fuses together the bone segments *(Figure 4.22d)*. Uncomplicated fractures take 8 to 12 weeks to heal. (Surgical procedures to help fractures heal are shown in Section 4.4.)

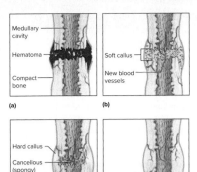

▶ **FIGURE 4.21**
Healing of Bone Fracture.

Word Analysis and Definition

S = Suffix   P = Prefix   R = Root   R/CF = Combining Form

WORD	PRONUNCIATION		ELEMENTS	DEFINITION
callus	**KAL**-us		Latin *hard skin*	Bony tissue that forms at a fracture site early in healing
cancellous	**KAN**-sell-us		Latin *lattice*	Bone that has a spongy or lattice-like structure
comminuted	**KOM**-ih-nyu-ted	S/ R/	-ed *pertaining to* comminut- *break into pieces*	A fracture in which the bone is broken into pieces
hematoma	he-mah-**TOH**-mah	S/ R/	-oma *tumor, mass* hemat- *blood*	Collection of blood that has escaped from blood vessels into tissue
osteoblast	**OSS**-tee-oh-blast	S/ R/CF	-blast *immature cell* oste/o- *bone*	A bone-forming cell
osteocyte	**OSS**-tee-oh-site	R/	-cyte *cell*	A bone-maintaining cell
pathologic fracture	path-oh-**LOJ**-ik **FRAK**-chur	S/ R/CF R/ S/ R/	-ic *pertaining to* path/o- *disease* -log- *to study* -ure *result of* fract- *to break*	Fracture occurring at a site already weakened by a disease process, such as cancer

Common Disorders of the Vertebral Column (LO 4.7)

The vertebral column, like any other body part, is susceptible to injury and disease. One common disorder of the vertebral column is **scoliosis**, an abnormal lateral curvature of the **spine** that occurs in both children and adults *(Figure 4.23)*. Abnormal curvature of the spine is more common in older people, particularly those with osteoporosis; in this case, the normal anteriorly concave curvature in the thoracic region (**kyphosis**) is exaggerated. An exaggerated lumbar curve is called **lordosis**.

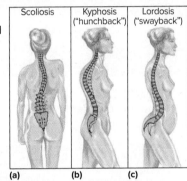

▶ **FIGURE 4.22**
Abnormal Spinal Curvatures.

Word Analysis and Definition

S = Suffix   P = Prefix   R = Root   R/CF = Combining Form

WORD	PRONUNCIATION		ELEMENTS	DEFINITION
kyphosis	kie-**FOH**-sis	S/ R/	-osis *condition* kyph- *humpback*	A normal posterior curve of the thoracic spine that can be exaggerated in disease
kyphotic (adj)	ki-**FOT**-ik	S/ R/CF	-tic *pertaining to* kyph/o- *humpback*	Pertaining to kyphosis
lordosis	lore-**DOH**-sis	S/ R/	-osis *condition* lord- *bend backward*	An exaggerated forward curvature of the lumbar spine
lordotic (adj)	lore-**DOT**-ik	S/ R/CF	-tic *pertaining to* lord/o- *bend backward*	Pertaining to lordosis
scoliosis	skoh-lee-**OH**-sis	S/ R/	-osis *condition* scoli- *crooked*	An abnormal lateral curvature of the vertebral column
scoliotic (adj)	**SKOH**-lee-**OT**-ik	S/ R/CF	-tic *pertaining to* scoli/o- *crooked*	Pertaining to scoliosis
whiplash	**WHIP**-lash	R/ R/	whip- *to swing* -lash *end of whip*	Symptoms caused by sudden, uncontrolled extension, and flexion of the neck, often in an automobile accident

Common Disorders of the Upper Extremity

Disorders of the Shoulder Girdle (LO 4.7)

As the result of the increased range of motion of this joint, the shoulder joint also is the most unstable joint and is liable to dislocation.

Shoulder separation is a dislocation of the acromioclavicular (AC) joint, often caused by a fall onto the point of the shoulder.

Shoulder dislocation occurs when the ball of the humerus slips out of the scapula's socket, usually anteriorly.

Shoulder subluxation occurs when the ball of the humerus slips partially out of position in the socket, and then moves back in.

Disorders of the Elbow Joint (LO 4.7)

When you bend your elbow, you can easily feel the olecranon that extends from the ulna. The olecranon can be easily fractured by a direct blow to the elbow or by a fall on a bent elbow.

The olecranon bursa is a thin, slippery sac between the skin and the posterior prominence of the olecranon bone. It contains a small amount of fluid to enable the skin to move freely over the bone. If the bursa becomes irritated or inflamed, fluid accumulates and **bursitis** occurs.

Tennis elbow is caused by overuse of the elbow joint or poor form when playing tennis or golf. The pain occurs when ligaments and muscle tendons around the joint tear. Treatment is rest, ice, anti-inflammatory and/or pain medication, massage, and stretching exercises.

When a child falls on an outstretched arm, the force of hitting the ground can be transmitted up the arm to cause a fracture of the elbow joint. This accounts for about 10% of all fractures in children.

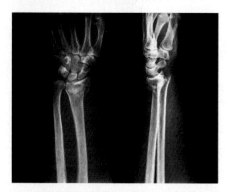

▲ FIGURE 4.23
X-Ray of Colles Fracture.

Puwadol Jaturawutthichai/Shutterstock

Disorders of the Wrist (LO 4.7)

A **Colles fracture** is a common fracture of the radius just above the wrist joint *(Figure 4.23)* that occurs when a person tries to break a fall with an outstretched hand.

Fracture of the scaphoid bone, the most common fracture of a carpal bone, also results from breaking a fall with an outstretched hand, but poor blood supply here makes healing slow and difficult.

Carpal tunnel syndrome is inflammation of the tendon synovial sheaths on the back of the wrist arising from repetitive movements such as computer keyboard operation.

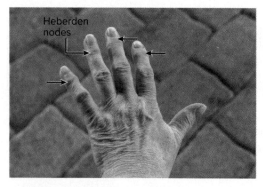

▲ FIGURE 4.24
Hand with Osteoarthritis.

Vincent Scherer/Alamy Images

Disease of Joints (LO 4.7)

Osteoarthritis (OA), often referred to as **degenerative joint disease (DJD)**, is caused by the breakdown and eventual destruction of cartilage in a joint. It develops as the result of wear and tear and is common in the hands, knees, and hips. Osteoarthritis in the hand joints occurs from wear and tear leading to deterioration of joint cartilage. Small bony spurs called **Heberden nodes** form over the joint *(Figure 4.24)*. OA can occur in joints.

Rheumatoid arthritis (RA), with destruction of joint surfaces, joint capsules, and ligaments, leads to noticeable deformity and joint instability *(Figure 4.25)*. RA is an autoimmune inflammatory disease that occurs mostly in women, between ages 40 and 60, and affects the synovial membrane lining the joints and tendons. Lumps known as **rheumatic nodules** form over the small joints of the hand and wrist.

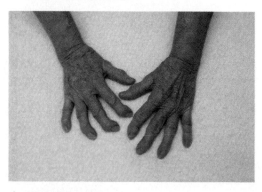

▲ FIGURE 4.25
Hands with Rheumatoid Arthritis.

Aaron Roeth Photography

WORD	PRONUNCIATION	ELEMENTS		DEFINITION
arthritis	ar-**THRI**-tis	S/ R/	-itis *inflammation* arthr- *joint*	Inflammation of a joint or joints
bursitis	burr-**SIGH**-tis	S/ R/	-itis *inflammation* burs- *bursa*	Inflammation of a bursa
Colles fracture	**KOL**-ez **FRAK**-chur		Abraham Colles, Irish surgeon, 1773–1843	Fracture of the distal radius at the wrist
deformity	dee-**FOR**-mih-tee	S/ P/ R/	-ity *condition* de- *change of* -form- *appearance, form*	A permanent structural deviation from the normal
degenerative	dee-**JEN**-er-a-tiv	S/ R/	-ive *quality of* degenerat- *deteriorate*	Relating to the deterioration of a structure
dislocation	dis-low-**KAY**-shun	S/ P/ R/	-ion *action, condition* dis- *apart, away from* -locat- *place*	Completely out of joint
Heberden node	**HEH**-ber-den NOHD		William Heberden, 1710–1801, English physician **node** Latin *a knot*	Bony lump on the terminal phalanx of the fingers in osteoarthritis
nodule	**NOD**-yule	S/ R/	-ule *little, small* nod- *node*	Small node or knotlike swelling
osteoarthritis	**OS**-tee-oh-ar-**THRIE**-tis	S/ R/CF R/	-itis *inflammation* oste/o- *bone* -arthr- *joint*	Chronic inflammatory disease of the joints with pain and loss of function
rheumatism	**RHU**-mat-izm	S/ R/	-ism *condition* rheumat- *a flow*	Pain in various parts of the musculoskeletal system
rheumatic (adj) rheumatoid arthritis	rhu-**MAT**-ik **RHU**-mah-toyd ar-**THRIE**-tis	S/ S/ S/ R/	-ic *pertaining to* -oid *resembling* -itis *inflammation* arthr- *joint*	Relating to or characterized by rheumatism Disease of connecting tissue, with arthritis as a major manifestation
subluxation	sub-luck-**SAY**-shun	S/ P/ R/	-ion *action, condition* sub- *under, below, slightly* -luxat- *dislocate*	An incomplete dislocation when some contact between the joint surfaces remains

Common Disorders of the Lower Extremity (LO 4.7)

Disorders of the Pelvic Girdle (LO 4.7)

Sacroiliac (SI) joint strain is a common cause of lower back pain. Unlike most joints, the SI joint is designed to move only 1/4 of an inch during weight-bearing and forward-bending movements. Its main function is to provide shock absorption for the spine.

Because stretching in the SI joint ligaments makes this joint overly mobile, it is susceptible to wear and tear, including painful arthritis. Another cause of pain in the SI joint is trauma, when tearing of the joint ligaments allows too much motion.

For temporary pain relief, a local anesthetic can be injected into the joint. Standard treatment involves **stabilizing** the joint with a **brace** and strengthening the lower back muscles with physical therapy. Occasionally, **arthrodesis** of the joint is necessary. This surgical procedure fuses the joint, rendering the joint immobile.

Diastasis symphysis pubis sometimes occurs during pregnancy. It is caused by excessive stretching of pelvic ligaments, which widens the joint between the two pubic bones. This leads to pain and difficulty in walking, climbing stairs, and turning over in bed. During pregnancy, however, hormones generally enable connective tissue in the SI joint area to relax so the pelvis can expand enough to allow birth without causing SI joint strain.

> **Keynote**
>
> The sciatic nerve lies directly behind the lower third of the SI joint. Many patients with SI joint strain will have pain radiating down the back of the leg.

Disorders and Injuries of the Hip Joint (LO 4.7)

A **hip pointer,** a common football-related injury, is a blow to the rim of the pelvis that leads to bruising of the bone and surrounding tissues.

Avascular necrosis of the femoral head is the death (necrosis) of bone tissue when the blood supply is cut off (avascular), usually as a result of trauma.

Fractures of the neck of the femur occur as a result of a fall, most commonly in elderly women with osteoporosis.

Injuries to the Knee Joint (LO 4.7)

Ligament injuries range from a **sprain** to a partial to complete tear (rupture). The anterior cruciate ligament (ACL) is the most commonly injured ligament in the knee *(Figure 4.26)*, particularly in football players and female athletes. The injury is often caused by a sudden **hyperflexion** of the knee joint when landing awkwardly on flat ground. Because of its poor vascular (blood) supply, the torn ligament does not heal and has to be surgically mended.

Other commonly injured major ligaments are the medial and lateral collateral ligaments and the posterior cruciate ligament.

Meniscus injuries result from a twist to the knee that tears the meniscus. The torn meniscus flips in and out of the joint as it moves, locking the knee and creating pain.

Patellar subluxation or dislocation produces an unstable, painful kneecap.

Prepatellar bursitis ("housemaid's knee" or "carpenter's knee") produces painful swelling over the bursa at the front of the knee and is seen in people who kneel for extended periods of time, like carpet layers.

Tendinitis of the patellar tendon results from overuse during activities like cycling, running, or dancing. Pain is felt where the tendon is inserted into the tibia, and this is treated with RICE (rest, ice, compression, elevation).

Disorders and Injuries of the Ankle and Foot (LO 4.7)

Podiatry is a health care specialty concerned with the diagnosis and treatment of disorders and injuries of the foot and toenails. A **podiatrist** is not a doctor of medicine (MD) but is a doctor of podiatric medicine (DPM).

Bunions, deformities that appear as swollen bones, often occur at the base of the big toe. A bunion is also called a **hallux valgus,** and it causes the metatarsophalangeal joint to misalign and stick out.

Pott fracture is a fracture of the fibula near the ankle, often accompanied by a fracture of the medial malleolus of the tibia.

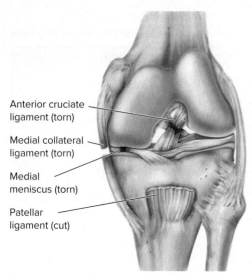

Anterior cruciate ligament (torn)

Medial collateral ligament (torn)

Medial meniscus (torn)

Patellar ligament (cut)

▲ **FIGURE 4.26**
Knee Injury to MCL and ACL.

Word Analysis and Definition

S = Suffix   P = Prefix   R = Root   R/CF = Combining Form

WORD	PRONUNCIATION		ELEMENTS	DEFINITION
avascular	a-**VAS**-cue-lar	S/ P/ R/	-ar *pertaining to* a- *without* -vascul- *blood vessel*	Without a blood supply
bunion	**BUN**-yun		French *bump*	A swelling at the base of the big toe
diastasis	die-**ASS**-tah-sis		Greek *separation*	Separation of normally joined parts
hallux valgus	**HAL**-uks **VAL**-gus	R/ R/	hallux *big toe* valgus *turn out*	Deviation of the big toe toward the medial side of the foot
hyperflexion	high-per-**FLEK**-shun	S/ P/ R/	-ion *action, condition* hyper- *excessive* -flex- *bend*	Flexion of a limb or part beyond the normal limits
necrosis necrotic (adj)	neh-**KROH**-sis neh-**KROT**-ik	 S/ R/CF	Greek *death* -tic *pertaining to* necr/o- *death*	Pathologic death of cells or tissue Pertaining to or affected by necrosis
podiatry podiatrist	poh-**DIE**-ah-tree poh-**DIE**-ah-trist	S/ R/ S/	-iatry *treatment* pod- *foot* -iatrist *practitioner*	The diagnosis and treatment of disorders and injuries of the foot Practitioner of podiatry
Pott fracture	**POT FRAK**-shur		Percival Pott, London surgeon, 1714–1788	Fracture of the lower end of the fibula, often with fracture of the tibial malleolus
rupture	**RUP**-tyur		Latin *break*	Break or tear of any body part
strain	**STRAIN**		Latin *to bind*	Overstretch or tear in a muscle or tendon
tendinitis *(also spelled tendonitis)*	ten-dih-**NYE**-tis	S/ R/	-itis *inflammation* tendin- *tendon*	Inflammation of a tendon

EXERCISES

 Case Report 4.2

You are . . .

. . . an **orthopedic** technologist working for Kenneth Stannard, MD, an **orthopedist** in the Fulwood Medical Group.

You are communicating with . . .

. . . Mrs. Amy Vargas, a 70-year-old homemaker, who tripped while walking down the front steps of her house. She has severe pain in her right hip and is unable to stand. An X-ray shows a hip fracture and marked **osteoporosis**. Dr. Stannard examined her in the Emergency Department, and Mrs. Vargas is being admitted for a hip replacement.

On questioning, Amy Vargas demonstrated many of the risk factors for **osteoporosis**, including family history, lack of exercise, cigarette smoking, inadequate diet, postmenopause, and advanced age.

A. Read *Case Report 4.2 to answer the following questions. Fill in the blanks.* **LO 4.2, 4.7, 4.8, 4.9, 4.10, and 4.11**

1. What diagnostic test did Mrs. Vargas have? _____

2. What bone disease did Mrs. Vargas have prior to her current condition? _____

3. Which joint is affected? _____

4. What type of surgeon is Dr. Stannard? _____

5. What surgical procedure will Dr. Stannard perform on Mrs. Vargas? _____

B. Read *Case Report 4.2 to answer the following questions. Select the correct answer to each question.* **LO 4.5, 4.7, and 4.11**

1. What is a risk factor?

   a. an inherited condition

   b. a characteristic, condition, or behavior that decreases the possibility of disease

   c. a characteristic, condition, or behavior that increases the possibility of disease

   d. a behavior that promotes wellness

2. Which of the following risk factors is one that is out of a person's control?

   a. lack of exercise   **c.** cigarette smoking

   b. inadequate diet   **d.** increasing age

3. Which bone disease contributed to causing her hip fracture?

   a. osteomyelitis   **c.** achondroplasia

   b. osteoporosis   **d.** sarcoma

4. What does it mean if this diagnosis is in her family history?

   a. people in her family are in poor health

   b. no one in her family has had the same problem

   c. other people in her family have had the same problem

C. Suffixes: *The combining form oste/o means bone, and it is the main element in each of the following terms. Choose the correct suffix to complete the term. Fill in the blanks.* **LO 4.1 and 4.7**

-genesis	-genic	-sarcoma	-penia	-malacia	-porosis	-myelitis

1. Disease caused by vitamin D deficiency   osteo/ _____
2. Low bone density   osteo/ _____
3. Porous, brittle, fragile bones   osteo/ _____
4. Most common malignant bone tumor   osteo/ _____
5. Rare genetic disorder producing easily fractured bones, often in utero   osteo/ _____
6. Inflammation of bone and bone marrow   osteo/ _____

Note: *The meaning of the combining form never changes. The addition of six different suffixes has helped you learn six new terms in orthopedic vocabulary!*

D. Place in order *the steps the body takes to heal a bone fracture. The first event will be "1", and the last event will be "4".* **LO 4.7**

_____ spongy bone

_____ allus

_____ compact bone

_____ hematoma

E. Match the description of the fracture *in the first column with the fracture it is describing in the second column. Refer to Table 4.1.* **LO 4.7**

Fracture Seen on the Film   **Type of Fracture**

_____ 1. Fracture at a right angle to the long axis of the radius   a. open fracture

_____ 2. Femur broken into two clean pieces   b. oblique fracture

_____ 3. Cancer patient with vertebral fracture   c. closed fracture

_____ 4. Broken ankle but no broken skin   d. transverse fracture

_____ 5. Diagonal fracture across the long axis of the femur   e. pathologic fracture

_____ 6. Fractured hand with bone fragments sticking out   f. displaced fracture

F. Deconstruct *the following medical terms into their basic elements. Then provide a brief definition for each term. Fill in the chart.* **LO 4.1, 4.2, and 4.7**

Medical Term	Prefix	Root/CF	Suffix	Definition of Medical Term
pathologic	1.	2.	3.	4.
osteoblast	5.	6.	7.	8.
comminuted	9.	10.	11.	12.

Note: *The meaning of the combining form never changes. The addition of six different suffixes has helped you learn six new terms in orthopedic vocabulary!*

I. Deconstruct *the following terms by filling in the blanks:* **LO 4.1, 4.7, and 4.11**

1. Metacarpophalangeal: _____ / _____ / _____ / _____
                              P   R, R/CF   R, R/CF   S

2. Osteoarthritis: _____ / _____ / _____
                       R, R/CF   R, R/CF   S

G. Select *the best choice after you have discounted the answers you know are not correct.* **LO 4.9**

1. Inflammation of the bone and joints:

   a. arthritis   b. osteoarthritis   c. necrosis   d. avascular

2. Hip pointer injury results from a blow to the:

   a. femur   b. sacrum   c. pelvis   d. pubic symphysis

H. Match *the correct medical term in column one with its meaning in column two.* **LO 4.5**

1. _____ cast   a. artificial body part

2. _____ arthroplasty   b. mold

3. _____ prosthesis   c. to fasten

4. _____ brace   d. joint fixation

5. _____ arthrodesis   e. joint repair

Section 4.4

Diagnostic and Therapeutic Procedures and Pharmacology for Bone Disorders

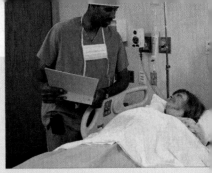

Rick Brady/McGraw Hill

The procedures and methods, other than clinical examination, that are used to assess, diagnose, and treat bone disorders, particularly bone cancer, can be complicated and expensive and have to be used with discretion. The treatments can also cause unpleasant side effects.

Diagnostic Procedures for Metabolic Bone Disorders
(LO 4.3 and LO 4.8)

- **Bone mineral density (BMD)** screening with dual-energy X-ray absorptiometry (**DEXA or DXA scan**) is used to diagnose and follow osteoporosis.
- **Nuclear bone scan** involves a radioactive substance injected into the bloodstream. From there, it travels into the bones and is detected by a special camera. It can show a bone infection, a fracture not clearly seen on X-ray, arthritis, and primary or metastatic cancer.
- **Blood tests** examine serum calcium, serum alkaline phosphate, and serum phosphate, which can be abnormal in metabolic bone disorders.
- **Bone biopsy** is the ultimate way to monitor and diagnose particular blood or marrow diseases as well as certain cancers.

Diagnostic Procedures for Bone Cancer (LO 4.3 and 4.8)

- **X-ray** shows the location, shape, and size of a bone tumor.
- **Nuclear bone scan** (described above).
- **Computed tomography (CAT or CT) scan** provides a series of detailed pictures of parts of the body, taken from different angles, that are computer-generated from multiple simultaneous X-rays. A CT offers better resolution than a standard X-ray.
- **Magnetic resonance imaging (MRI)** uses a strong magnet linked to a computer to create detailed pictures of body parts without using X-rays. An MRI produces higher resolution images than are possible by X-ray or CT.
- **Positron emission tomography (PET) scan** uses radioactive **glucose** that is injected into the bloodstream and a scanner that makes a computerized picture of body parts where the glucose is being used. Cancer cells can use more glucose than normal cells and can be detected by the scan.
- **Biopsy** can be a needle or **incisional** biopsy.

Diagnostic Procedures for Joint Disorders (LO 4.8)

- Clinical examination, joint X-ray **(radiology)**, and CT scan are first-line methods to determine the presence of a joint injury.
- **Arthrocentesis,** the aspiration of joint fluid, is used to establish the diagnosis of rheumatoid arthritis, gout, or acute arthritis with joint swelling.
- **Arthrography** is an X-ray of a joint after injection of a contrast medium (harmless dye) into the joint to make the inside details of the joint visible.
- **Diagnostic arthroscopy** is an exploratory procedure performed using an arthroscope to examine the internal compartment of a joint.

Keynotes

- Malignant tumors that begin in bone tissue are called primary bone cancer.
- Cancer that spreads to the bones from other organs and sites of the body, such as the lung, breast, or prostate, is called metastatic cancer.
- Primary bone cancer is uncommon.

Abbreviations

BMD	bone mineral density
CAT (CT)	computed tomography scan
DEXA (DXA)	dual energy x-ray absorptiometry
MRI	magnetic resonance imaging
PET	positron emission tomography
FDA	Food and Drug Administration

WORD	PRONUNCIATION	ELEMENTS		DEFINITION
arthrocentesis	AR-throw-sen-TEE-sis	S/ R/CF	-centesis *puncture* arthr/o- *joint*	Aspiration of fluid from a joint
arthrography	ar-THROG-rah-fee	S/ R/CF	-graphy *process of recording* arthr/o- *joint*	X-ray of a joint taken after the injection of a contrast medium into the joint
arthroscopy	ar-THROS-koh-pee	S/	-scopy *the process of using an instrument to examine visually*	Visual examination of the interior of a joint
arthroscope	AR-thro-skope	R/CF S/	arthr/o- *joint* -scope *instrument to examine visually*	Endoscope used to examine the interior of a joint
biopsy *(one of the "o"s is dropped from the spelling.)*	BI-op-see	S/ R/	-opsy *to view* bi/o- *life*	Process of removing tissue from a living person for laboratory examination
glucose	GLUE-kose	S/ R/	-ose *full of* gluc- *sugar, glucose*	The final product of carbohydrate digestion and the main sugar in blood
incision	in-SIZH-un	S/ R/	-ion *action, condition* incis- *cut into*	A cut or surgical wound
incisional (adj)	in-SIZH-un-al	S/	-al *pertaining to*	Pertaining to an incision

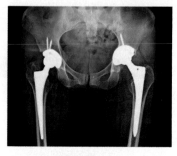

▲ **FIGURE 4.27**
Total Hip Replacement.
Colored X-ray of
prosthetic hip.

Tridsanu Thopet/Shutterstock

Therapeutic Procedures for Bone Disorders (LO 4.3 and 4.9)

- **Surgery** is a common treatment for many bone disorders. In bone cancer, the surgeon removes the entire tumor with margins that are negative for cancer cells. Modern surgical techniques have reduced the need for **amputation** in limb bone cancer. Surgical techniques used for specific bones, joints, and their disorders have been discussed previously in this chapter.

- **Chemotherapy** is the use of anticancer drugs, often in combinations, to kill cancer cells. Numerous drugs are available.

- **Radiotherapy** uses high-energy X-rays to kill cancer cells and is often used with surgery.

- **Cryosurgery** uses liquid nitrogen to freeze and kill cancer cells.

Therapeutic Procedures for Joint Disorders (LO 4.9)

- **Arthrocentesis** removes excess fluid from a joint, improving joint movement and relieving pain. Performed frequently for osteoarthritis.

- **Aspiration** of excess fluid from bursa sac.

- **Viscosupplementation** is the intra-articular injection of a gel-like hyaluronic acid liquid, acting like synovial fluid by lubricating the joint and reducing the pain caused by osteoarthritis.

- **Platelet-rich plasma (PRP) contains** a patient's concentration of platelets within a small amount of plasma. The PRP is injected into the injured site to repair torn ligaments and is currently being studied to determine its effectiveness in knee osteoarthritis.

- **Arthroscopy,** performed through an **arthroscope,** allows for visual examination of a joint. Procedures performed via arthroscopy include:

  - **Cartilage** repair of the shoulder, knee, ankle.

  - **Meniscus debridement,** suturing, partial and total **meniscectomy** of the knee.

- **Arthroplasty** repairs a joint by removing the diseased parts and replacing them with artificial parts made of titanium, other metals, and ceramics.

- **Total hip replacement (THP)** consists of replacing the femoral head and the hip socket (acetabulum) with a metal **prosthesis** *(Figure 4.27).*

- **Total knee arthroplasty (TKA)** *(Figure 4.28)* The lower end of the femur is replaced with a metal shell. The upper end of the tibia is replaced with a metal trough lined with plastic, and the back of the patella can be replaced with a plastic button.

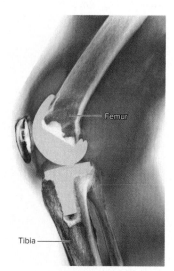

Femur

Tibia

▲ **FIGURE 4.28**
Colored X-Ray of Total
Knee Replacement.

Dr. P. Marazzi/Science Photo Library/
Brand X Pictures/Getty Images

Bone Fractures (LO 4.9)

The initial goal of fracture treatment is to join the ends of the bone at the break opposite each other so that they fit together as they did in the original bone. This is called **alignment** and is necessary to ensure that the bone heals.

External devices are frequently used to keep bones in alignment and include:

- **Slings** hold the arm in place while allowing some movement.

- **Splints** and **braces** immobilize the bone and allow for a small amount of movement.

- **Casts** immobilize the bone and prevent movement of the muscles that move the joint. They are made of plaster and fiberglass.

- **Arthrodesis** is the surgical fixation of a joint to prevent motion. Bone graft, wires, screws, or a plate can be used to stabilize the joint.

- **Fixation devices** are plates, screws, and rods used to reassemble bones with multiple fractures or bone fragments.

Word Analysis and Definition

S = Suffix   P = Prefix   R = Root   R/CF = Combining Form

WORD	PRONUNCIATION	ELEMENTS		DEFINITION
amputation (noun)	am-pyu-**TAY**-shun	S/ R/	-ation *a process* amput- *to prune, top off*	Process of removing a limb, part of a limb, a breast, or other projecting part
arthrodesis	ar-**THROW**-dee-sis	S/ R/CF	-desis *to fuse together* arthr/o- *joint*	Fixation or stiffening of a joint by surgery
arthroplasty	**AR**-throw-plas-tee	S/ R/CF	-plasty *reshaping by surgery* arthr/o- *joint*	Surgery to repair, as far as possible, the function of a joint
aspiration aspirate (verb)	as-pih-**RAY**-shun **AS**-pih-rate	S/ R/	-ion *process* aspirat- *to breathe on*	Removal by suction of fluid or gas from a body cavity
brace	BRACE		Old English *to fasten*	Appliance to support a part of the body in its correct position
chemotherapy	**KEY**-moh-**THAIR**-ah-pee	R/ R/CF	-therapy *medical treatment* chem/o- *chemical*	Treatment using chemical agents
cryosurgery	cry-oh-**SUR**-jer-ee	S/ R/CF R/	-ery *process of* cry/o- *icy cold* -surg- *operate*	Use of liquid nitrogen or argon gas in surgery to freeze and kill abnormal tissue
debridement	day-**BREED**-mon ("Mon" is the French pronunciation of *ment.*)	S/ P/ R/	-ment *action* de- *removal, out of* -bride- *rubble, rubbish*	The removal of injured or necrotic tissue
meniscectomy	men-ih-**SEK**-toh-me	S/ R/	-ectomy *surgical excision* menisc- *crescent, meniscus*	Excision (cutting out) of all or part of a meniscus
prosthesis prosthetic (adj)	**PROS**-thee-sis pros-**THET**-ik	S/ R/CF	Greek *addition* -ic *pertaining to* prosthet- *prosthesis*	An artificial part to remedy a defect in the body Pertaining to a prosthesis
radiology	ray-dee-**OL**-oh-jee	S/ R/CF	-logy *study of* radi/o- *radiation, X-rays*	The study of medical imaging
radiologist	ray-dee-**OL**-oh-jist	S/	-logist *one who studies, specialist*	Medical specialist in the use of X-rays and other imaging techniques
radiotherapy	**RAY**-dee-oh-**THAIR**-ah-pee	R/CF R/	radi/o- *X-ray, radiation* -therapy *medical treatment*	Treatment using radiation
stable stabilize	**STAY**-bell **STAY**-bill-ize	S/ R/	Latin *steady* -ize *action* stabil- *steady, fixed*	Steady, not varying To make or hold firm and steady

Pharmacology (LO 4.3 and 4.9)

Men and women over 50 who are receiving bone protective therapy are often advised to exercise regularly, take a daily regimen of 1,200 milligrams (mg) of calcium, 400 to 600 international units (IU) of vitamin D, and 15 minutes of real sun exposure several times each week. In addition, there are several FDA-approved medications available for treating osteoporosis.

Drug therapy for metabolic bone disorders includes, for osteoporosis, **estrogen replacement therapy (ERT)**, anti-estrogens, known as selective estrogen receptor modulators **(SERMs),** or bone-preserving medications such as **calcitonin**. A class of drugs called **bisphosphonates** prevents the loss of bone mass and is used in the treatment of osteoporosis, Paget disease, osteogenesis imperfecta, and any other condition that features bone fragility.

For patients at risk of fractures, several medications approved by the U.S. **Food and Drug Administration (FDA)** are available for the treatment of osteoporosis. Most inhibit osteoclast activity to reduce the rate of loss of bone (**resorption**), but some produce a direct increase in bone mass. As the turnover of bone is very slow, the time needed for assessing the effects of medications takes several years. Drugs that reduce the rate of bone resorption include estrogen, bisphosphonates, and calcitonin. **Bisphosphonates** (Alendronate *(Fosamax),* Risedronate *(Actonel),* and others) are poorly absorbed from the gastrointestinal tract and can be given intravenously. **Calcitonin** also decreases osteoclast activity and is available as a subcutaneous injection or nasal spray. Several other drugs are available in other countries and/or are undergoing clinical trials in the United States.

Medications to treat temporary joint pain, bursitis, and osteoarthritis are numerous. **Acetaminophen** reduces mild pain but does not affect inflammation or swelling. It is used in combination with aspirin and/or caffeine *(Excedrin)* as an **OTC** medicine, and with codeine or the narcotics hydrocodone *(Vicodin)* or oxycodone *(Percocet)* as prescription medications to treat severe pain. Nonsteroidal anti-inflammatory drugs **(NSAIDs)** such as ibuprofen *(Advil)* and naproxen *(Aleve)* work well for pain but can cause gastrointestinal problems and a potential increased risk of heart attacks and strokes.

Corticosteroids such as cortisone, prednisone, triamcinalone, and betamethsone, are used to reduce the pain and inflammation of severe osteoarthritis and are given orally or injected directly into the joint (**intra-articular**). Corticosteroids are also used to reduce inflammation in rheumatoid arthritis but do not slow the progression of the disease. **Disease modifying anti-rheumatic drugs (DMARDs)** such as methotrexate *(Trexall)* are effective in reducing the signs and symptoms of RA, and other DMARDs such as hydrochloroquine *(Plaquenil)* and sulfasalazine *(Azulfidine)* can be added to methotrexate to enhance its effects. **Tumor necrosis factor (TNF)** is produced in RA joints by synovial macrophages and lymphocytes to attack the joint tissues and TNF **inhibitors** such as abatacept *(Orencia)* and rituximab *(Rituxan)* slow or halt the destruction.

Abbreviations

DMARD	disease modifying anti-rheumatic drug
ERT	estrogen replacement therapy
FDA	Food and Drug Administration
IU	international unit(s)
NSAID	nonsteroidal anti-inflammatory drug
OTC	over the counter
SERM	selective estrogen receptor modulator
TNF	tumor necrosis factor

Word Analysis and Definition

S = Suffix   P = Prefix   R = Root   R/CF = Combining Form

WORD	PRONUNCIATION	ELEMENTS		DEFINITION
acetaminophen	ah-seat-ah-**MIN**-oh-fen		Generic drug name	Medication that modifies or relieves pain
bisphosphonate	bis-**FOSS**-foh-nate	S/ P/ R/ R/	-ate *composed of* bis- *two* -phos- *light* -phon- *sound*	Drug that delays the rate of bone resorption
calcitonin	kal-sih-**TONE**-in	S/ R/CF R/	-in *chemical compound* calci- *calcium* -ton- *tension, pressure*	Hormone that moves calcium from blood to bones
corticosteroid	**KOR**-tih-koh-**STEHR**-oyd	S/ R/CF R/	-oid *resembling* cortic/o- *cortisone* -ster- *steroid*	A hormone produced by the adrenal cortex
estrogen	**ESS**-troh-jen	S/ R/CF	-gen *produce, create* estr/o- *woman*	Generic term for hormones that stimulate female secondary sex characteristics
inhibit (verb) inhibitor (noun)	in-**HIB**-it in-**HIB**-it-or		Latin *to keep back*	To curb or restrain Agent that curbs or restrains
intra-articular	**IN**-trah-ar-**TIK**-you-lar	S/ P/ R/	-ar *pertaining to* intra- *inside* -articul- *joint*	Pertaining to the inside of a joint

EXERCISES

 Case Report 4.3

You are...

...an orthopedic technologist working with Kenneth Stannard, MD, at Fulwood Medical Center.

You are communicating with...

...Youseff Rabin a 17-year-old male who complains of severe pain in his right wrist. While playing soccer a few hours earlier, he fell. Youseff pushed his hand out to break his fall and heard his wrist snap, immediately experiencing pain. The wrist is now swollen and deformed.

T 98.2, P 92, R 15, BP 110/76. On examination, his right wrist is swollen and tender and has a dinner-fork **deformity**. An IV has been started, and he has been given 10 mg of morphine IV. An X-ray of the wrist has been ordered.

The X-ray of Youseff Rabin's wrist showed a **Colles fracture** of the radius, 1 inch above the end of the bone. Dr. Stannard applied a cast with the **distal** fragment of the fracture in palmar flexion and ulnar deviation. Mr. Rabin was sent home with Vicodin 500 mg **po** (by mouth), **prn** (pro re nata - as needed), for pain, and an appointment to return to the clinic in a week.

A. Read *Case Report 4.3 and then select the correct answer for the question or that completes the statement.*   **LO 4.3, 4.9, and 4.11**

1. Which of the following are Mr. Rabin's complaints?
   a. wrist snapped   b. fever   c. shortness of breath   d. severe pain

2. What is discovered on Mr. Rabin's physical examination?
   a. high blood pressure   b. swollen deformed wrist   c. fever   d. hematoma of fingers

3. IV is the abbreviation for the medical term:
   a. intravertebral   b. intervertebral   c. intravenous   d. intervenous

4. Morphine is given to treat Mr. Rabin's:
   a. low blood pressure   b. pain   c. swelling   d. fever

B. Read *Case Report 4.3 (continued) to select the correct answer to complete each statement.*   **LO 4.7, 4.8, and 4.11**

1. The specific type of fracture Mr. Rabin has is a _____ fracture.
   a. comminuted   b. Colles   c. open   d. greenstick

2. The presence of a fracture was confirmed by a(n):
   a. Vicodin   b. X-ray   c. cast   d. pronation

3. The treatment for the fracture was a(n):
   a. Vicodin   b. X-ray   c. cast   d. pronation

Abbreviations

po	per oral (bymouth)
prn	pro re nata (when necessary)

 Case Report 4.4

You are...

...a physical therapist assistant working in the physical therapy department of Fulwood Medical Center.

You are communicating with...

...Sandra Halpin, a 38-year-old female who is complaining of persistent low back pain on her left side. The pain began about two years previously, when she and her husband were moving and she was lifting heavy boxes. Her family physician has prescribed rest, back exercises, muscle relaxants, and painkillers, but she has experienced only mild relief.

On examination, she exhibits tenderness over the left sacroiliac joint, and when she presses her left knee to her chest, she experiences considerable pain over the **SI joint.** X-rays of the pelvis and hips, and an angle study of the SI joints, showed narrowing of the left SI joint space. A diagnosis of left sacroiliac joint strain has been made.

C. Read *Case Report 4.4 to select the correct answer the following questions.* **LO 4.9 and 4.11**

1. What is Sandra Halpin's chief complaint?

   a. prescription pain killers are not strong enough

   b. narrowing of the left SI joint space

   c. persistent low back pain on her left side

   d. left knee pain on standing

2. How did Ms. Halpin injure herself?

   a. lifting and moving heavy boxes

   b. pressing her left knee to her chest

   c. tripping on the stairs in front of her house

   d. overuse injury while exercising

3. Which of the following is a therapy prescribed by her physician to help Ms. Halpin's pain?

   a. acupuncture

   b. chiropractic manipulation

   c. deep tissue massage

   d. rest

4. What is Ms. Halpin's final diagnosis?

   a. subluxation of the left sacroiliac joint

   b. right sacroiliac joint strain

   c. left sacroiliac joint strain

   d. subluxation of the right sacroiliac joint

 Case Report 4.5

You are . . .

. . . an Emergency Medical Technician working in the Emergency Department of Fulwood Medical Center.

You are communicating with . . .

. . . Gail Griffith, a 17-year-old high school student and her mother, Ms. Cindy Griffith. Gail landed awkwardly after jumping for a ball during a basketball game.

Gail: "My knee kinda popped as I landed."

Gail had to be assisted off the court. In the Emergency Department, the knee was swollen and unstable. An MRI showed a partial tear of the medial **collateral** ligament, a complete **rupture** of the anterior **cruciate** ligament, and a partial tear of the medial **meniscus**. Gail decided to have surgery, even though full recovery will take 6 months to 1 year of rehabilitation.

Operative Report: Fulwood Medical Center

Patient: Gail Griffith, aged 17.

Preoperative Diagnosis: Traumatic **ACL** tear, medial collateral ligament tear, and tear of medial meniscus, right knee.

Postoperative Diagnosis: Same.

Procedure Performed: Arthroscopy, repair of medial collateral ligament, **ACL** reconstruction, repair of torn medial meniscus, right knee.

Operative Findings: A torn anterior cruciate ligament **(ACL)** of the femur with a tear of the posterior horn of the medial meniscus and tear of the medial collateral ligament.

D. Read *the Case Report 4.5 to select the correct answer for each question.* **LO 4.4, LO 4.8, 4.9, and 4.11**

1. What are Gail's symptoms when she presents to the Emergency Department?

   a. dislocated hip

   b. swollen and dislocated knee

   c. swollen and painful foot

   d. painful and dislocated ankle

2. What does MRI mean?

   a. multiple recurring images

   b. maximal reasonable intensity

   c. minimal recorded interference

   d. magnetic resonance imaging

3. As a diagnostic test, what did the MRI show? (choose all that apply)

   a. partial tear of the medial meniscus

   b. complete rupture of the anterior cruciate ligament

   c. complete rupture of the lateral collateral ligament

   d. partial tear of the medial collateral ligament

4. The meaning of collateral means situated:

    a. beneath   **c.** at the side

    b. in front of   **d.** behind

5. In her treatment plan, what will Gail be doing after surgery?

    a. limiting basketball practice for six months   **c.** six months to one year of rehabilitation

    b. limiting all after-school activities   **d.** two to six months of rehabilitation

6. What is the most severe of the injuries to Gail's knees?

    a. complete rupture of the lateral collateral ligament   **c.** partial tear of the medical meniscus

    b. complete rupture of the anterior cruciate ligament   **d.** partial tear of the medial collateral ligament

E. **Read** *Case Report 4.5 to select the correct answer(s) in the following questions.* **LO 4.3, 4.9, and 4.11**

1. Select all the structures that were torn in Gail's knee. (choose all that apply)

    a. medial meniscus   **d.** lateral collateral ligament

    b. posterior cruciate ligament   **e.** anterior cruciate ligament

    c. medial collateral ligament

2. In the abbreviation ACL, the "C" stands for:

    a. cross   **b.** collateral   **c.** cruciate   **d.** combined

3. Define the procedure performed.

    a. CT scan is taken of the knee to determine the ligament damage.

    b. Laser is aimed at the knee joint and the ligaments are fused.

    c. Incision is made into the knee joint and ligaments are sutured.

    d. Arthroscope is inserted into the joint and repairs are made through the scope.

4. Select all of the directional terms that are used in Case Report 4.5 (continued). (choose all that apply)

    a. medial   **d.** posterior

    b. collateral   **e.** collateral

    c. anterior

F. **Elements:** *Recognition of word elements will help you understand a medical term. For each of the following terms, identify the type of element shown in bold italics, and then define that element. Fill in the chart, and answer the questions below it.* **LO 4.1, 4.2, and 4.9**

    Remember: An element that begins a term is not necessarily a prefix!

Medical Term	Type of Element (P, R/CF, or S)	Meaning of Element	Meaning of Term
tendin*itis*	1.	2.	3.
*pre*patellar	4.	5.	6.
de*brid*ement	7.	8.	9.
*bur*sitis	10.	11.	12.
arthro*centesis*	13.	14.	15.

G. **Construct medical terms related to the bones of the pelvic girdle.** *Given the definition, complete the medical term with the correct word element. The first one has been done for you. Fill in the blanks.* **LO 4.1 and 4.9**

1. Study of medical imaging: _____ / _____
                                    R/CF   S

2. Surgical fixation of a joint: _____ / _____
                                    R/CF   S

3. Process of removing a limb: _____ / _____
                                    R/CF   S

4. Use of liquid nitrogen to freeze and kill abnormal tissue: _____ / _____
                                                    R/CF   S

H. Read *the answer choices for each question and immediately discard the ones you know are not correct. Select the correct answer in the remaining possibilities.*

LO 4.6 and 4.9

1. What can the physician do to provide temporary pain relief from SI joint strain?

   a. stretching

   b. a brace

   c. PT

   d. heat application

   e. local anesthetic injected into the joint

2. The expertise of a radiologist is in:

   a. skin diseases

   b. tissue study

   c. disorders of the brain

   d. interpreting X-rays

   e. lung conditions

3. Fixation or stiffening of a joint by surgery is called:

   a. arthroscopy

   b. arthroplasty

   c. arthrodesis

   d. arthrotomy

   e. none of these

4. What substance allows the SI joint to relax enough for delivery of a baby?

   a. lymph

   b. blood

   c. enzymes

   d. synovial fluid

   e. hormones

I. Match *the abbreviation in the first column with its correct application in the diagnosis and treatment of bone disorders described in the second column.*

LO 4.3 and 4.8

_____   **1** MRI

_____   **2.** CT scan

_____   **3.** BMD

_____   **4.** PET

_____   **5.** ERT

   a. provide detailed images of organs without the use of radiation

   b. determine the presence of osteoporosis

   c. used to determine the presence of cancer

   d. used to treat osteoporosis

   e. provide detailed images at different angles using X-rays

J. Identify *the diagnostic procedures to determine the presence of bone disorders including cancer.* **LO 4.8**

1. The physician wishes to definitively determine if a patient has a bone infection.

   a. X-ray

   b. DEXA scan

   c. nuclear bone scan

   d. CT scan

2. The gynecologist suspects that his patient has osteoporosis. He will order a:

   a. BMD

   b. bone biopsy

   c. MRI

   d. PET scan

3. It is necessary to decisively determine if the patient has osteomalacia. The physician should order a:

   a. BMD

   b. bone biopsy

   c. MRI

   d. PET scan

K. Construct *medical terms that are treatments used to treat bone disorders.* **LO 4.1 and 4.9**

1. Treatment using chemical agents: _____ / _____
                                        R/CF   R

2. Treatment using radiation: _____ / _____
                                  R/CF   R

3. Treatment that freezes and kills abnormal tissue: _____ / _____ / _____
                                       R/CF   R   S

4. Process of removing a limb: _____ / _____
                              R   S

L. Use terms related to pharmacology. *Using the terms provided, correctly complete the paragraph. Not all terms will be used. Fill in the blanks.* **LO 4.3, 4.7, 4.9, 4.10 and 4.11**

DMARD	podiatrist	RA	OTC	chiropractor	acetaminophen	calcitonin	corticosteroid

Ms. Walker made an appointment with a _____ for pain in her shoulder. She participates in high-intensity weightlifting and fitness training. She has been taking _____ medication to treat the pain; specifically, the medication _____ . She denies a personal or family history of _____ .

M. Construct medical terms related to the pharmacology of the skeletal system. *Insert the correct word element that completes each term. Fill in the blanks.* **LO 4.1 and 4.9**

1. Hormone that moves calcium from the blood to the bone: calci/_____/in

2. Hormone produced by the adrenal cortex: _____/ster/oid

3. Pertaining to the inside of a joint: intra-_____/ar

N. Pronunciation is important whether you are saying the word or listening to a word from a coworker. Identify the proper pronunciation of the following medical terms. Then, correctly spell the term. **LO 4.2**

1. The correct pronunciation for a fracture that is broken into pieces:
   a. IN-kom-plate   b. in-kom-**PLEET**   c. KOM-ih-nyu-ted   d. kom-you-**TATE**-ed
   Correctly spell the term: _____

2. The correct pronunciation for multiple bones joined by fibrocartilage:
   a. SIM-feh-sees   b. sim-**FEE**-sis   c. gom-**FOHS**-ees   d. gom-**FOH**-sis
   Correctly spell the term: _____

3. The correct pronunciation for the inflammation of a closed sac containing synovial fluid:
   a. burr-**SIGH**-tis   b. by-**YOUR**-sigh-tis   c. ar-**THRIE**-tis   d. **ARTH**-right-us
   Correctly spell the term: _____

4. The correct pronunciation for multiple openings through a structure:
   a. foh-**RAM**-in-ah   b. for-**AY**-men-ah   c. **KON**-dile   d. kon-**DILE**
   Correctly spell the term: _____

5. The correct pronunciation for the bones that form the bulging sides and roof of the cranium:
   a. pah-**RYE**-eh-tal   b. **PAIR**-ee-**EYE**-tal   c. ox-**IP**-it-al   d. ok-**SIP**-it-al
   Correctly spell the term: _____

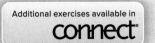
Additional exercises available in

Chapter Review exercises, along with additional practice items, are available in Connect!

5 Muscles and Tendons

CHAPTER

The Essentials of the Languages of Orthopedics and Rehabilitation

Rick Brady/McGraw Hill

Learning Outcomes

The **appendicular skeleton,** which includes the bones of the upper and lower limbs, is attached to the **axial skeleton** through joints and muscles. Understanding the terminology that identifies and describes the muscles and tendons of the limbs and trunk is vital to your knowledge of the human body. Information in this chapter provides correct medical terminology to:

LO 5.1 Use roots, combining forms, suffixes, and prefixes to construct and analyze (deconstruct) medical terms related to muscles and tendons and rehabilitation medicine.

LO 5.2 Spell and pronounce correctly medical terms related to muscles and tendons and rehabilitation medicine in order to communicate them with accuracy and precision in any health care setting.

LO 5.3 Define accepted abbreviations related to muscles and tendons and rehabilitation medicine.

LO 5.4 Relate the three different types of muscle to their structures, functions, and disorders.

LO 5.5 Identify and describe axial and appendicular muscles.

LO 5.6 Identify and describe muscular diseases and disorders.

LO 5.7 Describe diagnostic procedures used for diseases and disorders of the muscular system.

LO 5.8 Describe therapeutic methods and pharmacology for muscular diseases and disorders.

LO 5.9 Identify the goals of rehabilitation medicine and the health professionals involved in a rehabilitation program.

LO 5.10 Apply your knowledge of the medical terms of the muscles and tendons, their disorders and rehabilitation medicine to documentation, medical records, and medical reports and communication.

LO 5.11 Translate the medical terms of the muscles and tendons and their disorders and rehabilitation medicine into everyday language to communicate clearly with patients and their families.

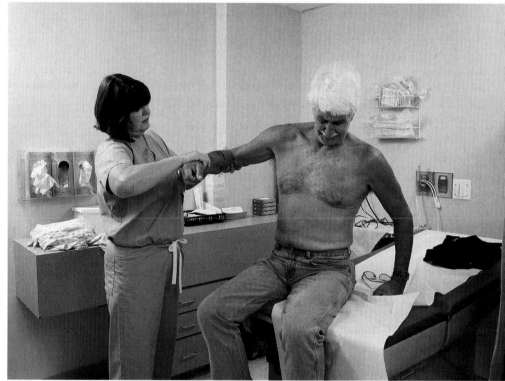

Rehabilitation programs involve a **multidisciplinary** team approach where each team member manages different rehabilitation activities. The members of a rehabilitation team include the following health professionals and their respective roles (see the Word Analysis and Definition [WAD] tables in this chapter for these terms):

- A **physiatrist**, often the team leader, is a physician specializing in physical medicine and rehabilitation.
- **Medical specialists** manage acute or chronic illnesses and pain.
- **Occupational therapists** practice occupational therapy **(OT)** to help improve a patient's activities of daily living **(ADLs)** and adapt to visual and other perceptual deficits.
- **Certified Occupational therapy assistants (COTAs)** assist occupational therapists.
- **Physical therapists** practice **physical therapy (PT)** to diagnose and treat injuries, disabilities, or other health conditions to improve a patient's **range of motion (ROM),** reduce pain, restore function, and prevent disability. Physical therapists are assisted by **restorative aids** and teach patients how to use these devices.
- **Physical therapy assistants (PTAs)** assist physical therapists.
- **Rehabilitation psychologists** and counselors are specialists who help patients undergoing rehabilitation and those with resulting disabilities to reclaim their sense of belonging, contributing to, and participating in the world around them.
- **Social workers** provide support and assistance with social issues, such as health insurance, care facilities, and employment.
- **Speech therapists** evaluate and treat communication, speech, and swallowing disorders.
- **Orthotists** make and fit orthopedic appliances (**orthotics**).
- **Nutritionists** evaluate and improve a patient's nutritional status.

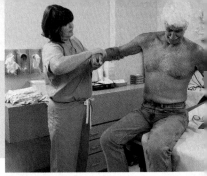

In Chapter 4, you learned how the bones of your skeleton support your body and how your joints provide mobility throughout your body. However, neither of these functions can occur without your **muscles**, which provide posture and movement.

Types, Functions, and Structure of Muscle (LO 5.4)

Types of Muscle (LO 5.4)

There are three types of **muscle**: **skeletal**, **cardiac**, and **smooth.** Skeletal muscles contract on demand to provide posture and locomotion. Cardiac and smooth muscle contract without conscious thought, cardiac muscle to power the heart contractions and smooth muscle to power the movement of food through the digestive system via **peristalsis**.

Functions and Structure of Skeletal Muscle (LO 5.4)

Functions of Skeletal Muscle (LO 5.4)

Skeletal muscles, which are attached to one or more bones, are also called **voluntary** muscles. This means that you have conscious control of your muscles, which perform your movements. Each muscle consists of bundles of muscle cells (often called **fibers** because of their length), blood vessels, and nerves. Connective tissue sheets hold your muscle fibers together and connect the muscles to your bones.

Your skeletal muscle has the following functions:

1. **Movement.** All skeletal muscles are attached to bones so when a muscle **contracts**, your bones move, too *(Figure 5.1)*. This allows for **active** movement when you walk, run, and work with your hands.

2. **Posture.** The **tone** of your skeletal muscles holds you upright when sitting, standing, or moving.

3. **Body heat.** When skeletal muscles contract, they produce the heat needed to maintain your body temperature.

4. **Respiration**. Skeletal muscles move the chest wall and diaphragm as you breathe.

5. **Communication.** Skeletal muscles enable you to speak, write, type, gesture, and smile.

Abbreviations

DC	Doctor of Chiropractic
DO	Doctor of Osteopathy
MD	Doctor of Medicine

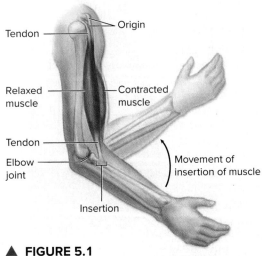

▲ **FIGURE 5.1**
Muscle Contraction to Flex the Elbow Joint.

WORD	PRONUNCIATION	ELEMENTS		DEFINITION
active activity	**ACK**-tiv ack-**TIV**-ih-tee	S/ R/	Latin *movement* -ity *condition, state* activ- *movement*	Causing action or change The state of being active
cardiac (adj)	**KAR**-dee-ak	S/ R/	-ac *pertaining to* cardi- *heart*	Involuntary, striated muscle found only in the heart.
contract	kon-**TRAKT**	P/ R/	con- *with, together* -tract *draw*	Draw together or shorten
fiber	**FIE**-ber		Latin *fiber*	A strand or filament
multidisciplinary	mul-tee-**DIS**-ih-plih-**NAIR**-ee	S/ P/ R/	-ary *pertaining to* multi- *many* -disciplin- *instruction*	Involving health care providers from more than one profession
muscle	**MUSS**-el		Latin *muscle*	A tissue consisting of cells that can contract
passive	**PASS**-iv		Latin *to endure*	Not active
peristalsis	pear-ih-**STAL**-sis	P/ R/	peri- *around* -stalsis *constrict*	Waves of alternate constriction and relaxation in a tube
skeletal (adj)	**SKEL**-eh-tal	S/ R/	-al *pertaining to* skelet- *skeleton*	Pertaining to the skeleton
smooth	SMOOTH		Old English *not rough*	Involuntary muscle, lacking striations, found in the walls of visceral organs and blood vessels.
tone	TONE		Greek *tone*	Tension present in resting muscles
voluntary muscle	**VOL**-un-tare-ee **MUSS**-el	S/ R/	-ary *pertaining to* volunt- *free will*	Muscle that is under the control of the will

Structure of Skeletal Muscle (LO 5.4)

Your skeletal muscle fibers are narrow and measure up to 1½ inches long. Bundles of these fibers create separate muscles, which are held in place by **fascia** *(Figure 5.2)*, a thick layer of connective tissue. Fascia extends beyond the muscle to form a **tendon**, which attaches to a bone's periosteum at the **origin** and **insertion** of the muscle.

Because skeletal muscle fibers contain **striations** (alternating dark and light bands of protein filaments responsible for muscle contraction), skeletal muscle can also be called **striated muscle**.

You have the same number of muscle fibers as an adult that you had in late childhood. Exercise and/or weightlifting will enlarge (**hypertrophy**) your muscles, increasing the thickness of your muscle fibers. If you neglect these muscles, they will shrink (**atrophy**).

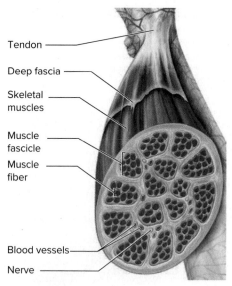

Tendon
Deep fascia
Skeletal muscles
Muscle fascicle
Muscle fiber
Blood vessels
Nerve

▲ **FIGURE 5.2**
Structure of Skeletal Muscle.

WORD	PRONUNCIATION		ELEMENTS	DEFINITION
atrophy	**A**-troh-fee	P/ R/	a- *without* -**trophy** *nourishment*	The wasting away or diminished volume of tissue, an organ, or a body part
hypertrophy	high-**PER**-troh-fee	P/ R/	**hyper**- *above, excessive* -**trophy** *nourishment*	Increase in size, but not in number, of an individual tissue element
fascia	**FASH**-ee-ah		Latin *a band*	Sheet of fibrous connective tissue
insertion insert (verb)	in-**SIR**-shun in-**SIRT**	S/ R/	-**ion** *action, condition* **insert**- *put together*	The insertion of a muscle is the attachment of a muscle to a more movable part of the skeleton, as distinct from the origin
origin	**OR**-ih-jin		Latin *source of*	Fixed source of a muscle at its attachment to bone
striated muscle	**STRIE**-ay-ted **MUSS**-el		**striated** Latin *stripe* **muscle** Latin muscle	Another term for skeletal muscle
striation	strie-**AY**-shun	S/ R/	-**ion** *action, condition* **striat**- *stripe*	Stripes
tendon	**TEN**-dun		Latin *sinew*	Fibrous band that connects muscle to bone

EXERCISES

A. Deconstruct *the following medical terms into their basic elements. Fill in the chart.* **LO 5.1**

Medical Term	Prefix	Root(s)/CF	Suffix
contract	1.	2.	3.
voluntary	4.	5.	6.
skeletal	7.	8.	9.

B. Meet chapter objectives *and use the correct medical terminology to answer the questions. Fill in the blanks.*   **LO 5.2 and 5.4**

1. Muscle cells are also referred to as muscle _____.

2. Skeletal muscle attaches to one or more _____.

3. Skeletal muscle is under conscious control; therefore, it is considered a _____ muscle.

4. Peristalsis is a function of _____ muscle.

C. Remembering *the meanings of word elements makes short work of defining medical terms. Select the correct answer.*   **LO 5.1**

1. The suffix -*itis* means: **a.** condition   **b.** disease   **c.** inflammation

2. Hyper- is a: **a.** suffix   **b.** prefix   **c.** root

3. The root *trophy*- means: **a.** condition   **b.** procedure   **c.** nourishment

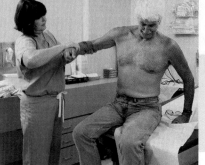

Muscles and Tendons of the Upper and Lower Extremities

Rick Brady/McGraw Hill

The muscles and tendons of your shoulders, arms, and hands are nearly always in motion. You shake hands, point your finger, turn doorknobs, and lift various objects throughout the course of any given day.

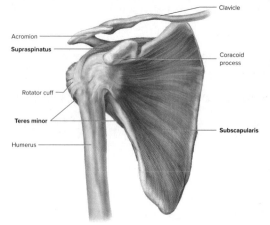

▲ **FIGURE 5.3**   Rotator Cuff Muscles (labeled in bold).

Shoulder Girdle (LO 5.5)

Your **pectoral** (shoulder) **girdle** connects your axial skeleton to your upper limbs and helps you to move these limbs. Without your shoulder girdle, you wouldn't be able to throw a ball, drive a car, or reach that top shelf of your closet or kitchen cabinet. In fact, you would not be able to move your upper limbs.

The muscles and tendons in your shoulder girdle get plenty of use. Four muscles that originate on your scapula wrap around the shoulder joint and fuse together. This fusion forms one large tendon (the **rotator cuff**), which is inserted into the humerus *(Figure 5.3)*. Your rotator cuff keeps the ball of the humerus tightly in the scapula's socket and provides the kind of strength needed by baseball pitchers.

Upper Arm and Elbow Joint (LO 5.4)

Your muscles connect your humerus (upper arm bone) to your shoulder girdle, vertebral column, and ribs. These muscles enable your arm to move freely at the shoulder joint. Your major anterior muscles (those at the front of your body) are the **deltoid** (shoulder muscle) and **pectoralis major** (chest muscle) *(Figure 5.4a)*. Among the major posterior muscles is the **latissimus dorsi**, found in your back *(Figure 5.4b)*.

Muscles that move your elbow joint and forearm originate on the upper arm bone or shoulder girdle and are inserted into the bones of your forearm. On the front of the arm, you have a group of three muscles *(Figure 5.4a)*–**biceps brachii**, **brachialis**, and **brachioradialis**. These muscles flex your forearm at the elbow joint and rotate your forearm and hand sideways or laterally (supination). A single muscle on the back of your arm (the **triceps brachii**) extends your elbow joint and forearm *(Figure 5.4b)*.

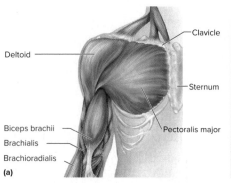
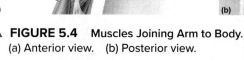

▲ **FIGURE 5.4**   Muscles Joining Arm to Body. (a) Anterior view.   (b) Posterior view.

Forearm, Wrist, and Hand (LO 5.4)

The muscles of your forearm are responsible for various movements. These muscles supinate and pronate your forearm (turning it upward and downward), flex and extend your wrist joint and hand, and move your hand medially and laterally (back and forth crossways). These terms of movement are detailed in Chapter 2.

Your forearm is bigger near the elbow because the forearm muscles are fleshy and bulky. Your wrist is much thinner because these muscles taper into tendons that pass over your wrist on the way to being inserted into your finger bones.

When you look at the palm of your hand, you'll see a prominent pad of muscles (the **thenar eminence**) at the base of your thumb *(Figure 5.5)*. A smaller pad of muscles (the **hypothenar eminence**) is located at the base of your little finger. The back of your hand is called the **dorsum**.

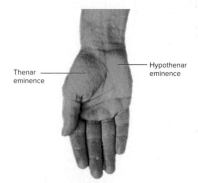

▲ **FIGURE 5.5**
Palmar Surface of the Hand.

Eric Wise

WORD	PRONUNCIATION	ELEMENTS		DEFINITION
biceps brachii	BYE-sepz BRAY-key-eye	P/ R/ R/CF	bi- *two* -ceps *head* brachi/i *of the arm*	A muscle of the arm that has two heads or points of origin on the scapula
brachialis	BRAY-kee-al-is	S/ R/	-alis *pertaining to* brachi- *arm*	Muscle that lies underneath the biceps and is the strongest flexor of the forearm
brachioradialis	BRAY-kee-oh-RAY-dee-al-is	S/ R/CF R/	-alis *pertaining to* brachi/o- *arm* -radi- *radius*	Muscle that helps flex the forearm
deltoid	DEL-toyd	S/ R/	-oid *resembling* delt- *triangle*	Large, fan-shaped muscle connecting the scapula and clavicle to the humerus
dorsum dorsal (adj) ventral (adj) *(opposite of dorsal)*	DOOR-sum DOOR-sal VEN-tral	S/ R/ R/	Latin *back* -al *pertaining to* dors- *back* ventr- *belly*	The back of any part of the body, including the hand Pertaining to the back of any part of the body Pertaining to the belly or situated nearer to the surface of the belly
latissimus dorsi	lah-TISS-ih-muss DOOR-sigh	S/ R/ R/	-imus *most* latiss- *wide* dorsi *of the back*	The widest (broadest) muscle in the back
pectoral pectoral girdle	PEK-tor-al PEK-tor-al GIR-del	S/ R/	-al *pertaining to* pector- *chest* girdle, Old English *encircle*	Pertaining to the chest Incomplete bony ring that attaches the upper limb to the axial skeleton
rotator cuff	roh-TAY-tor CUFF	S/ R/	-or *one who does* rotat- *rotate* cuff, Old English *band*	Part of the capsule of the shoulder joint
thenar eminence hypothenar eminence	THEE-nar EM-in-ens high-poh-THEE-nar EM-in-ens	R/ P/	eminence, Latin *stand out* thenar *palm* hypo- *below, smaller*	The fleshy mass at the base of the thumb The fleshy mass at the base of the little finger
triceps brachii	TRY-sepz BRAY-key-eye	P/ R/ R/CF	tri- *three* -ceps *head* brachi/i *of the arm*	Muscle of the arm that has three heads or points of origin

Muscles of the Hip and Thigh (LO 5.5)

Some of your body's most powerful muscles support your hip joint and move your thigh. These muscles originate on the pelvic girdle and are inserted into the femur. Among these prominent muscles are your three gluteal muscles, the gluteus—**maximus**, **medius**, and **minimus** *(Figure 5.6)* that abduct your thigh—and the **adductor** muscles that run down your inner thigh.

Thigh Muscles (LO 5.5)

Your thigh muscles move your knee joint and lower leg. Your anterior thigh (the front of your thigh) contains your large **quadriceps femoris** muscle. This muscle has four heads: the rectus femoris, vastus lateralis, vastus medialis, and the vastus intermedius (which lies beneath the rectus femoris). These four muscle heads join into the **quadriceps tendon** (which contains the patella) and continue as the patellar tendon to be inserted into the tibia *(Figure 5.7)*. The quadriceps muscle extends (straightens) the knee joint and, because of the lower leg's weight, it has to be a very strong muscle.

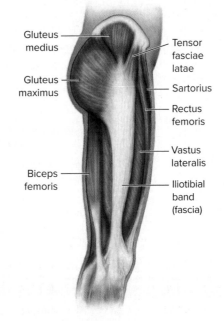

▲ **FIGURE 5.6**
Hip Joint.
Muscles of the hip and thigh, lateral view.

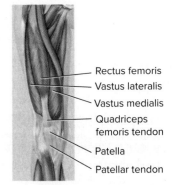

▲ **FIGURE 5.7**
Anterior Muscles of the Thigh.

> **FIGURE 5.8**
> Posterior Thigh Muscles.

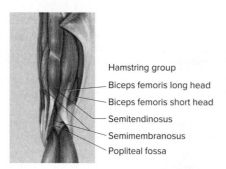

- Hamstring group
- Biceps femoris long head
- Biceps femoris short head
- Semitendinosus
- Semimembranosus
- Popliteal fossa

> **FIGURE 5.9**
> Muscles of Lower
> Leg and Foot.
> (a) Muscles of the
> front of the right leg.
> (b) Muscles of the
> back of the right leg.

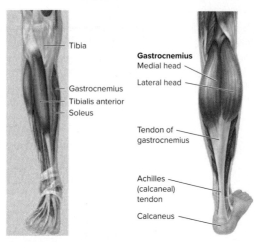

- Tibia
- Gastrocnemius
- Tibialis anterior
- Soleus

Gastrocnemius
- Medial head
- Lateral head
- Tendon of gastrocnemius
- Achilles (calcaneal) tendon
- Calcaneus

Your posterior (rear) thigh is composed mostly of your three **hamstring muscles**—the **biceps femoris, semimembranosus,** and **semitendinosus** *(Figure 5.8)*. These muscles flex (bend) your knee joint and rotate your leg. The hollow area at the back of your knee between your hamstring tendons is the **popliteal fossa**.

Muscles and Tendons of the Lower Leg, Ankle, and Foot (LO 5.5)

The muscles of your lower leg move your ankle, foot, and toes. Your front leg muscles bend your foot backward at the ankle and extend your toes. The side or lateral leg muscles turn your foot outward or evert it. Your back leg muscles plantar-flex your foot at the ankle, flex your toes, and turn in or invert your foot. The **gastrocnemius** muscle *(Figure 5.9b)*, located at the back of your leg, forms a large part of your calf. The distal end of this muscle joins the tendon of the smaller calf (soleus) muscle to create the **Achilles (calcaneal) tendon**, which is attached to the heel bone (**calcaneus**) *(Figure 5.9b)*. Together, your gastrocnemius muscle and Achilles tendon make it possible for you to "push off" when jumping or running. For more detailed foot movement descriptions, you may review the terms in Chapter 2.

Word Analysis and Definition

S = Suffix P = Prefix R = Root R/CF = Combining Form

WORD	PRONUNCIATION	ELEMENTS		DEFINITION
abduction abduct (verb)	ab-**DUCK**-shun ab-**DUKT**	S/ P/ R/	-ion *process, action* ab- *away from* -duct- *lead*	Action of moving away from the midline To move away from the midline
adductor	ah-**DUCK**-tor	S/ P/ R/	-or *that which does something* ad- *toward* -duct- *lead*	Muscle that moves the thigh toward the midline
adduction	ah-**DUCK**-shun	S/	-ion *action, condition*	Action of moving toward the midline
calcaneus calcaneal tendon *(same as **Achilles** tendon)* Achilles	kal-**KAY**-knee-us kal-**KAY**-knee-al ah-**KILL**-eeze	S/ R/	Latin *the heel* -eal *pertaining to* calcan- *calcaneus* mythical Greek warrior	The heel bone The tendon of the heel formed from gastrocnemius and soleus muscles and inserted into the calcaneus
gastrocnemius	gas-trok-**KNEE**-me-us	S/ R/	-ius *pertaining to* gastrocnem- *calf of leg*	Major muscle in back of the lower leg (the calf)
gluteus gluteal (adj)	**GLUE**-tee-us **GLUE**-tee-al	S/ R/	Greek *buttocks* -eal *pertaining to* glut- *buttocks*	Refers to one of three muscles in the buttocks Pertaining to the buttocks
maximus	**MAKS**-ih-mus		Latin *the biggest*	The gluteus maximus muscle is the largest muscle in the body, covering a large part of each buttock
medius	**MEE**-dee-us		Latin *middle*	The gluteus medius muscle is partly covered by the gluteus maximus
minimus	**MIN**-ih-mus		Latin *smallest*	The gluteus minimus is the smallest of the gluteal muscles and lies under the gluteus medius
hamstring	**HAM**-string		Old English *hollow of the knee* Old English *tendons*	Group of three muscles on the posterior side of the thigh that join at the back of the knee.
popliteal fossa	pop-**LIT**-ee-al **FOSS**-ah	S/ R/CF	-al *pertaining to* poplit/e- *ham, back of knee* fossa, Latin *trench, ditch*	The hollow at the back of the knee
quadriceps femoris	**KWAD**-rih-seps **FEM**-or-is	P/ R/ S/ R/	quadri- *four* -ceps *head* -is *belonging to, pertaining to* femor- *femur*	An anterior thigh muscle with four heads (origins)

EXERCISES

A. Construct *medical terms related to the muscles of the upper limb.*

Fill in the blanks.   **LO 5.1, 5.2, and 5.4**

1. Pertaining to the chest: _____/al

2. Part of the capsule of the shoulder joint: _____/or cuff

3. Point of attachment of a muscle to the more moveable part of the skeleton: _____/tion

B. Analyze *the underlined word or part of a word as your clue for the element in the correct term.*

Fill in the blanks.   **LO 5.2 and 5.4**

1. arm muscle with three heads: _____

2. triangular-shaped muscle: _____

3. widest muscle in the back: _____

4. arm muscle with two heads: _____

5. strongest flexor of the forearm: _____

6. A term meaning pertaining to the front.

   a. ventral   **b.** dorsal   **c.** posterior   **d.** lateral

7. A fluid-filled sac attached to a tendon describes:

   a. ganglia   **b.** pustule   **c.** cyst   **d.** bursa

C. Defining *the word element provides a clue to its meaning. Select the correct answer for each statement.*   **LO 5.1**

1. The prefix that means *four*:

   a. ad-   **b.** quadri-   **c.** ab-

2. The root that means *lead*:

   a. calcan-   **b.** femor-   **c.** glut-   **d.** duct-

3. The suffix that means *that which does something*:

   a. -is   **b.** -ion   **c.** -al   **d.** -or

4. The suffix *-ceps* means:

   a. trench, ditch   **b.** muscle   **c.** head   **d.** belong to

D. Identify medical terms that come from Latin. *Given the Latin meaning, insert the medical term that it is defining.*

Fill in the blanks.   **LO 5.2**

1. buttocks: _____

2. smallest: _____

3. the heel: _____

4. middle: _____

5. biggest: _____

Study Hint

To help remember the difference between the thenar eminence and the *hypothenar* eminence, focus on the prefix *hypo*, which can mean below or smaller. If you hold the hand open, palm facing you, with the thumb straight up, the *hypothenar* eminence is the fleshy mass at the base of the little finger, which is the smallest one on the hand.

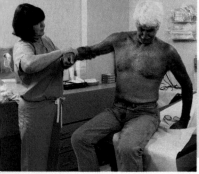

Rick Brady/McGraw Hill

Section 5.3

Disorders and Injuries of Muscles and Tendons

Disorders of Skeletal Muscles (LO 5.6)

Muscle disease and disorders are typically characterized by pain and muscle weakness.

Fibromyalgia affects muscles and tendons all over the body, causing chronic pain associated with fatigue and often resulting in cognitive or psychiatric symptoms. Its etiology is unknown. There are no laboratory tests for it and no specific treatment except pain management, physiotherapy, and stress reduction.

Injuries of Skeletal Muscles (LO 5.6)

Myopathies are diseases of skeletal muscles not caused by nerve disorders. This group of disorders causes the skeletal muscles to become weak or wasted. Most of these conditions last for a period of time, then go away.

- **Muscular dystrophy** is a general term for a group of hereditary, progressive disorders affecting skeletal muscles. **Duchenne muscular dystrophy (DMD)** is the most common, occurring in boys, who begin to have difficulty walking around the age of 3. Generalized muscle weakness and atrophy progress, and few live beyond 20 years. There is no effective treatment.

- **Inflammatory myopathies** are protective responses to injured tissues marked by redness, increased heat, swelling, and pain. **Dermatomyositis** and **polymyositis** are examples.

Muscle injury is very common and usually results from athletics or vocation.

Muscle soreness can result from vigorous exercise, particularly if your muscles are not used to it. Exercise increases the lactic acid in your muscle fibers, causing inflammation. However, the micro tears that occur when muscles are heavily worked are actually believed to be the cause of soreness after a good workout.

Muscle cramps are sudden, short, painful contractions of a muscle or group of muscles. The cause of these cramps is unknown. A poor diet that leads to low blood potassium, calcium, and magnesium levels; caffeine and tobacco use; and reduced blood supply may contribute to muscle cramps.

Muscle strains range from a simple stretch to a partial or complete tear in the muscle, tendon, or muscle-tendon combination.

A **sprain** is a stretch or tear of a ligament, often in the ankle, knee, or wrist.

Rhabdomyolysis is the breakdown of muscle fibers. This releases a protein pigment called myoglobin into the bloodstream. Causes of rhabdomyolysis include muscle trauma and severe exertion (marathon running).

Tenosynovitis is inflammation of the sheath that surrounds a **tendon.** It is usually related to repetitive use, occurs commonly in the wrist and hands in computer users, and is beginning to be seen in the thumbs of frequent texters. It produces pain, tenderness in the tendon, and difficulty in movement of a joint.

Bursitis, inflammation of the lubricating sac of the rotator cuff, can also be produced by overuse.

Rotator cuff tears (a frequent injury to the shoulder girdle) are caused by wear and tear from overuse in work situations or in certain sports, such as baseball, football, and golf. These tears can be partial or complete.

Tendonitis can occur at any site of the body where a tendon connects to a bone. Common forms of tendonitis:

- **Shoulder joint** tendonitis is caused when the rotator cuff and/or biceps tendon becomes inflamed from overuse.

- **Tennis elbow** occurs at the location where the upper arm and forearm muscle tendons are inserted into the upper arm bone just above the elbow joint. Small tears in these tendons at their attachments can be caused by trauma or overuse of the elbow joint.

- **Achilles tendonitis** results from a small stretch injury that causes the tendon to become swollen and painful; people prone to this injury are runners who suddenly increase their mileage.

Common Disorders of the Wrist and Hand (LO 5.6)

Because you use your hands and wrists almost constantly, your wrists can be prone to disorders and injuries.

Ganglion cysts are fluid-filled cysts on the back of the wrist, which result from irritation or inflammation of the synovial tendon sheaths in this area. These cysts usually disappear on their own.

Stenosing tenosynovitis is a painful inflammation of the synovial sheaths on the back of the wrist.

Carpal tunnel syndrome (CTS) develops on the front of the wrist and results from inflammation and swelling of overused tendon sheaths. Repetitive movements, like typing on a computer keyboard, can lead to CTS. A feeling of "pins and needles" or pain and loss of muscle power in the thumb side of the hand are common.

Word Analysis and Definition

S = Suffix   P = Prefix   R = Root   R/CF = Combining Form

WORD	PRONUNCIATION		ELEMENTS	DEFINITION
bursitis	burr-**SIGH**-tis	S/ R/	-itis *inflammation* burs- *bursa*	Inflammation of a bursa
cyst	**SIST**		Greek *fluid-filled sac*	An abnormal, fluid-containing sac
dermatomyositis	**DER**-mah-toh-**MY**-oh-site-is	S/ R/CF R/	-itis *inflammation* dermat/o- *skin* -myos- *muscle*	Inflammation of the skin and muscles
Duchenne muscular dystrophy	**DOO**-shen **MUSS**-kyu-lar **DISS**-troh-fee	 P/ R/	Guillaume Benjamin Duchenne, French neurologist, 1806–1875 dys- *bad, difficult* -trophy *nourishment*	A condition with symmetrical weakness and wasting of pelvic, shoulder, and proximal limb muscles
fibromyalgia	fie-broh-my-**AL**-jee-ah	S/ R/CF R/	-algia *pain* fibr/o- *fiber* -my- *muscle*	Pain in the muscle fibers
ganglion	**GANG**-lee-on		Greek *swelling*	Fluid-containing swelling attached to the synovial sheath of a tendon
myoglobin	**MY**-oh-**GLOW**-bin	S/ R/CF R/	-in *substance* my/o- *muscle* -glob- *globe*	Protein of muscle that stores and transports oxygen
myopathy	my-**OP**-ah-thee	S/ R/CF	-pathy *disease* my/o- *muscle*	Any disease of muscle
myositis	my-oh-**SIGH**-tis	S/	-sitis *inflammation*	Inflammation of muscle tissue
polymyositis	**POL**-ee-my-oh-**SIGH**-tis	P/ R/CF S/	poly- *many* -myos- *muscle* -itis *inflammation*	Inflammation of many voluntary muscles simultaneously.
rhabdomyolysis	**RAB**-doh-my-oh-**LIE**-sis or **RAB**-doh-my-**OL**-ih-sis	S/ R/CF R/CF	-lysis *destruction* rhabd/o- *rod-shaped* -my/o- *muscle*	Destruction of muscle to produce myoglobin
sprain	**SPRAIN**		root unknown	A wrench or tear in a ligament
stenosis	steh-**NOH**-sis		Greek *narrowing*	Narrowing of a passage
strain	**STRAIN**		Latin *to bind*	Overstretch or tear in a muscle or tendon
tendinitis (*also spelled* tendonitis)	ten-dih-**NYE**-tis	S/ R/	-itis *inflammation* tendin- *tendon*	Inflammation of a tendon
tenosynovitis	**TEN**-oh-sin-oh-**VIE**-tis	S/ R/CF R/	-itis *inflammation* ten/o- *tendon* - synov- *synovial membrane*	Inflammation of a tendon and its surrounding synovial sheath

EXERCISES

Case Report 5.1

You are

. . . an orthopedic technologist working with orthopedist Kenneth Stannard, MD, in Fulwood Medical Center.

You are communicating with

Mr. Bruce Adams, a 55-year-old construction worker who presents with persistent pain in his right shoulder.

Mr. Adams' pain began 3 or 4 months ago; it is worse at the end of the workday and when he lifts his arm above his head. During the past week, the pain has woken him from sleep and become more intense. Mr. Adams' primary care physician has given him anti-inflammatory and pain medication, advised him to rest his shoulder, and referred him to Dr. Stannard for further diagnosis and treatment. A physical examination shows that Mr. Adams' pain noticeably limits all the **passive** and **active** movements of his right shoulder, including his ability to lift weight.

When Dr. Stannard evaluated Mr. Adams, an MRI revealed a full-thickness tear of his **rotator cuff**. Mr. Adams has been scheduled for outpatient surgery to repair the tear.

A. Read *Case Report 5.1 to answer the following questions.*   **LO 5.1, 5.2, and 5.6**

1. What type of physician is Dr. Stannard? _____

2. Did Mr. Adams see another physician before seeing Dr. Stannard? _____

3. What is Mr. Adams's chief complaint? _____

4. The one word that describes "movement in which Dr. Stannard moves the arm while Mr. Adams does not contract his muscle" is termed: _____

B. Read *Case Report 5.1 to correctly answer the following questions. Fill in the blanks.*   **LO 5.2, 5.4, 5.6, 5.7, and 5.9**

1. What type of diagnostic test did Mr. Adams have? _____

2. What muscular structure was injured? _____

3. Mr. Adams experiences pain when he moves his arm because the muscles _____ (*insert or originate*) on the humerus.

4. Is Mr. Adams scheduled to spend the night in the hospital? _____

C. Select *the answer that correctly completes each statement.*   **LO 5.4**

1. Muscle that has decreased in size is said to have the condition of:
   a. edema   b. hypertrophy   c. atrophy   d. paralysis

2. Lifting heavy objects over a long period of time can result in muscle:
   a. polymyalgia   b. tenosynovitis   c. atrophy   d. hypertrophy

3. An overstretch or tear in a muscle is termed a:
   a. strain   b. fasciotomy   c. sprain   d. tenosynovitis

4. The symptoms of fibromyalgia include: (choose all that apply)
   a. pain in muscles   b. depression   c. pain in tendons   d. fatigue

5. Inflammation of the lubricating sac near a joint: _____/itis

6. Inflammation of the connective tissue that connects muscle to bone: _____/itis

7. *Fibro* is a: **a.** combining form   **b.** root   **c.** suffix

8. The root *my-* means: **a.** tendon   **b.** ligament   **c.** muscle

9. The suffix *-algia* means: **a.** inflammation   **b.** pain   **c.** swelling

D. *Match the medical term in the first column with its correct description in the second column.*   **LO 5.4**

_____ 1. thenar eminence	a. abnormal, fluid-filled sac		_____ 4. ventral	d. fleshy mass at the base of the thumb
_____ 2. hypothenar eminence	b. pertaining to the back		_____ 5. ganglion	e. pertaining to the front
_____ 3. dorsal	c. fluid-filled sac attached to a tendon		_____ 6. cyst	f. fleshy mass below the base of the little finger

Section 5.4

Physical Medicine and Rehabilitation (PM&R)

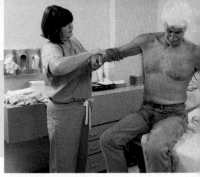

Rick Brady/McGraw Hill

Physical Medicine and Rehabilitation (PM&R) (LO 5.8)

PM&R health professionals are listed and defined at the beginning of this chapter.

Physical medicine and rehabilitation are also called **physiatry**. Its goal is to develop a comprehensive program to put together the different pieces of a person's life—medical, social, emotional, and **vocational**—after injury or disease. **PM&R** programs cover a wide spectrum, from prevention of injury in athletes to treating sports-related injuries in sports medicine to coping with complicated multiple traumas.

Rehabilitation Definitions (LO 5.3 and 5.8)

The following definitions of terms or phrases specific to rehabilitation will help you to understand more precisely the different kinds of rehabilitation in which you may be involved as a health professional.

Rehabilitation medicine focuses on function. Being able to function is essential to an individual's independence and ability to have a good quality of life.

Rehabilitation medicine is also involved with the **prevention** of function loss and the prevention of injury. In sports medicine, an example is the prevention of shoulder and elbow injuries often experienced by baseball pitchers.

Restorative rehabilitation restores a function that has been lost, such as after a hip fracture, hip replacement, or stroke. This process can be intense, but is usually short term.

Maintenance rehabilitation strengthens and maintains a function that is gradually being lost. It is less intense than restorative rehabilitation but often long term. Problems of senescence (old age), like difficulty with balance or flexibility, require this long-term approach.

Activities of daily living (ADLs) are the routine activities of personal care. The six basic ADLs are eating, bathing, dressing, grooming, toileting, and transferring. **Assistive devices** are designed to make ADLs easier to perform and help maintain the patient's independence. Examples of these devices include reachers and grabbers, easy-pull sock aids, long shoehorns, jar openers, and eating aids *(Figure 5.10)*. ADLs are also a measurement to assess **therapy** needs and monitor its effectiveness.

Instrumental activities of daily living (IADLs) relate to independent living. These activities include managing money, using a telephone, cooking, driving, shopping for groceries and personal items, and doing housework.

Amputations (LO 5.3 and 5.8)

Seventy-five percent of all amputations are performed on people over 65 years of age with **peripheral vascular disease (PVD)**. This includes complications from arteriosclerosis and diabetes. Most of these cases involve **below-the-knee amputations (BKAs).** On the other hand, war-time injuries, other physical trauma (e.g., crush injury), and infection may also require limb amputation.

Rehabilitation after amputation is an increasingly important component in rehabilitation programs. Immediately after surgery, the objectives of the rehabilitation team are to:

- Promote healing of the stump;
- Strengthen the muscles above the site of the amputation;
- Strengthen arm muscles to assist in ambulation or help with walking using a cane, crutches, or other assistive devices;
- Prevent **contractures** or tightening of the joints above the amputation (knee and hip for BKAs);
- Shrink the post-amputation stump with elastic cuffs or bandages to fit the socket of a temporary **prosthesis** *(Figure 5.11);* and
- Provide emotional, psychological, and family support.

Abbreviations

ADLs	activities of daily living
BKA	below-the-knee amputation
COTA	certified occupational therapy assistant
IADLs	instrumental activities of daily living
OT	occupational therapy
PM&R	physical medicine and rehabilitation
PVD	peripheral vascular disease

Keynote

- Coordinated multidisciplinary evaluation, management, and therapy add significantly to the chances of a good recovery.

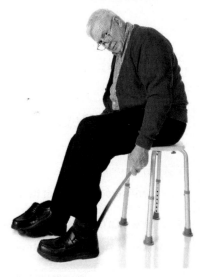

▲ **FIGURE 5.10**
Assistive Device for Dressing.

glenda/Shutterstock

▶ **FIGURE 5.11**
A Physical Therapist Explains to a Patient How to Use Her Prosthesis

Mood Board/Shutterstock

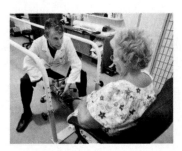

S = Suffix   P = Prefix   R = Root   R/CF = Combining Form

WORD	PRONUNCIATION	ELEMENTS		DEFINITION
amputation	am-pyu-**TAY**-shun	S/ R/	-ation *a process* amput- *prune*	Removal of a limb, part of a limb, or other projecting body part
assistive device	ah-**SIS**-tiv de-**VICE**	S/ R/ R/	-ive *nature of* assist- *aid, help* device *an appliance*	Tool, software, or hardware to assist in performing daily activities
contracture	kon-**TRAK**-chur	S/ R/	-ure *result of* contract- *pull together*	Muscle shortening due to spasm or fibrosis
occupational therapy	**OCK**-you-**PAY**-shun-al **THAIR**-ah-pee	S/ R/ R/	-al *pertaining to* occupation- *work* therapy *treatment*	Use of work and recreational activities to increase independent function
physiatry physiatrist	fih-**ZIE**-ah-tree fih-**ZIE**-ah-trist	 S/ R/ R/	Greek *science of nature* -ist *specialist* phys- *nature* -iatr- *treatment*	Physical medicine Specialist in physical medicine
physical medicine	**FIZ**-ih-cal **MED**-ih-sin	S/ R/	-al *pertaining to* physic- *body*	Diagnosis and treatment by means of remedial agents, such as exercises, manipulation, heat, etc.
prevention	pree-**VEN**-shun	S/ R/	-ion *action, condition* prevent- *prevent*	Process to prevent occurrence of a disease or health problem
prosthesis	**PROS**-thee-sis		Greek *an addition*	An artificial part to remedy a defect in the body
rehabilitation	**REE**-hah-bill-ih-**TAY**-shun	S/ P/ R/	-ion *action, condition* re- *again* -habilitat- *restore*	Therapeutic restoration of an ability to function as before
restorative rehabilitation	ree-**STOR**-ah-tiv **REE**-hah-bill-ih-**TAY**-shun	S/ R/	-ative *quality of* restor- *renew*	Therapy that promotes renewal of health and strength
vocation	voh-**KAY**-shun		Latin *a call, summons*	An occupation for which a person is trained or qualified to perform
vocational (adj)	voh-**KAY**-shun-al	S/	-al *pertaining to*	Pertaining to an occupation

EXERCISES

 Case Report 5.2

You are

. . . a **certified occupational therapist assistant** working in the Rehabilitation Unit at Fulwood Medical Center.

You are communicating with

. . . Mr. Ivan Postovich a 65-year-old print shop owner.

One year ago, Mr. Postovich had an elective left total-hip replacement for osteoarthritis. Four months later, he had a myocardial infarction. Two weeks ago, while on his exercise bike, he had a stroke. His right arm and leg were paralyzed, he lost his speech, and he had difficulty swallowing. He arrived in the Emergency Department within 90 minutes of the stroke and received **thrombolytic therapy** *(see Chapter 6).* Mr. Postovich is now receiving **physical therapy, occupational therapy,** and speech therapy in the inpatient Rehabilitation Unit. He is able to say some simple words and has begun to have voluntary movements in the affected arm and leg. Your roles are to help him regain function in his arm and leg and to monitor and record his progress.

A. Read *Case Report 5.2. Apply your knowledge of medical language to select the correct answer(s) for each question.* **LO 5.5 and 5.9**

1. Mr. Postovich needed a hip replacement due to:

   a. myocardial infarction   **b.** osteoarthritis   **c.** stroke   **d.** hemiplegia

2. What two major medical events did Mr. Postovich suffer recently? (choose two)

   a. stroke   **b.** muscle strain   **c.** rotator cuff tear   **d.** myocardial infarction

3. Which of the following are the goals of Mr. Postovich's rehabilitation? (choose all that apply)

   a. walk safely using an assistive device   **c.** restore his speech abilities

   b. prevent congestive heart failure   **d.** prevent a second stroke

4. Of his goals for rehabilitation, which one are you tasked with you helping him meet?

   a. walk safely using an assistive device   **c.** restore his speech abilities

   b. prevent congestive heart failure   **d.** prevent a second stroke

B. Deconstruct *the following medical terms into their word elements. Some terms will not have every element present. Fill in the chart.* **LO 5.1, 5.2, and 5.8**

Medical Term	Prefix	Root/CF	Suffix
therapeutic	1.	2.	3.
rehabilitation	4.	5.	6.
orthotic	7.	8.	9.
multidisciplinary	10.	11.	12.
orthotist	13.	14.	15.
assistive	16.	17.	18.

C. Deconstruct *the following terms:* **LO 5.1, 5.2, 5.6, and 5.8**

1. Prevention: _____ / _____
   R, R/CF   S

2. Contracture: _____ / _____
   R, R/CF   S

3. Restorative: _____ / _____
   R, R/CF   S

D. Identify *abbreviations that describe medical terms. Match the abbreviation in the first column to its correct description in the second column.* **LO 5.3**

_____   **1.** COTA   **a.** removal of the lower leg and foot

_____   **2.** ADL   **b.** a professional that assists people in improving their activities of daily living

_____   **3.** IADL   **c.** examples include toileting, brushing one's hair, brushing one's teeth

_____   **4.** PVD   **d.** examples include reachers, grabbers, and long shoehorns

_____   **5.** BKA   **e.** condition that is responsible for a large percentage of below-the-knee amputations

E. Utilize *the correct language of rehabilitation in the following paragraph. The word bank contains more terms than you need to use—some terms you may use more than once. When you have finished the exercise, proofread it again to see if it makes sense. Fill in the blanks.* **LO 5.2, 5.3, 5.8, and 5.9**

adapt	contracture	amputation(s)	prosthesis
amputee	assistive devices	elective	amputate
residual	PVD	assistive	protocol

Seventy-five percent of all (1) _____ are performed on patients over 65 years of age with (2) _____ complicating arteriosclerosis and diabetes. Loss of blood flow to a limb area produces necrotic tissue, which in time can become infected or gangrenous and makes the need for this procedure urgent, rather than (3) _____. _____ The decision to (4) _____ is a serious one and must be undertaken by a qualified surgeon.

The (5) _____ will require a physical therapist to help the patient learn to (6) _____ to the use of a (7) _____. Hopefully, there will be no muscle (8) _____ or (9) _____ pain after the surgery.

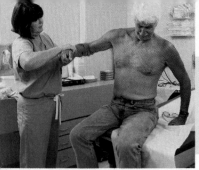

Rick Brady/McGraw Hill

Abbreviations

Bx	biopsy
CK	creatine kinase
CRP	C-reactive protein
CT	computed tomography
EMG	electromyography
MRI	magnetic resonance imaging
MSA	myositis specific antibodies

Section 5.5

Procedures and Pharmacology

Many different health professionals are involved in the diagnosis and treatment of disorders of muscles and tendons in their acute phase, primary care, and rehabilitation. It is essential to have a common language and understanding to ensure a high quality of patient care.

Diagnostic Procedures for Disorders of Muscles and Tendons (LO 5.7)

A medical history and physical examination are essential components of a diagnostic examination. Additional diagnostic tests include:

- **Blood tests.** Damaged muscles release **enzymes** such as **creatine kinase (CK)** and proteins such as myoglobin into the blood, and their levels can be measured. A C-reactive protein **(CRP)** is not specific for any disease process, but it indicates the presence of **inflammation**, and serial readings can be used to measure changes in inflammation.

- **Electromyography (EMG)** is a procedure in which an **electrode** needle is attached to the muscle to test, measure and record the electrical activity in that muscle as the muscle is contracted and relaxed.

- **Nerve conduction studies** also known as nerve conduction velocity testing are used to measure the speed at which motor or sensory nerves conduct impulses and also can show problems at the neuromuscular junction; for example, in myasthenia gravis.

- **Magnetic resonance imaging (MRI)** and **computed tomography (CT)** scan show detailed images of damage or disease in muscles.

- **Ultrasonography (US)** can identify tears and inflammation of tendons and involves no exposure to radiation, unlike MRI and CT scans.

- **Muscle biopsy (Bx)** is performed by removing a small piece of the abnormal muscle through a hollow needle or by small incision to be sent to the laboratory for examination and analysis.

- **Genetic testing** of blood or tissues can show the mutations in some of the genes that cause the different types of muscular dystrophy.

- **Myositis specific antibodies (MSA)** can confirm a diagnosis of **dermatomyositis** or **polymyositis.** Many of these antibodies have been identified and research is ongoing to define their significance.

WORD	PRONUNCIATION	ELEMENTS		DEFINITION
antibody	**AN**-tih-body	P/ R/	anti- *against* -body *substance*	Protein produced in response to an antigen
antimetabolite	**AN**-teh-meh-**TAB**-oh-lite	S/ P/ R/	-ite *pertaining to* anti- *against* -metabol- *change*	A substance that replaces or inhibits a specific part of a cell's normal metabolism
biopsy (**Note:** *one of the "o" 's is removed*)	**BY**-op-see	S/ R/	-opsy *to view* bio- *life*	Removal of a tissue from a living person for laboratory examination
corticosteroid	**KOR**-tih-koh-**STEHR**-oyd	S/ R/	-steroid *steroid* cortic/o- *from the cortex*	A hormone produced by the adrenal cortex
creatine kinase	**KREE**-ah-teen **KI**-nase	S/ R/ S/ R/	-ine *pertaining to* creat- *flesh* -ase *enzyme* kin- *motion*	Enzyme elevated in the plasma following heart muscle damage
electrode	ee-**LEK**-trode	S/ R/	-ode *way, road* electr- *electricity*	A device for conducting electricity
electromyography	ee-**LEK**-troh-my-**OG**-rah-fee	S/ R/CF R/CF	-graphy *process of recording* electr/o- *electricity* -my/o- *muscle*	Recording of electrical activity in a muscle
enzyme	**EN**-zime	P/ R/	en- *in* -zyme *fermenting*	Protein that induces change in other substances
immunosuppressive	**IM**-you-noh-suh-**PRESS**-iv	S/ R/CF R/	-ive *nature of* immun/o *immune response* -suppress- *press under*	Substance that causes failure of the immune system
inflammation	in-flah-**MAY**-shun	S/ P/ R/	-ation *process* in- *in* -flamm- *flame*	A basic complex of reactions in blood vessels and adjacent tissues in response to injury or abnormal stimulation
ultrasonography	**UL**-trah-soh-**NOG**-rah-fee	S/ P/ R/CF	-graphy *process of recording* ultra- *beyond* -son/o- *sound*	Delineation of deep structures using sound waves

Therapeutic Methods for Disorders of Muscles and Tendons (LO 5.8)

RICE (rest, ice, compression, and elevation) (*Figure 5.3*) is used in the acute phase for muscle and tendon strains and sprains (*Figure 5.12*).

- **Physical therapy (PT)** and **exercise** are important in the treatment of muscle diseases and involve **range of motion (ROM)** exercises to prevent contracture of joints, and exercises and resistance training to restore muscle mass and strength. **Physical therapists (PT)** create exercise plans while **physical therapy assistants (PTA)** work under the direction of the PT to assist the PT with the patient's rehabilitation process.

- There are no effective medications available for muscle cramps, although various supplementations may help relieve symptoms.

- **Medications** are used frequently in muscle diseases. Acetaminophen (*Tylenol*) and hydrocodone can be used for pain in the acute stages following injury, and nonsteroidal anti-inflammatory drugs (**NSAIDs**) are also often prescribed as part of the acute treatment regimen. For specific inflammatory myopathies, **oral corticosteroids** are often the first line of treatment, sometimes with the **anti-metabolite** drugs methotrexate. For patients who do not respond to standard treatments, **immunosuppressive** drugs can be used.

- **Surgical** treatments include **tendon reconstruction,** in which the two ends of a ruptured or torn tendon are **sutured** back together. In ligament injuries of the elbow joint in high-level, overhead-throwing athletes, such as baseball pitchers, reconstruction techniques and tendon grafting are often used with success.

- **Orthopedic appliances (orthotics)** such as braces and walkers are used during recovery from muscle and tendon injury.

Abbreviations

PT	physical therapy
ROM	range of motion
RICE	rest, ice, compression, and elevation

Keynote

Spasticity is a state of increased muscular tone with exaggeration of the tendon reflexes.

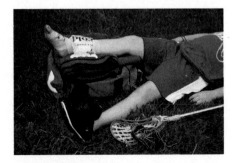

▲ **FIGURE 5.12**
RICE Treatment.

Rick Brady/McGraw Hill

WORD	PRONUNCIATION	ELEMENTS		DEFINITION
orthopedic (adj)	or-tho-**PEE**-dik	S/ R/CF R/	-ic *pertaining to* orth/o- *straight* -ped- *child*	Pertaining to the correction and cure of deformities and diseases of the musculoskeletal system; originally, most of the deformities treated were in children
orthopedist	or-tho-**PEE**-dist	S/	-ist *specialist*	Specialist in orthopedics
physical therapy *(also known as physiotherapy)* physiotherapy (syn)	**FIZ**-ih-cal **THAIR**-ah-pee **FIZ**-ee-oh-**THAIR**-ah-pee	S/ R/ R/ R/CF	-al *pertaining to* physic- *body* therapy *treatment* physi/o- *body*	Use of remedial processes to overcome a physical defect Another term for physical therapy
therapy	**THAIR**-ah-pee		Greek *medical treatment*	Systematic treatment of a disease, dysfunction, or disorder
therapeutic (adj)	**THAIR**-ah-**PYU**-tik	S/ R/	-ic *pertaining to* therapeut- *treatment*	Relating to the treatment of a disease or disorder
therapist	**THAIR**-ah-pist	S/ R/	-ist *specialist* therap- *treatment*	Professional trained in the practice of a particular therapy

Abbreviations

COX	cyclooxygenase enzymes
NSAID	nonsteroidal anti-inflammatory drug

Musculoskeletal Drugs (LO 5.8)

NSAIDs inhibit the two cyclooxygenase (**COX**) enzymes that are involved in producing the inflammatory process. They have **analgesic** and **antipyretic** effects and are used for treatment of tissue injury, pyrexia, rheumatoid arthritis, osteoarthritis, gout, and nonspecific joint and tissue pains. The three major **NSAIDs,** each of which is available OTC, are:

1. **Acetylsalicylic acid** (aspirin), which, in addition to the above effects and uses, also has an antiplatelet effect due to its inhibition of one of the COX enzymes; thus, it is often used in the prevention of heart attacks.

2. **Ibuprofen** *(Advil, Motrin,* and several other trade names), which acts by inhibiting both the COX enzymes, essential elements in the enzyme pathways involved in pain, inflammation, and fever. It is taken orally, but in 2009 an injectable form of ibuprofen *(Caldolor)* was approved for use. In some studies, ibuprofen has been associated with the prevention of Alzheimer and Parkinson diseases, but further studies are needed.

3. **Naproxen** *(Aleve* and many other trade names), which is taken orally once a day and also inhibits both the COX enzymes.

Acetaminophen (*Tylenol*), an active **metabolite** of phenacetin (not an NSAID), is a widely used OTC analgesic and antipyretic. It is used for the relief of minor aches and pains and is an **ingredient** in many cold and flu remedies.

Skeletal muscle relaxants are FDA approved for spasticity (baclofen, dantrolene, tizanidine) or for muscular conditions like multiple sclerosis (carisoprodol, chlorzoxazone, cyclobenzaprine, metaxalone, methocarbamol, orphenadrine). A commonly prescribed, specialized muscle relaxant, Carisoprodol (*Soma*), is known as a centrally acting muscle relaxant with additional pain-relieving properties because of its effect on the nervous system.

Anabolic steroids are similar to testosterone but have been altered so that their main effect is to cause skeletal muscle to hypertrophy. Although used illegally in many sports to increase muscle strength, their main use as a therapeutic agent is to restore muscle mass in patients who are recovering from significant muscle-affecting illness or injury. Steroids have noticeable, often irreversible side effects. These include stunted growth in adolescents, shrinking testes and reduced sperm counts, masculinization of women's bodies and over aggression. Long-term effects may be increased risk of heart attack and stroke, kidney failure, and liver tumors.

Word Analysis and Definition

S = Suffix   P = Prefix   R = Root   R/CF = Combining Form

WORD	PRONUNCIATION	ELEMENTS		DEFINITION
anabolic steroid	an-ah-**BOL**-ik **STER**-oyd	S/ R/ S/ R/	-ic *pertaining to* anabol- *to raise up* -oid *resembling* ster- *solid*	Prescription drug used by some athletes to increase muscle mass
analgesia	an-al-**JEE**-zee-ah	S/ P/ R/	-ia *condition* an- *without* -alges- *sensation of pain*	State in which pain is reduced
analgesic	an-al-**JEE**-zik	S/	-ic *pertaining to*	Agent that produces analgesia
antimetabolite	**AN**-teh-meh-**TAB**-oh-lite	S/ P/ R/	-ite *pertaining to* anti- *against* -metabol- *change*	A substance that replaces or inhibits a specific part of a cell's normal metabolism
antipyretic	**AN**-tee-pie-**RET**-ik	S/ P/ R/	-ic *pertaining to* anti- *against* -pyret- *fever*	Agent that reduces fever
ingredient	in-**GREE**-dee-ent	S/ P/ R/	-ent *end result, pertaining to* in- *in, into* -gredi- *to go*	An element in a mixture
metabolism	meh-**TAB**-oh-lizm	S/ R/	-ism *condition* metabol- *change*	The constantly changing physical and chemical processes in the cell
metabolite	meh-**TAB**-oh-lite	S/	-ite *associated with*	Any product of metabolism
orthotic	or-**THOT**-ik	S/ R/	-ic *pertaining to* orthot- *correct*	Orthopedic appliance to correct an abnormality
orthotist	or-**THOT**-ist	S/	-ist *specialist*	Specialist who makes and fits orthopedic appliances
statin	**STAH**-tin		Greek *stationary*	A class of drug used to lower blood cholesterol levels
thymectomy	thigh-**MEK**-toe-me	S/ R/	-ectomy *surgical excision* thym- *thymus gland*	Surgical removal of the thymus gland

EXERCISES

A. Determine the appropriate diagnostic test. *Read each scenario and determine which diagnostic test is indicated to support the diagnosis. Fill in the blanks. Not all answers will be used.*   **LO 5.3 and 5.8**

ESR   EMG   CK   Bx   MSA

1. The physician ordered a(n) _____ to determine the strength of muscular contraction in the patient with polio.

2. In order to support the diagnosis of myositis, a(n) _____ of the muscle tissue was ordered.

3. Dr. Novak sent a blood sample to the lab to have the medical technologist measure the _____ to determine if the patient had rhabdomyolysis.

4. The patient's blood was sent to the lab with an order for the medical technologist to measure the _____ in order to determine if the patient had a chronic inflammatory condition.

B. The following statement is written in the medical record. *Explain the meaning of the term in bold to your patient.*   **LO 5.7 and 5.10**

1. In order to diagnose the cause of a patient's muscle weakness, an **EMG** will be performed.

    a. test to measure the electrical activity of a muscle

    b. X-ray that views organs in different slices

    c. test to measure the presence of inflammatory substances in your blood

    d. examination of the genetic makeup of one's body

C. Select the correct medical term to complete the following questions. *Choose the correct answer.* LO 5.8

1. NSAIDS inhibit enzymes that are involved in the process.

    a. respiratory   b. digestive   c. urinary   d. pulmonary   e. inflammatory

2. The class of medication that treats muscle spasticity:

    a. COX inhibitor   b. analgesic   c. muscle relaxant   d. antipyretic

3. The analgesic listed that is NOT an NSAID:

    a. naproxen   b. ibuprofen   c. aspirin   d. paracetamol

4. An NSAID that is described as an effective pain reliever but can also be used long-term for its antiplatelet effects:

    a. orphenadrine   b. naproxen   c. acetaminophen   d. aspirin

5. A medication that lowers a fever is termed a(n):

    a. metabolite   b. antipyretic   c. ingredient   d. anti-inflammatory

D. Pronunciation is important whether you are saying the word or listening to a word from a coworker. Identify the proper pronunciation, of the following medical terms. Then, correctly spell the term. LO 5.1, 5.2, 5.6, and 5.7

1. The correct pronunciation for a breakdown of muscle fibers:

    a. rab-**DOH**-my-oh-**LIE**-sis   c. **RAB**-doh-my-**OL**-eye-sis

    b. **RAB**-doh-my-**OL**-ih-sis   d. rab-doh-**MY**-oh-**LIE**-sis

    Correctly spell the term: _____

2. The correct pronunciation for inflammation of a tendon and surrounding synovial sheath:

    a. **TEN**-oh-sine-oh-**VIE**-tis   c. **TEN**-oh-**SINE**-oh-vie-tis

    b. ten-**OH**-sine-oh-**VIE**-tis   d. **TEN**-oh-**SINE**-oh-**VIE**-tis

    Correctly spell the term: _____

3. The correct pronunciation for recording of electrical activity in a muscle:

    a. **EE**-lek-troh-my-og-**RAH**-fee   c. **UL**-trah-soh-**NOG**-rah-fee

    b. ee-**LEK**-troh-my-**OG**-rah-fee   d. ul-**TRAH**-soh-nog-**RAFEE**

    Correctly spell the term: _____

4. The correct pronunciation for the fibrous tissue that surrounds muscle and organs:

    a. **FIE**-ber   c. fash-**EE**-ah

    b. fie-**BER**   d. **FASH**-ee-ah

    Correctly spell the term: _____

5. The correct pronunciation for a condition that causes the muscles to shorten due to spasm:

    a. kon-**TRAK**-chur   c. **DERM**-at-oh-**MY**-oh-site-is

    b. **KON**-trak-tire   d. **DERM**-mah-toh-**MY**-oh-site-is

    Correctly spell the term: _____

6. Use of anabolic steroids can result in muscle:

    a. polymyalgia   c. atrophy

    b. strain   d. hypertrophy

    Correctly spell the term: _____

Additional exercises available in

connect

Chapter Review exercises, along with additional practice items, are available in Connect!

The Cardiovascular and Circulatory Systems

The Essentials of the Language of Cardiology

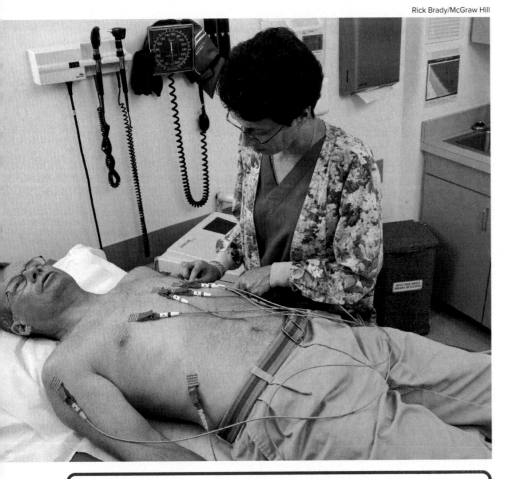

CHAPTER 6

Rick Brady/McGraw Hill

The health professionals involved in the diagnosis and treatment of problems with the cardiovascular system include the following:

- **Cardiologists** are medical doctors who specialize in disorders of the cardiovascular system.
- **Cardiothoracic surgeons** perform surgeries on the heart and other organs of the thoracic cavity.
- **Cardiovascular (cardiac) surgeons** are surgeons who specialize in surgery of the heart and the major blood vessels that surround the heart.
- **Vascular surgeons** specialize in the treatment of peripheral arteries and veins.
- **Cardiovascular technologists** and technicians assist physicians in the diagnosis and treatment of cardiovascular disorders.
- **Vascular technologists** are practitioners who assist physicians by performing diagnostic and monitoring procedures using ultrasound.
- **Cardiac sonographers** or echocardiographers are technologists who use ultrasound to observe the heart chambers, valves, and blood vessels.
- **Phlebotomists** or phlebotomy technicians assist physicians by drawing patient blood samples for laboratory testing.
- **Perfusionists** are highly trained health care professionals who operate the heart-lung machine during cardiac and other surgeries that require cardiopulmonary bypass.

Learning Outcomes

The health of a patient's heart—in fact, the entire cardiovascular system—will always be a factor in the diagnosis and treatment of any condition, no matter what discipline or setting you find yourself working in as a health professional. From routine blood pressure checks to ultrasounds to surgical procedures, the condition of a patient's cardiovascular system must be carefully monitored. In order to best understand, communicate, and document conditions affecting the heart, blood vessels, and blood, you need to be able to:

LO 6.1   Use roots, combining forms, suffixes, and prefixes to construct and analyze (deconstruct) medical terms related to the cardiovascular and circulatory systems.

LO 6.2   Spell and pronounce correctly medical terms and their plurals related to the cardiovascular and circulatory systems to communicate them with accuracy and precision in any health care setting.

LO 6.3   Define accepted abbreviations related to the cardiovascular and circulatory systems.

LO 6.4   Identify and describe the anatomy and physiology of the heart.

LO 6.5   Identify and describe the different circulatory systems.

LO 6.6   Identify and describe disorders and pathological conditions related to the cardiovascular system.

LO 6.7   Discuss the diagnostic and therapeutic procedures and pharmacologic agents used for cardiovascular and circulatory diseases and disorders.

LO 6.8   Identify health professionals involved in the care of patients with cardiovascular diseases and disorders.

LO 6.9   Apply your knowledge of the medical terms of the cardiovascular and circulatory systems to documentation, medical records, and medical reports.

LO 6.10   Translate the medical terms of the cardiovascular and circulatory systems into everyday language to communicate clearly with patients and their families.

Rick Brady/McGraw Hill

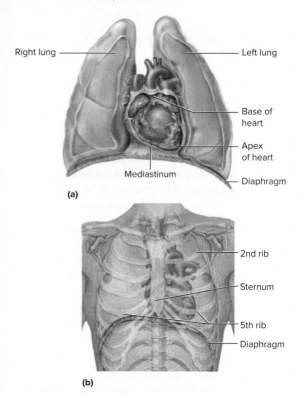

(a)

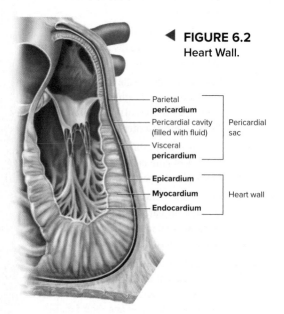

(b)

▲ **FIGURE 6.1** **Position of Heart in Thoracic Cavity.**
(a) Position of heart in mediastinum.
(b) Relationship of heart to sternum.

◀ **FIGURE 6.2**
Heart Wall.

Your heart is roughly the size of your fist, weighs approximately 8 to 10 ounces, and pumps around 2,000 gallons of blood each day. Your heart is always working. When your heart fails to work, your blood stops circulating, your tissues stop receiving oxygen and nutrients, your metabolic wastes accumulate, and your cells die.

Location of the Heart (LO 6.3 and 6.4)

The heart is located in the **thoracic cavity** between the lungs, in an area called the **mediastinum** *(Figure 6.1a)*. The heart is shaped like a blunt cone, pointing down and to the left. It rests at an angle with the majority of its mass to the left of the **sternum** *(Figure 6.1b)*.

Functions and Structure of the Heart (LO 6.4)

Functions of the Heart (LO 6.4)

In order to keep your body alive, your heart must work all the time, without stopping. Its three most important functions are to:

1. **Pump blood.** As your heart contracts, it generates pressure that moves your blood forward through your blood vessels.
2. **Route blood.** Your heart essentially has two pumps: one on the right side that sends blood through the **pulmonary** circulation of your lungs and back to the second pump on your left side, which sends blood through the **systemic** circulation of your body. Your heart valves make this one-way flow of blood possible.
3. **Regulate blood supply.** The changing metabolic needs of your tissues and organs—for example, when you exercise—are met by changes in the rate and force of your heart's contractions.

Structure of the Heart (LO 6.4)

The heart wall consists of three layers *(Figure 6.2)*:

1. **Endocardium**: Connective tissue lining the inside of your heart and in direct contact with blood.
2. **Myocardium**: **Cardiac** muscle cells that contract to enable your heart to pump blood.
3. **Epicardium**: An outer single layer of cells overlying a thin layer of connective tissue.

The **pericardium** is a double-layered connective tissue sac filled with fluid that surrounds and protects your heart. The **visceral** layer is the inner layer touching the heart, which folds over on itself, becoming the outer **parietal** layer.

WORD	PRONUNCIATION	ELEMENTS		DEFINITION
cardiac	**KAR**-dee-ak	S/ R/	-ac *pertaining to* cardi- *heart*	Pertaining to the heart
endocardium	EN-doh-**KAR**-dee-um	S/ P/ R/	-um *structure* endo- *inside* -cardi- *heart*	The inside lining of the heart
endocardial (adj)	EN-doh-**KAR**-dee-al	S/	-al *pertaining to*	Pertaining to the endocardium
epicardium	**EP**-ih-**KAR**-dee-um	S/ P/ R/	-um *structure* epi- *upon, above* -cardi- *heart*	The outer layer of the heart wall
epicardial (adj)	**EP**-ih-**KAR**-dee-al	S/	-al *pertaining to*	Pertaining to the epicardium
mediastinum	ME-dee-ass-**TIE**-num	S/ P/ R/	-um *structure* media- *middle* -stin- *partition*	Area between the lungs containing the heart, aorta, venae cavae, esophagus, and trachea
myocardium	**MY**-oh-**KAR**-dee-um	S/ R/CF R/	-um *structure* my/o- *muscle* -cardi- *heart*	Muscular layer of the heart
myocardial (adj)	my-oh-**KAR**-dee-al	S/	-al *pertaining to*	Pertaining to heart muscle
parietal (adj)	pah-**RYE**-eh-tal	S/ R/	-al *pertaining to* pariet- *wall*	Pertaining to the outer layer of the pericardium and the wall of any body cavity
pericardium (noun)	per-ih-**KAR**-dee-um	S/ P/ R/	-um *structure* peri- *around* -cardi- *heart*	A double layer of membranes surrounding the heart
pericardial (adj)	per-ih-**KAR**-dee-al	S/	-al *pertaining to*	Pertaining to the pericardium
pulmonary	**PULL**-moh-**NAIR**-ee	S/ R/	-ary *pertaining to* pulmon- *lung*	Pertaining to the lungs and their blood supply
sternum	**STIR**-num		Latin *the chest*	Long, flat bone forming the center of the anterior wall of the chest
thoracic cavity	**THOR**-ass-ik **KAV**-ih-tee	S/ R/	-ic *pertaining to* thorac- *chest* cavity, Latin *hollow*	Space within the chest containing the lungs, heart, esophagus, trachea, aorta, venae cavae, and pulmonary vessels
visceral (adj)	**VISS**-er-al	S/ R/	-al *pertaining to* viscer- *internal organs*	Pertaining to the internal organs
viscus viscera (pl)	**VISS**-kus **VISS**--er-ah		Latin *an internal organ*	Any single internal organ

The Heartbeat (LO 6.4)

The actions of the four heart chambers are coordinated. When the atria contract (atrial **systole**), the ventricles relax (ventricular **diastole**). When the atria relax (atrial diastole), the ventricles contract (ventricular systole). Then the atria and ventricles all relax briefly. This series of events is a complete cardiac cycle, or heartbeat.

Electrical Properties of the Heart (LO 6.3 and 6.4)

A small electrical current sustains your heartbeat rhythm through a conduction system *(Figure 6.3)*. Prior to the heart contraction, the electrical signal must be generated and conducted to the heart muscle. Here is how this conduction system works:

1. A small region of specialized muscle cells in the right atrium's **sinoatrial (SA) node** initiates the electrical signal that will cause your heartbeat. The SA node is the **pacemaker** of your heart's rhythm.

2. Electrical signals from the SA node spread out through the atria and rejoin at the **atrioventricular (AV) node.** The AV is the electrical gateway to the ventricles.

3. Electrical signals leave the AV node and travel to the ventricular myocardium where they stimulate the ventricular myocardium to contract, creating your heartbeat.

Abbreviations

AV	atrioventricular
SA	sinoatrial

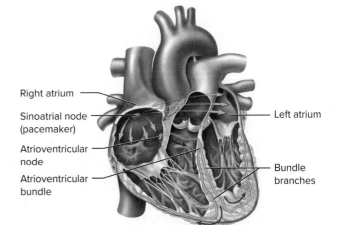

Right atrium

Sinoatrial node (pacemaker)

Atrioventricular node

Atrioventricular bundle

Left atrium

Bundle branches

▲ **FIGURE 6.3**   Cardiac Conduction System.

Word Analysis and Definition

S = Suffix   P = Prefix   R = Root   R/CF = Combining Form

WORD	PRONUNCIATION	ELEMENTS		DEFINITION
atrioventricular (AV)	A-tree-oh-ven-**TRICK**-you-lar	S/ R/CF R/	-ar *pertaining to* atri/o- *entrance, atrium* -ventricul- *ventricle*	Pertaining to both the atrium and the ventricle
diastole (noun) diastolic (adj)	die-**AS**-toe-lee die-as-**TOL**-ik	 S/ R/	Greek *dilation* -ic *pertaining to* diastol- *diastole*	Dilation of heart cavities, during which they fill with blood Pertaining to diastole
sinoatrial (SA) node	sigh-noh-**AY**-tree-al NODE	S/ R/CF R/	-al *pertaining to* sin/o- *sinus* -atri- *atrium*	The center of modified cardiac muscle fibers in the wall of the right atrium that acts as the pacemaker for the heart rhythm
sinus rhythm	**SIGH**-nus **RITH**-um		sinus Latin *channel, cavity* rhythm Greek *to flow*	The normal (optimal) heart rhythm arising from the sinoatrial node
systole (noun) systolic (adj)	**SIS**-toe-lee sis-**TOL**-ik	 S/ R/	Greek *contraction* -ic *pertaining to* systol- *systole, contraction*	Contraction of the heart muscle Pertaining to systole

Blood Flow through the Heart (LO 6.4)

Your heart *(Figures 6.4 and 6.5)* has four chambers through which your blood flows. These chambers are the:

1. Right **atrium**
2. Right **ventricle**
3. Left atrium
4. Left ventricle

Your right and left atria are separated by a thin muscle wall called the **interatrial septum**. Your right and left ventricles are divided by a thicker muscle wall called the **interventricular septum**. These septa prevent blood from flowing directly between the right and left sides of the heart. The heart has two sets of valves: the atrioventricular (A/V) valves and the semilunar valves.

- **AV valves** control blood flow between the atria and ventricles. They are open only when the atria are in systole, during ventricular diastole.

- **Semilunar valves** control blood flow between the right ventricle and pulmonary artery, and between the left ventricle and aorta. Semilunar valves open when the ventricles are in systole, during atrial diastole.

You have four valves that work together to ensure the correct flow of blood through your heart; on the right side are the **tricuspid** and **pulmonary** valves, and on the left side are the **mitral (bicuspid)** and **aortic** valves *(Figure 6.4).*

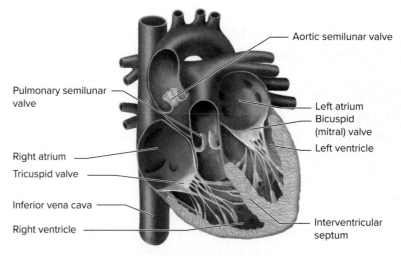

▲ **FIGURE 6.4**   Anatomy of the Heart.

Word Analysis and Definition

S = Suffix   P = Prefix   R = Root   R/CF = Combining Form

WORD	PRONUNCIATION		ELEMENTS	DEFINITION
atrium atria (pl) atrial (adj)	**A**-tree-um **A**-tree-ah **A**-tree-al	S/ R/ S/	-um *structure* atri- *entrance, atrium* -al *pertaining to*	Chamber where blood enters the heart on both the right and left sides Pertaining to the atrium
bicuspid	by-**KUSS**-pid	S/ P/ R/	-id *having a particular quality* bi- *two* -cusp- *point*	Having two points; a bicuspid heart valve has two flaps
deoxygenation deoxygenate (v)	dee-**OCK**-se-je—**NAY**-shun dee-**OCK**-se-je-nate	S/ P/ R/ S/	-ation *process* de- *without, removal from* -oxygen- *oxygen* -ate *composed of, pertaining to*	The removal of oxygen from a liquid (blood) To remove oxygen from a liquid (blood)
interatrial	**IN**-ter-**AY**-tree-al	S/ P/ R/	-al *pertaining to* inter- *between* -atri- *atrium*	Between the atria of the heart
interventricular (IV)	**IN**-ter-ven-**TRIK**-you-lar	S/ P/ R/	-ar *pertaining to* inter- *between* -ventricul- *ventricle*	Between the ventricles of the heart
mitral	**MY**-tral		Latin *turban*	Shaped like the headdress of a Catholic bishop
septum septa (pl)	**SEP**-tum **SEP**-tah		Latin *partition*	A thin wall dividing two cavities
tricuspid	try-**KUSS**-pid	S/ P/ R/	-id *having a particular quality* tri- *three* -cusp- *point*	Having three points; a tricuspid heart valve has three flaps
vena cava venae cavae (pfl)	**VEE**-nah **KAY**-vah **VEE**-nee **KAY**-vee	R/CF R/	ven/a *vein* cava *cave*	One of the two largest veins in the body The two largest veins in the body (superior and inferior venae cavae)
ventricle	**VEN**-trih-kel		Latin *small belly*	Chamber of the heart (pumps blood) or a cavity in the brain (produces cerebrospinal fluid)

EXERCISES

 ## Case Report 6.1

You are

. . . a cardiovascular technologist (CVT) employed by the **Cardiology** Department at Fulwood Medical Center. You have been called to the Emergency Department (ED) to perform an **electrocardiogram (ECG** or **EKG),** STAT.

You are communicating with

. . . Mr. Hank Johnson, a 64-year-old owner of a printing company. Eight months ago, he had a left total hip replacement. In the past 3 months, Mr. Johnson has returned to his daily workouts. This morning, while riding his exercise bike, he felt a tightness in his chest, but continued cycling. He developed pain in the center of his chest, radiating down his left arm and up into his jaw, and became **diaphoretic**. His personal trainer called 911. You perform the ECG and the automatic report describes various abnormalities with "ST elevation". As you remove the **electrodes**, Mr. Johnson complains that he is feeling faint and having difficulty breathing (dyspnea). You are the only person in the room.

A **myocardial infarction** (heart attack) is what was happening to Mr. Johnson when he first began having chest discomfort. The changes on the ECG showed this event. A doctor should be called.

For Mr. Johnson in the Emergency Department, the ECG (EKG) indicated that he was having an MI affecting the anterior wall of his left ventricle. The cardiovascular technician, who did not want to leave the patient alone, used the call system to obtain nursing and medical help.

A. Read *Case Report 6.1 and correctly answer the following questions. Fill in the blanks.*
LO 6.2, 6.3, 6.7, and 6.8

1. The following abbreviations all appear in the Case Report. Demonstrate your understanding of the abbreviations by providing the terms they represent.

   a. ECG _____

   b. ED _____

   c. CVT _____

B. Read *Case Report 6.1 and answer the following questions. Select the correct answer.* **LO 6.3, 6.4, 6.6, and 6.7**

1. Which specific place in Mr. Johnson's heart was affected by his MI?

   a. posterior wall of his left ventricle

   b. anterior wall of his left ventricle

   c. anterior wall of his right ventricle

   d. posterior wall of his left ventricle

2. What does an MI do to the living tissue in Mr. Johnson's heart?

   a. increases oxygen delivery to myocardial cells

   b. causes death to myocardial cells

   c. produces myocardial hypertrophy

   d. results in valve insufficiency

3. The device that indicated that Mr. Johnson was having an MI is the:

   a. echocardiograph

   b. automatic electronic defibrillator

   c. electrocardiogram

   d. patient call system

C. Read *Case Report 6.1 and correctly answer the following questions. Fill in the blanks.* **LO 6.1, 6.2, 6.3, 6.5, 6.6, and 6.7**

1. Based on the patient's ECG, what was his final diagnosis? _____

2. What is the abbreviation for this condition? _____

3. **Deconstruct** *Mr. Johnson's diagnosis. If the term does not have a particular element, insert N/A. Fill in the blanks.*

_____ / _____ / _____
    R/CF   R/CF   S

_____ / _____ / _____
      P   R/CF   S

D. Construct medical terms. *Provide the correct part to the term to correctly complete each sentence.* **LO 6.1 and 6.4**

1. The inside heart is termed the _____ /cardium.

2. The muscular part of the heart is termed the _____ /cardium.

3. The outer layer of the heart is termed the _____ /cardium.

4. The area between the upper chambers of the heart is termed inter/_____ /ar.

5. The area between the lower chambers of the heart is termed inter/_____ /ar.

E. Match *the correct element to its meaning.* **LO 6.1**

_____ **1.** atri/o   **a.** without

_____ **2.** -ar   **b.** contraction

_____ **3.** -ia   **c.** middle

_____ **4.** systol   **d.** entrance

_____ **5.** media-   **e.** condition

_____ **6.** a-   **f.** pertaining to

F. Spelling: *The following terms commonly occur in the cardiology department. Select the correct choice for the documentation.* **LO 6.2 and 6.4**

1. Blood in the pulmonary arteries is (deoxyginated/deoxygenated).

2. Her (sysstolic/systolic) blood pressure is dangerously high.

3. The (viscus/visceral) pericardium touches the heart.

4. The heart chamber is contracting during (systole/sysastole).

5. The (sinoatrial/synoatrial) node is the pacemaker for the heart rhythm.

G. Define *the words in bold using the correct medical term. Use the terms related to the function and structure of the heart to correctly complete each statement.*
LO 6.2, 6.4, and 6.5

The right side of the heart pumps blood through arteries to the **lungs** to pick up oxygen. The left side of the heart pumps blood through arteries to deliver oxygenated blood to the organs of each body **system.**

1. The right side of the heart pumps blood to the _____ circulation.

2. The left side of the heart pumps blood to the _____ circulation.

When learning how to ride a bike, children might first learn to ride a **three**-wheeled tricycle, and then learn to ride a **two**-wheeled bicycle.

When learning blood flow through the heart, students usually start with the right side of the heart and trace flow to the left side of the heart.

3. Blood returns from the systemic circulation and passes through the right-sided _____ /cuspid valve.

4. Blood returns from the pulmonary circulation and passes through the left-sided _____ /cuspid valve.

H. Plurals of medical terms *follow established rules. Apply these rules and change the singular form of each term to its plural form.* **LO 6.2**

1. Singular: **atrium** Plural: _____

2. Singular: **septum** Plural: _____

3. Singular: **vena cava** Plural: _____

4. Singular: **ventricle** Plural: _____

I. Meet lesson objectives *and use the language of cardiology to answer the following questions.* **LO 6.2 and 6.4**

1. Name the four chambers in the heart. _____

2. List the four valves in the heart. _____

3. What is the function of a valve? _____

4. What is the purpose of the systemic circulation? _____

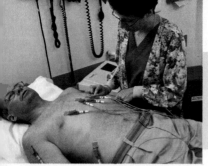

Rick Brady/McGraw Hill

Circulatory System (LO 6.5)

The circulatory system is made up of three categories of blood vessels:

• **arteries:** carry blood away from the heart

• **capillaries:** vessels that allow for gases, nutrients, and wastes to leave and enter the blood

• **veins:** carry blood back to the heart

There are two major **circulations:** the **pulmonary** and the **systemic** *(see Figure 6.6):*

1. The **pulmonary circulation** carries **deoxygenated** blood from the heart to the lungs *(see Chapter 8),* In the lungs, the carbon dioxide (CO_2) waste material from the body's tissues is exchanged for oxygen (O_2) from inhaled air *(Figure 6.5).* This **oxygenated** blood then travels through the pulmonary veins back to the left side of the heart.

2. The **systemic circulation** begins with the largest artery, the **aorta,** and ends with the largest veins, the **superior** and **inferior venae cavae.** Supplies oxygenated blood to every organ except the lungs, and then returns deoxygenated blood to the heart, which pumps it into the pulmonary circulation.

Functions of the Circulatory System (LO 6.5)

The circulatory system has the following three functions:

• **Transportation.** It carries oxygen, nutrients, hormones, and enzymes that **diffuse** from the blood into the cells. Waste products and carbon dioxide diffuse back from the cells into the circulatory system and are carried to the lungs, liver, and kidney for excretion.

• **Homeostasis maintenance.** The systemic circulation directs blood flow to the tissues to enable them to meet their metabolic needs.

• **Blood pressure regulation.** In the systemic circulation, the arteries' ability to expand and contract in coordination with the systole and diastole of the heartbeat maintains a steady flow of blood and blood pressure to the tissues.

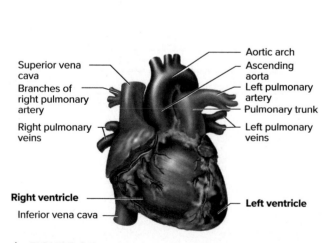

Superior vena cava
Branches of right pulmonary artery
Right pulmonary veins
Aortic arch
Ascending aorta
Left pulmonary artery
Pulmonary trunk
Left pulmonary veins
Right ventricle
Inferior vena cava
Left ventricle

▲ **FIGURE 6.5**
External Anatomy of the Heart: Frontal View.

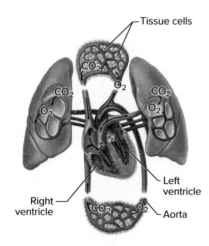

Tissue cells
CO_2
CO_2
O_2
CO_2
O_2
O_2
Right ventricle
CO_2
O_2
Left ventricle
Aorta

▲ **FIGURE 6.6**
Systemic and Pulmonary Circulations.

Blood Supply to Heart Muscle (LO 6.5)

Because your heart beats continually and forcefully, it requires an abundant supply of oxygen and nutrients. To meet this need, your cardiac muscle has its own blood circulation called the **coronary circulation** *(Figure 6.7)*. This system of arteries arises directly from the root of the **aorta**.

Arterioles, Capillaries, and Venules (LO 6.5)

Blood leaves the left ventricle through the aorta, the systemic circulation's largest artery. As the arteries branch farther away from the heart and distribute blood to specific organs, they become smaller, muscular vessels called **arterioles**. By contracting and relaxing, these arterioles are the primary controllers that help the body direct the amount of blood that the organs and structures receive.

From the arterioles, the blood flows into **capillaries** and **capillary beds** *(Figure 6.8)*. Red blood cells flow in single file through the small capillaries.

From the capillaries, tiny **venules** accept the blood and merge to form veins. The veins form reservoirs for blood. At any moment, 60% to 70% of the total blood volume is contained in the venules and veins.

Systemic Venous Circulation (LO 6.5)

There are three major types of veins:

1. **Superficial**, such as those you can see under the skin of your arms and hands;

2. **Deep**, which run parallel to arteries and drain the same tissues that the arteries supply; and

3. **Venous sinuses**, which are in the head and heart and have specific functions.

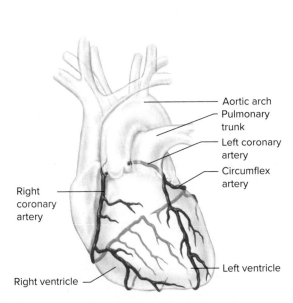

▲ **FIGURE 6.7** Coronary Arterial Circulation.

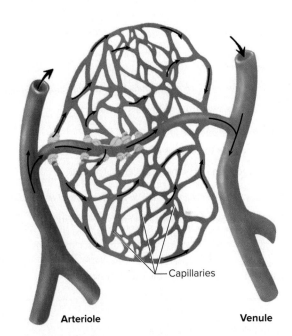

▲ **FIGURE 6.8** Capillary Bed.

Word Analysis and Definition

WORD	PRONUNCIATION		ELEMENTS	DEFINITION
aorta	a-**OR**-tuh		Greek *lift up*	Main trunk of the systemic arterial system
aortic (adj)	a-**OR**-tik	S/	-ic *pertaining to*	Pertaining to the aorta
		R/	aort- *aorta*	
artery	**AR**-ter-ee		Greek *artery*	Thick-walled blood vessel carrying oxygenated blood away from the heart
arterial	ar-**TEER**-ee-al	S/	-al *pertaining to*	Pertaining to an artery
		R/	arteri- *artery*	
arteriole	ar-**TEER**-ee-ole	S/	-ole *small*	Small terminal artery leading into the capillary network
		R/	arteri- *artery*	
capillary	**KAP**-ih-lair-ee	S/	-ary *pertaining to*	Minute blood vessel between the arterial and venous systems
capillaries	**KAP**-ih-lair-eez	R/	capill- *hairlike structure*	
coronary circulation	**KOR**-oh-nair-ee	S/	-ary *pertaining to*	Blood vessels supplying the heart muscle
	SER-kyu-**LAY**-shun	R/	coron- *crown, coronary*	
		S/	-ion *action, condition*	
		R/	circulat- *circular route*	
diffuse (verb)	di-**FUZE**		Latin *to pull in different directions*	To disseminate or spread out
homeostasis	hoh-mee-oh-**STAY**-sis	S/	-stasis *stand still*	Maintaining the stability, or equilibrium, of a system or the body's internal environment
		R/CF	home/o- *the same*	
vein	**VANE**		Latin *vein*	Blood vessel carrying blood toward the heart
venous (adj)	**VEE**-nuss	S/	-ous *pertaining to*	Pertaining to a vein
		R/	ven- *vein*	
venule	**VEN**-yule or **VEEN**-yule	S/	-ule *small*	Small vein leading from the capillary network

Exercises

A. Build *your knowledge of the elements and terms that make up the language of the cardiovascular system. Fill in the blanks.* **LO 6.2 and 6.6**

1. A small vein leading away from a capillary network: _____ .

2. To disseminate or spread out: _____

3. State of equilibrium in the body is called _____ .

4. The two largest veins in the body are collectively called _____ .

B. Construct *the correct medical term to match the definition. If the term does not have a particular element, insert N/A. Fill in the blanks.* **LO 6.1, 6.2, and 6.7**

1. Minute blood vessel between the arterial and venous systems:

_____ / _____ / _____

          P   R/CF   S

2. Small terminal artery leading into the capillary network:

_____ / _____ / _____

          P   R/CF   S

3. State of equilibrium in the environment:

_____ / _____ / _____

          P   R/CF   S

4. Small vein leading from the capillary network:

_____ / _____ / _____

          P   R/CF   S

Section 6.3

Disorders and Diseases of the Heart and Circulatory System

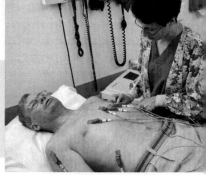

Rick Brady/McGraw Hill

Disorders of the Heart (LO 6.6)

Abnormal Heart Rhythms (LO 6.5 and 6.6)

Sinus rhythm is the term used to describe a normal heartbeat, where normal electrical conduction leads to a ventricular rate of about 60 to 80 beats per minute. A heart rate slower than 60 is called **bradycardia** *(Figure 6.9).* A heart rate faster than 100 is called **tachycardia** *(Figure 6.10).* An abnormal cardiac rhythm is called an **arrhythmia** or a **dysrhythmia.**

Six types of arrhythmias are commonly seen:

1. **Premature beats** occur most often in elderly people and are usually associated with caffeine and stress.

2. **Atrial fibrillation (A-fib)** occurs when the two atria quiver rather than contract correctly to pump blood. This causes blood to pool in the atria and sometimes clot.

3. **Ventricular tachycardia (V-tach)** is a rapid heartbeat occurring in the ventricles often resulting in loss of pulse.

4. **Ventricular arrhythmias** include:

   a. **Premature ventricular contractions (PVCs),** which result when extra impulses arise from a ventricle; and

   b. **Ventricular fibrillation (V-fib),** which occurs when the ventricles lose control, quivering instead of pumping.

5. **Heart block** occurs when interference in cardiac electrical conduction prevents atrial contractions from coordinating with ventricular contractions.

6. **Palpitations** are brief but unpleasant sensations of a rapid or irregular heartbeat. They can be brought on by exercise, anxiety, and stimulants like caffeine.

Abbreviations

A-fib	atrial fibrillation
PVC	premature ventricular contraction
V-fib	ventricular fibrillation
V-tach	ventricular tachycardia

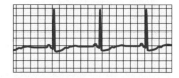

▲ **FIGURE 6.9**
Bradycardia.

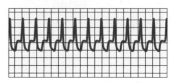

▲ **FIGURE 6.10**
Tachycardia.

Word Analysis and Definition

S = Suffix   P = Prefix   R = Root   R/CF = Combining Form

WORD	PRONUNCIATION		ELEMENTS	DEFINITION
arrhythmia (**Note:** *double "rr"*)	a-**RITH**-me-ah	S/ P/ R/	-ia *condition* a- *without* -rrhythm- *rhythm*	Condition when the heart rhythm is abnormal
bradycardia	**BRAYD**-ee-**KAR**-dee-ah	S/ R/ P/	-ia *condition* -card- *heart* brady- *slow*	Condition of slow heart beat
dysrhythmia (**Note:** *single "r"*)	dis-**RITH**-me-ah	S/ P/ R/	-ia *condition* dys- *bad, difficult* -rhythm- *rhythm*	An abnormal heart rhythm
murmur	**MUR**-mur		Latin *low voice*	Abnormal heart sound heard with a stethoscope when a valve closes or opens abnormally
fibrillation	fi-brih-**LAY**-shun	S/ R/	-ation *a process* fibrill- *small fiber*	Uncontrolled quivering or twitching of the heart muscle
palpitation	pal-pih-**TAY**-shun	S/ R/	-ation *a process* palpit- *throb*	Forcible, rapid beat of the heart felt by the patient
tachycardia	**TAK**-i h-**KAR**-dee-ah	S/ R/ P/	-ia *condition* -card- *heart* tachy- *rapid*	Condition of rapid heart beat
vital signs (VS)	**VI**-tal SIGNS		vital Latin *life* signs Latin *mark*	A procedure during a physical examination in which temperature (T), pulse (P), respirations (R), and blood pressure (BP) are measured to assess general health and cardiorespiratory function

Disorders of Heart Valves (LO 6.3 and 6.6)

The heart valves can malfunction in two basic ways. Malfunctions most often occur in the heart's left side.

1. **Stenosis**: The valve cannot open fully, and its opening is narrowed (constricted). Because blood cannot flow freely through the valve, it accumulates in the chamber behind the valve, causing an increase in pressure in the region immediately prior to the stenosis.

2. **Incompetence** or **insufficiency** is a condition where the heart valve cannot close fully, allowing blood to leak or **regurgitate** (flow back) through the valve to the heart chamber from which it came.

Mitral valve stenosis can occur following rheumatic fever or as a result of a birth defect. Because the blood cannot flow freely through the valve, the left atrium experiences a constant accumulation of excess blood and becomes dilated (enlarged). Eventually, chronic heart failure results.

Mitral valve prolapse (MVP) occurs when the cusps of the valve bulge back into the left atrium when the left ventricle contracts. This allows blood to flow back into the atrium.

Aortic valve stenosis is common in the elderly when the valves become calcified due to atherosclerosis. Blood flow into the systemic circulation is diminished, leading to dizziness and fainting. The left ventricle dilates, **hypertrophies**, ceases to beat strongly, and ultimately fails.

Aortic valve insufficiency initially produces few symptoms other than a **murmur**. Eventually the left ventricle is unable to cope with the excess volume of blood and fails. (*Figure 6.11* enables you to review the locations of the valves and chambers.)

Cor pulmonale is failure of the right ventricle to pump properly. Almost any chronic lung disease causing low blood oxygen (hypoxia) can cause this disorder. Malfunctions of the valves on the right side of the heart are much less common than those on the left side.

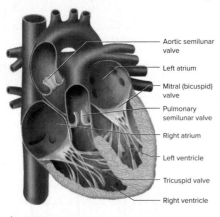

Aortic semilunar valve

Left atrium

Mitral (bicuspid) valve

Pulmonary semilunar valve

Right atrium

Left ventricle

Tricuspid valve

Right ventricle

▲ **FIGURE 6.11** Heart Valves.

Word Analysis and Definition

S = Suffix P = Prefix R = Root R/CF = Combining Form

WORD	PRONUNCIATION	ELEMENTS		DEFINITION
cardiomegaly	KAR-dee-oh-MEG-ah-lee	S/ R/CF	-megaly *enlargement* cardi/o- *heart*	Enlargement of the heart
cardiomyopathy	KAR-dee-oh-my-OP-ah-thee	S/ R/CF R/CF	-pathy *disease* cardi/o -*heart* -my/o- *muscle*	Disease of the heart muscle, the myocardium
cor pulmonale	KOR pul-moh-NAH-lee	 S/ R/	cor Latin *heart* -ale *pertaining to* pulmon- *lung*	Right-sided heart failure arising from chronic lung disease
endocarditis (**Note:** The extra "i" from the root *cardi* is dropped when joined to the suffix *-itis.*)	EN-doh-kar-DIE-tis	S/ P/ R/	-itis *inflammation* endo- *within* -cardi- *heart*	Inflammation of the lining of the heart
exudate	EKS-you-date	S/ P/ R/	-ate *pertaining to* ex- *out of* -sud- *sweat*	Fluid that has passed out of a tissue or capillaries as a result of inflammation or injury
hypertrophy (can be a noun or a verb)	high-PER-troh-fee	P/ R/	hyper- *above, excessive* -trophy *development*	Increase in size, but not in number, of an individual tissue element
incompetence (**Note:** *Same as insufficiency*)	in-KOM-peh-tense	S/ P/ R/	-ence *quality of* in- *not* -compet- *strive together*	Failure of a valve to close completely
insufficiency (**Note:** *Same as incompetence*)	in-suh-FISH-en-see	S/ P/ R/CF	-ency *quality of* in- *not* -suffic/i- *enough*	Lack of completeness of function; e.g., a heart valve that fails to close properly
myocarditis (**Note:** The extra "i" from the root *cardi* is dropped when joined to the suffix *-itis.*)	MY-oh-kar-DIE-tis	S/ R/CF R/	-itis *inflammation* my/o- *muscle* -cardi- *heart*	Inflammation of the heart muscle
pericarditis (**Note:** The extra "i" from the root *cardi* is dropped when joined to the suffix *-itis.*)	PER-ih-kar-DIE-tis	S/ P/ R/	-itis *inflammation* peri- *around* -cardi- *heart*	Inflammation of the pericardium, the covering of the heart
prolapse	pro-LAPS		Latin a *falling*	An organ slips out of its normal position
regurgitate	ree-GUR-jih-tate	S/ P/ R/	-ate *pertaining to* re- *back* -gurgit- *flood*	To flow backward; e.g., blood through a heart valve
stenosis	ste-NOH-sis	S/ R/CF	-sis *abnormal condition* sten/o- *narrow*	Narrowing of a canal or passage, e.g., of a heart valve
tamponade	tam-poh-NAID	S/ R/	-ade *a process* tampon- *plug*	Pathologic compression of an organ, such as the heart

Disorders of the Heart Wall (LO 6.3 and 6.6)

Endocarditis is an inflammation of the heart's internal lining, which is usually secondary to an infection elsewhere. Certain bacterial or fungal infections, intravenous drug use, and a pre-existing heart valve abnormality are main causes of endocarditis.

Myocarditis is an inflammation of the heart muscle. Although a rare condition overall, myocarditis can be caused by a bacterial, viral, or fungal infection.

Pericarditis is inflammation of the covering (pericardium) of the heart. The inflammation causes an **exudate** (pericardial effusion) to be released into the pericardial space between the two layers of the pericardium. This interferes with the heart's ability to contract and expand normally, which reduces cardiac output **(CO)** and leads to a life-threatening condition called **cardiac tamponade.**

Cardiomyopathy is a weakening of the heart muscle that causes inadequate pumping. This causes the heart to enlarge (**cardiomegaly**) and leads to heart failure.

Coronary Artery Disease (CAD) (LO 6.3 and 6.5)

Coronary artery disease occurs when the coronary arteries supplying blood to the myocardium are constricted by **atherosclerotic plaques** called **atheroma** (compare *Figure 6.12a to 6.12b*. This reduces the blood supply to the cardiac muscle. Platelet clumping can occur on the plaque and form a blood clot **(coronary thrombosis). Atherosclerosis** is the most common form of **arteriosclerosis** (hardening of the arteries) and can lead to **arteriosclerotic** heart disease **(ASHD).**

Angina pectoris (pain in the chest on exertion) is often the first symptom of a reduced oxygen supply to the myocardium. **Myocardial infarction (MI)** is the death of myocardial cells, caused by the lack of blood supply **(ischemia)** when an artery eventually becomes blocked **(occluded).** Signs of a MI include **diaphoresis** and pain radiating up the jaw and arm. Along with chest pain, most individuals also experience dizziness and nausea. If the ischemia is not reversed within 4 to 6 hours, the myocardial cells die **(necrosis).**

Shock is a life-threatening condition that occurs when the body is not getting sufficient blood flow; this can damage multiple organs. A classification of shock includes:

- **Cardiogenic shock** occurs when the heart fails to pump blood effectively through the body's organs and tissues.
- **Hypovolemic shock** occurs from a loss of blood volume, often due to excessive bleeding (hemorrhage) or dehydration.
- **Anaphylactic shock** is caused by a severe allergic reaction.
- **Septic shock** is caused by a severe infection.
- **Neurogenic shock** is associated with damage to the nervous system.

Cardiac arrest is the sudden cessation of cardiac activity that often results from **anoxia** (lack of oxygen in the body tissues). Most patients show **asystole** (no heartbeat) on the cardiac monitor after the heart's rhythm disturbance worsens *(Figure 6.13).* Immediate cardiopulmonary resuscitation **(CPR)** is required for patients in cardiac arrest.

Abbreviation

CO   cardiac output

Keynotes

- Risk factors for CAD include:
  - Heredity
  - Age
  - Obesity
  - Lack of exercise
  - Tobacco
  - Diabetes mellitus
  - Stress
  - High blood pressure
  - Elevated serum cholesterol
- All these risk factors—except heredity and age—can be reduced by lifestyle changes.

Abbreviations

ASHD	arteriosclerotic heart disease
CAD	coronary artery disease
MI	myocardial infarction
CPR	cardiopulmonary resuscitation

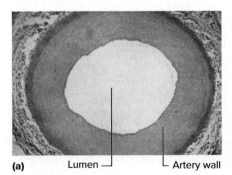

(a) Lumen ⌐ ⌐ Artery wall

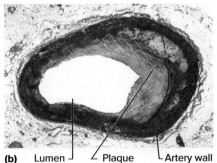

(b) Lumen ⌐ ⌐ Plaque ⌐ Artery wall

▲ **FIGURE 6.12** Arterial Structure.
(a) Normal coronary artery.
(b) Advanced atherosclerosis.

a. Choksawatdikorn/Shutterstock b. Kateryna Kon/Shutterstock

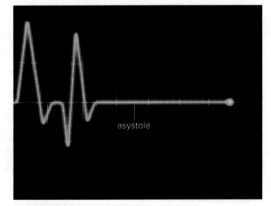

asystole

▲ **FIGURE 6.13** Electrocardiogram (ECG) Showing Asystole.

angelhell/iStock/Getty Images

WORD	PRONUNCIATION		ELEMENTS	DEFINITION
angina pectoris	an-**JUH**-nuh **PEK**-tor-iss		**angina** Greek *strangling* **pectoris** Latin *chest*	Condition of severe pain in the chest due to coronary heart disease
anoxia (noun)	an-**OCK**-see-ah	S/ P/ R/	**-ia** *condition* **an-** *without* **-ox-** *oxygen*	Without oxygen
anoxic (adj)	an-**OCK**-sik	S/	**-ic** *pertaining to*	Pertaining to or suffering from lack of oxygen
arteriosclerosis	ar-**TIER**-ee-oh-skler-**OH**-sis	S/ R/CF R/CF	**-sis** *abnormal condition* **arteri/o-** *artery* **-scler/o-** *hardness*	Hardening of the arteries
arteriosclerotic (adj)	ar-**TIER**-ee-oh-skler-**OT**-ik	S/	**-tic** *pertaining to*	Pertaining to or affected by arteriosclerosis
asystole	a-**SIS**-toe-lee	P/ R/CF	**a-** *without* **-systol/e** *contraction*	Absence of the heart's electrical activity and contractions
atheroma (plaque)	**ATH**-er-**OH**-mah	S/ R/	**-oma** *tumor, mass* **ather-** *porridge, gruel*	Fatty deposit in the lining of an artery
atherosclerosis	**ATH**-er-oh-skler-**OH**-sis	S/ R/CF R/CF	**-sis** *abnormal condition* **ather/o-** *porridge, gruel* **-scler/o-** *hardness*	Hardening of the arteries due to atheroma (plaque)
cardiogenic	**KAR**-dee-oh-**JEN**-ik	S/ R/CF R/	**-ic** *pertaining to* **cardi/o-** *heart* **-gen-** *produce*	Of cardiac origin
diaphoresis (noun)	**DIE**-ah-foh-**REE**-sis	S/ R/	**-esis** *condition* **diaphor-** *sweat*	Sweat, perspiration, or sweaty
diaphoretic (adj)	**DIE**-ah-foh-**RET**-ic	S/	**-etic** *pertaining to*	Pertaining to sweat or perspiration
hypovolemia	**HIGH**-poh-vo-**LEE**-me-ah	S/ S/ P/ R/	**-emia** *a blood condition* **-emic** *pertaining to a blood condition* **hypo-** *below* **-vol-** *volume*	Decreased blood volume in the body
hypovolemic (adj)	**HIGH**-poh-vo-**LEE**-mik	S/	**-ic** *pertaining to*	Pertaining to a decreased blood volume in the body
infarct	in-**FARKT**	P/ R/	**in-** *in* **-farct-** *area of dead tissue*	Area of tissue cell death resulting from an abnormal decrease in blood supply
infarction	in-**FARKT**-shun	S/	**-ion** *action, condition*	Sudden blockage of an artery
ischemia	is-**KEY**-me-ah	S/ R/	**-emia** *a blood condition* **isch-** *to keep back*	Lack of blood supply to a tissue
ischemic (adj)	is-**KEY**-mik	S/	**-emic** *pertaining to a blood condition*	Pertaining to or affected by the lack of blood supply to a tissue
necrosis	neh-**KROH**-sis	S/ R/	**-osis** *condition* **necr-** *death*	Pathologic death of cells or tissue
necrotic (adj)	neh-**KROT**-ik	S/	**-tic** *pertaining to*	Pertaining to or affected by necrosis (death)
occlude (verb)	oh-**KLUDE**		Latin *to close*	To close, plug, or completely obstruct
occlusion (noun)	oh-**KLU**-zhun			A complete obstruction
plaque	PLAK		French a *plate*	Patch of abnormal tissue
thrombosis	throm-**BOH**-sis	S/ R/	**-osis** *abnormal condition* **thromb-** *clot*	Formation of a clot (thrombus)

Keynotes

- Hypertension is the major cause of heart failure, stroke, and kidney failure.
- The risk factors for hypertension are:
  - Overweight
  - Alcohol
  - Lack of exercise
  - Tobacco
  - Stress
- All these risk factors can be reduced by lifestyle changes.

Abbreviation

HTN   hypertension

Hypertensive Heart Disease (LO 6.3 and 6.6)

Hypertension (HTN), the most common cardiovascular disorder in this country, affects more than half of the adult population. It results from a prolonged elevated blood pressure in the arteries which forces the ventricles to work harder to pump blood.

High blood pressure is indicated by a blood pressure reading of 130/80 mmHg (millimeters of mercury) or higher. A normal blood pressure is below 120/80 mmHg. The top number, or systolic reading, reflects the blood pressure when the heart is contracting. The bottom number, or diastolic reading, reflects the blood pressure when the heart is relaxed between contractions.

Primary or **essential hypertension** is the most common type of hypertension. Its cause (etiology) is unknown (**idiopathic**).

Secondary hypertension results from other diseases like kidney disease, atherosclerosis, and hyperthyroidism.

Malignant hypertension is a rare, severe, life-threatening form of hypertension that involves a sudden extreme increase in blood pressure causing organ damage. Aggressive intervention is mandatory to quickly reduce the blood pressure.

Congestive Heart Failure (CHF) (LO 6.3 and 6.6)

CHF occurs when the heart is unable to produce enough cardiac output to meet the body's metabolic needs, and the blood backs up to congest the lungs. The most common conditions leading to CHF are:

- Cardiac ischemia
- Severe hypertension
- Valvular regurgitation
- Aortic stenosis
- Cardiomyopathy

Congenital Heart Disease (CHD) (LO 6.3 and 6.6)

CHD is the result of an abnormal development of the heart in the fetus. Common **congenital** defects or abnormalities can usually be surgically repaired, and can include the following:

1. **Atrial septal defect (ASD)** is a hole in the interatrial septum *(Figure 6.14).*
2. **Ventricular septal defect (VSD)** is a gap in the interventricular septum *(Figure 6.14).*
3. **Patent ductus arteriosus (PDA)** is a pathway between the pulmonary artery and aorta that arises from a failure of the ductus arteriosus (a normal blood vessel in the fetus) to close within 24 hours of birth.
4. **Coarctation of the aorta** is a narrowing of the aorta anywhere along its length. This causes **hypertension** in the arms prior to the narrowing and **hypotension** in the lower limbs and organs (like the kidney) beyond the narrowing.
5. **Tetralogy of Fallot (TOF)** is a **syndrome** in which four congenital heart defects prevent enough blood from reaching the lungs. TOF occurs in about 5 out of every 10,000 newborns. Babies and children with TOF have episodes of **cyanosis** and are often called "blue babies." Treatment is with open heart surgery soon after birth or in infancy.

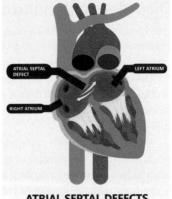

ATRIAL SEPTAL DEFECTS

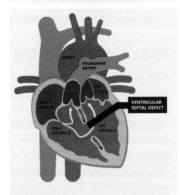

VENTRICULAR SEPTAL DEFECT

▲ **FIGURE 6.14** Atrial and Ventricular Septal Defects.

Pepermpron/Shutterstock

Word Analysis and Definition

S = Suffix   P = Prefix   R = Root   R/CF = Combining Form

WORD	PRONUNCIATION	ELEMENTS		DEFINITION
coarctation	koh-ark-**TAY**-shun	S/ R/	-ation *process* coarct- *press together, narrow*	Constriction or stenosis, particularly of the aorta
congenital	kon-**JEN**-ih-tal	S/ P/ R/	-al *pertaining to* con- *together, with* -genit- *bring forth*	Present at birth, either inherited or due to an event during gestation up to the moment of birth
cyanosis	sigh-ah-**NO**-sis	S/ R/	-osis *condition* cyan- *dark blue*	Blue discoloration of the skin, lips, and nail beds due to low blood oxygen
defect	**DEE**-fect		Latin *to lack*	An absence, malformation, or imperfection
hypertension	**HIGH**-per-**TEN**-shun	S/ P/ R/	-ion *condition, action* hyper- *excessive* -tens- *pressure*	Persistent high arterial blood pressure
hypotension	**HIGH**-poh-**TEN**-shun	P/	hypo- *low*	Persistent low arterial blood pressure
idiopathic	**ID**-ih-oh-**PATH**-ik	S/ R/CF R/	-ic *pertaining to* idi/o- *unknown* -path- *disease*	Pertaining to a disease of unknown etiology
patent ductus arteriosus (PDA) (Note: This term is composed only of roots.)	**PAY**-tent **DUK**-tus ar-**TIER**-ee-**OH**-sus		patent Latin *lie open* ductus Latin *leading* arteriosus Latin *artery*	An open, direct channel between the aorta and the pulmonary artery in the newborn
syndrome	**SIN**-drohm	P/ R/	syn- *together* -drome *running*	Combination of signs and symptoms associated with a particular disease process
tetralogy of Fallot (TOF)	te-**TRA**-loh-jee of fah-**LOW**	P/ R/	tetra- *four* -logy *study of* Etienne-Louis Fallot, French physician, 1850–1911	Set of four congenital heart defects occurring together

Abbreviations

DVT   deep vein thrombosis
PVD   peripheral vascular
        disease

Keynote

• Disorders of the systemic arterial
  and venous systems are grouped
  under the term peripheral vascular
  disease (PVD).

Disorders of Veins (LO 6.3 and 6.6)

Our veins and arteries can be prone to certain disorders, such as a DVT experienced by patients with PVD. **Phlebitis** is an inflammation of a vein. There are many causes for phlebitis, including venous infections and the presence of an intravenous (IV) catheter.

Thrombophlebitis is an inflammation of the lining of a vein, allowing clots (**thrombi**) to form.

Deep vein thrombosis (DVT) is a thrombus formation in a deep vein. The increased pressure in the capillaries due to back pressure from the blocked blood flow in the veins creates a collection of fluid in the tissues called **edema**.

A major complication of thrombus (clot) formation is that a piece of the clot can break off (**embolus**) and be carried in the bloodstream to another organ where it can block blood flow (**thromboembolism**). The embolus often lodges in the lungs, causing a pulmonary embolus and decreasing circulation to the lungs *(see Chapter 8)*.

Varicose veins are superficial veins that have lost their elasticity and appear swollen and tortuous *(Figure 6.15)*. Their valves become incompetent, and blood flows backward and pools. Smaller, more superficial varicose veins are called spider veins. **Collateral** circulations develop to take the blood through alternative routes.

Disorders of Arteries (LO 6.3 and 6.6)

An **aneurysm** is a localized **dilation** of an artery, and this commonly occurs in the abdominal aorta *(Figure 6.16)*.

Aneurysms can **rupture**, leading to severe bleeding and hypovolemic shock.

Intracranial aneurysms are an important cause of bleeds into the cranial cavity and brain tissue.

Thromboangiitis obliterans (Buerger disease) is an inflammatory disease of the arteries with clot formation, usually in the legs. The occlusion of arteries and impaired circulation lead to intermittent pain when walking **(claudication),** and a person will often limp to compensate.

Raynaud's disease is characterized by episodes of spasm (following exposure to cold) of the small arteries supplying the fingers, hands, and feet. It can be associated with connective tissue disorders like scleroderma and lupus.

Carotid artery disease affects the carotid arteries—the two major arteries supplying the brain, which can be affected by arteriosclerosis and the deposition of plaque, placing the patient at risk for a stroke.

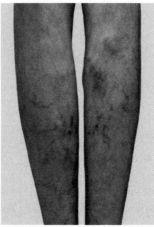

▲ **FIGURE 6.15** Varicose
Veins of the Leg.

Marina113/iStock/Getty Images

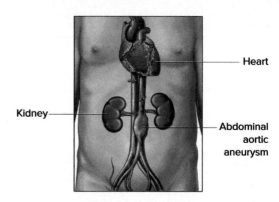

▲ **FIGURE 6.16** Diagram of an Abdominal
Aortic Aneurysm.

Word Analysis and Definition

WORD	PRONUNCIATION	ELEMENTS		DEFINITION
aneurysm	**AN**-yur-izm		Greek *dilation*	Circumscribed dilation of an artery or cardiac chamber
claudication	klaw-dih-**KAY**-shun	S/ R/	-ation *process* claudic- *limping*	Intermittent leg pain often causing limping
collateral	koh-**LAT**-er-al	S/ P/ R/	-al *pertaining to* col- *before* -later- *at the side*	Situated at the side, often to bypass an obstruction
edema edematous (adj)	ee-**DEE**-mah ee-**DEM**-ah-tus	S/ R/	Greek *swelling* -tous *pertaining to* edema- *swelling, edema*	Excessive accumulation of fluid in cells and tissues Pertaining to or marked by edema
pitting edema	**PIT**-ing ee-**DEE**-mah			Edema that maintains indentations made by applying pressure to the area for a time
embolus emboli (pl)	**EM**-boh-lus **EM**-boh-lie		Greek *plug, stopped*	Detached piece of thrombus, a mass of bacteria, quantity of air, or foreign body that blocks a blood vessel
peripheral	peh-**RIF**-er-al	S/ R/	-al *pertaining to* peripher- *outer part*	Pertaining to the periphery or an external boundary
phlebitis	fleh-**BIE**-tis	S/ R/	-itis *inflammation* phleb- *vein*	Inflammation of a vein
thromboembolism	**THROM**-boh-**EM**-boh-lizm	S/ R/CF R/	-ism *condition* thromb/o- *clot* -embol- *plug*	A piece of detached blood clot (embolus) blocking a distant blood vessel
thrombophlebitis	**THROM**-boh-fleh-**BIE**-tis	S/ R/CF R/	-itis *inflammation* thromb/o- *clot* -phleb- *vein*	Inflammation of a vein with clot formation
thrombus thrombi (pl) thrombosis	**THROM**-bus **THROM**-bie throm-**BOH**-sis	R/ S/	Latin *clot* thromb- *clot* -osis *condition*	A clot attached to a diseased blood vessel or heart lining Formation of a thrombus
varix varices (pl) varicose (adj)	**VAIR**-iks **VAIR**-ih-seez **VAIR**-ih-kose	S/ R/	Latin *dilated vein* -ose *full of* varic- *varicosity; dilated, tortuous vein*	Dilated, tortuous vein Characterized by or affected with varices

EXERCISES

 ## Case Report 6.2

You are

. . . a certified medical assistant **(CMA)** working for Dr. Lokesh Bannerjee, a cardiologist at Fulwood Medical Center.

You are communicating with

. . . Mrs. Martha Jones. You are documenting her medical record after Dr. Bannerjee interviewed and examined her.

Mrs. Martha Jones, who has been referred to Dr. Bannerjee's cardiovascular clinic, has several circulatory problems related to her diabetes and obesity. She was diagnosed previously with hypertension, **CAD,** and diabetic retinopathy. She now has severe pain in her legs when walking. Doppler studies and angiograms showed significant blockage of blood flow due to arteriosclerosis of the large arteries in her legs. This blockage produces the pain when walking (intermittent claudication) and is part of her peripheral vascular disease **(PVD).**

The ulcers on the edges of her big toes are a result of thickening capillary walls and arterioles; this has led to poor circulation in her feet. Mrs. Jones's uncontrolled diabetes has caused these problems.

In addition, in her left leg's venous (vein) system, the tender cord-like lesion is due to **thrombophlebitis** of a superficial vein. A venogram showed a deep vein thrombosis **(DVT).**

Fulwood Medical Center
Consultation Request and Report Form

Patient's Name: Jones, MARTHA   Age: 52
To: Dr. LoKESH BANNERJEE   Department: Cardiology
From: Dr. Susan Lee   Department: Primary Care
Patient's Location: Fulwood MEDICAL CENTER
Type of Consultation Desired:
☐ Consultation Only
☐ Consultation and follow Jointly
☒ Accept in Transfer
Referring Diagnoses: CLAUDICATION, POSSIBLE DVT
Reason for Consultation: Severe pain in both legs on walking

Signature: _____ Date: 2/21/09   Time 1105 hrs
Consultation Report: by Lokesh Bannerjee
Chief complaint: Pt. c/o severe pain in both legs on walking about 100 yards or climbing a flight of stairs. Pain is so severe she must stop and wait 5 mins. before she can go on. For the past two weeks she has noticed soreness and hardness along a vein in her left calf.
Past medical history: Known type 2 diabetic with hypertension, CAD, diabetic retinopathy, and OA of her hips and knees. Several episodes of ketoacidosis and one of pulmonary edema. Bariatric surgery performed 8 months prior at 275 lbs.
Medications: metformin, verapamil, propanolol, Mevacor
Allergies: NKA
Physical examination: Ht: 5'2" Wt: 210 lbs. BP: 170/100 sitting. P: 80, regular. Both feet show slight pitting edema and skin is pale, cold, and dry. Small ulcer on lateral margin of each big toe. Varicosities, both legs. Tender cord in superficial vein of left calf. Flexion of left foot produces pain in left calf. Chest clear. Heart sounds unremarkable. No loss of sensation in legs or feet.
Impression: 1. varicose veins, both legs.
             2. severe claudication, both legs.
             3. probable deep vein thrombosis, left leg
             4. possible peripheral neuropathy
             5. H/o diabetes type 2, CAD, hypertension, retinopathy, OA
Plan: Admit patient to cardiology unit stat for IV heparin and conversion to oral anticoagulant therapy with Coumadin. Doppler studies, venogram, and angiogram have been ordered.

Signature: _____ Date 2/21/09   Time 1250 hrs

ORDER # **267116** ANDRUS CLINI-REC ®PRIMARY CARE CHARTING SYSTEM • © BIBBERO SYSTEMS, INC. • PETALUMA, CA
TO REORDER CALL TOLL FREE: (800) BIBBERO (800-242-9330)   MFG IN U.S.A.

A. Read *Case Report 6.2 and answer the following questions. Select the correct answer.*   **LO 6.6 and 6.8**

1. Which of the following are Mrs. Jones's symptoms? (choose all that apply)

   a. severe pain in legs while sitting

   b. severe pain in legs when walking 100 yards

   c. severe pain in legs when climbing stairs

   d. pain in her left calf

   e. chest pain on exertion

2. Which of the following are diseases and conditions that Mrs. Jones is suffering from? (choose all that apply)

   a. hypertension   b. pulmonary embolism   c. osteoarthritis   d. type 1 diabetes mellitus   e. gout

3. Why did Mrs. Jones have bariatric surgery?

   a. diabetic retinopathy   b. osteoarthritis   c. obesity   d. hypertension

4. What is the purpose of anticoagulant therapy?

   a. to prevent the formation of blood clots

   b. to make the heart beat slower

   c. treat the diabetes mellitus

   d. lower the blood pressure

5. Of the studies ordered, which one uses ultrasound?

   a. angiogram   b. venogram   c. Doppler studies   d. IV anticoagulant therapy

6. What is pitting edema?

   a. a finger that is pressed into a swollen area leaves an indentation in the tissue

   b. swelling that moves toward the feet when a person is standing upright

   c. swelling around a wound that indents into the surrounding tissue

   d. small pockets of swelling that are distributed throughout body

B. **Apply the language** *of cardiology in the following documentation. Be sure to use the correct form (noun, adjective) of the term. There is only one best answer for each blank.* **LO 6.2, 6.7, and 6.8**

cardiologist   **cardiovascular**   **cardiology**

1. The _____ Department sent a specialist to examine the patient in the Emergency Department because of his symptoms. The _____ ordered an angioplasty, which found that the patient had three obstructed arteries in his heart, so the _____ surgeon prepared to operate immediately.

C. **Apply** *the language of the cardiovascular system. Select the best answer to complete each statement.* **LO 6.1 and 6.6**

1. The suffix tells you that **thrombophlebitis** is a(n)

   a. puncture   b. inflammation   c. excision   d. vein

2. **Collateral** means

   a. at the front   b. in the middle   c. at the side

3. The combining form *phleb/o-* means

   a. artery   b. vein   c. capillary

4. The combining form *scler/o-* describes a

   a. softening   b. clotting   c. hardening   d. constriction

5. The symptom of **edema** is a

   a. rash   b. swelling   c. lesion

6. **Aneurysm** describes a blood vessel that is

   a. dilated   b. constricted   c. collapsed   d. obstructed

7. The roots tell you that **thromboembolism** is a(n)

   a. clot or plug   b. tear or rupture   c. swelling or lesion   d. vein or artery

8. The combining form *thromb/o-* means

   a. clot   b. lump   c. plug   d. vein

D. **Use your knowledge** *of the language of cardiology to match the description in the left column with the correct medical term in the right column. Match the term to its correct meaning.* **LO 6.4 and 6.6**

_____	1. Weakening of heart muscle	a. prolapse
_____	2. Inflammation that causes exudates	b. cardiomegaly
_____	3. Cusps of valve bulge back into atrium	c. cor pulmonale
_____	4. Constricted valve opening	d. pericarditis
_____	5. Failure of right ventricle to pump properly	e. stenosis
_____	6. Cardiomyopathy can be the cause	f. cardiomyopathy

E. Spell *the term that correctly completes each statement.*   **LO 6.2 and 6.6**

1. The MVP caused the blood to _____ into the left atrium.

2. In heart disease, the left ventricle can _____ in an effort to increase CO.

3. Right heart failure is termed _____.

4. Inflammation of the tissue lining the inside of the heart is termed _____.

F. Precision *in communication and documentation is required for patient safety in health care. Match the term in the first column with its correct definition in the second column.*   **LO 6.6 and 6.9**

_____   **1.** arteriosclerosis   **a.** fatty deposit in an artery

. _____   **2.** atherosclerosis   **b.** hardening of an artery due to a fatty deposit

_____   **3.** atheroma   **c.** hardening of an artery

G. Abbreviations *need to be used carefully so that you communicate exactly what is necessary. Match the abbreviation to the correct condition it describes.*   **LO 6.3, 6.4, 6.6, and 6.9**

_____   **1.** ASD   **a.** force of blood pushing on the vessel walls

_____   **2.** TOF   **b.** artery remains open instead of normally closing after birth

_____   **3.** VSD   **c.** chronic elevated blood pressure

_____   **4.** PDA   **d.** congenital heart defect that is made up of four congenital abnormalities

_____   **5.** CHF   **e.** abnormal opening between the atria

_____   **6.** BP   **f.** abnormal opening between the ventricles

_____   **7.** HTN   **g.** heart is unable to pump enough blood to meet the body's needs

H. Spelling: *The following terms commonly occur in the cardiology department. Select the correct choice for the documentation.*   **LO 6.2 and 6.6**

1. An (arhythmia/arrhythmia) has been confirmed with the EKG.

2. The (murrmur/murmur) was detected during ventricular (dyastole/diastole).

3. Cardiac (dysrrhythmia/dysrhythmia) can be a symptom of a serious underlying condition.

4. A sign of Buerger disease is (claudication/cluadication).

5. A traveling thrombus is an (embulos/embolus).

Diagnostic and Therapeutic Procedures and Pharmacology of the Heart and Circulatory Systems

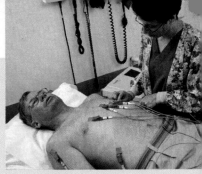

Rick Brady/McGraw Hill

Cardiovascular Diagnostic Procedures (LO 6.3 and 6.7)

Phlebotomists are health care professionals that obtain blood for diagnostic purposes.

A **lipid profile** helps determine the risk of CAD and comprises:

- Total cholesterol;
- High-density **lipoprotein (HDL)** ("good cholesterol");
- Low-density lipoprotein (**LDL**) ("bad cholesterol"); and
- **Triglycerides**.

Troponin I and **T** are part of a protein complex in muscle that is released into the blood during a muscle injury. Troponin I is found in heart muscle but not in skeletal muscle, which makes it a highly sensitive indicator of a recent MI.

Noninvasive Diagnostic Tests (LO 6.3, 6.7, and 6.9)

Several diagnostic tests are used to measure heart health.

The pulse is always part of a clinical examination because it can provide information about heart rate, heart rhythm, and the state of the arterial wall by **palpation** *(Figure 6.17)*. The most easily accessible artery is the radial artery at the wrist, where the pulse is usually taken.

Blood pressure (BP) is measured using a **sphygmomanometer** and a **stethoscope,** usually at the **brachial artery** *(Figure 6.17)*. Blood pressure is measured to help identify whether a person is at risk for heart disease or stroke. Blood pressure is the result of the blood exerting its force on arterial walls as it is pumped around the circulatory system by the left ventricle.

Auscultation occurs when heart sounds are heard via a **stethoscope** during the cardiac cycle. The "lub-dub, lub-dub" sounds heard through a stethoscope are made by the heart valves snapping as they close. If there is an abnormality, such as blood flowing against a restriction (e.g., a stenosed or incompetent valve), it may produce an extra, abnormal sound called a murmur.

Electrocardiography is the process of recording the electricity passing through the heart muscle by using electrodes placed on the skin. The **electrodes** connect to an **electrocardiograph,** which then amplifies the electrical changes to record an **electrocardiogram (ECG or EKG)** in the form of five waves *(Figure 6.18)*. The ECG waves are labeled P, Q, R, S, and T.

Keynote

- Vital signs (VS) measure temperature (T), pulse (P), respiration (R), and blood pressure (BP) to assess cardiorespiratory function.

Abbreviations

CVT	cardiovascular technologist
ECG or EKG	electrocardiogramh
ED	emergency department
HDL	high-density lipoprotein
LDL	low-density lipoprotein
STAT	immediately

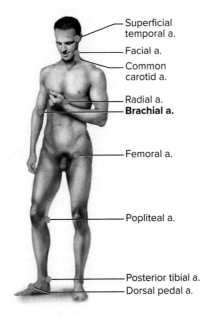

▲ **FIGURE 6.17** Arterial Pulses—9 locations (a. = artery).

Labels: Superficial temporal a.; Facial a.; Common carotid a.; Radial a.; **Brachial a.**; Femoral a.; Popliteal a.; Posterior tibial a.; Dorsal pedal a.

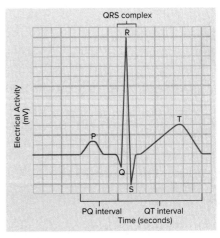

▲ **FIGURE 6.18** Normal Electrocardiogram.

Labels: QRS complex; R; P; Q; S; T; PQ interval; QT interval; Time (seconds); Electrical Activity (mV)

It is common during an **emergency department (ED)** visit for patients who present with chest pain to have various diagnostic procedures ordered as **STAT.** When certain specialized diagnostic testing is needed, a specially trained **cardiovascular technologist (CVT)** may be called upon to perform an ultrasound of the heart, known as an echocardiogram.

A **Holter monitor** is a smaller single-lead electrograph device *(Figure 6.19)*. The device continuously records ECG data on a digital recording device as the person works, plays, and rests for 24 to 48 hours. The patient keeps a diary of all symptoms and activities so that the data on the monitor can be correlated with symptoms and activities. The electrograph sends the data electronically to the monitoring company.

Smartphone apps providing at-home ECGs are being evaluated for their effectiveness compared to a standard 12-lead ECG.

Color Doppler ultrasonography uses high-frequency sound (ultrasound) waves to evaluate cardiac valve function and to show different rates of blood flow through the heart and blood vessels.

A **venogram** is a radiograph (X-ray record) of a vein. It is used to view the blood flow through the veins.

Cardiac stress testing is an exercise tolerance test that raises your heart rate through exercise (like walking on an inclined treadmill) and monitors its effect on cardiac function. **Nuclear imaging** of the heart, which involves the injection of a radioactive substance, can be used with the stress test.

Echocardiography uses ultrasound waves to study cardiac function.

Magnetic resonance imaging (MRI) can produce detailed images of the heart and identify sections of cardiac muscle that are not receiving an adequate blood supply.

Abbreviation

MRI   magnetic resonance
        imaging

Invasive Diagnostic Tests (LO 6.3 and 6.7)

Cardiac catheterization detects pressure and blood flow patterns in the heart. A thin tube is inserted into a vein or artery and is then threaded into the heart under X-ray guidance.

A **coronary angiogram** uses a contrast dye injected during cardiac catheterization to identify coronary artery blockages.

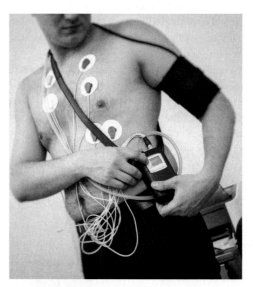

▲ **FIGURE 6.19**
Holter Monitor.

Lena Ivanova/Shutterstock

WORD	PRONUNCIATION		ELEMENTS	DEFINITION
angiogram	**AN**-jee-oh-gram	S/ R/CF	-gram *a record* angi/o- *blood vessel*	Radiograph obtained after injection of radiopaque contrast material into blood vessels
angiography	**AN**-jee-**OG**-rah-fee	S/	-graphy *process of recording*	Radiography of blood vessels after injection of contrast material
auscultation	aws-kul-**TAY**-shun	S/ R/	-ation *process* auscult- *listen to*	Diagnostic method of listening to body sounds with a stethoscope
brachial	**BRAY**-kee-al	S/ R/	-al *pertaining to* brachi- *arm*	Pertaining to the arm
catheter	**KATH**-eh-ter		Greek *to send down*	Hollow tube to allow passage of fluid into or out of a body cavity, organ, or vessel
catheterize (verb)	**KATH**-eh-teh-**RIZE**	S/ R/	-ize *action* catheter- *catheter*	To introduce a catheter
catheterization (noun)	**KATH**-eh-ter-ih-**ZAY**-shun	S/	-ization *process of inserting*	Introduction of a catheter
Doppler	**DOP**-ler		Johann Doppler, Austrian mathematician and physician, 1803–1853	Diagnostic instrument that sends an ultrasonic beam into the body
echocardiography	**EK**-oh-kar-dee-**OG**-rah-fee	S/ R/CF R/CF	-graphy *process of recording* ech/o- *sound wave* -cardi/o- *heart*	Ultrasound recording of heart function
electrocardiogram (ECG, EKG)	ee-lek-troh-**KAR**-dee-oh-gram	S/ R/CF R/CF	-gram *a record* electr/o- *electricity* -cardi/o- *heart*	Record of the electrical signals of the heart
electrocardiograph electrocardiography	ee-lek-troh-**KAR**-dee-oh-graf ee-**LEK**-troh-kar-dee-**OG**-rah-fee	S/ S/	-graph *to record* -graphy *process of recording*	Machine that produces the electrocardiogram The method of recording and the interpretation of electrocardiograms
electrode	ee-**LEK**-trode	S/ R/	-ode *way, road* electr- *electricity*	A device for conducting electricity
lipid	**LIP**-id		Greek *fat*	General term for all types of fatty compounds
lipoprotein	**LIE**-poh-pro-teen	R/CF R/	lip/o- *fat* -protein *protein*	Bonding of molecules of fat and protein
profile	**PRO**-file	S/ R/	pro- *forward* -file *contour, line*	A set of characteristics which determine the structure of a group
palpate (verb) palpation (noun)	**PAL**-pate pal-**PAY**-shun	S/ R/	Latin *touch, stroke* -ion *action, condition* palpat- *touch, stroke*	To examine with the fingers and hands Examination with the fingers and hands
phlebotomist	fleh-**BOT**-oh-mist	S/ R/CF R/	-ist *specialist in* phleb/o- *vein* -tom- *incise, cut*	Person skilled in taking blood from veins
phlebotomy	fleh-**BOT**-oh-me	S/	-tomy *surgical incision*	Withdrawing blood from a vein through a needle or catheter
sphygmomanometer	**SFIG**-moh-mah-**NOM**-ih-ter	S/ R/CF R/CF	-meter *instrument to measure* sphygm/o- *pulse* -man/o- *pressure*	Instrument for measuring arterial blood pressure
stethoscope	**STETH**-oh-skope	S/ R/CF	-scope *instrument to examine* steth/o- *chest*	Instrument for listening to respiratory and cardiac sounds
triglyceride	try-**GLISS**-eh-ride	S/ P/ R/	-ide *having a particular quality* tri- *three* -glycer- *sweet, glycerol*	Lipid containing three fatty acids
venogram	**VEE**-noh-gram	S/ R/CF	-gram *recording* ven/o- *vein*	Radiograph of veins after injection of radiopaque contrast material

Treatment Procedures (LO 6.3, 6.7, and 6.8)

Cardiologists treat heart problems that usually do not require surgery: catheterization, stent placement, and angioplasty.

Cardiovascular surgeons perform surgeries on the heart: coronary artery bypass grafting (CABG), heart valve repair or replacement, and correction of congenital heart defects.

Cardiopulmonary resuscitation (CPR) is given when a person's heart is no longer beating in a coordinated manner, and therefore there is no pulse. CPR is given by a trained professional, such as an **Emergency Medical Technician–Paramedic (EMT-P),** or by any trained person.

Heart transplant: The heart of a recently deceased person (donor) is transplanted into the recipient after the recipient's diseased heart has been removed.

Treatment for Myocardial Infarction (LO 6.3 and 6.7)

The most immediate need in the treatment of MI is to get blood and oxygen to the affected myocardium. This can be attempted in several ways:

1. **Injection of clot-busting (thrombolytic) drugs:** These drugs are injected within 3½ hours of the MI to dissolve the **thrombus**.

2. **Artery-cleaning angioplasty (percutaneous transluminal coronary angioplasty, or PTCA):** A balloon-tipped **catheter** is guided to the blockage site and inflated. The inflated balloon expands the artery from the inside by compressing the plaque against the artery's walls.

3. **Rotational atherectomy:** A high-speed rotational device is used to "sand" away calcified plaque.

4. **Stent placement:** To reduce the likelihood that the artery will close up again (occlude), a wire-mesh tube, or **stent**, is placed inside the vessel. **Drug-eluting** stents are covered with a special medication to help keep the artery open.

5. **Coronary artery bypass graft (CABG):** Healthy blood vessels harvested from the leg, chest, or arm are used to bypass (detour) the blood around blocked coronary arteries. A heart-lung bypass machine operated by a cardiac **perfusionist** may be used during this procedure.

Treatment for Arrhythmias (LO 6.3 and 6.7)

Arrhythmias can be treated with medications, but some patients require mechanical **pacemakers**. Pacemakers consist of a battery, electronic circuits, and computer memory in addition to sensors to generate electronic signals. These signals are carried along thin, insulated wires to the heart muscle. Pacemakers are ideal for patients with a very slow heart rate (bradycardia).

In emergency situations, external **defibrillation** is performed through **automated external defibrillators,** or **AEDs** *(Figure 6.20).* AEDs send an electric shock to the heart in order to stop the heart temporarily so that a normal contraction rhythm can resume.

People with life-threatening arrhythmias may need **an implantable cardioverter defibrillator (ICD),** which senses abnormal rhythms. An ICD gives the heart a small electric shock (less energy than external defibrillation) to return its rhythm to normal.

Defibrillation is the controlled delivery of energy to the heart during any phase of the cardiac cycle used in emergency situations. **Cardioversion** is the delivery of lower levels of energy synchronized to the large R waves of the QRS complex and is mostly used for A-fib or flutter and V-tach.

Radiofrequency ablation uses a catheter with an electrode in its tip that is guided into the heart to destroy cells from which abnormal cardiac rhythms are originating.

Valve Replacement (LO 6.3 and 6.7)

When a valve replacement is necessary, there are two types of artificial valves available:

1. Mechanical or **prosthetic** valves, which are made from metal alloys and plastics; or

2. **Tissue** valves, which can come from a pig or cow, a human cadaver (dead person), or a patient's own pericardium.

A transcatheter aortic valve replacement (**TAVR**) is a relatively common procedure that does not require open-heart surgery and replaces a damaged aortic valve with a biological donor valve from the heart tissue of a cow or pig.

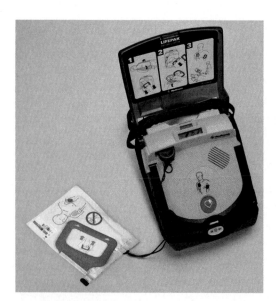

▲ **FIGURE 6.20**
Automatic External Defibrillator.

Rick Brady/McGraw Hill

Treatment for Peripheral Vascular Disorders (LO 6.3 and 6.7)

Varicose veins can be treated with laser technology and **sclerotherapy,** where a solution that scars (**scleroses**) the veins is injected into them.

Aneurysm repair consists of excision of the aneurysm and replacement with a synthetic graft.

Plaques within a carotid artery wall are compressed by angioplasty and stenting or surgically removed via an **endarterectomy.**

Word Analysis and Definition

S = Suffix   P = Prefix   R = Root   R/CF = Combining Form

WORD	PRONUNCIATION	ELEMENTS		DEFINITION
ablation	ab-**LAY**-shun	S/ P/ R/	-ion *process* ab- *take away* -lat- *to take*	Removal of a tissue to destroy its function
angioplasty	**AN**-jee-oh-**PLAS**-tee	S/ R/CF	-plasty *surgical repair* angi/o- *blood vessel*	Repair or unblocking of a blood vessel through surgery
atherectomy	ath-er-**EK**-toe-me	S/ R/	-ectomy *surgical excision* ather- *porridge, gruel*	Surgical removal of the atheroma
cardiologist	kar-dee-**OL**-oh-jist	S/ R/CF	-logist *one who studies, specialist* cardi/o- *heart*	A medical specialist in the diagnosis and treatment of the heart (cardiology)
cardiology	kar-dee-**OL**-oh-jee	S/	-logy *study of*	Medical specialty of diseases of the heart
cardiopulmonary resuscitation (CPR)	**KAR**-dee-oh-**PUL**-mo-nair-ee ree-sus-ih-**TAY**-shun	S/ R/CF R/ S/ R/-	-ary *pertaining to* cardi/o- *heart* -pulmon- *lung* -ation *a process* resuscit- *revive from apparent death*	The attempt to restore cardiac and pulmonary function
cardiovascular	**KAR**-dee-oh-**VAS**-kyu-lar	S/ R/CF R/	-ar *pertaining to* cardi/o- *heart* -vascul- *blood vessel*	Pertaining to the heart and blood vessels
cardioversion	**KAR**-dee-oh-**VER**-zhun	S/ R/CF	-version *change* cardi/o- *heart*	Restoration of a normal heart rhythm by electric shock or medications
defibrillation	dee-fib-rih-**LAY**-shun	S/ P/ R/	-ation *process* de- *from, out of* -fibrill- *small fiber*	Restoration of normal cardiac activity in life-threatening cardiac arrhythmias
defibrillator	dee-**FIB**-rih-lay-tor	S/	-ator *instrument*	Instrument for defibrillation
excision	eck-**SIZH**-un	S/ R/	-ion *action* excis- *cut out*	Surgical removal of part or all of a structure
implantable	im-**PLAN**-tah-bul	S/ P/ R/	-able *capable* im- *in* -plant- *insert*	A device that can be inserted into tissues
pacemaker	**PACE**-may-ker	S/ R/	-maker *one who makes* pace- *step*	Device that regulates cardiac electrical activity
percutaneous	**PER**-kyu-**TAY**-nee-us	S/ P/ R/	-ous *pertaining to* per- *through* -cutane- *skin*	Passage through the skin, in this case, by needle puncture
perfusion	per-**FYU**-zhun	S/ R/	-ion *action* perfus- *to pour*	The act of forcing blood to flow through a lumen or a vascular bed
perfusionist	per-**FYU**-zhun-ist	S/	-ist *specialist*	Specialist in operation of heart-lung machine
prosthesis (noun)	pros-**THEE**-sis		Greek *an addition*	A manufactured substitute for a missing or diseased part of the body
prosthetic (adj)	pros-**THET**-ik	S/ R/	-ic *pertaining to* prosthet- *artificial part*	Pertaining to a prosthesis
stent	STENT		Charles Stent, English dentist, 19th century	Wire-mesh tube used to keep arteries open
thrombolytic (adj)	throm-boh-**LIT**-ik	S/ R/CF	-lytic *pertaining to destruction* thromb/o- *blood clot*	Able to dissolve or break up a blood clot
thrombolysis	throm-**BOH**-lih-sis	S/	-lysis *dissolve*	Dissolving of a thrombus (clot)

Cardiac Pharmacology (LO 6.4 and 6.9)

Clinically, there are eight types of cardiac drugs in use:

1. **Anticoagulants** are drugs that reduce susceptibility to blood clot formation *see Chapter 7*. This can help prevent deep vein thrombosis (DVT), pulmonary embolism, myocardial infarction (MI), and stroke.

   Warfarin (Coumadin) and heparin are anticoagulants in frequent use. *Dabigatran* (Pradaxa) and related drugs are newer anticoagulants. Aspirin prevents platelets from clumping together as part of clot formation and is used to help prevent heart or artery diseases and strokes.

2. **Chronotropic drugs** alter the heart rate. Positive chronotropic drugs such as epinephrine (adrenaline), norepinephrine, and atropine increase the heart rate. Negative chronotropic drugs, such as quinidine, procainamide, lidocaine, and propranolol, slow the heart.

3. **Inotropic drugs** can also be positive and negative. Positive inotropic drugs increase the force of the ventricular contraction to increase cardiac output when the function is impaired, as in congestive heart failure, cardiogenic shock, and cardiomyopathy. Digitalis and its derivatives, digoxin and digitoxin, are the most effective positive inotropic drugs.

   Negative inotropic drugs decrease the strength of the ventricular contraction and are used for treating hypertension, angina, and heart attacks. Beta blockers (beta-adrenergic-blocking agents) and calcium-channel blockers are examples of negative inotropic drugs.

4. **Antiarrhythmic drugs** change the electrical properties of the myocardial cells to restore a normal rate and rhythm to the heart beat. Beta blockers, which can reduce the strength and rate of myocardial contractions, are used in treating arrhythmias.

5. **Vasoconstrictor drugs** contract the smooth muscle in blood vessels, which increases both arterial and venous blood pressures—hence, they are also called **pressor drugs.**

6. **Vasodilator drugs** relax smooth muscle in arterioles, which leads to a drop in blood pressure. Therefore, they are used in treating hypertension, angina, and congestive heart failure. Organic nitrates dilate coronary arteries. An example is nitroglycerin, which can be given **sublingually** for rapid action lasting for 30 minutes or via transdermal patches, which last 12 hours. There are a number of types of vasodilators, including **angiotensin-converting enzyme (ACE)** inhibitors, angiotensin II receptor blockers, and calcium-channel blockers.

7. **Diuretics** indirectly affect the heart by stimulating urine production, thus reducing the fluid volume with which the heart has to cope. Examples include furosemide (Lasix) and **thiazides.**

8. **Lipid-regulating drugs** inhibit the progression of atherosclerosis by lowering "bad cholesterol," or low-density lipoprotein (LDL), and/or increasing "good cholesterol," or high-density lipoprotein (HDL). Statins also lower LDL but carry a risk of muscle damage. Fibrates and niacin lower triglycerides.

Abbreviation

ACE	angiotensin-converting enzyme

Word Analysis and Definition

S = Suffix   P = Prefix   R = Root   R/CF = Combining Form

WORD	PRONUNCIATION	ELEMENTS		DEFINITION
antiarrhythmic	AN-tee-a-RITH-mik	S/ P/ R/	-ic *pertaining to* anti- *against* -rrhythm- *rhythm*	Pertaining to restoring a normal cardiac rhythm
anticoagulant	AN-tee-koh-AG-you-lant	S/ P/ R/	-ant *forming* anti- *against* -coagul- *clump*	Substance that prevents clotting
chronotropic	KRONE-oh-TROH-pic	S/ R/CF	-tropic *change* chron/o- *time*	Affecting the rate of rhythmic movements—in this case, the heart rate
diuretic	die-you-RET-ic	S/ P/ R/	-ic *pertaining to* di- *through* -uret- *urination*	Agent that increases urine output
inotropic	IN-oh-TROH-pic	S/ R/	-tropic *change* ino- *sinew*	Affecting the contractility of cardiac muscle
lipid	LIP-id		Greek *fat*	General term for fatty compounds
pressor	PRESS-or		Latin *to press*	Producing increased blood pressure
sublingual	sub-LING-wal	S/ P/ R/	-al *pertaining to* sub- *beneath* -lingu- *tongue*	Underneath the tongue
vasoconstrictor	VAY-so-con-STRIK-tor	S/ R/CF R/	-or *that which does something* vas/o *blood vessel* -constrict- *narrow*	Agent that reduces the diameter of a blood vessel
vasodilator	VAY-so-die-LAY-tor	R/	-dilat- *widen, open up*	Agent that increases the diameter of a blood vessel

EXERCISES

 Case Report 6.3

You are

. . . an Emergency Medical Technician-Paramedic (EMT-P) called to the gymnasium of Fulwood University

You are communicating with

. . . Danny Gitlin, a 21-year-old guard on the university basketball team.

Danny lost consciousness during a strenuous practice. He had no pulse but was revived by the coach, who used an automatic external **defibrillator (AED)**. Danny had never lost consciousness before, but he has noticed episodes of rapid **palpitations** after games. On examination, he is fully conscious and appears to be fit. His pulse is 70 but irregular in rate and force. His blood pressure is 110/65 mmHg. He has no known family history of heart disease.

The physical findings on Danny Gitlin suggested a **cardiomyopathy**, which was confirmed by echocardiography. Exercise testing (a cardiac stress test), with close medical supervision, produced a ventricular arrhythmia that returned to normal after conclusion of the test. Danny was treated with beta blockers and restricted to nonstrenuous sports.

A. Read *Case Report 6.3 and correctly answer the following questions. Select the correct answer to complete the statement or answer the question.* **LO 6.3, 6.7, 6.8, and 6.9**

1. When a person *loses consciousness,* they:

   a. are not aware of their surroundings and cannot be aroused   **c.** have no pulse

   b. appear to be asleep and are easily aroused   **d.** have a have a rapid heartbeat

2. What seems to be the trigger for causing his symptoms?

   a. high temperature   **b.** increased physical activity   **c.** dehydration   **d.** lack of exercise

3. How might Danny describe his *palpitations?*

   a. "I have times that I black out and forget what has happened."   **c.** "I have a dizzy feeling that makes me feel like I will faint."

   b. "I feel like my heart quits beating for a moment."   **d.** "My heart beats hard and feels like it is beating out of my chest."

4. Which of the following describes an AED?

   a. blood pressure is measured by a machine   **c.** machine displays the electrical activity of the heart

   b. the heart rate is counted by a computer   **d.** machine determines when to deliver an electrical shock to the heart

B. Construct *the correct medical terms to match the definitions given. If a term does not have a particular element, insert N/A on that blank. Fill in the blanks.* **LO 6.1, 6.3, 6.4, and 6.7**

1. Forceful, rapid beat of the heart

   _____ / _____ / _____

              P   R/CF   S

2. Uncontrolled heart muscle twitching

   _____ / _____ / _____

              P   R/CF   S

3. Device that restores uncontrolled twitching of cardiac muscle to normal rhythm

   _____ / _____ / _____

              P   R/CF   S

4. Implanted device that regulates cardiac electrical activity

   _____ / _____ / _____

              P   R/CF   S

5. Instrument for listening to respiratory and cardiac sounds:

_____ / _____ / _____
           P   R/CF   S

6. Pertaining to the arm:

_____ / _____ / _____
           P   R/CF   S

7. Instrument for measuring arterial blood pressure:

_____ / _____ / _____
           R/CF   R/CF   S

C. **Use the correct abbreviation** _from the provided list to complete each statement. Not all choices will be used. Fill in the blanks._   **LO 6.3, 6.6, 6.7, and 6.9**

    CABG   ECG   HDL   LDL   MRI   PTCA

1. The blood tests revealed that Ms. Nugrak's good cholesterol, her _____ , was high.

2. Mr. Tervo will undergo a _____ to open the occluded coronary artery.

3. The _____ showed that Mr. Welch's heart has normal electrical activity.

4. The _____ was high, which may place a person at risk of developing coronary artery disease.

D. **Determine the type of condition** _that is treated with a particular procedure._   **LO 6.6 and 6.7**

1. Coronary artery bypass grafting

    a. arrhythmia   **b.** occluded coronary artery

2. Radiofrequency ablation

    a. arrhythmia   **b.** occluded coronary artery

3. Cardioversion

    a. arrhythmia   **b.** occluded coronary artery

4. Percutaneous transluminal coronary angioplasty

    a. arrhythmia   **b.** occluded coronary artery

E. **Deconstruct** _the medical terms in this chart into their basic elements and give the meaning of the term. Fill in the blanks._   **LO 6.1**

Medical Term	Prefix	Root, Root/CF	Suffix
inotropic	1.	2.	3.
diuretic	4.	5.	6.
anticoagulant	7.	8.	9.
sublingual	10.	11.	12.
antiarrhythmic	13.	14.	15.

F. **Construct terms** _using word elements. The roots/combining forms are important when describing the effects of cardiac medications. Given the definition, provide the missing combining form element. Enter it as one term, for example: sclero_   **LO 6.1 and 6.7**

1. A medication that affects the heart rate. _____/tropic

2. A medication that affects the contractility of the heart: _____/tropic

3. A medication that is placed under the tongue: sub/ _____/al

4. A medication that increases urine output: di/ _____/ic

G. **Singulars and plurals,** *nouns and adjectives: Terms from the WAD can all be correctly inserted into the following paragraph of radiology documentation. Fill in the blanks.* **LO 6.2, 6.6, and 6.7**

veins   varicosities   varix   vein   varicose   varices   venogram   venous

1. A _____ performed on this patient's left saphenous and popliteal _____ .

   Abnormalities: One slightly engorged and dilated _____ at the midpoint of the saphenous _____ and several _____ at the terminal end of the popliteal vein where _____ blood is pooling.

   Diagnosis: _____ veins. These _____ need immediate attention by a vascular surgeon.

H. **Proper pronunciation of terms is key to verbal communication.** *Choose the answer that correctly completes each statement.* **LO 6.1 and 6.2**

1. In the combining form *brachi/o,* the vowel i is pronounced like the vowel in:

   a. key   b. eye   c. sick   d. rate

2. When pronouncing the term *popliteal,* emphasis is put on the syllable:

   a. pop   b. lit   c. ee   d. al

3. The first syllable in the term *carotid* sounds like the first syllable in the term:

   a. cat   b. carrot   c. cousin   d. cake

I. **Pronunciation is important whether you are saying the word or listening to a word from a coworker.** Identify the proper pronunciation of the following medical terms. Then correctly spell the term. **LO 6.1, 6.2, 6.4, and 6.6**

1. The correct pronunciation for a small vein leading away from a capillary network:

   a. vay-NYOU-el   c. VEN-yule

   b. veen-UHL   d. VANE-yule-ah

   Correctly spell the term: _____

2. The correct pronunciation for an agent that affects the heart rate:

   a. IN-oh- TROH-pik   c. KRONE-oh-TROH-pik

   b. IN-oh-troop- IK   d. KROON-oh-troop- IK

   Correctly spell the term: _____

3. The correct pronunciation for an enzyme elevated in the plasma following heart muscle damage:

   a. KREE-ah-teen KI-nase   c. try-GLISS-eh-ride

   b. creat-in-KI-nase   d. try-GLICE-er-ide

   Correctly spell the term: _____

4. The correct pronunciation for the surgical removal of the atheroma:

   a. an-JEEO-plast-er-EE   c. ath-er-EK-toh-mee

   b. AN-jee-oh-PLAS-tee   d. ATHREK-to-mee

   Correctly spell the term: _____

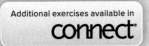
Additional exercises available in
connect

Chapter Review exercises, along with additional practice items, are available in Connect!

The Blood, Lymphatic, and Immune Systems

The Essentials of the Languages of Hematology and Immunology

Learning Outcomes

In order to be able to communicate intelligently with members of the health care team and to appropriately document the medical care for patients with diseases and disorders of the blood, lymphatic, and immune systems, you first need to be familiar with the anatomy, physiology, and medical terminology of hematology. This chapter will provide you with information that enables you to:

LO 7.1 Use **roots, combining forms, suffixes,** and prefixes to construct and analyze (deconstruct) medical terms related to the blood, lymphatic, and immune systems.

LO 7.2 Spell and pronounce correctly medical terms and their plurals related to the blood, lymphatic, and immune systems to communicate them with accuracy and precision in any health care setting.

LO 7.3 Define accepted abbreviations related to the blood, lymphatic, and immune systems.

LO 7.4 Relate the functions of blood to its components.

LO 7.5 Relate the structure of major types of white blood cells and platelets to their function.

LO 7.6 Identify the different ABO and Rh blood groups, their roles, and effects.

LO 7.7 Relate the structure of the lymphatic system and its organs to its functions.

LO 7.8 Describe the structure and functions of the immune system and the roles, methods, and effects of immunization.

LO 7.9 Describe and differentiate blood disorders, lymphatic disorders, autoimmune disorders, and major types of infection.

LO 7.10 Describe the diagnostic laboratory studies, therapeutic procedures, and pharmacologic agents used in blood and immune disorders.

LO 7.11 Identify health professionals involved in the care of patients with blood and lymphatic disorders.

LO 7.12 Apply your knowledge of the medical terms of the blood, lymphatic, and immune systems to documentation, medical records, and medical reports.

LO 7.13 Translate the medical terms of the blood, lymphatic, and immune systems into everyday language to communicate clearly with patients and their families.

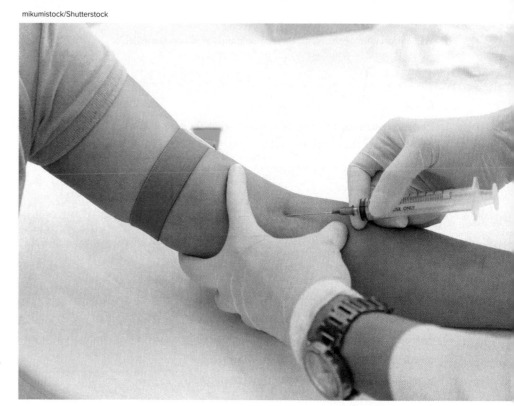

mikumistock/Shutterstock

The health professionals involved in the diagnosis and treatment of problems with the blood, lymphatic, and immune systems include the following:

- **Hematologists** are physicians who specialize in the diagnosis, treatment, and prevention of blood and bone marrow diseases.
- **Immunologists** and **allergists** are physicians who specialize in immune system disorders, such as allergies, asthma, and immunodeficiency and autoimmune diseases.
- **Epidemiologists** are medical scientists involved in the study of epidemic diseases and how they are transmitted and controlled.
- **Medical** or **clinical laboratory** technicians, also known as technologists, scientists perform routine testing procedures on body fluids, blood, and other tissues using microscopes, computers, and other laboratory equipment.
- **Immunology technologists** are certified laboratory technicians with a special interest in immunology who generally work alongside medical researchers.
- **Transfusion technicians** are certified technicians who deal with all phases of blood transfusions.
- **Phlebotomists** assist physicians by drawing patient blood samples for laboratory testing.

Components and Functions of Blood

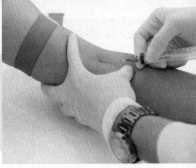

mikumistock/Shutterstock

The average-sized adult carries about 5 liters (10 pints) of blood in the body at all times.

Components of Blood (LO 7.3 and 7.4)

Blood is a type of connective tissue that consists of cells contained in a liquid **matrix**. If a blood specimen is collected in a tube and centrifuged, the cells of the blood separate out and fill the bottom 45% of the tube (*see Figure 7.1*). Red blood cells (**RBCs**) make up 99% of the formed elements; white blood cells (**WBCs**) and **platelets** make up the remainder of this sample. The **hematocrit (Hct)** is the percentage of total blood volume composed of red blood cells. Note that whole blood, when separated into formed elements, can be subdivided further into additional categories and other smaller elements.

Plasma—a clear, yellowish liquid that is 91% water—makes up the remaining 55% of the blood sample in the tube. Plasma is a **colloid**, a liquid that contains floating particles, most of which are plasma proteins. **Nutrients**, waste products, hormones, and enzymes are dissolved in plasma for transportation. When blood clots, and the solid clot is removed, **serum** remains. Serum is a clear, yellowish fluid that contains all the blood proteins not used in clotting and all the electrolytes, antibodies, antigens, and hormones that are carried in blood.

Keynote

- Blood serum is identical to plasma except for the absence of clotting proteins.

Abbreviations

Hct	hematocrit
RBC	red blood cell
WBC	white blood cell

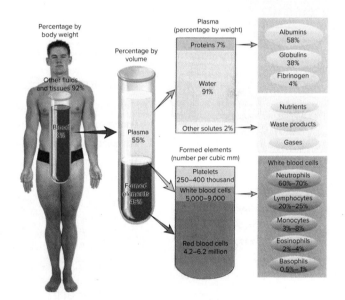

▲ **FIGURE 7.1** Components of Blood.

(Adult male body - anterior view): Eric Wise

Word Analysis and Definition

S = Suffix   P = Prefix   R = Root   R/CF = Combining Form

WORD	PRONUNCIATION		ELEMENTS	DEFINITION
colloid	**COLL**-oyd	S/ R/	-oid *resembling* coll- *glue*	Liquid containing suspended particles
matrix	**MAY**-triks		Latin mater *mother*	Substance that surrounds and protects cells, is manufactured by the cells, and holds cells together
nutrient nutrition nutritionist	**NYU**-tree-ent nyu-**TRISH**-un nyu-**TRISH**-un-ist	S/ R/ S/	Latin *to nourish* -ion *action, condition* nutrit- *nourishment* -ist *specialist*	Constituent of food necessary for the body to function normally The study of food and liquid requirements for normal function of the human body A person who specializes in the study of food and liquid requirements for normal function of the human body
plasma	**PLAZ**-mah		Greek *something formed*	Fluid, noncellular component of blood
platelet (*Also called* thrombocyte.)	**PLAYT**-let	S/ R/	-let *little, small* plate- *flat*	Small particle involved in the clotting process
serum	**SEER**-um		Latin *whey*	Fluid remaining after removal of blood cells and the formation of a clot

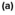
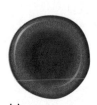

Abbreviations

CO_2	carbon dioxide
Hb or Hgb	hemoglobin
NO	nitric oxide
O_2	oxygen
PMNL	polymorphonuclear leukocyte

Functions of Blood (LO 7.4)

Your blood travels throughout your body while performing a number of important functions. Your blood:

1. **Maintains your body's homeostasis** *(see Chapter 2).*

2. **Transports nutrients, vitamins, and minerals** from your digestive system and storage areas to your organs and cells. Examples of nutrients are glucose and amino acids *(see Chapter 9).*

3. **Transports waste products** from your cells and tissues to your liver and kidney for excretion. These waste products include creatinine, urea, bilirubin, and lactic acid.

4. **Transports hormones,** like insulin and thyroxine *(see Chapter 12),* from your endocrine glands to target cells.

5. **Transports gases,** like oxygen and carbon dioxide *(see Chapter 8),* to and from your lungs and cells.

6. **Protects against foreign substances, including microorganisms and toxins.** Cells and chemicals in your blood are an important part of your immune system's protective properties.

7. **Forms clots.** Clots provide protection against blood loss. Clotting is the first step in tissue repair and restoration of normal function.

Structure and Functions of Red Blood Cells (Erythrocytes) (LO 7.5)

Structure of RBCs (Erythrocytes) (LO 7.5)

Each RBC is a disk with raised edges that are thicker than the flattened center *(Figure 7.2).* This biconcave surface area enables a more rapid flow of gases into and out of the cell.

The main component of RBCs is **hemoglobin (Hb)**, which gives the cells and blood their red color. Hb is composed of the iron-containing pigment **heme** bound to a protein called globin. The rest of the red blood cell consists of the cell membrane, water, electrolytes, and enzymes. Mature RBCs do not have a nucleus.

Functions of RBCs (Erythrocytes) (LO 7.3 and 7.5)

The functions of the RBCs are to:

1. **Transport oxygen (O_2),** in combination with hemoglobin, throughout the body, from the lungs to the cells;

2. **Transport carbon dioxide (CO_2)** from the tissue cells to the lungs for excretion; and

3. **Transport nitric oxide (NO),** a gas produced by the lining cells of blood vessels that signals smooth muscle to relax, throughout the body.

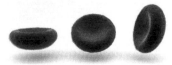

(a)

(b)

▲ **FIGURE 7.2**
Red Blood Cells.
(a) Top view. (b) Side view.

7.2b: ClaudioVentrella/iStock/Getty Images

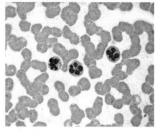

▲ **FIGURE 7.3**
Neutrophils Are Granulocytes.

JOSE LUIS CALVO MARTIN & JOSE ENRIQUE GARCIA-MAURIÑO MUZQUIZ/iStock/Getty Images

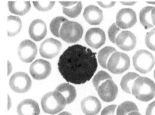
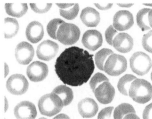

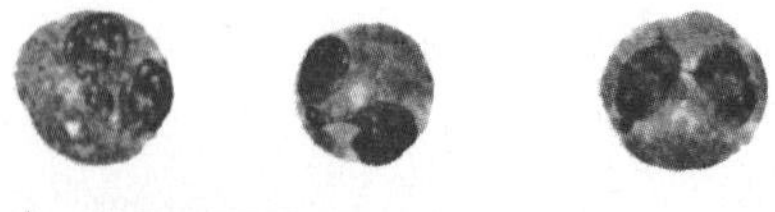

▲ **FIGURE 7.4**
Eosinophils Are Granulocytes.

toeytoey2530/iStock/Getty Images

▲ **FIGURE 7.5**
Basophils Are Granulocytes.

Alvin Telser/McGraw Hill

Types and Functions of White Blood Cells (Leukocytes)
(LO 7.3 and 7.5)

The types of white blood cells **(WBCs)** can be categorized as **granulocytes** or **agranulocytes.** Granulocytes contain granular cytoplasm, made up of secreting granules, which are sites for enzyme and chemical production. Agranulocytes do not contain cytoplasmic granules.

Granulocytes (LO 7.3 and 7.5)

1. **Neutrophils** *(Figure 7.3),* also called **polymorphonuclear leukocytes (PMNLs),** are normally 55% to 65% of the total WBC count. These cells ingest bacteria, fungi, and some viruses. In **neutropenia,** the number of neutrophils is decreased. In **neutrophilia,** the number is increased.

2. **Eosinophils** *(Figure 7.4)* are normally 2% to 4% of the total WBC count. They leave the bloodstream to enter tissue that is undergoing an allergic response. In allergic reactions, the number and percentage of eosinophils increase.

3. **Basophils** *(Figure 7.5)* are normally less than 1% of the total WBC count. Basophils migrate to damaged tissues to release histamine (which increases blood flow) and heparin (which prevents blood clotting).

Agranulocytes (LO 7.3 and 7.5)

4. **Monocytes** *(Figure 7.6)* are the largest blood cells and are normally 3% to 8% of the total WBC count. Monocytes leave the bloodstream and become **macrophages** that ingest bacteria, dead neutrophils, and dead cells in the tissues.

5. **Lymphocytes** *(Figure 7.7)* are the smallest white blood cells and compose 25% to 35% of the total WBC count. Lymphocytes are produced in red bone marrow and migrate through the bloodstream to lymphatic tissues—lymph nodes, tonsils, spleen, and thymus—where they multiply.

There are two main types of lymphocytes:

a. **B cells** differentiate into plasma cells, which are stimulated by bacteria or toxins to produce antibodies or immunoglobulins (**Ig**).

b. **T cells** attach directly to foreign antigen-bearing cells like bacteria, which they kill with toxins they secrete.

Abbreviation

Ig   immunoglobulin

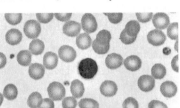

▲ **FIGURE 7.6**
Monocytes Are Agranulocytes.

Alvin Telser/McGraw Hill

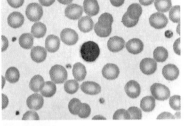

▲ **FIGURE 7.7**
Lymphocytes Are Agranulocytes.

jarun011/iStock/Getty Images

Word Analysis and Definition

S = Suffix   P = Prefix   R = Root   R/CF = Combining Form

WORD	PRONUNCIATION	ELEMENTS		DEFINITION
agranulocyte	a-**GRAN**-you-loh-site	S/ P/ R/CF	-cyte *cell* a- *without, not* -granul/o- *granule*	A white blood cell without any granules in its cytoplasm
basophil	**BAY**-so-fill	S/ R/CF	-phil *attraction* bas/o- *base*	A basophil's granules attract a basic blue stain in the laboratory
eosinophil	ee-oh-**SIN**-oh-fill	S/ R/CF	-phil *attraction* eosin/o- *dawn*	An eosinophil's granules attract a rosy-red color on staining
erythrocyte	eh-**RITH**-roh-site	S/ R/CF	-cyte *cell* erythr/o- *red*	Red blood cell (RBC)
granulocyte	**GRAN**-you-loh-site	S/ R/CF	-cyte *cell* granul/o- *small grain*	A white blood cell that contains multiple small granules in its cytoplasm
heme	**HEEM**		Greek *blood*	The iron-based component of hemoglobin that carries oxygen
hemoglobin	**HE**-moh-**GLOW**-bin	R/CF R/	hem/o- *blood* -globin *protein*	Red-pigmented protein that is the main component of red blood cells
leukocyte leucocyte (syn) (Note: *Either spelling is acceptable.*)	**LOO**-koh-site	S/ R/CF	-cyte *cell* leuk/o- *white*	Another term for a white blood cell
lymphocyte	**LIM**-foh-site	R/ R/CF	-cyte *cell* lymph/o- *lymph*	Small white blood cell with a large nucleus
monocyte	**MON**-oh-site	R/ P/	-cyte *cell* mono- *single*	Large white blood cell with a single nucleus
neutrophil	**NEW**-troh-fill	S/ R/CF	-phil *attraction* neutr/o- *neutral*	Neutrophils' granules take up purple stain equally, whether the stain is acid or alkaline
polymorphonuclear	**POL**-ee-more-foh-**NEW**-klee-ar	S/ P/ R/CF R/	-ar *pertaining to* poly- *many* -morph/o- *shape* -nucle- *nucleus*	White blood cell with a multilobed nucleus

Hemostasis (LO 7.3 and 7.5)

Hemostasis, the control of bleeding, is important in maintaining **homeostasis,** the state of the body's equilibrium. Uncontrolled bleeding can offset the body's balance by decreasing blood volume and lowering blood pressure.

Platelets (also called **thrombocytes**) play a key role in hemostasis. They have no nucleus and are minute fragments of large bone marrow cells consisting of a small amount of granular cytoplasm surrounded by a plasma membrane.

Hemostasis is achieved through a three-step process:

1. **Vascular spasm,** an immediate but temporary constriction of the injured blood vessels.

2. **Platelet plug formation,** an accumulation of platelets that bind themselves together and adhere to surrounding tissues. The binding and adhesion of platelets are mediated through **von Willebrand factor (vWF),** a protein produced by the cells lining the blood vessels.

3. **Blood coagulation** is the process of going through **prothrombin** and **thrombin** to the formation of a blood clot that traps blood cells, platelets, and tissue fluid in a network of **fibrin** *(Figure 7.8).*

After a blood clot forms, platelets adhere to strands of fibrin and contract to pull the fibers and the edges of the broken blood vessel together. **Fibroblasts** invade the clot to produce a fibrous connective tissue that seals the blood vessel.

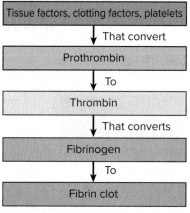

▲ **FIGURE 7.8**
Blood Coagulation.

Word Analysis and Definition

S = Suffix   P = Prefix   R = Root   R/CF = Combining Form

WORD	PRONUNCIATION		ELEMENTS	DEFINITION
coagulant	koh-**AG**-you-lant	S/ R/	-ant *forming, pertaining to* coagul- *clot, clump*	Substance that causes clotting
coagulation	koh-ag-you-**LAY**-shun	S/	-ation *process*	Process of blood clotting
fibrin	**FIE**-brin		Latin *fiber*	Stringy protein fiber that is a component of a blood clot
fibroblast	**FIE**-broh-blast	S/ R/CF	-blast *immature cell* fibr/o- *fiber*	Cell that forms collagen fibers
hemostasis (**Note:** *Homeostasis has a very different meaning.*)	he-moh-**STAY**-sis	S/ R/CF	-stasis *control, stop* hem/o- *blood*	Control of or stopping bleeding
prothrombin	pro-**THROM**-bin	S/ P/ R/	-in *substance* pro- *before* -thromb- *blood clot*	Protein formed by the liver and converted to thrombin in the blood-clotting mechanism
thrombocyte (*also called platelet*)	**THROM**-boh-site	S/ R/CF	-cyte *cell* thromb/o- *blood clot*	Another name for a platelet
von Willebrand	**VON WILL**-eh-brand		E.A. von Willebrand, Finnish physician, 1870–1949	

Blood Groups and Transfusions (LO 7.3 and 7.8)

Red Cell Antigens (LO 7.3 and 7.8)

Antigens are molecules that exist on the surfaces of red blood cells. **Antibodies** are present in the plasma. Each antibody can combine with only a specific antigen.

The antigens on the surfaces of the cells have been categorized into groups. Two of these groups–the **ABO** and **Rh** blood groups–are the most important.

ABO Blood Group (LO 7.3 and 7.8)

The two major antigens on the cell surface are antigen A and antigen B.

A person with only antigen A has *type A* blood.

A person with only antigen B has *type B* blood.

A person with both antigen A and antigen B has *type AB* blood.

A person with neither antigen has *type O* blood and is considered a universal donor, able to give blood to any other person.

Specific antibodies are synthesized in the plasma during the first 8 months after birth:

- Whenever antigen A is absent, anti-A antibody is produced.
- Whenever antigen B is absent, anti-B antibody is produced.

Figure 7.9 shows the different combinations of antigens and antibodies in the different blood types.

Rh Blood Group (LO 7.3 and 7.8)

If an Rh antigen is present on the red cell surface, the blood is said to be Rh-positive (Rh+). This is common, as about 85% of people are Rh-positive. If there is no Rh antigen on the surface, the blood is Rh-negative (Rh−), which is the case for the other 15% of the population.

Abbreviations

ABO   blood group system
Rh   rhesus

Keynotes

- All blood groups (A, B, AB, O) are inherited.
- Rh factor is an antigen on the surface of a red blood cell. Its presence or absence is inherited.

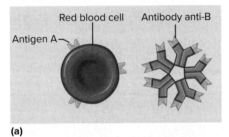

(a)

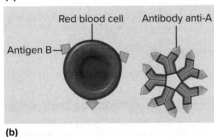

(b)

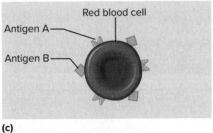

(c)

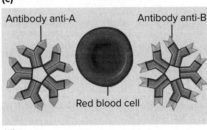

(d)

▲ **FIGURE 7.9**
(a) Type A blood. (b) Type B blood. (c) Type AB blood. (d) Type O blood.

Word Analysis and Definition

S = Suffix   P = Prefix   R = Root   R/CF = Combining Form

WORD	PRONUNCIATION	ELEMENTS		DEFINITION
antibody antibodies (pl)	**AN**-tee-bod-ee	P/ R/	anti- *against* -body *substance, body*	Protein produced in response to an antigen
antigen	**AN**-tee-gen	P/ R/	anti- *against* -gen *produce, create*	Substance capable of triggering an immune response
Rhesus factor	**REE**-sus **FAK**-tor		Greek *mythical king of Thrace*	Antigen on surface of red blood cells of Rh+ individuals; it was first identified in Rhesus monkeys

EXERCISES

Case Report 7.1

You are

. . . a medical assistant employed by Susan Lee, MD, a primary care physician at Fulwood Medical Center.

You are communicating with

. . . Ms. Luisa Sosin, a 47-year-old woman who presented a week ago with fatigue, lethargy, and muscle weakness. A physical examination revealed paleness (pallor) of her skin, a pulse rate of 90, and a respiratory rate of 20. Dr. Lee referred her for extensive blood work. She also determined that Ms. Sosin had been taking aspirin and **NSAIDs** (nonsteroidal anti-inflammatory drugs) for the past 6 months for lower back pain. Ms. Sosin's laboratory reports show an **iron-deficiency anemia.** You are responsible for documenting her examination and care.

A. Read *Case Report 7.1. Select the answer that correctly completes the statement or answers the question.* **LO 7.4, 7.9, 7.10, 7.11, and 7.12**

1. The lab results showed an abnormality in Ms. Sosin's:

   a. platelets   **b.** albumin   **c.** red blood cells   **d.** white blood cells   **e.** plasma

2. How might have Ms. Sosin described her fatigue?

   a. "My heart beats very rapidly."   **c.** "It is difficult to breathe."

   b. "I feel tired all of the time."   **d.** "I have episodes of dizziness."

3. The diagnostic test that Dr. Lee ordered was:

   a. computed tomogram   **b.** sonography   **c.** electrocardiography   **d.** blood work   **e.** bone marrow biopsy

4. What is your role in Ms. Sosin's care?

   a. proper documentation   **c.** diagnosing her condition

   b. drawing the blood for testing   **d.** filling her prescription

Case Report 7.2

You are

. . . an emergency medical technician (EMT) working in the Fulwood Medical Center Emergency Department.

You are communicating with

. . . Janis Tierney, a 17-year-old high school student who presents with fainting at school. She is pale. Her pulse is 109 and her blood pressure is 92/54. She tells you that she is having a menstrual period with excessive bleeding. Her physical examination is otherwise unremarkable. She has a history of easy bruising and recurrent nosebleeds, and an episode of severe bleeding after a tooth extraction. Janis has a deficiency of **von Willebrand factor (vWF).** Her platelets are unable to stick together, and a platelet plug cannot form in the lining of her uterus to help end her menstrual flow.

B. Read *Case Report 7.2 to answer the following questions. Select the correct answer to each question.* **LO 7.9, 7.12, and 7.13**

1. Why is Janis Tierney in the Emergency Department at Fulwood Medical Center?

   a. bruising, tachycardia   **b.** menstrual period with excessive bleeding   **c.** pallor and nosebleeds   **d.** fainting at school

2. What is causing her blood-related issues?

   a. deficiency of von Willebrand factor   **c.** lack of oxygen in the blood

   b. excessive white blood cells   **d.** deficient number of platelets

3. Which of the following are Janis Tierney's symptoms?

   a. fatigue   **b.** menstrual period with excessive bleeding   **c.** palpitations   **d.** increased pain with activity

4. What blood-related issues does she have in her medical history? (choose all that apply)

    a. she is pale   **b.** easy bruising   **c.** recurrent nosebleeds   **d.** fainting   **e.** hypertension

5. Translate into medical language: "her blood clotting cells are unable to stick together"

    a. thrombocytopenia   **b.** anemia   **c.** inability to coagulate   **d.** pancytopenia

C. Match *the definition in column 1 with the correct medical term in column 2. Fill in the blanks.*   **LO 7.4 and 7.5**

    _____ **1.** substance causing clotting   **a.** platelet

    _____ **2.** the last step in the process of blood coagulation   **b.** plasma

    _____ **3.** fluid remaining after removal of clot   **c.** coagulant

    _____ **4.** fluid noncellular component of blood   **d.** fibrin clot

    _____ **5.** also called a thrombocyte   **e.** serum

D. Using the medical terms *related to white blood cells, match the correct term in column one to its meaning in column two. Fill in the blanks.*   **LO 7.4 and 7.9**

    _____   **1.** eosinophil   **a.** largest blood cells

    _____   **2.** leukocyte   **b.** white blood cell with a multilobed nucleus

    _____   **3.** basophil   **c.** white blood cell

    _____   **4.** monocyte   **d.** releases histamine in damaged tissues

    _____   **5.** polymorphonuclear   **e.** involved in an allergic response

G. Provide the abbreviation *for each given definition. Fill in the blanks.*   **LO 7.3 and 7.8**

1. A group of cells that include those that fight infection, produce antibodies, or respond to allergens: _____

2. A lab test that reports the percentage of each type of white blood cell: _____

3. Proteins that are produced by B cells: _____

4. Type of leukocyte that ingests bacteria: _____

H. Test *your knowledge of blood, blood groups, and Rh factor by selecting the correct answer to the following questions.*   **LO 7.1 and 7.6**

1. A person with both antigen A and antigen B will have:

    a. blood type O

    b. blood type A

    c. blood type B

    d. blood type AB

2. Blood is said to be Rh-positive if the:

    a. Rh antigen is present on the RBC surface

    b. Rh antibody is present in the blood type

    c. Rh antibody is present in the plasma

    d. Rh antigen is present on the WBCs

    e. blood type is AB

3. A person with type B blood has B _____.

    a. antigens

    b. antibodies

4. A person with type A blood has _____.

    a. anti-A antibodies

    b. anti-B antibodies

    c. no antigens

Lymphatic System

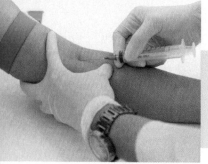

Abbreviation

Ab   antibody

As part of your body's defense mechanisms, the lymphatic system and its fluid provide surveillance and protection against foreign materials.

Lymphatic System (LO 7.7)

You live in a world surrounded with chemicals and disease-causing organisms waiting for a chance to enter your body and harm you. Your body has three lines of defense mechanisms against foreign organisms **(pathogens)**, cells (cancer), or molecules **(pollutants** and **allergens).**

1. **Physical defense mechanisms** include your skin and mucous membranes; chemicals in your perspiration, saliva, and tears; hairs in your nostrils; and cilia and mucus to protect your lungs. The physical defense mechanisms are further discussed in the individual body system chapters.

2. **Humoral defense mechanisms** *(see Lesson 7.3),* based on antibodies **(Abs).** These are found in body fluids and bind to bacteria, toxins, and extracellular viruses, tagging them for destruction.

3. **Cellular defense mechanisms,** based on defensive cells (lymphocytes). These directly attack suspicious cells like cancer cells, transplanted tissue cells, or cells infected with viruses or parasites.

The lymphatic system has three functions:

1. **Absorb** excess **interstitial** fluid and return it to the bloodstream;
2. **Remove** foreign chemicals, cells, and debris from the tissues; and
3. **Absorb** dietary lipids from the small intestine *(see Chapter 9).*

The lymphatic system *(Figure 7.10)* has three components:

1. A network of thin **lymphatic** capillaries and vessels, similar to blood vessels, that penetrates the **interstitial spaces** (spaces between tissues) of nearly every tissue in the body except cartilage, bone, red bone marrow, and the central nervous system;

2. A group of tissues and organs that produce **immune cells;** and

3. **Lymph**, a clear colorless fluid similar to blood plasma but with a composition that varies throughout the body. It flows through the network of lymphatic capillaries and vessels.

The **lymphatic network** begins with lymphatic capillaries that are closed-ended tubes nestled among **blood capillary networks** *(Figure 7.11).* The lymphatic capillaries are designed to let interstitial fluid enter so it can become lymph. In addition, bacteria, viruses, cellular debris, and traveling cancer cells can enter the lymphatic capillaries with the interstitial fluid. The lymphatic capillaries converge to form the larger **lymphatic collecting vessels,** which resemble small veins and have one-way valves. They travel alongside veins and arteries. Collecting vessels can continue into lymphatic trunks or into lymph nodes.

▼ **FIGURE 7.10**
The Lymphatic System.

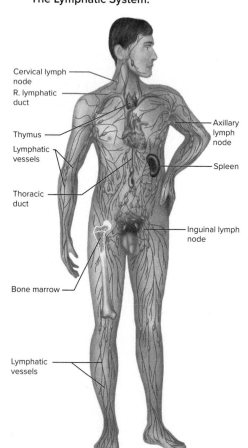

Cervical lymph node
R. lymphatic duct
Thymus
Lymphatic vessels
Thoracic duct
Bone marrow
Lymphatic vessels

Axillary lymph node
Spleen
Inguinal lymph node

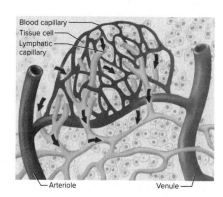

Blood capillary
Tissue cell
Lymphatic capillary

Arteriole   Venule

◀ **FIGURE 7.11**
Lymphatic Flow.

WORD	PRONUNCIATION	ELEMENTS		DEFINITION
absorb (verb)	ab-**SORB**		Latin *to swallow*	To take in
afferent (**Note:** *These are opposite terms.*)	**AFF**-eh-rent	S/ R/	-ent *pertaining to* affer- *move toward the center*	Moving toward a center
allergen (**Note:** *The duplicate letter "g" is omitted.*) allergic (adj) allergy	**AL**-er-jen ah-**LER**-jik **AL**-er-jee	S/ R/ R/ S/ S/	-gen *create* all- *other, strange* -erg- *work* -ic *pertaining to* -ergy *process of working*	Substance creating a hypersensitivity (allergic) reaction Pertaining to or suffering from an allergy Hypersensitivity to a particular allergen
efferent	**EFF**-eh-rent	S/ R/	-ent *end result, pertaining to* effer- *move away from the center*	Moving away from a center
immune	im-**YUNE**		Latin *protected from*	Protected from an infectious disease
interstitial	in-ter-**STISH**-al	S/ R/	-al *pertaining to* interstiti- *space between cells*	Pertaining to spaces between cells in an organ or tissue
lymph	LIMF		Latin *clear, spring water*	A clear fluid collected from tissues and transported by lymph vessels to the venous circulation
lymphatic (adj) lymphoid (adj)	lim-**FAT**-ik **LIM**-foyd	S/ R/ S/	-atic *pertaining to* lymph- *lymph* -oid *resembling*	Pertaining to lymph or the lymphatic system Resembling lymphatic tissue
node	NOHD		Latin *a knot*	A circumscribed mass of tissue
pathogen	**PATH**-oh-jen	S/ R/CF	-gen *produce, create, form* path/o- *disease*	A disease-causing microorganism
pollutant	poh-**LOO**-tant	S/ R/	-ant *pertaining to* pollut- *unclean*	Substance that makes an environment unclean or impure

Lymph Nodes (LO 7.2 and 7.10)

At irregular intervals, the collecting vessels enter into the lymph nodes *(Figure 7.12)* via afferent lymph vessels. There are hundreds of lymph nodes stationed all over the body *(Figure 7.10)*, concentrated in the neck, axilla, and groin. Lymph nodes are bundles of **lymphoid** tissue with the functions of filtering impurities from the lymph and alerting the immune system to the presence of pathogens.

The lymph moves slowly through the nodes, which filter the lymph and remove any foreign matter. Macrophages in the lymph nodes ingest and break down foreign matter and display its fragments to T cells. This alerts the immune system to the presence of an invader. Lymph leaves the nodes when it enters into the **efferent** collecting vessels. All these lymph vessels move lymph toward the thoracic cavity.

Collecting vessels merge into **lymphatic trunks** that drain lymph from a major body region. These lymphatic trunks then merge into two large **lymphatic ducts**—the thoracic duct on the left and the right lymphatic duct, which empty into the subclavian veins beneath the collarbone. *(Figure 7.10)*.

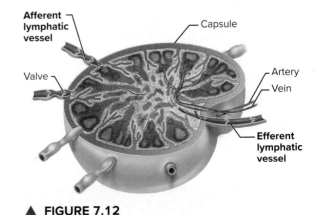

▲ **FIGURE 7.12**
Lymph Node.

Lymphatic Tissues and Cells (LO 7.2 and 7.10)

In some organs, lymphocytes and other cells form dense clusters called lymphatic **follicles**. These are constant features in the lymph nodes, the tonsils, and the ileum (part of the small intestine).

Lymphatic tissues are composed of a variety of cells that include:

- **T lymphocytes (T cells):** The "T" stands for thymus, which is where these cells develop and mature. T lymphocytes make up 75% to 85% of body lymphocytes.

- **B lymphocytes (B cells):** These cells mature in the bone marrow. B lymphocytes make up 15% to 25% of lymphocytes. They respond to a specific antigen and become plasma cells to produce antibodies **(immunoglobulins, Ig)** that immobilize, neutralize, and prepare the specific antigen for destruction. Macrophages that have developed from monocytes ingest and destroy antigens, tissue debris, **bacteria**, and other foreign matter through a process known as phagocytosis.

Keynote

- Tissues that are the first line of defense against pathogens—for example, the airway passages—have lymphatic tissue in the submucous layers to help protect against invasion.

Lymphatic Organs (LO 7.2 and 7.10)

Spleen (LO 7.2 and 7.10)

The **spleen**, a highly vascular and spongy organ, is the largest lymphatic organ. It is located in the left upper quadrant of the abdomen, below the diaphragm and lateral to the kidney *(Figure 7.13)*.

The functions of the spleen are to:

- **Phagocytose (consume)** bacteria and other foreign materials.
- **Phagocytose old, defective erythrocytes** and platelets.
- **Initiate an immune response** when antigens are found in the blood.
- **Serve as a reservoir** for erythrocytes and platelets.

Tonsils and Adenoids (LO 7.2 and 7.10)

The **tonsils** *(see Chapter 8)* are two masses of lymphatic tissue located at the entrance to the upper part of the throat (the oropharynx) that entrap inhaled and ingested pathogens. **Adenoids** are similar tissues on the posterior wall of the upper pharynx or nasopharynx *(see Chapter 8)*. The tonsils and adenoids form lymphocytes and antibodies, trap bacteria and viruses, and drain them into the tonsillar lymph nodes for elimination. Both the tonsils and the adenoids can also become infected and are commonly removed during childhood.

Thymus (LO 7.2 and 7.10)

The thymus, a small organ of the immune system located in the center of the upper chest, has both endocrine *(see Chapter 12)* and lymphatic functions. T lymphocytes develop and mature in the thymus and are released into the bloodstream. The thymus is largest in infancy *(Figure 7.14a)* and reaches its maximum size at puberty. It then shrinks *(Figure 7.14b)* and is eventually replaced by fibrous and fatty (adipose) tissue.

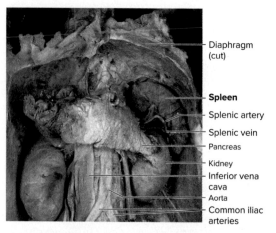

- Diaphragm (cut)
- **Spleen**
- Splenic artery
- Splenic vein
- Pancreas
- Kidney
- Inferior vena cava
- Aorta
- Common iliac arteries

▲ **FIGURE 7.13** Position of Spleen.

Dennis Strete/McGraw Hill

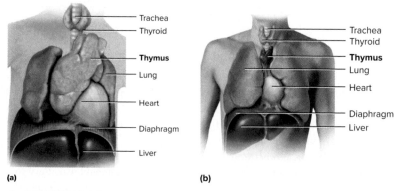

(a) — Trachea, Thyroid, **Thymus**, Lung, Heart, Diaphragm, Liver

(b) — Trachea, Thyroid, **Thymus**, Lung, Heart, Diaphragm, Liver

▲ **FIGURE 7.14** Thymus.
(a) Large thymus in infant. (b) Adult thymus.

Word Analysis and Definition

S = Suffix   P = Prefix   R = Root   R/CF = Combining Form

WORD	PRONUNCIATION	ELEMENTS		DEFINITION
adenoid	ADD-eh-noyd	S/ R/	**-oid** *resemble* **aden-** *gland*	Single mass of lymphoid tissue in the midline at the back of the throat
bacterium bacteria (pl)	bak-**TEER**-ee-um bak-**TEER**-ee-ah		Greek *a staff*	A unicellular, simple, microscopic organism
follicle	FOLL-ih-kull		Latin *a small sac*	Spherical mass of cells containing a cavity; or a small cul-de-sac, such as a hair follicle
immunoglobulin	IM-you-noh-**GLOB**-you-lin	S/ R/CF R/	**-in** *chemical compound, substance* **immun/o-** *immune* **-globul-** *globular, protein*	Specific protein evoked by an antigen. All antibodies are immunoglobulins
spleen	SPLEEN		Greek *spleen*	Vascular, lymphatic organ in left upper quadrant of abdomen
thymus	THIGH-mus		Greek *sweetbread*	Endocrine gland located in the mediastinum
tonsil	TON-sill		Latin *tonsil*	Mass of lymphoid tissue on either side of the throat at the back of the tongue

Immune System (LO 7.11 and 7.13)

The immune system is a group of specialized cells in different parts of the body that recognize and neutralize foreign substances. It is the **third line of defense** listed earlier in this chapter. When the immune system is weak, it allows pathogens, including the viruses that cause common colds and flu, and cancer cells, to successfully invade the body.

Three characteristics distinguish **immunity** from the first two lines of defense of physical and cellular mechanisms:

1. **Specificity**: The immune response is directed against a specific pathogen. Immunity to one pathogen does not grant immunity to others. Specificity has one disadvantage; if a virus or a bacterium changes a component of its genetic code, it then becomes a new organism to the immune system. This **mutation** occurs, for example, with bacteria in response to antibiotics and in HIV's response to anti-HIV drugs **(development of resistance).**

2. **Memory:** When exposure to the same pathogen occurs again, the immune system recognizes the pathogen and has its responses ready to act quickly.

3. **Discrimination:** The immune system learns to recognize agents (antigens) that represent **"self"** and agents (antigens) that are **"nonself"** (foreign). Most of this recognition is developed prior to birth. A variety of disorders occur when this discrimination breaks down. They are known as **autoimmune disorders.**

An antigen is any molecule that triggers an immune response. Most antigens are unique in their structure. It is this uniqueness that enables your body to distinguish its own (self) molecules from foreign (nonself) molecules.

Immunology is the study of the immune system. An **immunologist** is a medical specialist who is involved in the study and research of the immune system, and in treating immune system disorders.

Immunity (LO 7.11)

Immunity is the state of being able to resist a specific infectious disease. It is classified biologically into two types, although these often respond to the same antigen:

1. **Cellular (cell-mediated) immunity:** This is a direct form of defense based on the actions of lymphocytes to attack foreign and diseased cells and destroy them. The many different types of T cells, B cells, and macrophages described in the previous lesson of this chapter are involved in this style of attack *(Figure 7.15).*

2. **Humoral (antibody-mediated) immunity:** This is an indirect form of attack that employs antibodies produced by plasma cells, which have been developed from B cells. Immunoglobulins are antibodies present in blood plasma and body secretions that bind to an antigen and tag it for destruction.

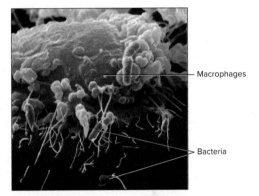

Macrophages

Bacteria

▲ **FIGURE 7.15** Macrophage Phagocytoses Bacteria. Filamentous extensions of a macrophage cell snare the bacteria and draw them to the surface of the cell where they are engulfed into the macrophage.

Eye of Science/Science Source

Word Analysis and Definition

S = Suffix   P = Prefix   R = Root   R/CF = Combining Form

WORD	PRONUNCIATION		ELEMENTS	DEFINITION
discrimination	DIS-krim-ih-**NAY**-shun	S/ P/ R/	-ation *process* dis- *away from* -crimin- *distinguish*	Ability to distinguish between different things
immunity	im-**YUNE**-ih-tee	S/ R/	-ity *condition* immun- *immune*	State of being protected
immunologist	im-you-**NOL**-oh-jist	S/	-logist *one who studies, specialist*	Medical specialist in immunology
immunology	im-you-**NOL**-oh-jee	S/	-logy *study of*	The science and practice of immunity and allergy
mutation	myu-**TAY**-shun		Latin *to change*	Change in the chemistry of a gene
nonself	awe-toe-im-**YUNE**	P/	non- *no, not*	In immunology, pertaining to foreign antigens
self		R/ Old English *one's own person*	-self *self*	In immunology, pertaining to the body's own antigens
specific	speh-**SIF**-ik	S/ R/	-ic *pertaining to* specif- *species*	Relating to a particular entity
specificity (Note: Has two suffixes.)	spes-ih-**FIS**-ih-tee	S/	-ity *condition, state*	State of having a specific, fixed relation to a particular entity
toxin toxicity	**TOK**-sin toks-**ISS**-ih-tee	S/ R/	Greek *poison* -ity *state, condition* toxic- *poison*	Poisonous substance formed by a cell or organism The state of being poisonous

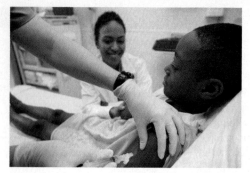

ERproductions Ltd/Blend Images LLC

Complement Fixation (LO 7.2 and 7.11)

The complement system is a group of 20 or more proteins continually present in blood plasma. Immunoglobulins bind to foreign cells, initiating the binding of **complement** to the cell and leading to its destruction.

Immunization (LO 7.2 and 7.11)

Immunization is the preventive method of stimulating the immune system without exposing the body to an infection. An agent **(vaccine)** composed of the antigenic components of a killed or **attenuated** microorganism or its inactivated **toxins** is injected into the body. **Vaccination** is a crucial step in keeping our population healthy. For example, vaccination has eradicated smallpox worldwide. However, if we stop vaccinating against smallpox, our population will again be susceptible to smallpox outbreaks. The same concept applies to the diseases in childhood immunizations *(Table 7.1)*.

Table 7.1 Recommended Immunizations for Persons Aged 0 to 6 Years

Hepatitis A (HepA)	Hepatitis B (HepB)
Rotavirus (RV)	Influenza (Yearly)
Inactivated poliovirus (IPV)	Varicella (chickenpox)
Diphtheria, tetanus, pertussis (DTaP)	Pneumococcal (PCV)
Measles, mumps, rubella (MMR)	Coronavirus disease 2019 (COVID-19)
Hemophilus influenza type b (Hib)	

Source: Centers for Disease Control and Prevention, 2023.

Word Analysis and Definition

S = Suffix   P = Prefix   R = Root   R/CF = Combining Form

WORD	PRONUNCIATION		ELEMENTS	DEFINITION
attenuate (verb)	ah-**TEN**-you-ate	S/ R/	-ate *composed of, pertaining to* attenu- *weaken*	Weaken the ability of an organism to produce disease
attenuated (adj)	ah-**TEN**-you-a-ted	S/	-ated *pertaining to a condition*	Weakened
complement	**KOM**-pleh-ment		Latin *that which completes*	Group of proteins in serum that finishes off the work of antibodies to destroy bacteria and other cells
humoral immunity	**HYU**-mor-al im-**YUNE**-ih-tee	S/ R/ S/ R/	-al *pertaining to* humor- *fluid* -ity *condition* immun- *immune*	Defense mechanism arising from antibodies in the blood
immunize (verb)	**IM**-you-nize	S/ R/	-ize *affect in a specific way* immun- *immune*	To cause to be resistant to an infectious disease
immunization (noun)	**IM**-you-nih-**ZAY**-shun	S/	-ization *process of inserting or creating*	Administration of an agent to provide immunity
vaccinate (verb)	**VAK**-sin-ate	S/ R/	-ate *pertaining to, composed of* vaccin- *vaccine, giving a vaccine*	To administer a vaccine
vaccination vaccine	vak-sih-**NAY**-shun **VAK**-seen	S/	-ation *process* Latin *related to a cow*	Administration of a vaccine Preparation to generate active immunity

EXERCISES

 ## Case Report 7.3

You are

. . . laboratory technician working the night shift at Fulwood Medical Center.

You are communicating with

. . . Mr. Michael Cowan, a 40-year-old homeless man and drug addict, who has presented to the Emergency Department with a high fever, with no obvious cause.

You have been called to the emergency room to take blood from Mr. Cowan. You insert the needle into an **antecubital** vein, but he starts jerking his arm around and trying to get off the gurney. In the struggle, the needle comes out of the vein and pricks your hand through your glove.

You immediately flush and clean your wound, report the incident, seek immediate medical attention, and go through your initial medical evaluation. However, because of your possible exposure to Mr. Cowan's blood, it is essential that you have knowledge about your own immune system and its response to a potential infection. This will help you to make informed decisions about your treatment and future employment.

A. Analyze *Case Report 7.3 and select the correct answer to complete each statement.* **LO 7.9 and 7.11**

1. What is the purpose of flushing the wound?

   a. Hydrate the skin   **b.** Replace any lost blood   **c.** Remove pathogens from the wound   **d.** Water is a natural antibiotic

2. Mr. Cowan's high fever is most likely due to:

   a. an infection   **b.** heatstroke   **c.** an allergic reaction   **d.** cardiac arrest

3. If you have been exposed to a pathogen, your body will react to it by creating:

   a. haptens   **b.** erythrocytes   **c.** mutations   **d.** antibodies

B. Construct *the correct medical terms that match the definitions given. If a term does not have a particular element, insert N/A for that blank. Fill in the blanks.* **LO 7.1 and 7.9**

1. substance that makes the environment unclean or impure:

   _____ / _____ / _____
         P   R/CF   S

2. substance creating a hypersensitivity reaction:

   _____ / _____ / _____
        R/CF   R/CF   S

3. resembling lymphatic tissue:

   _____ / _____ / _____
         P   R/CF   S

4. a disease-causing microorganism:

   _____ / _____ / _____
         P   R/CF   S

5. hypersensitivity to a particular allergen:

   _____ / _____ / _____
        R/CF   R/CF   S

C. Precision *in usage is important if you want to communicate correct information. These six terms all contain a common root/combining form. Insert the correct term in each sentence.* **LO 7.2, 7.8, and 7.11**

immune   **immunology**   **immunity**   **immunologist**   **immunization**   **immunize**

1. One who specializes in (the study of the science of immunity and allergy) _____ is termed an (type of specialist) _____ .

2. The _____ system is a group of specialized cells in different parts of the body that recognize foreign substances and neutralize them.

3. We need to _____ young children before they start school.

4. A prior (injection) _____ obtained before she went overseas boosted her (status of being immune) _____ to the disease.

D. Demonstrate *your understanding of anatomy and function of the lymphatic system. Select the correct answer to each question.*   **LO 7.4, 7.5, and 7.7**

1. Where are the interstitial spaces located?

   a. in the capillary bed   **b.** between blood vessels   **c.** between tissues   **d.** between cells

   e. within the blood vessels

2. Lymph is similar to what other body fluid?

   a. spinal fluid   **b.** sputum   **c.** urine   **d.** blood plasma

3. Which of the following are functions of the lymphatic system? (choose all that apply)

   a. eliminate excess bilirubin from the blood

   b. absorb interstitial fluid and return it to the bloodstream

   c. remove foreign chemicals, cells, and debris from tissues

   d. absorb dietary lipids from the small intestine

4. Which of the following tissues lack lymphatic capillaries and vessels in the interstitial spaces? (select all that apply)

   a. cartilage   **b.** bone   **c.** pancreas   **d.** central nervous system

   e. red bone marrow

5. Where in the body are the major concentrations of lymph nodes?

   a. neck, chest, groin   **b.** axilla, chest, abdomen   **c.** neck, axilla, abdomen   **d.** neck, axilla, groin

   e. chest, abdomen, groin

6. What substance enters lymphatic capillaries to become lymph?

   a. blood plasma   **b.** interstitial fluid   **c.** red bone marrow   **d.** lymphocytes   **e.** mucus

E. *Answer the following questions by selecting the best choice.*   **LO 7.1, 7.3, and 7.10**

1. In the term *adenoid* one of the elements means:

   a. tissue   **b.** organ   **c.** gland

2. The correct plural of bacterium is:

   a. bacteria   **b.** bacteriae   **c.** bacteriums

3. In addition to referring to a lymph follicle, the term *follicle* can also apply to:

   a. digits   **b.** bones   **c.** hair

4. What do *tonsil* and *adenoid* have in common?

   a. lymphatic tissue   **b.** connective tissue   **c.** adipose tissue

5. Immunoglobulin can also be considered:

   a. tissue collection   **b.** pathogen   **c.** antibody

6. The suffix in the term *adenoidectomy* implies:

   a. surgical excision   **b.** surgical fixation   **c.** surgical incision

7. A microscopic organism is:

   a. bacteria   **b.** follicle   **c.** bacterium

8. The spleen is located in the:

   a. ABG   **b.** RLQ   **c.** LUQ

9. The specific protein evoked by an antigen is:

   a. bacterium   **b.** enzyme   **c.** immunoglobulin

10. The element meaning *enlargement* is:

   a. megaly   **b.** ectomy   **c.** oid

F. Decide *if the statement is true or false. Select T if the statement is true. Select F if the statement is false.*   **LO 7.9**

1. Opportunistic infections occur when the immune system is strong.   T   F

2. The immune system is composed of specific organs that fight infections.   T   F

3. An autoimmune disorder develops when a person's immune system recognizes an agent as "self."   T   F

4. Immunity to one pathogen grants immunity to others.   T   F

5. A bacterium or virus develops resistance when a person's immune system is weakened.   T   F

G. Each of these questions *requires a one-word answer. Think carefully before writing the answers.*   **LO 7.2 and 7.12**

1. Ability to distinguish between different things: _____

2. Change in the chemistry of a gene produces a: _____

3. A molecule that triggers a response: _____

H. Patient Education. Select the statement that correctly explains functions of immunity.   **LO 7.12 and 7.13**

1. Explain to your patient how immunization works to protect the body.

   a. "An immunization contains live microorganisms that cause you to develop the infection so that components of the immune system prevent repeated infections."

   b. "An immunization contains killed microorganisms or toxins that do not cause infection but stimulate components of the immune system to protect you from repeat infections."

   c. "An immunization is a type of medication that heightens the awareness of the immune system for foreign invaders."

   d. "An immunization is a type of medication that strengthens the immune system so that it can do its job more effectively."

2. Explain what the complement system does for the body.

   a. "Complement is a type of cell-mediated immunity involving lymphocytes that attack foreign and diseased cells and destroy them."

   b. "Complement is a type of immunization to protect a person against infection."

   c. "Complement refers to a group of 20 or more immunoglobulins that are present in a vaccine."

   d. "Complement is a group of 20 or more proteins that bind to foreign cells, leading to their destruction."

3. Your patient has asked you what agglutinate means. How would you explain the concept to your patient?

   a. "Agglutinate refers to the destruction of foreign cells."

   b. "Agglutinate refers to cells sticking together to form clumps."

   c. "Agglutinate refers to the clumping together of platelets due to an allergic reaction"

   d. "Agglutinate refers to destruction of microorganisms following an immunization."

I. Identify the meanings of the word elements. *Select the answer that correctly completes each statement.*   **LO 7.1**

1. The root attenu- means:

   a. clumping   **c.** fluid

   b. inject   **d.** weaken

2. The suffix -ity means:

   a. source   **c.** condition

   b. process   **d.** pertaining to

3. The suffix -tion means:

   a. weaken   **c.** condition

   b. process   **d.** pertaining to

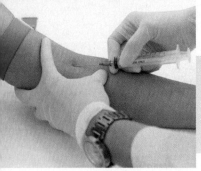

Section 7.3

Disorders of Blood and Blood Components

Disorders of the Blood

Disorders of Red Blood Cells (LO 7.3 and 7.9)

Anemia is a condition where the number of RBCs or amount of hemoglobin contained in each RBC is reduced. Both of these conditions reduce the blood's oxygen-carrying capacity, causing **hypoxia** and producing shortness of breath **(SOB)** and fatigue. Anemia produces **pallor** (pale color) because of the deficiency of the red-colored **oxyhemoglobin,** the combination of oxygen and hemoglobin.

The different types of anemia include:

- **Iron-deficiency anemia** is caused by chronic bleeding such as from the gastrointestinal tract due to long-term use of aspirin and other painkillers. Other causes of iron-deficiency anemia can be heavy menstrual bleeds or a diet deficient in iron.

- **Pernicious anemia (PA)** is due to **vitamin** B_{12} deficiency. It is caused by a shortage of intrinsic factor, which is normally secreted by cells in the stomach lining *(see Chapter 9)* and binds with B_{12}. This complex is absorbed into the bloodstream. Without B_{12}, hemoglobin cannot form. The number of red cells decreases, hemoglobin concentration decreases, and the size of the red cells increases.

- **Sickle cell anemia** is a genetic disorder found most commonly in African Americans. Here, the production of abnormal hemoglobin causes the RBCs to form a rigid sickle shape *(Figure 7.16)*. The abnormal cells **agglutinate** (clump together) and block small capillaries. This creates intense pain in the **hypoxic** tissues (a sickle cell crisis) and can lead to stroke, kidney failure, and heart failure. **Sickle cell trait** is a minor form of this disease and rarely has any symptoms.

- **Hemolytic anemia** is caused by excessive destruction of normal and abnormal RBCs. **Hemolysis** (the destruction of RBCs) can result from toxic substances, entering the bloodstream such as snake and spider venoms, mushroom toxins, and overdoses of drugs. Trauma to RBCs by hemodialysis or heart-lung machines, or an incompatible blood transfusion, can also cause hemolysis.

- **Aplastic anemia** is a condition in which the bone marrow is unable to produce sufficient new cells of all types—red cells, white cells, and platelets. It can be associated with exposure to radiation, benzene, and certain drugs.

- **Polycythemia** is an overproduction of RBCs by the bone marrow. The cause is unknown, but is often seen in cases of chronic hypoxemia.

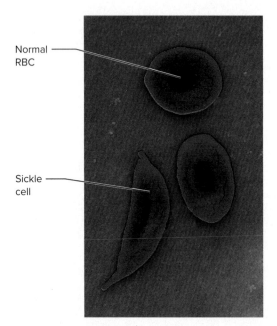

Normal RBC

Sickle cell

▲ **FIGURE 7.16** Sickle Cell Disease.

WORD	PRONUNCIATION	ELEMENTS		DEFINITION
agglutinate (verb)	ah-GLUE-tin-ate	S/ P/ R/	-ate composed of, pertaining to ag- (ad-) to -glutin- stick	Stick together to form clumps
agglutination (noun)	ah-glue-tih-NAY-shun	S/	-ation process	Process by which cells or other particles adhere to each other to form clumps
anemia	ah-NEE-me-ah	P/ R/	an- without -emia a blood condition	Decreased number of red blood cells
anemic (adj)	ah-NEE-mik	S/	-emic pertaining to a condition of the blood	Pertaining to or suffering from anemia
aplastic anemia	a-PLAS-tik ah-NEE-me-ah	S/ P/ R/ P/ R/	-tic pertaining to a- without -plas- formation an- without -emia blood condition	Condition in which the bone marrow is unable to produce sufficient red cells, white cells, and platelets
hemoglobinopathy	HE-moh-GLOW-bin-OP-ah-thee	S/ R/CF R/CF	-pathy disease hem/o- blood -globin/o- protein	Disease caused by the presence of an abnormal hemoglobin in red blood cells
hemolysis	he-MOL-ih-sis	S/ R/CF	-lysis destruction hem/o- blood	Destruction of red blood cells so that hemoglobin is liberated
hemolytic (adj)	he-moh-LIT-ik	S/ R/	-ic pertaining to -lyt- destroy	Pertaining to the destruction of red blood cells
hypoxia (Note: The duplicate letter "o" is omitted.) hypoxic (adj)	high-POCK-see-ah high-POCK-sik	S/ P/ R/ S/	-ia condition hypo- below, deficient -ox- oxygen -ic pertaining to	Below-normal levels of oxygen in tissues, gases, or blood Deficient in oxygen
hypoxemia	HIGH-pok-SEE-mee-ah	S/ P/ R/	-emia blood condition hyp(o)- below -ox- oxygen	Decreased levels of oxygen in the blood
oxyhemoglobin	OCK-see-he-moh-GLOW-bin	R/ R/CF R	oxy- oxygen hem/o blood -globin protein	Combination of hemoglobin and oxygen
pallor	PAL-or		Latin paleness	Paleness of the skin
pernicious anemia	per-NISH-us ah-NEE-me-ah	S/ P/ R/ P/ R/	-ous pertaining to per- through -nici- lethal an- without -emia a blood condition	Chronic anemia due to lack of vitamin B_{12}
polycythemia	POL-ee-sigh-THEE-me-ah	S/ P/ R/	-hemia blood condition poly- many, much -cyt- cell	A disease of bone marrow, excess production of RBCs
trait	TRAYT		Latin an extension	A discrete characteristic that has a known quality
vitamin (Note: The duplicate letter "a" is omitted. It was originally thought that all vitamins were amines.)	VYE-tah-min	S/ R/	-amin(e) nitrogen-containing substance vita- life	Essential organic substance necessary in small amounts for normal cell function

Erythroblastosis Fetalis

If an Rh-negative person receives a transfusion of Rh-positive blood, anti-Rh antibodies will be produced. This can cause RBC clumping (agglutination) and destruction (hemolysis).

If an Rh-negative woman and an Rh-positive man conceive an Rh-positive child *(Figure 7.17a),* the placenta normally prevents **maternal** and **fetal** blood from mixing. However, at birth or during a **miscarriage,** fetal cells can enter the mother's bloodstream. These Rh-positive cells stimulate the mother's tissues to produce Rh antibodies *(Figure 7.17b).*

If the mother becomes pregnant with a second Rh-positive fetus, her Rh antibodies can cross the **placenta** and agglutinate and hemolyze the fetal red cells *(Figure 7.17c).* This causes hemolytic disease of the newborn **(HDN,** or **erythroblastosis fetalis).**

Abbreviation

HDN	hemolytic disease of the newborn

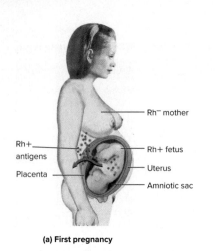
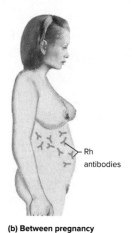
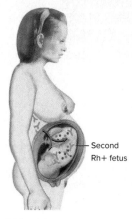

(a) First pregnancy   (b) Between pregnancy   (c) Second pregnancy

Hemolytic disease of the newborn due to Rh incompatibility can be prevented. The Rh-negative mother giving birth to an Rh-positive child should be given Rh-immune globulin (RhoGAM).

Other causes of hemolytic disease in newborns include ABO **incompatibility,** incompatibility in other blood group systems, hereditary **spherocytosis,** and infections acquired before birth.

▲ **FIGURE 7.17** Hemolytic Disease of the Newborn.
(a) First pregnancy. (b) Between pregnancies. (c) Second pregnancy.

Word Analysis and Definition

S = Suffix   P = Prefix   R = Root   R/CF = Combining Form

WORD	PRONUNCIATION	ELEMENTS		DEFINITION
erythroblastosis fetalis	eh-**RITH**-roh-blast-**OH**-sis fee-**TAH**-lis	S/ R/CF R/ S/ R/	-osis *condition* erythr/o- *red* -blast- *immature cell* -is *belonging to* fetal- *fetus*	Erythroblastosis fetalis is a hemolytic disease of the newborn (HDN)
fetus	**FEE**-tus		Latin *offspring*	Human organism from the end of the eighth week after conception to birth
fetal (adj)	**FEE**-tal	S/ R/	-al *pertaining to* fet- *fetus*	Pertaining to the fetus
incompatible	in-kom-**PAT**-ih-bul	S/ P/ R/	-ible *can do* in- *not* -compat- *tolerate*	Substances that interfere with each other physiologically
incompatibility	in-kom-**PAT**-ih-bil-i-tee	S/	-ibility *able to do*	The quality of being incompatible
maternal	mah-**TER**-nal	S/ R/	-al *pertaining to* matern- *mother*	Pertaining to or derived from the mother
miscarriage	mis-**KAIR**-aj	P/	mis- *not, incorrect* -carriage Old English *to carry*	Spontaneous expulsion of the products of pregnancy before fetal viability
placenta	plah-**SEN**-tah		Latin *a cake*	Organ that allows metabolic exchange between the mother and the fetus
spherocyte	**SFEAR**-oh-site	R/CF R/	spher/o- *sphere* -cyte *cell*	A spherical cell
spherocytosis	**SFEAR**-oh-site-**OH**-sis	S/	-osis *condition*	Presence of spherocytes in blood

Keynote

• Leukocytosis describes excessive amounts of white blood cells and often indicates the presence of an infection.

Disorders of White Blood Cells (LO 7.3 and 7.5)

A normal cubic millimeter (mm^3) of blood contains 5,000 to 10,000 white blood cells. In **leukocytosis**, the total WBC count exceeds 101,000 per cubic millimeter. Other conditions that increase the WBC count beyond the normal range include:

• Allergic reactions, which increase the number of eosinophils;

• Typhoid fever, malaria, and tuberculosis, which increase the number of monocytes; and

• Bacterial infections increase the number of lymphocytes.

• Viral infections often cause a decrease in the overall white blood cell count, known as **leukopenia.**

Infectious mononucleosis most commonly occurs in the 15- to 25-year-old population. Its cause—the **Epstein-Barr virus (EBV)**—is a very common virus and a member of the herpes family. EBV is transmitted by an exchange of saliva, such as when kissing.

Leukemia is cancer of the blood-forming tissues and produces a high number of leukocytes and their precursors. The **leukemic** cells multiply, taking over the bone marrow and causing a deficiency of normal red blood cells, white blood cells, and platelets. This makes the patient anemic and vulnerable to infection and bleeding.

In **leukopenia**, the WBC count drops below 5,000 cells per cubic millimeter of blood. Leukopenia is seen in viral infections like measles, mumps, chickenpox, poliomyelitis, and AIDS.

In **pancytopenia**, the erythrocytes (red blood cells), leukocytes (white blood cells), and thrombocytes (platelets) in the circulating blood are all noticeably reduced. This can occur with autoimmune disease, various genetic disorders, or cancer chemotherapy.

Word Analysis and Definition

S = Suffix   P = Prefix   R = Root   R/CF = Combining Form

WORD	PRONUNCIATION	ELEMENTS		DEFINITION
leukemia	loo-**KEE**-mee-ah	S/ R/	-emia *a blood condition* leuk- *white*	Disease when the blood is taken over by white blood cells and their precursors
leukemic (adj)	loo-**KEE**-mik	S/	-emic *pertaining to a blood condition*	Pertaining to or affected by leukemia
leukocytosis	**LOO**-koh-sigh-**TOH**-sis	S/ R/CF	-osis *condition* leuk/o- *white*	An excessive number of white blood cells
leukopenia	loo-koh-**PEE**-nee-ah	S/	-penia *deficiency*	A deficient number of white blood cells
mononucleosis	**MON**-oh-nyu-klee-**OH**-sis	S/ P/ R/	-osis *condition* mono- *single* -nucle- *nucleus*	Presence of large numbers of specific, diagnostic mononuclear leukocytes
neutropenia	**NEW**-troh-**PEE**-nee-ah	S/ R/CF	-penia *deficiency* neutr/o- *neutral*	A deficiency of neutrophils
neutrophilia	**NEW**-troh-**FILL**-ee-ah	S/	-philia *attraction*	An increase in neutrophils
pancytopenia	**PAN**-site-oh-**PEE**-nee-ah	S/ P/ R/CF	-penia *deficiency* pan- *all* -cyt/o- *cell*	Deficiency of all types of blood cells

Disorders of Coagulation (Coagulopathies) (LO 7.3 and 7.9)

There are several disorders that can prevent the blood from clotting properly, and these can lead to further health problems.

- **Hemophilia**, in its classical form (hemophilia A), is a disease males inherit from their mothers. It results from a deficiency of the coagulation factor named **factor VIII.**

- **Von Willebrand disease (vWD)**—the most common hereditary bleeding disorder—is a protein deficiency of the factor VIII complex **(vWF)** that is different from the factor deficiency involved in hemophilia.

- **Disseminated intravascular coagulation (DIC)** occurs when a severe bacterial infection activates the clotting mechanism simultaneously throughout the cardiovascular system. Small clots form and obstruct blood flow into tissues and organs, particularly the kidney, leading to renal failure.

- **Thrombus** formation **(thrombosis)** is a clot that forms attachment to a diseased or damaged area on the walls of blood vessels or the heart. If part of the thrombus breaks loose and moves through the circulation, it is called an **embolus.**

- **Thrombocytopenia** is a deficiency of platelets.

- **Purpura** is bleeding into the skin from small arterioles that produces a larger individual lesion than the tiny red spots or **petechiae** from capillary bleeds *(Figure 7.18a and b)*. **Bruises** (or ecchymoses) are leaks of blood from all types of blood vessels. A raised area of bruising is known as a **hematoma.**

- **Idiopathic thrombocytic purpura (ITP)** occurs when the immune system destroys the body's platelets. An acute, self-limiting form of the disease occurs in children; a chronic form affects adults.

Abbreviations

DIC	disseminated intravascular coagulation
EBV	Epstein-Barr virus
ITP	idiopathic thrombocytopenic purpura
vWD	von Willebrand disease

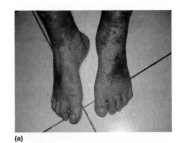

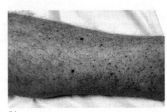

▶ **FIGURE 7.18** Subsurface Bleeding.
(a) Purpura. (b) Petechiae.

7.10a: LoyFah4158/Shutterstock
7.10b: TisforThan/Shutterstock

(a)

(b)

Word Analysis and Definition

S = Suffix   P = Prefix   R = Root   R/CF = Combining Form

WORD	PRONUNCIATION	ELEMENTS		DEFINITION
ecchymosis	EK-i-MO-sis	S/ P/ R/	-osis *condition of* ec- *out, outside* -chym- *juice*	Small hematoma resulting from a bruise
embolus	EM-boh-lus		Greek *plug, stopper*	Detached piece of thrombus, a mass of bacteria, quantity of air, or foreign body that blocks a blood vessel
hematoma (*also called* bruise)	he-mah-**TOE**-mah	S/ R/	-oma *mass, tumor* hemat- *blood*	Collection of blood that has escaped from vessels into surrounding tissues
hemophilia	he-moh-**FILL**-ee-ah	S/ R/CF	-philia *attraction* hem/o- *blood*	An inherited disease from a deficiency of clotting factor VIII
petechia petechiae (pl)	peh-**TEE**-kee-ah peh-**TEE**-kee-ee		Latin *spot on the skin*	Pinpoint capillary hemorrhagic spot in the skin
purpura	**PUR**-pyu-rah		Greek *purple*	Skin hemorrhages that are red initially and then turn purple
thrombocytopenia	**THROM**-boh-site-oh-**PEE**-nee-uh	S/ R/CF R/CF	-penia *deficiency* thromb/o- *blood clot* -cyt/o- *cell*	Deficiency of platelets in circulating blood

EXERCISES

 Case Report 7.4

You are

. . . an emergency medical technician–paramedic (EMT-P) working in the Level One Trauma Unit at Fulwood Medical Center.

You are communicating with

. . . Ms. Joanne Rodi, an 18-year-old student, who has been admitted to the unit from the operating room. Ms. Rodi has had surgery for multiple fractures sustained in a car accident. She is receiving a blood **transfusion**. You document that her temperature has risen to 102.8°F, her respirations have risen to 24 per minute, and she has chills. You take her blood pressure, and it has fallen to 95/602. What is your next step?

In Joanne Rodi's case, she has type A blood and by mistake received type AB blood, the red cells of which agglutinated in the presence of her anti-B antibodies. Your immediate response is to stop the transfusion, replace it with a saline **infusion**, call your supervisor, and notify the doctor.

A. Select *the correct term in bold that completes each statement*   **LO 7.1, 7.9, and 7.10**

1. It is the _____ on the erythrocyte that determines a person's blood type.

      antigen   **antibody**

2. It is _____ that contains antibodies that seek out antigens.

      red blood cells   **plasma**

3. The doctor ordered a(n) _____ of packed red blood cells.

      infusion   **transfusion**

4. The aspirin inhibited _____ , leading to an increased loss of blood.

      thrombus   **thrombosis**

5. The _____ of normal saline increased the patient's blood volume.

      infusion   **transfusion**

B. Fill in the blanks *with the correct medical term related to the disorders of coagulation.*   **LO 7.2, 7.9, and 7.12**

1. A decrease in the number of thrombocytes in the circulating blood: _____

2. A thrombus that has detached and lodged in another blood vessel: _____

3. A pinpoint hemorrhage: _____

4. Multiple pinpoint hemorrhages: _____

5. Skin hemorrhages that at first appear red and then turn purple: _____

C. Read *Fill in the blanks.*   **LO 7.1 and 7.2**

_____ 1. trans-	**a.** to pour
_____ 2. anti-	**b.** glue
_____ 3. -fusion	**c.** against
_____ 4. -glutin	**d.** across
_____ 5. -gen	**e.** produce

D. A suffix *completes a medical term. The element* leuk *or* leuk/o *remains the same in each term below. Fill in the blanks.*   **LO 7.1 and 7.9**

-penia   **-cyte**   **-cytosis**   **-emia**   **-ic**

1. An excessive number of white blood cells is: _____

2. The disease when the blood is taken over by the WBCs is: _____

3. Another term for a white blood cell is: _____

4. A deficient number of white blood cells is: _____

5. Pertaining to leukemia: _____

E. Explain the disorder erythroblastosis fetalis. *Select the correct answer to complete the statement or answer the question.*   **LO 7.3 and 7.8**

1. In the medical term **erythroblastosis fetalis,** the condition affects which component of the blood?

   a. white blood cells   **b.** plasma   **c.** coagulation   **d.** red blood cells

2. In the medical condition **erythroblastosis fetalis,** who is harmed: the mother or the baby?

   a. mother   **b.** baby

3. In order for **erythroblastosis fetalis** to occur, the mother must have blood that is:

   a. type A   **b.** type B   **c.** type O   **d.** Rh-   **e.** Rh+

4. The trigger for **erythroblastosis fetalis** to occur is a baby with blood that is:

   a. type A   **b.** type B   **c.** type O   **d.** Rh-   **e.** Rh+

5. It is impossible for the first child to have this condition.

   a. True   **b.** False

F. Use your knowledge *of medical terminology to answer the following questions. Fill in the blanks.*   **LO 7.9 and 7.13**

1. What is the medical term for *red blood cells clumping together?* _____

2. What is more common: being Rh+ or Rh- ? _____

3. The abbreviation for erythroblastosis fetalis is: _____

4. Transferring of blood from donor to recipient: _____

5. The medication containing Rhesus immune globulin given to mothers to prevent erythroblastosis fetalis: _____

G. Identify *the meanings of the word elements that construct medical terms. Select the correct answer.*   **LO 7.1**

1. The suffix in the term *hypoxia* means:

    a. blood   **b.** oxygen   **c.** deficient   **d.** condition

2. The combining form in the term *erythrocyte* means:

    a. red   **b.** white   **c.** cell   **d.** disc

3. The suffix in the term *hemoglobinopathy* means:

    a. pertaining to   **b.** condition of   **c.** disease   **d.** protein

4. The prefix in the term *polycythemia* means:

    a. cell   **b.** blood condition   **c.** many   **d.** through

5. The root in the term *pernicious* means:

    a. lethal   **b.** cell   **c.** small   **d.** crescent

H. Fill *in the correct disorder that matches the description.*   **LO 7.2, 7.3, 7.5, and 7.9**

1. numbers of RBCs reduced: _____

2. bone marrow produces an excess of erythrocytes: _____

3. genetic disorder found most commonly in African Americans: _____

4. disease caused by the presence of an abnormal hemoglobin in red blood cells: _____

5. disorder caused by vitamin B_{12} deficiency:

Disorders of the Lymphatic and Immune Systems

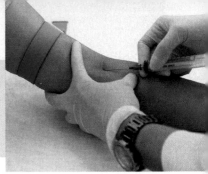

mikumistock/Shutterstock

Disorders of the Lymphatic System (LO 7.10)

Physicians routinely feel the accessible lymph nodes in the neck **(cervical nodes)**, axilla (armpit) **(axillary nodes)**, and groin **(inguinal nodes)** for enlargement and tenderness, which indicate disease in the tissues drained by the lymph nodes.

Cancerous lymph nodes are enlarged, firm, and usually painless. Infections in the lymph nodes cause them to be swollen and tender to the touch, a condition called **lymphadenitis**. All lymph node enlargements are collectively called **lymphadenopathy**.

Lymphoma is a malignant growth **(neoplasm)** of the lymphatic organs, usually the lymph nodes. Like many cancers, associated symptoms can be fever, night sweats, fatigue, and weight loss. Lymphomas are grouped into two categories by microscopic examination of affected lymphatic tissues:

1. **Hodgkin lymphoma**, or **Hodgkin disease:** The cancer spreads in an orderly manner to adjoining lymph nodes. This enables the disease to be staged depending on how far it has spread; and

2. **Non-Hodgkin lymphomas:** These occur much more frequently than Hodgkin lymphoma. They include some 30 different disease entities in 10 different subtypes.

Tonsillitis, inflammation of the tonsils and adenoids, occurs mostly in infancy and childhood. The infection can be viral or bacterial, usually streptococcal. It produces enlarged, tender lymph nodes under the jaw.

Splenomegaly, an enlarged spleen, is not a disease in itself but the result of an underlying disorder. But when the spleen enlarges, it traps and stores an excessive number of blood cells and platelets **(hypersplenism)**, reducing the number of blood cells and platelets in the bloodstream.

Ruptured spleen is a common complication from car accidents or other trauma when the abdomen and rib cage are damaged. Intra-abdominal bleeding from the ruptured spleen can be extensive, with a dramatic fall in blood pressure.

Lymphedema is localized, brawny (does not easily pit on finger pressure), minimally pitting fluid retention within the underlying tissues when lymphatic drainage is abnormal. It can be caused by a compromised lymphatic system, often after surgery or radiation therapy. It can also be primary, where the cause is unknown.

Keynote

- Lymphedema is the result of fluid retention within the underlying tissues when lymphatic drainage is abnormal.

WORD	PRONUNCIATION	ELEMENTS		DEFINITION
axillary (adj)	**AK**-sill-air-ee	S/	-ary *pertaining to*	Pertaining to the armpit
		R/	axill- *armpit*	
cervical (adj)	**SER**-vih-kal	S/	-al *pertaining to*	Pertaining to the cervix or to the neck region
		R/	cervic- *neck*	
hypersplenism (Note: *One "e" in this term*)	high-per-**SPLEN**-izm	S/	-ism *condition*	Condition in which the spleen removes blood components at an excessive rate
		P/	hyper- *excessive*	
		R/	-splen- *spleen*	
inguinal (adj)	**IN**-gwin-al	S/	-al *pertaining to*	Pertaining to the groin
		R/	inguin- *groin*	
lymphadenitis	lim-**FAD**-eh-**NEYE**-tis	S/	-itis *inflammation*	Inflammation of a lymph node(s)
		R/CF	lymphaden/o- *lymph node*	
lymphadenopathy	lim-**FAD**-eh-**NOP**-ah-thee	S/	-pathy *disease*	Any disease process affecting a lymph node(s)
lymphangiogram	lim-**FAN**-jee-oh-gram	S/	-gram *recording*	Radiographic images of lymph vessels and nodes following injection of contrast material
		R/CF	lymphangi/o- *lymphatic vessels*	
lymphedema	**LIMF**-eh-**DEE**-mah	R/	lymph- *lymph*	Tissue swelling due to lymphatic obstruction
		R/	-edema *edema*	
lymphoma	lim-**FOH**-mah	S/	-oma *tumor, mass*	Any neoplasm of lymphatic tissue
		R/	lymph- *lymphatic system, lymph*	
Hodgkin	**HOJ**-kin		Thomas Hodgkin, British physician, 1798–1866	Hodgkin lymphoma is marked by chronic enlargement of lymph nodes spreading to other nodes in an orderly way
neoplasm (noun)	**NEE**-oh-plazm	P/	neo- *new*	A new growth, either a benign or malignant tumor
		R/	-plasm *to form*	
splenomegaly	sple-noh-**MEG**-ah-lee	S/	-megaly *enlargement*	Enlarged spleen
		R/CF	splen/o- *spleen*	
tonsillitis	ton-sih-**LIE**-tis	S/	-itis *inflammation*	Inflammation of the tonsils
		R/	tonsill- *tonsil*	

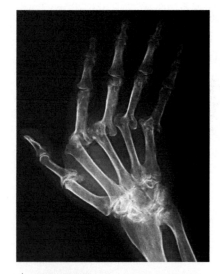

▲ **FIGURE 7.19**   Arthritic Hand. X-ray of the hand of a patient with severe rheumatoid arthritis.

ZEPHYR/SPL/Alamy Stock Photo

Disorders of the Immune System (LO 7.11)

The immune system is prone to very serious disorders, from allergic reactions to life-threatening infections.

Hypersensitivity is an excessive immune response to an antigen that would normally be tolerated. In most allergic (hypersensitivity) reactions, allergens (antigens) stimulate the cells to produce **histamine**. The symptoms produced by these changes include edema, mucus hypersecretion and congestion, watery eyes, and hives **(urticaria).**

Hypersensitivity includes:

- **Allergies**—reactions to environmental antigens like pollens, molds, dusts, foods, and drugs.
- **Autoimmune disorders**—abnormal reactions to your own tissues.
- **Alloimmune disorders**—reactions to tissues transplanted from another person.

Anaphylaxis is an acute, immediate, and severe allergic reaction which if left untreated may result in anaphylactic shock. Epinephrine is the first-line treatment of anaphylaxis, itching, and hives.

Anaphylactic shock is more severe and is characterized by difficulty in breathing (dyspnea) due to bronchiole constriction, circulatory shock, and even death. It is a life-threatening medical emergency.

Asthma is a disease of inflammation triggered by allergens, listed above, and by air pollutants, drugs, and emotions. Airway smooth muscles contract, causing bronchoconstriction (bronchospasm), leading to the wheezing and coughing of asthma.

Autoimmune disorders are an over-vigorous response of the immune system. Here, the immune system fails to distinguish self-antigens from foreign antigens. These self-antigens produce autoantibodies that attack the body's own tissues. This type of response occurs, for example, in lupus erythematosus, type 1 diabetes, multiple sclerosis, rheumatoid arthritis *(Figure 7.19)*, and psoriasis.

Immunodeficiency disorders are a deficient response of the immune system where it does not react adequately. These disorders are classified into three categories:

1. **Congenital (inborn) disorders** are caused by a genetic abnormality that is often sex-linked, with boys affected more often than girls. An example is **inherited combined immunodeficiency disease,**

characterized by an absence of both T cells and B cells. These children are very susceptible to **opportunistic** infections and must live in protective sterile enclosures.

2. **Immunosuppression** is a common side effect of corticosteroids used in treatment of inflammatory disorders, to prevent transplant rejection, and in chemotherapy treatment for cancer.

3. **Acquired immunodeficiency** results from diseases like **acquired immunodeficiency syndrome (AIDS),** which involves a severely depressed immune system from infection with the human immunodeficiency virus **(HIV).**

HIV and AIDS (LO 7.11)

HIV is one of a group of viruses known as **retroviruses.** Like other viruses, it can replicate only inside a living host cell and it invades helper T cells and cells in the upper respiratory tract and CNS. Inside the cell, the virus can stay **dormant** for months or years. When it is activated (AIDS), the new viruses emerge from the dying host cell and attack more cells. This dormant phase **(incubation)** can range from a few months to 12 years.

As the virus destroys more and more cells, the body cannot produce antibodies. Symptoms appear, including chills, fever, night sweats, fatigue, weight loss, and lymphadenitis. Opportunistic infections by bacteria, viruses, and fungi can occur. These infections include toxoplasmosis, pneumocystis, tuberculosis, herpes simplex, cytomegalovirus, and candidiasis. Cancers can also invade, and a form of skin cancer called **Kaposi sarcoma** *(Figure 7.20)* is common.

HIV survives poorly outside the human body. It is destroyed by laundering, dishwashing, chlorination, and the use of disinfectants, alcohol, and germicidal skin cleansers.

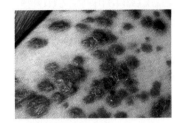

▲ **FIGURE 7.20** Lesions of Kaposi Sarcoma, a Malignancy That Is a Complication of AIDS.

National Institutes of Health/Stocktrek Images/Getty Images

Keynotes

- Common food and drug allergens are peanuts, milk, eggs, wheat, shellfish, penicillin and related antibiotics, and sulfa drugs.
- HIV is found in blood, semen, vaginal secretions, saliva, tears, and breast milk of infected mothers.
- The most common means of transmission of HIV are:
  - Sexual intercourse (vaginal, oral, anal).
  - Shared needles for drug use.
  - Contaminated blood products. (All donated blood is now tested for HIV.)
  - Transplacental transmission, from an infected mother to her fetus.

Abbreviations

AIDS — acquired immunodeficiency syndrome

HIV — human immunodeficiency virus

Word Analysis and Definition

S = Suffix   P = Prefix   R = Root   R/CF = Combining Form

WORD	PRONUNCIATION	ELEMENTS		DEFINITION
alloimmune	AL-oh-im-**YUNE**	P/ R/	all/o- *other, strange* -immune *immunity*	Immune reaction directed against foreign tissue
autoimmune	awe-toe-im-**YUNE**	P/ R/	auto- *self, same* -immune *protected*	Immune reaction directed against a person's own tissue
anaphylaxis	AN-ah-fih-**LAK**-sis	P/ R/	ana- *excessive* -phylaxis *protection*	Immediate severe allergic response
anaphylactic (adj)	AN-ah-fih-**LAK**-tik	S/ R/	-tic *pertaining to* -phylac- *protect*	Pertaining to anaphylaxis
asthma	**AZ**-mah		Greek *asthma*	Episodes of breathing difficulty due to narrowed or obstructed airways.
asthmatic (adj)	az-**MAT**-ik	S/ R/	-atic *pertaining to* asthm- *asthma*	Suffering from or pertaining to asthma.
dormant	**DOR**-mant	S/ R/	-ant *forming* dorm- *sleep*	Inactive
histamine	**HISS**-tah-mean	R/ R/	hist- *derived from histidine* -amine *nitrogen- containing substance*	Compound liberated in tissues as a result of injury or an immune response
hypersensitivity	**HIGH**-per-sen-sih-**TIV**-ih-tee	S/ P/ R/	-ity *condition* hyper- *excessive* -sensitiv- *feeling*	Exaggerated abnormal reaction to an allergen
immunodeficiency	**IM**-you-noh-dee-**FISH**-en-see	S/ R/CF R/	-ency *quality, state of* immun/o- *immune response* -defici- *failure, lacking*	Failure of the immune system
immunosuppression	**IM**-you-noh-suh-**PRESH**-un	S/ R/	-ion *action, condition* -suppress- *press under*	Failure of the immune system caused by an outside agent
incubation	in-kyu-**BAY**-shun	S/ R/	-ation *process* incub- *lie on, hatch*	Process to develop an infection
Kaposi sarcoma	Kah-**POH**-see sar-**KOH**-mah		Moritz Kaposi, Hungarian dermatologist, 1837–1902	A skin cancer often seen in AIDS patients
opportunistic	**OP**-or-tyu-**NIS**-tik	S/ R/	-istic *pertaining to* opportun- *take advantage of*	An organism or a disease in a host with lowered resistance
retrovirus	**REH**-troh-**VIE**-rus	P/ R/	retro- *backward* -virus *poison*	Virus with an RNA core
urticaria	ur-tee-**KARE**-ee-ah		Latin *nettle*	Rash of itchy wheals (hives)

Infection (LO 7.12)

Microbes (microorganisms) are everywhere—in the air, water, and soil and all over our bodies, where they are considered **normal flora**. These normal microorganisms are found on your skin, in your nose and respiratory tract, and in your mouth and digestive tract. Your brain and cardiovascular system, however, are microbe-free **(sterile).**

If microorganisms other than the normal flora invade the body, they become pathogens, which cause an **infection**. Pathogens include bacteria, viruses, fungi, and parasites. When pathogens spread from person to person, they are said to be **contagious**. If the infection harms the body, it creates an **infectious disease**. Bacterial, viral, fungal, and parasitic infections are all caused by pathogens.

Bacterial Infections (LO 7.12)

Thousands of different bacteria can cause infections. Bacteria are single-celled microorganisms that reproduce by dividing. Frequently seen bacteria include:

- **Staphylococcus ("staph")**, which can be harmless when present on the skin's surface but causes infections in wounds or other normally sterile places, like in a joint or the peritoneum;
- **Streptococcus ("strep")**, which is a common cause of sore throats;
- **Pneumococcus,** which is a common cause of pneumonia; and
- **Coliform** bacteria that normally live in the GI tract but cause infections elsewhere, such as the urinary tract.

Drug-resistant pathogens (DRPs) are now considered common in the healthcare environment. Methicillin-resistant *Staphylococcus aureus* **(MRSA)** is a type of bacteria that is resistant to the antibiotics normally used to treat staph infections. MRSA infections occur most frequently in hospitals **(nosocomial** infection), but are now being seen in community health care facilities as community-associated MRSA **(CA-MRSA).**

Clostridium difficile (C. diff) infection is a growing problem in health care facilities, and the infection kills 14,000 people in America alone each year. When **broad-spectrum** antibiotics, such as clindamycin, have destroyed normal gut flora, *C. diff* can take over the gut and release toxins, causing severe diarrhea and abdominal pain that can be difficult to treat and life threatening or fatal.

Carbapenem-resistant Enterobacteriaceae **(CRE)** is a lethal "superbug" occurring in American hospitals and responsible for about 9,300 infections and 610 deaths every year. The antibiotic carbapenem is considered a last-resort antibiotic for bacteria that have not responded to other antibiotics. In several cases, the CRE has been found in duodenoscopes, the complex design of which makes them difficult to clean and sterilize. The most recently discovered CRE has been given the name Carbapenem-resistant *Acinetobacter baumannii* (CRAB) and is considered a multi-drug resistant infection.

Viral Infections (LO 7.12)

Viruses are the smallest of the microorganisms. They cannot be seen under an ordinary light **microscope** but are visible through an electron microscope. Viruses spread from person to person through coughs, sneezes, and unwashed hands.

Viruses cause specific childhood diseases like measles (rubeola), German measles (rubella), chickenpox (varicella), and mumps. They cause upper respiratory infections *(see Chapter 8)*, including modern respiratory infections like **severe acute respiratory syndrome (SARS), avian influenza (bird flu),** and **West Nile virus (WNV).** WNV is a seasonal **epidemic** in North America that flares up in the summer and fall.

Coronavirus disease 2019 (COVID-19) is a highly contagious viral infection that caused a global pandemic in 2020. Although this virus is primarily a respiratory infection, its effects on the body were much more severe than other respiratory viruses due to its ability to quickly reproduce. Until vaccination was available, many people died as a result of this virus.

Fungal Infections (LO 7.12)

Many fungi are "good fungi," for example, the mushrooms that you eat and the yeasts that ferment beer and bread. Penicillin is derived from a fungus. The most common pathogenic fungi are those that cause skin infections *(see Chapter 3).*

Opportunistic fungi are normally harmless, but like their name, they pounce on any opportunity to cause disease. People who are on prolonged doses of antibiotics, are receiving chemotherapy or immunosuppressive therapy, or have diabetes mellitus or AIDS are especially susceptible.

Keynotes

- Viral diseases do not respond to antibiotics.
- Nosocomial infections (hospital-acquired infections) are becoming increasingly common and lethal.
- Handwashing is the most important factor in preventing the transmission of infections.

Abbreviations

CA-MRSA	community-associated methicillin-resistant *Staphylococcus aureus*
COVID-19	Coronavirus Disease 2019
CRAB	Carbapenem-resistant Acinetobacter baumannii
CRE	carbapenem-resistant *Enterobacteriaceae*
MRSA	methicillin-resistant *Staphylococcus aureus*
SARS	severe acute respiratory syndrome
WNV	West Nile virus

Parasitic Infections (LO 7.12)

Parasites are organisms that live on or in another organism and steal nourishment from their host. In many rural areas of the world, parasites are **endemic**.

Malaria is caused by a parasite that is transmitted from person to person by a single mosquito bite.

Pinworms are the most common parasite in America. Pinworm eggs are introduced into the body through the mouth and hatch in the intestine. The young worms migrate to the anus, where the female deposits her eggs. These eggs can be transferred unknowingly by the fingers from the anus or from infected bedding, to the mouth of the same child or to another child.

Word Analysis and Definition

S = Suffix   P = Prefix   R = Root   R/CF = Combining Form

WORD	PRONUNCIATION		ELEMENTS	DEFINITION
broad-spectrum	broad-**SPECK**-trum		broad Latin *wide* spectrum Latin *image*	An antibiotic with a wide range of activity against a variety of organisms
Clostridium difficile (also known as *Clostridiodes difficile*)	klah-**STRID**-ee-um **DIFF**-ih-seal	S/ R/	-ium *structure* clostrid- *spindle*	Gram-positive spore-forming bacteria that causes antibiotic-associated diarrhea.
contagious	kon-**TAY**-jus	S/ P/ R/	-ious *pertaining to* con- *with, together* -tag- *touch*	Infection can be transmitted from person to person or from a person to a surface to a person
endemic	en-**DEM**-ik	S/ P/ R/	-ic *pertaining to* en- *in* -dem- *the people*	Pertaining to a disease always present in a community
epidemic	ep-ih-**DEM**-ik	P/	epi- *above, upon*	Pertaining to an outbreak in a community of a disease or a health-related behavior
pandemic	pan-**DEM**-ik	P/	pan- *all*	Pertaining to a disease attacking the population of a whole country or the world
normal flora	**NOR**-mal **FLOR**-uh		Latin *flower*	Microorganisms covering the exterior and interior surfaces of a healthy animal and under normal circumstances do not cause disease
infect (verb) infection (noun)	in-**FEKT** in-**FEK**-shun	S/ R/	Latin *invade internally* -ion *condition, action* infect- *internal invasion*	To invade an organism by a microorganism Invasion of the body by disease-producing microorganisms
infectious (adj)	in-**FEK**-shus	S/	-ious *pertaining to*	Capable of being transmitted to a person; or a disease caused by the action of a microorganism
microbe	**MY**-krohb	P/ R/	micro- *small* -be *life*	Short for microorganism
microorganism	**MY**-kroh-**OR**-gan-izm	S/ R/	-ism *process* -organ- *organ, instrument*	Any organism too small to be seen by the naked eye
microscope	**MY**-kroh-skope	P/ R/	micro- *small* -scope *instrument for viewing*	Instrument for viewing something small that cannot be seen in detail by the naked eye
microscopic (adj) microscopy	**MY**-kroh-**SKOP**-ik my-**CROSS**-koh-pee	S/ S/	-ic *pertaining to* -scopy *to examine, to view*	Visible only with the aid of a microscope Investigation of minute objects through a microscope
nosocomial	noh-soh-**KOH**-mee-al	S/ R/CF R/	-ial *pertaining to* nos/o- *disease* -com- *take care of*	Acquired while in the hospital
sterile (adj) sterility	**STER**-ill steh-**RIL**-ih-tee	S/ R/	Latin *barren* -ity *state, condition* steril- *barren*	Unable to fertilize or reproduce Inability to reproduce

EXERCISES

 Case Report 7.5

You are

. . . a medical assistant working with Susan Lee, MD, in her primary care clinic.

You are communicating with

. . . Ms. Anna Clemons, a 20-year-old restaurant server, who is a new patient. She has noticed a lump in the left side of her neck. On questioning, you learn that Ms. Clemons has lost about 8 pounds in the past couple of months, has felt tired, and has had some night sweats. Her vital signs are normal. There are two firm, enlarged **lymph nodes** in her left neck in front of the **sternocleidomastoid** muscle (the long muscle in the side of the neck that extends up to the base of the skull behind the ear). Physical examination is otherwise unremarkable.

Ms. Anna Clemons has cancerous nodes in her neck. They were caused not by metastatic cancer but by a cancer of the lymph nodes called **Hodgkin lymphoma**.

A. Read *Case Report 7.5 to answer the following questions. Select the correct answer to complete each statement or answer each question.* **LO 7.3, 7.12, and 7.13**

1. Which of the following are Ms. Clemons' symptoms? (choose all that apply)

   a. weight loss   **b.** night sweats   **c.** hypertension   **d.** muscular pain   **e.** ear ache

2. What is present on physical examination of the patient?

   a. tenderness on the left side of her neck   **c.** two firm, enlarged lymph nodes in the left side of her neck

   b. swelling on the left side of the neck   **d.** bulging of the sternocleidomastoid muscle

3. What was the status of the patient's VS?

   a. below normal   **b.** above normal   **c.** normal   **d.** not recorded

4. What is the best description of a node?

   a. enlarged lymph gland   **b.** cancerous growth   **c.** circumscribed mass of tissue   **d.** benign growth   **e.** thickened fluid

B. Review *Case Report 7.5 to answer the following questions. Select the correct answer to each question.* **LO 7.2, 7.9, 7.10, and 7.12**

1. Which medical term in the Case Report signifies that the nodes are *malignant*? _____

2. Lymph nodes in the neck are termed _____ lymph nodes. _____

3. Is Ms. Clemons' cancer a primary or secondary cancer site? _____

C. Elements *remain your best tool for understanding the meaning of a term. Match the meaning of the definition in column 1 with the correct element in column 2.* **LO 7.1 and 7.10**

_____ **1.** groin   **A.** lymphangio

_____ **2.** lymph node   **B.** gram

_____ **3.** tumor, mass   **C.** inguin

_____ **4.** recording   **D.** oma

_____ **5.** lymph vessels   **E.** lymphadeno

D. Deconstruct medical terms into their elements. *Deconstruct each term using the slashed lines.* **LO 7.1 and 7.9**

1. lymphadenitis: _____/_____
                    R   S

2. hypersplenism: _____/_____/_____
                 P   R   S

3. neoplastic: _____/_____/_____
             P   R   S

4. lymphadenectomy: _____/_____/_____
             R/CF   R   S

E. Build *more medical vocabulary for the language of immunology. Complete the construction of each term by using the following elements to fill in the blanks. There are more answers than you need.* **LO 7.1 and 7.9**

defici-   allo-   -suppress-   -sensitiv-   -ion   hyper-   incub-   -osis   -phylaxis   -ic   -ency   dorm-

1. exaggerated, abnormal reaction to an allergen: _____/_____/ity

2. inactive: _____/ant

3. process to develop an infection: _____/ation

4. failure of the immune system: immuno /_____/_____

5. immune reaction toward a foreign tissue: _____/immune

F. Identify the meaning of the word elements. *Given the term, identify the correct definition of the indicated word element.* **LO 7.1 and 7.9**

1. In the term retrovirus, the root means:

   a. poison   **b.** cancer   **c.** process   **d.** nettle

2. In the term hypersensitivity, the root means:

   a. condition   **b.** allergen   **c.** feeling   **d.** inflammation

3. In the term dormant, the suffix means:

   a. forming   **b.** take advantage   **c.** pertaining to   **d.** sleep

4. In the term opportunistic, the root means:

   a. forming   **b.** take advantage of   **c.** press   **d.** backward

G. Correct usage *of the appropriate grammatical form of a medical term is the mark of an educated professional. Practice your language of immunology in the following sentences. Fill in the blanks.* **LO 7.2, 7.9, and 7.10**

1. infect   infection   infectious

   This patient has a rarely seen (a) _____. Please refer her to the (b) _____ disease specialist.

2. bacterium   bacteria   bacterial

   The (a) _____ streptococcus causes (b) _____ infections in the throat.

3. sterile   sterility   sterilize

   An autoclave is used to (a) _____ instruments.

   If the (b) _____ of an instrument is in question, it should not be used.

   The term (c) _____ can also mean *unable* to *reproduce.*

H. Use the language of immunology *and select the best answer.* **LO 7.2 and 7.13**

1. What agent causes infections in wounds and joints?

   a. staph

   b. pneumococcus

   c. heme

2. What term is the same as "microbe free"?

   a. opportunistic

   b. anemic

   c. sterile

3. MRSA occurs most frequently in:

   a. prisons

   b. schools

   c. hospitals

4. Another name for microbes is:

   a. normal flora

   b. bacteria

   c. pollutants

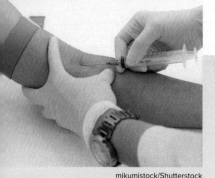

Section 7.5

Diagnostic and Therapeutic Procedures and Pharmacology for the Blood, Lymphatic, and Immune Systems

CBC	complete blood count
DIFF	differential white blood cell count
ITP	idiopathic thrombocytic purpura
MCV	mean corpuscular volume
PT	prothrombin time
PTT	partial thromboplastin time
TPA	tissue plasminogen activator

Diagnostic Procedures for Blood Disorders (LO 7.3, 7.4, 7.5, 7.6, 7.7, 7.9, and 7.11)

The patient's medical and family histories and physical examination are important tools in diagnosing blood disorders.

The study of the blood and its disorders—the red and white blood cells within the blood, their proportions, and their overall cell health—is called **hematology. A hematologist** is a physician specialist who is trained in this area.

- A **complete blood count (CBC)** gives important information about the types and numbers of cells in the blood, enabling diagnosis of the cause of such symptoms as weakness, fatigue, and bruising. Included in the CBC is the number of red blood cells; a low count may indicate anemia whereas a higher than normal count may indicate polycythemia. If the total amount of hemoglobin in the blood and the **hematocrit** are both low in the CBC, anemia is present. A red blood cell **index,** the **mean corpuscular volume (MCV),** shows the average size of the red blood cells. If the cells are small **(microcytic),** the most common cause is an iron-deficiency anemia. If the cells are large **(macrocytic),** a possible cause is pernicious anemia.

- A **white blood cell (WBC) count** is usually included in a CBC along with the numbers and types of the different WBCs, a **WBC differential (DIFF).** These tests give the pathologists and clinicians who read the tests critical information about the body's response to infection, **toxic** medicines, chemicals, and allergens and show many other conditions, such as leukemia.

- Also included in a CBC is the number of platelets. A low platelet count can indicate **idiopathic thrombocytopenic purpura (ITP).** There are more than a dozen coagulopathies (bleeding disorders), and the diagnostic procedures to determine the cause of a patient's abnormal bleeding include the CBC, International Normalized Ratio (INR), **prothrombin time (PT), and partial thromboplastin time (PTT),** which help define where deficiencies might lie in the clotting process. The combination of all these tests is called a **coagulation panel.**

- Other diagnostic procedures for blood disorders include a **blood smear,** in which a drop of blood is smeared on a slide, stained, and examined under a microscope to determine the size and shape of RBCs, WBCs, and platelets. A **bone marrow aspiration (biopsy)** is a procedure used to define the production of the different blood cells. For example, in disorders of the lymphatic system, the essential diagnostic procedure is biopsy of an enlarged lymph node. This can be followed by X-rays, CT scans, and MRI scans to determine the spread of a disease such as lymphoma.

- A **transfusion** of blood or packed red blood cells replaces lost red blood cells to restore the blood's oxygen-carrying capacity. **Autologous** donation and transfusion occur when people donate their own blood ahead of time to be given back to them if necessary during a surgical procedure.

WORD	PRONUNCIATION	ELEMENTS		DEFINITION
aspiration	as-pih-**RAY**-shun	S/ R/	-ion *process* aspirat- *to breathe on*	Removal by suction of fluid or gas from a body cavity
autologous	awe-**TOL**-oh-gus	P/ R/	auto- *self, same* -logous *relation*	Blood transfusion with the same person as donor and recipient—self-transfusion
coagulopathy coagulopathies (pl)	koh-ag-you-**LOP**-ah-thee	S/ R/CF	-pathy *disease* coagul/o *clotting*	Disorder of blood clotting
corpuscle corpuscular (adj)	**KOR**-pus-ul kor-**PUS**-kyu-lar	S/ R/ S/	-cle *small* corpus- *body* -ar *pertaining to*	A red blood cell Pertaining to a red blood cell
hematocrit (Hct)	he-**MAT**-oh-krit	S/ R/CF	-crit *to separate* hemat/o- *blood*	Percentage of red blood cells in the blood
hematology hematologist	he-mah-**TOL**-oh-jee he-mah-**TOL**-oh-jist	S/ R/CF S/	-logy *study of* hemat/o- *blood* -logist *one who studies, specialist*	Medical specialty of the blood and its disorders Specialist in hematology
index indices (pl)	**IN**-deks **IN**-dih-seez		Latin *one that points out*	A standard indicator of measurement
infusion	in-**FYU**-zhun	P/ R/	in- *in* -fusion *to pour*	Introduction intravenously of a substance other than blood
macrocyte macrocytic (adj)	**MACK**-roh-site mack-roh-**SIT**-ik	P/ S/ S/	macro- *large* -cyte *cell* -ic *pertaining to*	Large red blood cell Pertaining to a large red blood cell
microcyte microcytic (adj)	**MY**-kroh-site my-kroh-**SIT**-ik	P/ R/ S/	micro- *small* -cyte *cell* -ic *pertaining to*	Small red blood cell Pertaining to a small red blood cell
occult blood	oh-**KULT BLUD**		occult Latin *to hide*	Blood that cannot be seen in the stool but is positive on a fecal occult blood test
transfusion	trans-**FYU**-zhun	P/ R/	trans- *across* -fusion *to pour*	Transfer of blood or a blood component from donor to recipient

Diagnostic Procedures for the Lymphatic and Immune Systems (LO 7.9)

Immunoassays rely on the ability of an antibody to recognize and bind to a specific antigen and produce a measurable response. In some cases they can use an antigen to detect for the presence of antibodies, and again produce a measurable response. A wide range of medical tests are immunoassays.

Immunodiagnostics uses an antigen-antibody reaction as a diagnostic tool; an antigen is used to detect antibodies to a pathogen; an antibody is used to detect an antigen of a pathogen in a patient's specimen. Very small amounts of biochemical substances can be detected when antibodies specific for a desired antigen are **conjugated** with a radiolabel, fluorescent label, or a color-forming enzyme and used as a "probe" to detect it.

Applications include pregnancy testing, dipstick analysis, and **enzyme-linked immunosorbent assay (ELISA)**. ELISA uses antibodies and enzymes linked to color-changing dyes to detect specific antibodies and chemicals. ELISA is used to diagnose HIV, West Nile virus, malaria, tuberculosis, and rotavirus in feces, as well as in drug screening.

In **agglutination tests,** a particle such as a latex bead or a **bacterium** is coupled to a **reagent** antigen or antibody and the resulting particle **complex** is mixed with the specimen (e.g., serum or CSF). If the target antibody or antigen is present in the specimen, it attaches to the particle complex and produces agglutination.

A **complement fixation** test measures the amount of an antibody in the serum or CSF to viral and fungal infections such as coccidioidomycosis.

Diagnostic tests for allergies include:

- **nasal smears** to check the amount of eosinophils in the nose.
- **skin tests** to measure the level of IgE antibodies in response to allergens that are injected under the skin or applied with a small scratch. A reaction appears as a small reddened (flare) and/or raised (wheal) area.
- **blood tests** measure IgE antibodies to specific allergens in the blood. A **radioallergosorbent test (RAST)** uses a **radioimmunoassay** to detect the specific IgE antibodies.
- **Challenge testing** is performed by an allergist, who administers a very small amount of an allergen orally or by inhalation and monitors its effect.

High blood levels of IgA are found in multiple myeloma, autoimmune diseases such as rheumatoid arthritis and systemic lupus erythematosus *(see Chapter 3)*, and cirrhosis of the liver *(see Chapter 9)*. Low levels of IgA occur in some types of leukemia and in nephrotic syndrome *(see Chapter 13)*.

High blood levels of IgG can indicate a chronic infection, such as HIV and in chronic hepatitis and multiple sclerosis. Low levels are found in some types of leukemia and in nephrotic syndrome.

High blood levels of IgE are also found in patients with parasitic infections or those with allergic asthma.

Lymphoma (LO 7.9)

Diagnostic procedures used to determine lymphoma include a biopsy of an enlarged node, X-rays, CT, and MRI scans, a **lymphangiogram,** and a bone marrow biopsy.

Word Analysis and Definition

S = Suffix   P = Prefix   R = Root   R/CF = Combining Form

WORD	PRONUNCIATION		ELEMENTS	DEFINITION
allergist	**AL**-er-jist	S/ R/ R/	-ist *specialist* all- *other, strange* -erg- *work*	Specialist in hypersensitivity reactions
bacterium bacteria (pl)	bak-**TEER**-ee-um bak-**TEER**-ee-ah		Greek a *staff*	A unicellular microorganism that multiplies by cell division
complex	**KOM**-pleks		Latin *woven together*	A stable combination of two or more compounds in the body
conjugate (verb)	**KON**-joo-gate	S/ P/ R/	-ate *composed of, pertaining to* con- *together* -jug- *yoke*	To join together, usually in pairs.
immunoassay	**IM**-you-no-**ASS**-ay	R/CF R/	immun/o- *immune* -assay *evaluate*	Biochemical test that uses the reaction of an antibody to its antigen to measure the amount of a substance in a liquid
immunodiagnostics	**IM**-you-no-die-ag-**NOSS**-tiks	S/ R/CF R/	-ics *pertaining to* immun/o- *immune* -diagnost- *decision*	A diagnostic process using antigen-antibody reactions
lymphangiogram	lim-**FAN**-jee-oh-gram	S/ R/CF	-gram *recording* lymphangi/o- *lymphatic vessels*	Radiographic images of lymph vessels and nodes following injection of contrast material
radioallergosorbent	**RAY**-dee-oh-ah-**LUR**-go-**SOAR**-bent	S/ R/CF R/CF R/	-ent *end result* radi/o- *radiation* -allerg/o- *allergy* -sorb- *suck in*	A radioimmunoassay to detect IgE-bound allergens responsible for tissue hypersensitivity
radioimmunoassay	**RAY**-dee-oh-im-you-no-**ASS**-ay	R/CF R/	-immun/o- *immune* -assay *evaluate*	Immunoassay of a substance that has been radioactively labeled
reagent	ree-**A**-jent	P/ R/	re- *again, back* -agent *doing*	Any substance added to a solution of another substance to examine, produce, or measure another substance

Therapeutic Procedures for Blood Disorders (LO 7.4, 7.5, 7.6, 7.7, and 7.9)

In anemia, treatment consists of replacing any deficiency in the production of hemoglobin, such as with iron or vitamin B_{12} supplementation. With certain stages of kidney disease, the hormone necessary for red bone marrow production of blood cells is not produced adequately, requiring hormone supplementation. For hemolytic and aplastic anemias, the treatment is to define and remove the toxin, drug, or radiation source that is causing the destruction of, or inability of the bone marrow to produce, red cells. A **bone marrow transplant** is the transfer of bone marrow from an **aspirated** healthy, compatible donor to a patient with aplastic anemia, leukemia, lymphoma, or other disease.

Therapeutic Procedures and Pharmacology for the Lymphatic and Immune Systems (LO 7.9)

Immunotherapy, also called **biologic therapy,** is designed to boost the body's natural defenses against cancer by using substances either made in the laboratory or made by the body to enhance or restore immune system function. This form of therapy can stop or slow the growth of cancer cells, and stop cancer from metastasizing.

The types of immunotherapy include:

- **Monoclonal antibodies,** made in the laboratory, can attach to cancer cells to flag them so that macrophages in the body's immune system can recognize and destroy them. Two pathways inside cells that cancers use to evade the immune system have been identified and named PD-1/PD-L1 and CTLA-4. These pathways can be blocked with antibodies called **immune checkpoint inhibitors** to allow the body's immune system to respond to the cancer. Immune checkpoint inhibitors ipilimumab *(Yervoy),* nivolumab *(Opdivo),* and pembrolizumab *(Keytruda)* have been shown to improve overall patient survival in advanced melanoma.

- **Interferons** are a nonspecific immunotherapy given at the same time as other cancer treatments such as chemotherapy or radiation therapy. An interferon called **interferon alpha** made in a laboratory is the most common type of interferon used in cancer treatment.

- **Interleukins** are also a nonspecific immunotherapy used to treat kidney and skin cancers, including melanoma.

Human immunoglobulins are given by injection to confer passive (temporary) immunity that provides immediate protection lasting several weeks. There are two types:

- **Human normal immunoglobulin (HNIG)** made from the plasma of about 1,000 unselected donors to provide antibodies against hepatitis A, rubella, measles, and other viruses found in the general population.

- **Hyperimmune specific immunoglobulins** are made from selected donors and provide antibodies individually against hepatitis B, varicella zoster, rabies, tetanus, and cytomegalovirus.

Word Analysis and Definition

S = Suffix   P = Prefix   R = Root   R/CF = Combining Form

WORD	PRONUNCIATION	ELEMENTS		DEFINITION
adenoidectomy	ADD-eh-noy-DEK-toh-me	S/ R/ S/	-ectomy *surgical excision* aden- *gland* -oid *resemble*	Surgical removal of the adenoid tissue
biologic	BI-oh-LOJ-ik	S/ R/CF R/	-ic *pertaining to* bio- *life* -log- *study of*	Pertaining to the study of life and living organisms
immunotherapy	IM-you-noh-THAIR-ah-pee	R/ R/CF	immun/o- *immune response* -therapy *treatment*	Treatment to boost immune system function
interferon	in-ter-FEER-on	S/ P/ R/	-on *on* inter- *between* -fer- *to strike*	A small protein produced by T-cells in response to infection
interleukin	IN-ter-LOO-kin	S/ P/ R/	-in *chemical* inter- *between* leuk- *white*	A group of cytokines synthesized by white blood cells
lymphadenectomy	lim-FAD-eh-NECK-toe-me	S/ R/	-ectomy *surgical excision* lymphaden- *lymph node*	Surgical excision of a lymph node(s)
monoclonal	MON-oh-KLOH-nal	S/ P/ R/	-al *pertaining to* mono- *one* -clon- *cutting used for propagation*	Derived in the laboratory from a protein from a single colony of cells
splenectomy (Note: *Single "e" in splen*)	sple-NECK-toe-me	S/ R/	-ectomy *surgical excision* splen- *spleen*	Surgical removal of the spleen
transplant	TRANZ-plant	P/ R/	trans- *across* -plant *insert, plant*	To transfer from one tissue or organ to another

Lymphatic Therapy (LO 7.9)

Careful observation to **chemotherapy, radiation,** and bone marrow transplantation is considered based on the rate of growth of Hodgkin and Non-Hodgkin's lymphoma cancer cells.

Regional lymphadenectomy removes several lymph nodes from an area.

Radical lymphadenectomy removes all the lymph nodes from an area to detect the presence of cancer cells.

Compression garments and treatments, and massage are used for lymphedema. There is no cure.

Antibiotics treat strep throat and tonsillitis. Recurrent tonsillitis may be treated with a **tonsillectomy** and **adenoidectomy.**

Splenectomy is most often performed for a ruptured spleen and painful splenomegaly.

Abbreviation

INR	International Normalized Ratio

Pharmacology for Blood Disorders (LO 7.3, 7.4, 7.5, 7.6, 7.7, and 7.9)

Anticoagulants used to reduce or prevent blood clotting include:

- **Aspirin,** which reduces platelet **adherence** and is used in small 81 mg doses to reduce the incidence of heart attack.

- **Heparin,** which prevents prothrombin and fibrin formation and is given **parenterally;** its dose is monitored by activated partial thromboplastin time (aPTT).

- **Warfarin** *(Coumadin),* which inhibits the synthesis of prothrombin and others to act as an **anticoagulant.** It prevents prothrombin and fibrin formation. It is given by mouth and its dose is monitored by prothrombin times (PTs), which are reported as an **International Normalized Ratio** (INR).

- **Dabigatran etexilate** *(Pradaxa)* and **rivaroxaban** *(Xarelto),* which inhibit the synthesis of thrombin and are given by mouth to reduce the risk of **embolism** and stroke in patients with nonvalvular atrial fibrillation *(see Chapter 10).* **Idarucizumab** *(Praxbind injection)* is available for patients using *Pradaxa* when reversal of its anticoagulant effects is needed for emergency surgery, for urgent procedures, or in life-threatening or uncontrolled bleeding.

- **Streptokinase,** derived from hemolytic streptococci, which dissolves the fibrin in blood clots. Given intravenously within 3 to 4 hours of a heart attack, it is often effective in dissolving a clot that has caused the heart attack.

Recombinant Factor VIII, developed through **recombinant DNA** technology, is the main medication used to treat hemophilia A. It is given intravenously through a vein in the arm or a port in the chest. **Desmopressin acetate** *(DDAVP)* is a synthetic version of **vasopressin** that helps stop bleeding in patients with mild hemophilia.

Pernicious anemia is treated initially with injections of vitamin B_{12}, and then the vitamin B_{12} can be given through a nasal gel.

Eltrombopag *(Promacta)* is available for pediatric patients with idiopathic thrombocytopenic purpura (ITP) who have not responded to corticosteroids, immunoglobulins, or splenectomy.

Most leukemias in both adults and children are treated with **chemotherapy,** often with added radiation therapy and a stem cell transplant.

Word Analysis and Definition

S = Suffix P = Prefix R = Root R/CF = Combining Form

WORD	PRONUNCIATION		ELEMENTS	DEFINITION
adhere adherence	add-**HEER** add-**HEER**-ents	 S/ R/	Latin *to stick to* -ence *forming, quality of* adher- *stick to*	To stick to something The act of sticking to something
anticoagulant	**AN**-tee-koh-**AG**-you-lant	P/ R/ S/	anti- *against* -coagul- *clot, clump* -ant *forming, pertaining to*	Substance that prevents clotting
chemotherapy	**KEE**-moh-**THAIR**-ah-pee	R/CF R/	chem/o- *chemical* -therapy *treatment*	Treatment using chemical agents
embolism	**EM**-boh-lizm		Greek *a plug or patch*	A plug of tissue or air from afar that obstructs a blood vessel
parenteral	pah-**REN**-ter-al	S/ P/ R/	-al *pertaining to* par- *abnormal* -enter- *intestine*	Administering medication by any means other than the GI tract
recombinant DNA	ree-**KOM**-bin-ant **DEE**-en-a	S/ P/ R/	-ant *forming* re- *again* -combin- *combine*	Deoxyribonucleic acid (DNA) altered by inserting a new sequence of DNA into the chain
streptokinase	strep-toh-**KIE**-nase	P/ R/	strepto- *curved* -kinase *enzyme*	An enzyme that dissolves clots
vasopressin (also called antidiuretic hormone)	vay-so h-**PRESS**-in	S/ R/CF R/	-in *chemical compound* vas/o- *blood vessel* -press- *close, press*	Pituitary hormone that constricts blood vessels and decreases urinary output

Pharmacology for Immune Disorders (LO 7.9)

Immunosuppressant Drugs (LO 7.9)

Immunosuppressant drugs inhibit or prevent activity of the immune system and are used to prevent the rejection of transplanted organs and tissues, treat autoimmune diseases, and help control long-term allergic asthma. There are four main types of immunosuppressant drugs:

- **Glucocorticoids,** which suppress cell-mediated immunity and protect through enhancing T-cell and interfering with macrophages, and by stimulating cells to secrete **cytokines.**

- **Cytostatics,** which inhibit cell division. Cyclophosphamide *(Cytoxan),* an **alkylating** agent, is probably the most potent immunosuppressant and works by blocking cellular DNA production. Methotrexate, an **antimetabolite,** interferes with the **synthesis** of nucleic acids and is used in the treatment of autoimmune diseases. Azathioprine *(Imuran)* is the main immunosuppressive **cytotoxic** substance and is used to control transplant rejection reactions.

- **Antibodies** can be used as quick immunosuppressive therapy and are described above in sections on monoclonal antibodies and immunoglobulins.

- **Calcineurin** is a phosphatase that stimulates the growth and differentiation of T-cells. **Calcineurin inhibitors** such as ciclosporin *(Sandimmune),* tacrolimus *(Prograf),* and sirolimus *(Rapamune)* are used in the prevention and treatment of transplant rejection reactions and work by preventing cell-mediated immunity inflammation.

HIV Drugs (LO 7.9)

Antiretroviral treatment (ART) medications do not cure HIV, but instead decrease the amount of HIV in the blood, letting infected people live a longer healthier life, and decrease the risk of passing HIV to another person. Medication must be taken daily or the amount of HIV in the blood will increase.

Initial regimens consist of three or more classes of antiretroviral drugs. Combination medications deliver this combination in one tablet: bictegravir/tenofovir alafenamide/emtricitabine *(Biktarvy)*, and dolute gravir/abacavir/lamivudine *(Triumeq).*

Influenza Drugs (LO 7.9)

Oseltamivir phosphate *(Tamiflu)* can be used to prevent the flu or to treat the flu within 48 hours of the onset of symptoms.

Zanamivir *(Relenza)* is an orally inhaled white powder that can be taken to prevent influenza infection during a flu outbreak.

WORD	PRONUNCIATION	ELEMENTS		DEFINITION
alkylation	al-kih-**LAY**-shun	S/ R/	-ation *process* alkyl- *alkali*	Introduction of a side chain into a compound
antimetabolite	**AN**-tih-meh-**TAB**- oh-lite	S/ P/ R/	-ite *resembling* anti- *against* -metabol- *change*	A substance that antagonizes another substance
antiretroviral	**AN**-tee-**RET**-roh-**VIE**-ral	P/ P/ R/ S/	anti- *against* -retro- *backward* -vir- *virus* -al *pertaining to*	Drug that fights infection by a virus
calcineurin	kal-see-**NYUR**-in	S/ R/CF R/	-in *chemical* calc/i- *calcium* -neur- *nerve*	A chemical that stimulates the growth and differentiation of T-cels
cytokine	**SIGH**-toh-kine	S/ R/CF	-kine *movement* cyt/o- *cell*	A hormone-like protein that regulates the intensity of an immune response
cytostatic	**SIGH**-toh-**STAT**-ik	S/ R/CF R/	-ic *pertaining to* cyt/o- *cell* -stat- *stop*	Inhibiting cell division
cytotoxic	**SIGH**-toh-**TOK**-sik	S/	-toxic *able to kill*	Destructive to cells
immunosuppressant	**IM**-you-noh-soo-**PRESS**-ant	S/ R	-ant *forming, pertaining to* -suppress- *to stop*	An agent that interferes with or prevents the immune response
immunoglobulin	**IM**-you-noh-**GLOB**-you-lin	S/ R/CF R/	-in *chemical* immun/o- *immune response* -globul- *protein*	Specific protein (antibody) generated by an antigen
inhibitor	in-**HIB**-ih-tor	S/ R/	-or *that which does* inhibit- *restrain*	An agent that restrains a chemical action

EXERCISES

A. Interpret abbreviations. *Given the abbreviation, choose what the diagnostic test is measuring.* Select the correct answer to complete each statement. **LO 7.3, 7.4, 7.5, and 7.10**

1. WBC differential

   a. number of leukocytes   **b.** measure of inflammation   **c.** types of leukocytes   **d.** average red blood cell size

2. PT

   a. evaluates bleeding and clotting disorders   **c.** counts the number of platelets

   b. hemoglobin amount per erythrocyte   **d.** determines presence of bone cancer

3. MCV

   a. measures amount of iron in the blood   **c.** reports the average size of red blood cells

   b. determines amount of hemoglobin per erythrocyte   **d.** used to monitor anticoagulation therapies

B. Deconstruct *the following terms into their elements. If a term does not have a particular element, insert N/A.*   **LO 7.1 and 7.2**

1. parenteral: _____ / _____ / _____

P   R/CF   S

2. coagulopathy: _____ / _____ / _____

P   R/CF   S

3. corpuscular: _____ / _____ / _____

P   R/CF   S

4. transplant: _____ / _____ / _____

P   R/CF   S

5. aspiration: _____ / _____ / _____

P   R/CF   S

C. Describe the action of medications as they relate to hematology. *Place the anticoagulant with the action it uses to prevent or reduce the formation of clots.* **LO 7.2 and 7.10**

Pradaxa   aspirin   *Coumadin*   streptokinase   *Xarelto*   heparin (has two actions, use the term twice)

Dissolves fibrin in blood clots	Decreases platelet adherence	Inhibits synthesis of prothrombin	Inhibits synthesis of thrombin
1.	2.	3.	5.
		4.	6.
			7.

D. Match the therapy in the first column to the disorder it treats in the second column. *Fill in the blanks.* **LO 7.4, 7.5, 7.9, and 7.10**

_____ 1. Vitamin B$_{12}$

_____ 2. *Promacta* (eltrombopag)

_____ 3. desmopressin acetate

_____ 4. Recombinant Factor VIII

a. idiopathic thrombocytopenic purpura

b. mild hemophilia

c. pernicious anemia

d. hemophilia A

E. Immunoglobulin (Ig) levels are used to support the diagnosis of lymphatic system disorders. Match the Ig levels in the first column with the condition it is associated with in the second column. **LO 7.3 and 7.9**

_____ 1. increased IgE antibodies

_____ 2. increased IgG antibodies

_____ 3. decreased IgG antibodies

a. HIV infection

b. leukemia

c. parasitic infections

F. Choose the correct test used in the diagnosis of conditions caused by immune system disorders. **LO 7.3 and 7.9**

1. The test used to detect the presence of HIV infection:

   a. ELISA   b. RAST   c. challenge testing   d. Ig levels

2. Patient inhales allergens to see if they cause an allergic reaction:

   a. skin test   b. blood test   c. challenge testing   d. agglutination testing

3. Measures the amount of antibody present in cerebrospinal fluid or serum:

   a. RAST   b. complement fixation test   c. ELISA   d. challenge testing

G. Identify the action of the drug based on a word element that it contains. *Being able to pick out and define word elements can help you determine the meaning of the word. Select the answer that correctly completes each statement.* **LO 7.10**

1. A medication that would provide antibodies to persons to prevent viral infections:

   a. cytostatic   b. glucocorticoid   c. human normal immunoglobulin   d. monoclonal antibodies

2. A medication that would inhibit cell division:

   a. cytostatic   b. calcineurin   c. interleukin   d. interferon

H. Categorize medications of immunotherapy. *Match the medication in the first column with the disorder it is used to treat in the second column.* **LO 7.10**

_____ 1. interleukin

_____ 2. interferons

_____ 3. monoclonal antibodies

a. treat kidney and skin cancers

b. flag cancer cells for macrophages

c. given alongside chemotherapy and radiation therapy

I. Categorize immunosuppressant drugs. *Match the medication in the first column with the disorder it is used to treat in the second column.* **LO 7.10**

_____ 1. methotrexate

_____ 2. tacrolimus (*Prograf*)

_____ 3. glucocorticoid

_____ 4. cyclophosphamide (*Cytoxan*)

a. interferes with nucleic acids as a means to treat autoimmune diseases

b. most potent immunosuppressant

c. given to reduce inflammation

d. prevents and treats transplant rejection reactions

J. Pronunciation is important whether you are saying the word or listening to a word from a coworker. Identify the proper pronunciation of the following medical terms. Correctly spell the term. **LO 7.2, 7.9, and 7.10**

1. The correct pronunciation for the property of glowing in ultraviolet light:

   a. **RAY**-dee-oh- im-**YUNE**-ass-ay

   b. **RAY**-dee-oh-im-you-no-**ASS**-ay

   c. **FLOR**-ess-ent

   d. flor-**ESS**-ent

   Correctly spell the term: _____

2. The correct pronunciation for the surgical removal of the spleen:

   a. ton-sigh-**LEK**-tuh-mee

   b. ton-sih-**LEK**-toh-mee

   c. sple-**NEK**-toh-mee

   d. splee-**NEK**-toh-mee

   Correctly spell the term: _____

3. The correct pronunciation for a malignant tumor originating in connective tissue:

   a. **SAR**-koh-mah

   b. sark-oh-**MOH**

   c. try-**GLISS**-eh-ride

   d. try-**GLICE**-er-ide

   Correctly spell the term: _____

4. The correct pronunciation for a disease-causing organism:

   a. tok-**SIK**

   b. **TOK**-sik

   c. **PATH**-oh-jen

   d. path-**OH**-jen

   Correctly spell the term: _____

5. The correct pronunciation for the term that means to ingest foreign particles and cells:

   a. **SIGH**-tuh-tok-sik

   b. sigh-toh-**TOK**-sik

   c. **FAYG**-oh-sigh-**TOH**-sis

   d. **FAG**-oh-site-**OH**-seez

   Correctly spell the term: _____

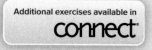
Additional exercises available in
connect

Chapter Review exercises, along with additional practice items, are available in Connect!

The Respiratory System

The Essentials of the Language of Pulmonology

CHAPTER 8

Rick Brady/McGraw Hill

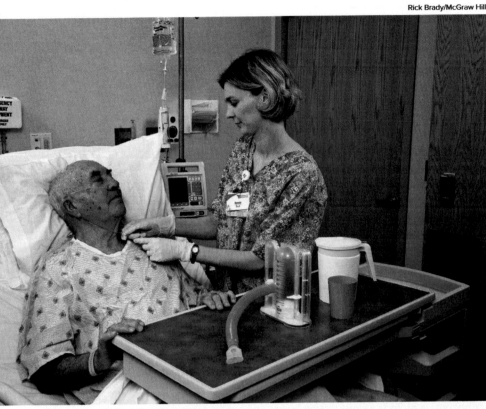

Learning Outcomes

In order to provide optimal care to patients with respiratory conditions, and to, determine what is causing symptoms and signs, and communicate with the other health professionals involved in the care of these patients care, you need to be able to:

LO 8.1 Use roots, combining forms, suffixes, and prefixes to construct and analyze (deconstruct) medical terms related to the respiratory system.

LO 8.2 Spell and pronounce correctly medical terms related to the respiratory system in order to communicate with accuracy and precision in any health care setting.

LO 8.3 Define accepted abbreviations related to the respiratory system.

LO 8.4 Relate the structures of the upper respiratory tract to their functions.

LO 8.5 Relate the structures of the lower respiratory tract to their functions.

LO 8.6 Identify and describe disorders and pathological conditions related to the respiratory system.

LO 8.7 Explain the diagnostic and therapeutic procedures and pharmacologic agents used for disorders of the respiratory system.

LO 8.8 Identify health professionals involved in the care of patients with pulmonary diseases and disorders.

LO 8.9 Apply your knowledge of the medical terms of the respiratory system to documentation, medical records, and medical reports.

LO 8.10 Translate the medical terms of the respiratory system into everyday language to communicate clearly with patients and their families.

In your future career, being able to communicate comfortably, accurately, and effectively with the health professionals involved in the diagnosis and treatment of respiratory problems is key. You may work directly and/or indirectly with one or more of the following:

- **Pulmonologists** are physicians who specialize in the diagnosis and treatment of lung/pulmonary conditions.
- **Registered respiratory therapists (RRT) or respiratory care practitioners** assist physicians in evaluating, treating, and caring for patients who have respiratory disorders. They also supervise RT technicians.
- **Respiratory therapy (RT) technicians** assist physicians and RRTs in evaluating, monitoring, and treating patients with respiratory disorders.
- **Sleep technologists** are trained in sleep technology and sleep medicine. These technologists assist sleep specialists in the assessment, monitoring, management, and follow-up care of patients with sleep disorders.

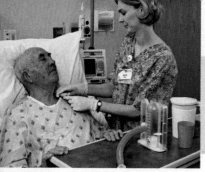

Section 8.1

Introduction to the Respiratory System

Keynotes

- On December 14, 1799, President George Washington died of an obstructed airway due to acute epiglottitis.

- Croup occurs in children aged 3 months to 5 years.

- Heavy smokers and drinkers have a 200 times greater risk of developing cancer of the larynx.

Abbreviations

O_2	oxygen
RRT	registered respiratory therapist

Organization of the Respiratory System

The respiratory system can be organized according to structure and function. Structurally, the respiratory tract is divided into an upper respiratory tract and a lower respiratory tract. Functionally, the respiratory tract is divided into the conduction and respiration areas.

Structural Organization (LO 8.4 and 8.5)

The **respiratory tract** *(Figure 8.1)* has six connected elements:

1. **Nose**
2. **Pharynx**
3. **Larynx**
4. **Trachea**
5. **Bronchi** and **bronchioles**
6. **Alveoli**

Functional Organization (LO 8.4 and 8.5)

Respiration has two components:

- **Ventilation**, which is the bulk movement of air and its gases into **(inspiration)** and out of **(expiration)** the lungs; and

- The **exchange of gases** between air and blood, and between blood and interstitial fluids.

Functions of the Respiratory System (LO 8.4 and 8.5)

Your respiratory system is responsible for the following key functions:

1. **Exchange of gases:** All of your body cells need oxygen and produce carbon dioxide. Your respiratory system allows oxygen from the air to enter the blood and carbon dioxide to leave the blood and enter the air.

2. **Regulation of blood pH:** Regulation occurs by changing carbon dioxide levels in the blood.

3. **Protection:** The respiratory system protects against foreign bodies and against some microorganisms.

4. **Voice production:** Movement of air across the vocal cords makes voice **phonation** and sound possible.

5. **Olfaction:** The 12 million receptor cells for smell are in a quarter-sized patch of epithelium. These are located in the **olfactory region** *(Figure 8.2),* the extreme superior region of the nasal cavity. Each cell has 10 to 20 hair-like structures called **cilia** that project into the nasal cavity in a thin mucous film.

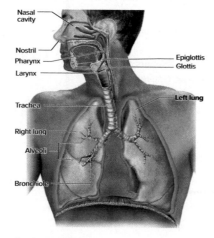

▲ **FIGURE 8.1**
The Respiratory System.

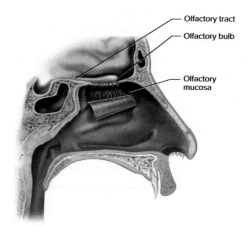

▲ **FIGURE 8.2**
Olfactory Region of the Nose.

Word Analysis and Definition

WORD	PRONUNCIATION	ELEMENTS		DEFINITION
alveolus alveoli (pl) alveolar (adj)	al-**VEE**-oh-lus al-**VEE**-oh-lie al-**VEE**-oh-lar	 S/ R/	Latin *hollow sac* -ar *pertaining to* alveol- *air sac*	Terminal element of respiratory tract where gas exchange occurs Pertaining to the alveoli
bronchus bronchi (pl) bronchiole	**BRONG**-kuss **BRONG**-kie **BRONG**-key-ole	 S/ R/CF	Greek *windpipe* -ole *small* bronch/i- *bronchus*	One of two subdivisions of the trachea Increasingly smaller subdivisions of bronchi
cilium cilia (pl)	**SILL**-ee-um **SILL**-ee-ah		Latin *eyelash*	Hairlike motile projection from the surface of a cell
expiration (**Note:** *The "s" is deleted from the root spirat because the prefix ex already has the "s" sound.*)	**EKS**-pih-**RAY**-shuni	S/ P/ R/	-ion *action, condition, process of* ex- *out* -spirat- *breathe*	Breathe out
inspiration (**Note:** *The opposite of expiration*)	in-spih-**RAY**-shun	S/ P/ R/	-ion *action, condition, process of* in- *into* -spirat- *breathe*	Breathe in
larynx	**LAH**-rinks		Greek *larynx*	Organ of sound production
olfaction olfactory (adj)	ol-**FAK**-shun ol-**FAK**-toh-ree	S/ S/ R/	-ion *action, condition, process of* -ory *having the function of* olfact- *smell*	Sense of smell Relating to the sense of smell
oxygen	**OCK**-si-jen	S/ R/	-gen *create* oxy- *oxygen*	The gas essential for life
pharynx pharyngeal (adj)	**FAH**-rinks fah-**RIN**-jee-al	 S/ R/	Greek *throat* -eal *pertaining to* pharyng- *pharynx*	Tube from the back of the nose to the larynx. Pertaining to the pharynx
pulmonary pulmonology pulmonologist	**PULL**-moh-**NAIR**-ee **PULL**-moh-**NOL**-oh-jee **PULL**-moh-**NOL**-oh-jist	S/ R/ S/ R/CF S/	-ary *pertaining to* pulmon- *lung* -logy *study of* pulmon/o- *lung* -logist *one who studies, specialist*	Pertaining to the lungs Study of the lungs, or the medical specialty of disorders of the lungs Specialist in treating disorders of the lungs
respiration respiratory (adj)	**RES**-pih-**RAY**-shun **RES**-pih-rah-tor-ee	S/ P/ R/ S/	-ation *a process, formed from* re- *again* -spir- *to breathe* -atory *pertaining to, produced by*	Process of breathing; fundamental process of life used to exchange oxygen and carbon dioxide Pertaining to respiration
trachea trachealis (adj)	**TRAY**-kee-ah tray-kee-**AY**-lis	 S/ R/	Greek *windpipe* -alis *pertaining to* trache- *trachea*	Air tube from the larynx to the bronchi Pertaining to the trachea

EXERCISES

 Case Report 8.1

You are

. . . an advanced-level **registered respiratory therapist (RRT)** working with **pulmonologist** Tavis Senko, MD, in the Acute Respiratory Care unit of Fulwood Medical Center.

You are communicating with

. . . Mr. Jude Jacobs, a 68-year-old white, retired, mail carrier, who has chronic obstructive pulmonary disease **(COPD)** and is on continual **oxygen (O_2)** by nasal cannula. He has smoked two packs of cigarettes per day throughout his adult life.

Last night, he was unable to sleep because of increased shortness of breath **(SOB)** and cough. He had to sit upright in bed in order to breathe. His cough produces yellow **sputum**.

Mr. Jacobs' vital signs are temperature **(T)** 101.6°, pulse **(P)** 98, respirations **(R)** 36, and blood pressure **(BP)** 150/90. On examination, he is **cyanotic** and frightened, and he is on oxygen by nasal cannula. Air entry is diminished in both lungs, and there are **rales** (crackles) at the bases of both lungs.

You have been ordered to draw blood for arterial blood gases **(ABGs)** and to measure the amount of air entering and leaving his lungs by using **spirometry**.

Mr. Jacobs' forced expiratory volume was reduced at 65% of normal due to obstructive disease from chronic smoking. While continuing his oxygen therapy, his arterial oxygen levels were at 85% of normal.

Study Hint

Frequent errors are made on test questions regarding the term *pleural,* meaning *pertaining to the pleura.* It is not spelled "plural," which means *more than one.* Be especially careful when dealing with this term, and always check your spelling. Both terms sound alike, are spelled differently, and have very different meanings. *The right answer (pleural) is wrong if it is spelled "plural."* Don't lose points on a test because of carelessness.

A. Read *Case Report 8.1 before answering the questions. Fill in the blanks.*
   LO 8.8, 8.9, and 8.10

1. In Case Report 8.1, the type of physician that is responsible for Mr. Jacobs's care

   is a: _____ .

2. The device that is delivering oxygen therapy to Mr. Jacobs

   is: _____ .

3. The device that measures that amount of air entering and leaving Mr. Jacobs's lungs

   is a: _____ .

4. Which test ordered for Mr. Jacobs involves drawing his blood? (Provide the

   abbreviation) _____

5. The material that Mr. Jacobs brought up from is lung is termed: _____ .

6. The medical term in Case Report 8.1 that indicates that his skin has a blue color is: _____ .

Section 8.2

Upper Respiratory Tract

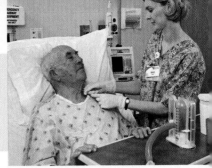

Your upper respiratory tract consists of your nose, pharynx, and larynx. It is the first site that brings air and its pollutants inside your body.

The Nose (LO 8.4)

When you breathe in air through your nose, the air goes through the nostrils (**nares**) into the nasal cavity. Internal hairs guard the nares to prevent large particles from entering your body.

The nasal **septum** divides the nasal cavity into right and left compartments. The **palate** forms the floor of the nose as well as the roof of the mouth *(Figure 8.3)*. The **paranasal, frontal,** and **maxillary sinuses** *(Chapter 4)* open into the nose.

Functions of the Nose (LO 8.4)

The nose serves as an important part of the respiratory system in several ways:

1. **Passageway for air** to enter or leave the body.

2. **Air cleanser:** The nasal hairs and the mucus (secreted by the nasal mucous membrane) trap particles of dust and solid pollutants.

3. **Air moisturizer:** It adds moisture to the air. Moisture is secreted by the nasal mucosa (mucous membrane) and from tears that drain into the nasal cavity through the nasao lacrimal duct *(see Chapter 11)*.

4. **Air warmer:** The blood flowing through the nasal cavity beneath the mucous membrane lining also warms the air. This prevents damage from cold to the more fragile lower respiratory passages.

5. **Sense of smell (olfaction):** The olfactory region recognizes some 4,000 separate smells *(see previous pages)*.

The Pharynx (LO 8.4)

Your pharynx is a muscular funnel that receives air from the nasal cavity, and food and drink from the oral cavity. It is divided into three regions *(Figure 8.4)*:

1. **Nasopharynx:** Located at the back of the nose and above the soft palate and uvula. The posterior surface contains the pharyngeal **tonsil (adenoid).** Only air moves through this region;

2. **Oropharynx:** Located at the back of the mouth, and below the soft palate and above the epiglottis. It contains two sets of tonsils called the palatine and lingual tonsils. Air, food, and drink all pass through this region; and

3. **Laryngopharynx:** Located below the tip of the epiglottis. It is the pathway to the esophagus. Only food and drink normally pass through the laryngopharynx.

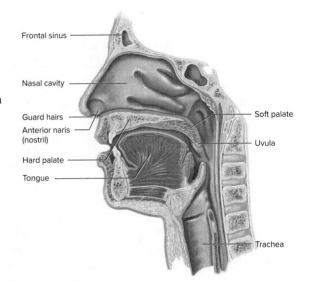

▲ **FIGURE 8.3**
Upper Respiratory Tract.

Frontal sinus · Nasal cavity · Guard hairs · Anterior naris (nostril) · Hard palate · Tongue · Soft palate · Uvula · Trachea

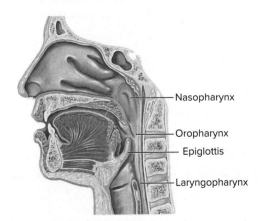

▲ **FIGURE 8.4**
Regions of the Pharynx.

Nasopharynx · Oropharynx · Epiglottis · Laryngopharynx

The Larynx (LO 8.4)

The flow of inhaled air moves on from your pharynx to your **larynx**. The upper opening into the larynx from the oropharynx is called the **glottis**. The spoon-shaped **epiglottis** guards the glottis. When you swallow food, your tongue pushes down the epiglottis to close the glottis and direct the food into the esophagus behind it *(Figure 8.5)*. The thyroid cartilage, or the Adam's apple, forms the anterior and lateral walls of the larynx. Inside the larynx, two pairs of horizontal ligaments—your **vocal** cords *(Figures 8.6 and 8.7)*—stretch across the lateral walls and enable sounds (phonation) to be made as air passes between them.

Functions of the Larynx (LO 8.4)

Two major roles of your larynx are:

1. Maintaining an open passage for the movement of air to and from the trachea *(Figure 8.6)*, and

2. Producing sounds through the vocal cords.

Sound Production Air moving past the vocal cords makes them vibrate to produce sound (phonation). The force of the air moving past the vocal cords determines the loudness of the sound. Muscles in the cords pull them closer together with varying degrees of tautness *(Figure 8.7)*. A high-pitched sound is produced by taut cords, and a low-pitched sound is made by more relaxed cords. Cis gender males' vocal cords are longer and thicker than those of females. They vibrate more slowly and produce lower-pitched sounds.

The crude sounds produced by the larynx are transformed into words by the actions of the pharynx, tongue, teeth, and lips.

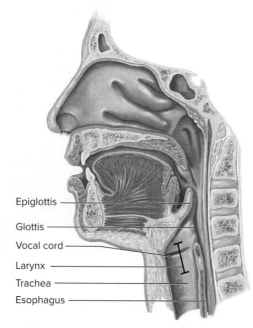

▲ **FIGURE 8.5**
Larynx Location.

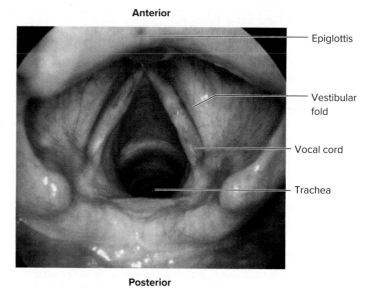

▲ **FIGURE 8.6**
View of Larynx Using a Laryngoscope.

CNRI/Science Source

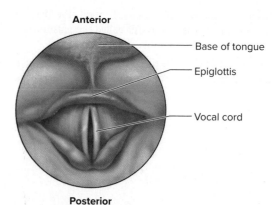

▲ **FIGURE 8.7**
Vocal Cords Pulled Close and Taut.

WORD	PRONUNCIATION		ELEMENTS	DEFINITION
acute	ah-**KYUT**		Latin *sharp*	Disease of sudden onset
adenoid	**ADD**-eh-noyd	S/ R/	-oid *resembling* aden- *gland*	Single mass of lymphoid tissue in the midline at the back of the throat
chronic	**KRON**-ik		Greek *time*	A persistent, long-term disease
epiglottis	ep-ih-**GLOT**-is	P/ R/	epi- *above* -glottis *mouth of windpipe*	Leaf-shaped plate of cartilage that shuts off the larynx during swallowing
frontal	**FRUNT**-al	S/ R/	-al *pertaining to* front- *front of*	Pertaining to the front
glottis	**GLOT**-is		Greek *opening of larynx*	The opening from the oropharynx into the larynx
laryngopharynx	lah-**RING**-oh-**FAIR**-rinks	R/CF R/	laryng/o- *larynx* -pharynx *pharynx, throat*	Region of the pharynx below the epiglottis that includes the larynx
maxilla maxillae (pl)	mak-**SILL**-ah mak-**SILL**-ee		Latin *jawbone*	Upper jawbone, containing right and left maxillary sinuses
maxillary (**Note:** the extra "a" is dropped when joined to the suffix -*ary*)	**MAK**-sih-lair-ee	S/ R/	-ary *pertaining to* maxilla- *maxilla*	Pertaining to the maxilla
naris nares (pl) nasal	**NAH**-ris **NAH**-rees **NAY**-zal	S/ R/	Latin *nostril* -al *pertaining to* nas- *nose*	Nostril Pertaining to the nose
nasopharynx nasopharyngeal (adj)	**NAY**-zoh-**FAH**-rinks **NAY**-zoh-fah-**RIN**-jee-al	R/CF R/ S/ R/CF	nas/o- *nose* -pharynx *pharynx, throat* -eal *pertaining to* -pharyng- *pharynx, throat*	Region of the pharynx at the back of the nose and above the soft palate Pertaining to the nasopharynx
oropharynx oropharyngeal (adj)	**OR**-oh-fah-rinks **OR**-oh-fah-**RIN**-jee-al	R/CF R/ S/ R	or/o- *mouth* -pharynx *pharynx, throat* -eal *pertaining to* -pharyng- *pharynx, throat*	Region at the back of the mouth between the soft palate and the tip of the epiglottis. Pertaining to the oropharynx
palate	**PAL**-at		Latin *palate*	Roof of the mouth, floor of the nose
paranasal	**PAIR**-ah-**NAY**-zal	S/ P/ R/	-al *pertaining to* para- *adjacent to* -nas- *nose*	Adjacent to the nose
septum septa (pl)	**SEP**-tum **SEP**-tah		Latin *partition*	Thin wall separating two cavities or tissue masses
sinus	**SIGH**-nus	R/	Latin *cavity* sinus- *sinus*	Cavity or hollow space in a bone or other tissue
tonsil	**TON**-sill		Latin *tonsil*	Mass of lymphoid tissue on either side of the throat at the back of the tongue
vocal	**VOH**-kal	S/ R/	-al *pertaining to* voc- *voice*	Pertaining to the voice

EXERCISES

A. Elements: *Work with elements to build your knowledge of the language of pulmonology. One element in each of the following medical terms is boldfaced.*

Identify the type of element (P, R, CF, or S) in column 2; then provide the meaning of that element in column 3.   **LO 8.1**

Medical Term   **Type of Element**   **Meaning of Element**

1. **nas**al   _____   _____

2. **para**nasal   _____   _____

3. sinu**sitis**   _____   _____

B. Plural versions of Greek and Latin terms. *Not all plural terms end in "s." Provide the plural form of the following terms.*   **LO 8.1 and 8.2**

1. **septum:** _____

2. **naris:** _____

3. **sinus:** _____

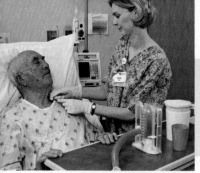

Section 8.3

Lower Respiratory Tract

Abbreviation

CO_2 carbon dioxide

Once the air you inhale has passed through the upper airway and many of the pollutants and impurities have been filtered out, the major needs still remain: to get oxygen (O_2) into the blood and remove carbon dioxide (CO_2) from the blood. To make this possible, the inhaled air has to travel into the alveoli of the lungs, where these exchanges can occur.

Trachea (LO 8.4)

The flow of inhaled air now moves into your trachea (windpipe). This is a rigid tube that descends from the larynx and divides into the two main bronchi *(Figure 8.8)*, each of which serves as airways going to your right and left lungs.

The Lungs (LO 8.4 and 8.5)

Your two lungs are the main organs of respiration and are located in the thoracic cavity. Each lung is a soft, spongy, cone-shaped organ with its **base** resting on the **diaphragm** and its top **(apex)** above and behind the clavicle. Its outer convex, costal surface presses against the **rib cage.** Its inner concave surface presses against the chest region **(mediastinum).**

The right lung has three **lobes:** superior, middle, and inferior. The left lung has two lobes; superior and inferior *(Figure 8.8a)*. Each lobe is separated from the others by **fissures.**

Lung Parenchyma (LO 8.4 and 8.5)

As airways taper into smaller **bronchioles, alveoli** begin to appear and form the gas exchange portion of lung tissue known as parenchyma. The **parenchyma** describes the functional units of lung tissue in which oxygen and carbon dioxide are exchanged with blood via adjacent pulmonary capillaries.

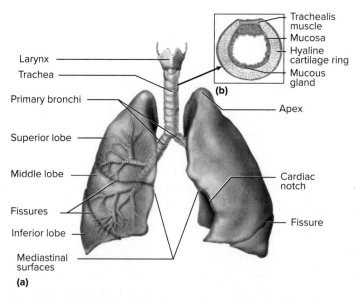

▲ **FIGURE 8.8**
Lower Respiratory Tract.
(a) Gross anatomy. (b) C-shaped tracheal cartilage.

Tracheobronchial Tree (LO 8.4 and LO 8.5)

The tracheobronchial tree is an upside-down, tree-like structure that conducts air in your chest. It comprises the trachea, bronchi, and bronchial tubes. As inhaled air continues down the respiratory tract, the main bronchi divide into a **lobar** (secondary) bronchus for each lobe. Each secondary bronchus then divides into tertiary (third) bronchi that supply **segments** of each lobe *(Figure 8.9)*. These divisions create branch-like airways.

Bronchioles and Alveoli (LO 8.4 and LO 8.5)

These tertiary bronchi further divide into bronchioles, which in turn eventually divide into several thin-walled alveoli. Each **alveolus** is a thin-walled sac supported by a thin, semipermeable **respiratory membrane**. This membrane allows the exchange of gases with the surrounding pulmonary capillary network.

The Pleura (LO 8.4 and LO 8.5)

The **pleura** is a double-layered **serous** membrane that covers the surface of both lungs. The space between these two layers is called the **pleural cavity,** which contains a thin film of lubricant fluid. This lubricant enables the lungs to expand (inspiration) and deflate (expiration) with minimal friction.

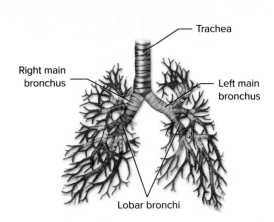

▲ **FIGURE 8.9**
Latex Cast of the Tracheobronchial Tree.

Mechanics of Respiration (LO 8.4 and LO 8.5)

A resting adult breathes 10 to 15 times per minute and **inhales** about 500 mL of air during inspiration and **exhales** it during expiration. The mission is to get air into and out of the alveoli so that oxygen can enter the bloodstream and carbon dioxide can exit.

Your diaphragm does most of the work. In inspiration, it drops down and flattens to expand the thoracic cavity and reduce the pressure in the airways. The external intercostal muscles also help by lifting the chest wall up and out to further expand the thoracic cavity *(Figure 8.10a)*.

Expiration is a process of letting go. The diaphragm and the intercostal muscles relax, and the thoracic cavity springs back to its original size *(Figure 8.10b)*.

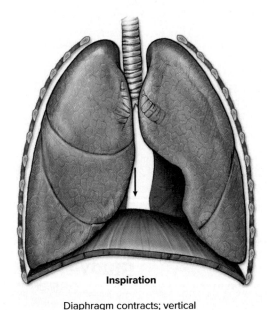

Inspiration

Diaphragm contracts; vertical dimensions of thoracic cavity increase.

(a)

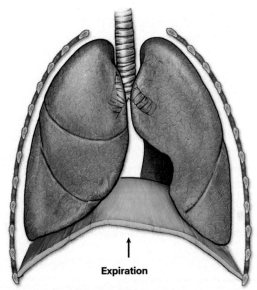

Expiration

Diaphragm relaxes; vertical dimensions of thoracic cavity decrease.

(b)

▲ **FIGURE 8.10**
Inspiration and Expiration.

S = Suffix   P = Prefix   R = Root   R/CF = Combining Form

WORD	PRONUNCIATION		ELEMENTS	DEFINITION
apex	AY-peks		Latin *summit or tip*	Tip or end of cone-shaped structure, such as the bottom of the heart or top of the lung
base	BASE		Latin or Greek *basis*	Structurally it is the lower part or bottom of the area opposite the apex. Referring to pH, greater than 7.0
cavity cavities (pl)	KAV-ih-tee KAV-it-ees	S/ R/	-ity *state, condition* cav- *hollow space*	A hollow space or body or compartment
diaphragm diaphragmatic (adj)	DIE-ah-fram DIE-ah-frag-**MAT**-ik	 S/ R/CF	Greek *diaphragm* -tic *pertaining to* diaphragm/a- *diaphragm*	The muscular sheet separating the abdominal and thoracic cavities Pertaining to the diaphragm
exhale	EKS-hail	P/ R/	ex- *out* -hale *breathe*	Breathe out
fissure fissures (pl)	FISH-ur	S/ R/	-ure *process, result of* fiss- *split*	Deep furrow or cleft
inhale	IN-hail	P/ R/	in- *in* -hale *breathe*	Breathe in
lobe lobar (adj)	LOBE LOW-bar	 S/ R/	Greek *lobe* -ar *pertaining to* lob- *lobe*	Subdivision of an organ or other part Pertaining to a lobe
mediastinum mediastinal (adj)	ME-dee-ass-**TIE**-num ME-dee-ass-**TIE**-nal	S/ P/ R/ S/	-um *structure* media- *middle* -stin- *partition* -al *pertaining to*	Area between the lungs containing the heart, aorta, venae cavae, esophagus, and trachea Pertaining to the mediastinum
membrane membranous (adj)	MEM-brain MEM-brah-nus	 S/ R/	Latin *parchment* -ous *pertaining to* membran- *cover, skin*	Thin layer of tissue covering a structure or cavity Pertaining to a membrane
parenchyma	pah-**REN**-ki-mah		Greek *to pour in*	The specific functional cells of a gland or organ (e.g., the lung) that are supported by the connective tissue framework
pleura pleurae (pl) pleural (adj)	PLUR-ah PLUR-ee PLUR-al	 S/ R/	Greek *rib* -al *pertaining to* pleur- *pleura*	Membrane covering the lungs and lining the ribs in the thoracic cavity Pertaining to the pleura
pleural cavity	PLUR-al	S/ R/	-al *pertaining to* pleur- *pleura* Latin *hollow*	Pertaining to the space that surrounds the lungs
respiratory membrane	RES-pih-rah-tor-ee MEM-brain	S/ P/ R/	-atory *pertaining to, produced by* re- *again* -spir- *to breathe* Latin *parchment*	A thin, semipermeable membrane between the alveoli and the pulmonary capillaries
segment	SEG-ment		Latin *to cut*	A section of an organ or structure
serous	SEER-us		Latin *serum*	Thicker and less transparent than water

EXERCISES

A. Provide the term *being described using the language of pulmonology.*   LO 8.2, 8.4, and 8.5

1. The top of the lung is termed the: _____

2. The bottom of the lung is termed the: _____

3. Which lung has three lobes, the right or the left? _____

4. Each lung lobe is separated by a: _____

5. The serous membrane that covers the surface of the lungs is called the: _____

Study Hint

The English word *breath* describes a noun and is the air you inhale and exhale. ("Take a deep breath.") The English word *breathe* has an "e" on the end of it and is the verb meaning to *inhale and exhale.* ("She was unable to breathe.")

B. Precision in communication *means using the correct form of the medical term, as well as the correct spelling. Test your knowledge of plurals, adjectives, and spelling with this exercise. Select the correct choice.*   **LO 8.4, 8.5, and 8.10**

1. The area between the lungs containing the heart, aorta, venae cavae, esophagus, and trachea is the:
   a. mediastenum   b. medisternum   c. mediastinum   d. midiasternum

2. The patient was diagnosed with _____ pneumonia.
   a. lobe   b. lobular   c. lobar   d. lumbar

3. Is the term for the functional cells of an organ.
   a. perenchyma   b. parenchyma   c. perinchkima   d. perenkima

4. Because there is a hilum in each lung, collectively they are referred to as the:
   a. hilla   b. hila   c. hilia   d. hilea

5. The muscle separating the abdominal and thoracic cavities is the:
   a. diaphram   b. diaphragm   c. diahragm   d. diapragm

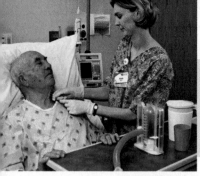

Disorders of the Respiratory System

Disorders of the Upper Respiratory Tract

Disorders of the Nose (LO 8.4)

A **common cold** is a viral upper respiratory infection (**URI**). It is contagious and easily transmitted in airborne droplets through coughing and sneezing. There is no proven effective treatment.

Rhinitis, also called **coryza**, is an acute inflammation of the nasal mucosa, which is usually viral.

Allergic rhinitis affects 15% to 20% of the population. The mucous membranes of the nose, pharynx, and sinuses swell and produce a clear, watery discharge. Treatment entails defining and removing the allergy-causing agent.

Sinusitis is an infection of the paranasal sinuses, often following a viral upper respiratory tract infection. It can also be part of an allergic response.

A **deviated nasal septum** occurs when the partition between the two nostrils is pushed to one side, leading to a partially obstructed airway in one nostril.

Nasal polyps are benign growths arising from the mucosa of the nasal cavity or a sinus.

Epistaxis (a nosebleed) is bleeding from the septum of the nose, usually as a result of trauma.

Disorders of the Pharynx (LO 8.4 and 8.7)

Snoring occurs regularly in 25% of normal adults and is most common in overweight males. It worsens with age. Snoring noises are made at the back of the mouth and nose where the tongue and upper pharynx meet the soft palate and uvula *(Figure 8.11)*.

Obstructive sleep apnea (**OSA**) can cause an obstruction by the soft tissues at the back of the nose and mouth. This leads to frequent episodes of gasping for breath, followed by complete cessation of breathing (**apnea**). These episodes reduce the level of oxygen in the blood (**hypoxemia**), making the heart pump harder. If this problem goes untreated for several years, it can cause hypertension and cardiac enlargement.

Pharyngitis is an acute or chronic infection involving the pharynx, tonsils, and uvula. It is usually viral in children. Increasing air humidity and getting extra rest are effective treatments.

Tonsillitis is usually a viral infection of the tonsils in the oropharynx. In less than 20% of cases, this infection is caused by a streptococcus. A rapid strep test and throat culture are used to identify the strep sore throat or pharyngitis.

Disorders of the Larynx (LO 8.4 and 8.6)

Laryngitis is an inflammation of the mucosal lining of the larynx, which produces hoarseness and sometimes progresses to a loss of voice.

Epiglottitis is an inflammation of the epiglottis and is seen most commonly in children between the ages of 2 and 7. It is preventable by vaccine.

Croup (**laryngotracheobronchitis**) is a group of viral diseases causing an inflammation and obstruction of the upper airway. It's most common in persons between ages 3 months and 5 years. In severe cases, a child makes a high-pitched, squeaky, inspiratory noise called **stridor**.

Papillomas, or polyps, are benign tumors of the larynx due to overuse or irritation.

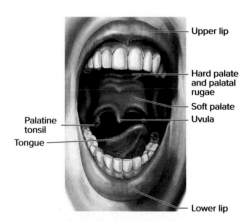

Upper lip
Hard palate and palatal rugae
Soft palate
Uvula
Palatine tonsil
Tongue
Lower lip

▲ **FIGURE 8.11**
Soft Tissues at the Back of the Mouth.

WORD	PRONUNCIATION	ELEMENTS		DEFINITION
apnea	AP-nee-ah	P/ R/	a- *without* -pnea *breathe*	Absence of spontaneous respiration
coryza (*also called* rhinitis)	koh-RYE-zah		Greek *catarrh*	Acute inflammation of the mucous membrane of the nose
croup (*also called* laryngotracheobronchitis)	KROOP		Old English *to cry out loud*	Infection of the upper airways in children characterized by a barking cough
epiglottitis	ep-ih-glot-EYE-tis	S/ R/	-itis *inflammation* -glott- *mouth of windpipe*	Inflammation of the epiglottis
epistaxis	ep-ih-STAK-sis	S/ P/ R/	-is *pertaining to* epi- *above, upon* -stax- *fall in drops*	Nosebleed
hypoxemia	high-pock-SEE-me-ah	S/ P/ R/	-emia *condition of the blood* hyp- *below* -ox- *oxygen*	Low oxygen level in arterial blood
hypoxia (noun)	high-POCK-see-ah	S/	-ia *condition*	Decreased below normal levels of oxygen in tissues, gases, or blood
hypoxic (adj)	high-POCK-sik	S/	-ic *pertaining to*	Deficient in oxygen
laryngotracheobronchitis (*also called* croup)	lah-RING-oh-TRAY-kee-oh-brong-KIE-tis	S/ R/CF R/CF R/	-itis *inflammation* laryng/o- *larynx* -trache/o -*trachea* -bronch- *bronchus*	Inflammation of the larynx, trachea, and bronchi
laryngitis	lah-rin-JEYE-tis	S/ R/CF	-itis *inflammation* laryng/o- *larynx*	Inflammation of the larynx
papilla papillae (pl) papilloma	pah-PILL-ah pah-PILL-ee pap-ih-LOH-mah	 S/ R/CF	Latin *small pimple* -oma *tumor, mass* papill/o- *pimple*	Any small projection Benign projection of epithelial cells
pharyngitis	fair-in-JIE-tis	S/ R/	-itis *inflammation* pharyng- *pharynx, throat*	Inflammation of the pharynx
polyp	POL-ip		Latin *many feet*	Any mass of tissue that projects outward
rhinitis (*also called* coryza)	rye-NIE-tis	S/ R/	-itis *inflammation* rhin- *nose*	Acute inflammation of the nasal mucosa
sinusitis	sigh-nu-SIGH-tis	S/ R/	-itis *inflammation* sinus- *sinus*	Inflammation of the lining of a sinus
stridor	STRY-door		Latin *a harsh, creaking sound*	High-pitched noise made when there is a respiratory obstruction in the larynx or trachea
tonsillitis (Note: double "ll")	ton-sih-LIE-tis	S/ R/	-itis *inflammation* tonsill- *tonsil*	Inflammation of the tonsils

Disorders of the Lower Respiratory Tract (LO 8.4, 8.5, and 8.6)

Common Signs and Symptoms of Respiratory Disorders

(LO 8.4, 8.5, and 8.6)

The common signs and symptoms of respiratory disorders are often visible and audible, and they include the following:

1. **Cough** is triggered by irritants in the respiratory tract. Irritants include cigarette smoke, infection, or tumors, as in lung cancer. A productive cough produces **sputum**, which can be swallowed or **expectorated**. Bloody sputum is called **hemoptysis**. Thick, yellow **(purulent)** sputum indicates infection. A **nonproductive** cough is usually dry and hacking or a cough that does not result in sputum or expectoration.

   Abnormal amounts of mucus arising from the upper respiratory tract and expectorated or coughed up are called **phlegm**.

2. **Dyspnea,** or the sensation of shortness of breath **(SOB),** can occur from exertion or, in severe disorders, during rest when all the respiratory muscles are used to exchange only a small volume of air.

3. **Cyanosis** is seen when the blood has increased levels of **unoxygenated hemoglobin** and has a characteristic dark red-blue color.

4. **Changes in the breathing rate** may occur. **Eupnea** is the normal, easy respiration (average 10 to 15 breaths per minute) in a resting adult. Both **tachypnea** (rapid breathing) and **hyperpnea** (breathing deeper and more rapidly than normal) are signs of respiratory difficulty, as is **bradypnea** (slow breathing).

5. **Sneezing** is caused by irritants in the nasal cavity.

6. **Hiccups** are reflex spasms of the diaphragm. The etiology is unknown, and there is no specific medical cure.

7. **Yawning** is a reflex that originates in the brainstem in response to hypoxia, boredom, or sleepiness. The exact mechanisms are not known.

Abbreviation

SOB   Shortness of Breath

WORD	PRONUNCIATION	ELEMENTS		DEFINITION
bradypnea (opposite of tachypnea)	brad-ip-NEE-ah	P/ R/	brady- slow -pnea breathe	Slow breathing
cough	KAWF		Middle English to shout	Forceful expulsion of air from the lungs, occurring immediately after a closed glottis
cyanosis	sigh-ah-NO-sis	S/ R/	-osis condition cyan- dark blue	Blue discoloration of the skin, lips, and nail beds due to low levels of oxygen in the blood
cyanotic (adj)	sigh-ah-NOT-ik	S/ R/CF	-tic pertaining to cyan/o- dark blue	Pertaining to or marked by cyanosis
deoxygenated	de-OCK-suh-je-nay-ted	S/ P/ R/	-ated pertaining to a condition de- without, removal -oxygen- oxygen	Not combined with oxygen
dyspnea	disp-NEE-ah	P/ R/	dys- bad, difficult -pnea breathe	Difficult breathing
eupnea	yoop-NEE-ah	P/ R/	eu- normal, good -pnea breathe	Normal breathing
expectorate	ek-SPEK-toh-rate	S/ P/ R/	-ate pertaining to ex- out -pector- chest	Cough up and spit out mucus from the respiratory tract
hemoglobin	HEE-moh-GLOH-bin	R/CF R/	hem/o- blood -globin protein	Red-pigmented protein that is the main component of red blood cells
hemoptysis	he-MOP-tih-sis	R/CF S/	hem/o- blood -ptysis spit	Bloody sputum
hyperpnea	high-perp-NEE-ah	P/ R/	hyper- excessive -pnea breathe	Deeper and more rapid breathing than normal
productive cough	proh-DUC-tiv KAWF		Latin bring forth Middle English to shout	Cough resulting in matter being brought up from the airways or lungs
nonproductive	NON-proh-DUC-tiv	P/ R/	non- no, not -productive produce	Cough that does not result in matter brought up from the airways or lungs
phlegm	FLEM		Greek flame	Abnormal amounts of mucus expectorated from the respiratory tract
purulent	PURE-you-lent	S/ R/	-ulent abounding in pur- pus	Showing or containing pus
tachypnea (opposite of bradypnea)	tak-ip-NEE-ah	P/ R/	tachy- rapid -pnea breathe	Rapid breathing

Disorders of the Lower Respiratory Tract (LO 8.5 and 8.6)

There are a number of disorders that are specific to your lower respiratory tract. These disorders are described below.

Acute bronchitis can be viral or bacterial, leading to the production of excess mucus with some obstruction of airflow. It resolves without significant residual damage to the airway.

Acute respiratory distress syndrome (ARDS) is sudden, life-threatening lung failure caused by a variety of underlying conditions such as major trauma or sepsis. The alveoli fill with fluid and collapse, preventing adequate gas exchange and resulting in hypoxemia.

Asthma is a disorder with recurrent acute episodes of bronchial obstruction. This results from a constriction of bronchi and bronchioles **(bronchoconstriction), hypersecretion** of mucus, and inflammatory swelling of the airway lining. Between attacks, breathing can be normal. The etiology of asthma is an inflammatory response to substances like pollen, animal dander, or the feces of dust mites.

Bronchiectasis is the abnormal widening (dilation) of the small airways to medium-sized airways due to repeated infections. The damaged, dilated bronchi accumulate secretions, making them prone to further infections and increased damage.

Bronchiolitis is a viral inflammation of the smaller airways (bronchioles) that most commonly affects younger children and infants. In severe cases, this disease can cause respiratory distress, leading to a need for mechanical ventilation.

Chronic bronchitis is a long-term form of airway inflammation and is the most common obstructive disease, caused by cigarette smoking or repeated episodes of acute bronchitis. Along with excess mucus production, cilia are destroyed. A pattern develops, involving chronic cough, dyspnea, and recurrent acute infections.

In advanced chronic bronchitis, hypoxia and **hypercapnia** (excess carbon dioxide) occur and heart failure follows.

Abbreviation

ARDS	adult respiratory distress syndrome

Chronic infections of the lung parenchyma are the result of prolonged exposure to pathogens or occupational irritant dusts or droplets. These disorders are known by different names according to the cause or description of the abnormality. Certain levels of dust or particle inhalation overwhelm the airways' particle-clearing abilities. The dust particles accumulate in the alveoli and parenchyma, leading to **fibrosis.** Coal worker's **pneumoconiosis,** also known as "black lung," is caused by inhalation of coal dust. **Asbestosis** results from inhaling fibrous asbestos particles and can lead to a cancer in the pleura called **mesothelioma.** Silicosis, also known as "stonecutters' disease," is caused by inhalation of silica particles. **Anthracosis** from coal dust particles is called "coal miners' disease." (**Anthrax** is a different disease, caused by toxins produced by the anthrax bacillus.)
Sarcoidosis is an uncommon disorder where lesions form across the body also causing fibrosis (scarring) of the lung parenchyma.

Chronic obstructive pulmonary disease (COPD) is a common, progressive and deadly disease. Smoking is the most common risk factor for COPD, although exposure to pollutants can also cause the condition. A history of cigarette smoking *(Figure 8.12),* with chronic cough and sputum production, is followed by increasing dyspnea and need for oxygen. Right-sided heart failure (cor pulmonale, *see Chapter 6*) may occur due to pulmonary hypertension and a continuous backup of excess blood into the right ventricle.

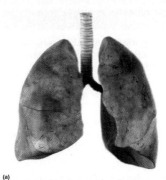
(a)

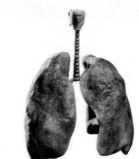
(b)

▶ **FIGURE 8.12** Whole Lungs.
(a) Lungs of a Non-smoker.
(b) Lungs of a Smoker.
SCIEPRO/Science Photo Library/Getty Images

Word Analysis and Definition

S = Suffix   P = Prefix   R = Root   R/CF = Combining Form

WORD	PRONUNCIATION		ELEMENTS	DEFINITION
asthma	AZ-mah		Greek *asthma*	Episodes of breathing difficulty due to narrowed or obstructed airways from inflammation
asthmatic (adj)	az-**MAT**-ik	S/ R/	-atic *pertaining to* asthm- *asthma*	Pertaining to or suffering from asthma
bronchiectasis	brong-key-**ECK**-tah-sis	S/ R/CF	-ectasis *dilation* bronch/i- *bronchus*	Chronic dilation of the bronchi following inflammatory disease or infection
bronchiolitis	brong-key-oh-**LYE**-tis	S/ R/CF	-itis *inflammation* bronchiol/o *bronchus*	Inflammation of the small bronchioles
bronchitis	brong-**KI**-tis	S/ R/	-itis *inflammation* bronch- *bronchus*	Inflammation of the bronchi
bronchoconstriction	**BRONG**-koh-kon-**STRIK**-shun	S/ R/CF R/	-ion *action, condition* bronch/o- *bronchus* -constrict- *to narrow*	Reduction in diameter of a bronchus
bulla bullae (pl)	**BULL**-ah **BULL**-ee		Latin *bubble*	Bubble-like dilated structure
cystic fibrosis (CF)	**SIS**-tik fie-**BRO**-sis	S/ R/ S/ R/	-ic *pertaining to* cyst- *cyst* -osis *abnormal condition* fibr- *fiber*	Genetic disease in which excessive viscid mucus obstructs passages, including bronchi
edema	eh-**DEE**-mah	S/	*Greek swelling*	Excessive accumulation of fluid in cells and tissues
emphysema	em-fih-**SEE**-mah	P/ R/	em- *in, into* -physema *blowing*	Enlargement of respiratory bronchioles and alveoli with destruction of airspace walls
hypercapnia	**HIGH**-per-**KAP**-nee-ah	S/ P/ R/	-ia *condition* hyper- *excessive* -capn- *carbon dioxide*	Abnormal increase of carbon dioxide within the bloodstream
hypersecretion	**HIGH**-per-seh-**KREE**-shun	S/ P/ R/	-ion *action, condition* hyper- *excessive* -secret- *secrete*	Excessive secretion of mucus (or enzymes or waste products)
sputum	**SPYU**-tum		Latin *to spit*	Matter coughed up and spat out by individuals with respiratory disorders
viscosity viscous (adj) *(cf.* viscus, *any internal organ)*	viss-**KOS**-ih-tee **VISS**-kus	S/ R/	-ity *condition* viscos- *viscous, sticky*	The resistance of a fluid to flow Sticky fluid that is resistant to flow

Keynotes

- Worldwide, 65 million people are affected by moderate to severe COPD.
- In 2019, 16 million Americans are affected by moderate to severe COPD.
- Alabama, Tennessee, Kentucky, and West Virginia have the highest incidence of COPD.

Abbreviations

CF	cystic fibrosis
CHF	congestive heart failure
COPD	chronic obstructive pulmonary disease
COVID-19	Coronavirus disease 2019
IRDS	Infant respiratory distress syndrome

Coronavirus disease 2019 (COVID-19) is a highly contagious coronavirus that primarily affects the lung parenchyma. This infectious disease typically leads to respiratory symptoms similar to pneumonia or acute respiratory distress syndrome in patients in high-risk categories. Patients with severe cases of COVID-19 require hospitalization and mechanical ventilation due to respiratory failure.

Cystic fibrosis (CF) is a genetic disorder caused by an increased **viscosity** (thickness and stickiness) of secretions from the pancreas, salivary glands, liver, intestine, and lungs. In the lungs, a very thick mucus obstructs the airways and causes repeated infections. Many CF patients require frequent hospitalizations and experience early death.

Infant respiratory distress syndrome (IRDS) is seen in premature babies whose lungs have not matured enough to produce surfactant, a detergent-like substance secreted in the lungs to decrease surface tension of alveoli. The alveoli passively collapse during expiration, and mechanical ventilation is needed to keep them open.

Lung abscess can be a complication of bacterial pneumonia or cancer. Long-term antibiotics are used, and partial or full surgical excision of the abscess may be necessary.

Lung cancer is primarily caused by smoking and is the third most common cancer type in the United States. A major portion of lung cancers arise in the mucous membranes of the larger bronchi and are called **bronchogenic carcinomas.** A subgroup of bronchogenic carcinomas called adenocarcinoma accounts for 30% to 50% of all lung cancers and is the most common in women. The lung cancer typically obstructs the airways and can spread into the surrounding lung tissues, metastisizing to the lymph nodes, liver, brain, and bone.

Pleurisy, an inflammation of the pleurae, can be a complication of pneumonia. This condition makes breathing painful because the outer parietal pleura is very pain-sensitive. The inflammation often leads to fluid accumulating in the pleural cavity. This is a **pleural effusion.** If the pleural effusion contains pus, the condition is called **empyema.** If it contains blood, the condition is called **hemothorax.**

Pneumonia *(Figure 8.13)* is an acute infection of the alveoli and lung parenchyma (functional gas exchange unit of the lung). Pneumonia is mostly caused by bacteria or viruses. The alveoli become filled with inflammatory fluid, decreasing the exchange of oxygen and carbon dioxide. **Lobar pneumonia** is an infection limited to one lung lobe. **Bronchopneumonia** is an infection in the bronchi that spreads to the alveoli.

When a segment or lobe of the lung becomes airless as a result of the infection, the lung is considered to be **consolidated.** When an area of the lung collapses as a result of bronchial obstruction, this is called **atelectasis.**

Pneumothorax is the entry of air into the pleural cavity *(Figure 8.14)*. The cause can be unknown, called a **spontaneous pneumothorax,** but it often results from trauma when a fractured rib, sharp object or bullet lacerates the pleura. A **tension pneumothorax** describes progressive build up of air and pressure within the pleural space, usually as a result of non-penetrating chest wall injury such as when lung tissue is ruptured or punctured from within.

Pulmonary edema describes the collection of fluid in the lung tissues and alveoli. It commonly results from left ventricular dysfunction or mitral valve disease progressing to congestive heart failure **(CHF).**

Pulmonary emphysema is a type of obstructive lung disease primarily affecting the alveoli. The septa between the alveoli and other surrounding interstitial tissue are destroyed, forming large sacs of trapped air **(bullae).** There is a loss of surface area for gas exchange.

Pulmonary tuberculosis is a highly contagious, infectious disease of the lungs that requires prolonged treatment and results in chronic latent infection.

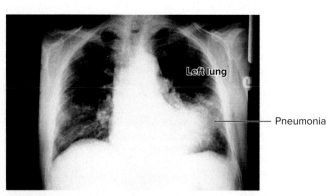

▲ **FIGURE 8.13**   Chest X-ray of Patient with Pneumonia in the Lower Lobe of the Left Lung.

Anthony Ricci/Shutterstock

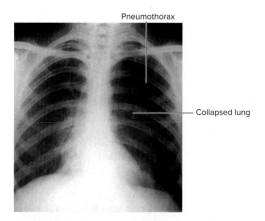

▲ **FIGURE 8.14**   Left Pneumothorax. There are no lung markings seen in the area of the pneumothorax.

Zephyr/Science Source

WORD	PRONUNCIATION		ELEMENTS	DEFINITION
abscess	**AB**-sess		Latin *a going away*	A collection of pus
adenocarcinoma	**ADD**-eh-noh-kar-sih-**NOH**-mah	S/ R/CF R/	-oma *tumor* aden/o- *gland* -carcin- *cancer*	A cancer arising from glandular epithelial cells
anthracosis	an-thra-**KOH**-sis	S/ R/	-osis *condition* anthrac- *coal*	Lung disease caused by the inhalation of coal dust
anthrax	**AN**-thraks		Greek *carbuncle*	A severe, malignant infectious disease
asbestosis	as-bes-**TOE**-sis	S/ R/	-osis *condition* asbest- *asbestos*	Lung disease caused by the inhalation of asbestos particles
atelectasis	at-el-**ECK**-tah-sis	S/ R/	-ectasis *dilation* atel- *incomplete*	Collapse of part of a lung
bronchogenic	**BRONG**-koh-**JEN**-ik	S/ R/CF	-genic *creation* bronch/o- *bronchus*	Arising from a bronchus
bronchopneumonia	**BRONG**-koh-new-**MOH**-nee-ah	S/ R/CF R/	-ia *condition* bronch/o- *bronchus* -pneumon- *air, lung*	Acute inflammation of the walls of smaller airways with spread to lung parenchyma
consolidate (v) consolidated (adj) consolidation	kon-**SOL**-i-date kon-**SOL**-i-day-tid kon-**SOL**-i-day-shun	 S/ S/	Latin *to make solid* -ed *pertaining to* -ion *process*	Making firm or solid An aerated tissue that has become firm or solid Area of solid tissue that was once aerated
effusion	eh-**FYU**-shun		Latin *pouring out*	Collection of fluid that has escaped from blood vessels into a cavity or tissues
empyema	**EM**-pie-**EE**-mah	S/ P/ R/	-ema *quality of, quantity of* em- *in, into* -py- *pus*	Pus in a body cavity, particularly in the pleural cavity
fibrosis	fie-**BROH**-sis	S/ R/CF	-sis *condition* fibr/o- *fiber*	Repair of dead tissue cells by formation of fibrous tissue
hemothorax	he-moh-**THOR**-ax	R/CF R/	hem/o- *blood* -thorax *chest*	Blood in the pleural cavity
mesothelioma	**MEEZ**-oh-thee-lee-**OH**-mah	S/ P/ R/CF	-oma *tumor, mass* meso- *middle* -thel/i -*lining*	Cancer arising from the cells lining the pleura or peritoneum
pleurisy	**PLUR**-ih-see	S/ R/	-isy *inflammation* pleur- *pleura*	Inflammation of the pleura
pneumoconiosis pneumoconioses (pl)	new-moh-koh-nee-**OH**-sis new-moh-koh-nee-**OH**-seez	S/ R/CF R/	-osis *condition* pneum/o- *lung, air* -coni- *dust*	Fibrotic lung disease caused by the inhalation of different dusts
pneumonia pneumonitis (*same as* pneumonia)	new-**MOH**-nee-ah new-moh-**NI**-tis	S/ R/ S/	-ia *condition* pneumon- *lung, air* -itis *inflammation*	Inflammation of the lung parenchyma (tissue)
pneumothorax	new-moh-**THOR**-ax	R/CF R/	pneum/o- *air, lung* -thorax *chest*	Air in the pleural cavity
sarcoidosis (**Note:** *Two suffixes*)	sar-koy-**DOH**-sis	S/ S/ R/	-osis *condition* -oid- *resembling* sarc- *flesh*	Granulomatous lesions of the lungs and other organs; cause is unknown
silicosis	sil-ih-**KOH**-sis	S/ R/	-osis *condition* silic- *silicon, glass*	Fibrotic lung disease from inhaling silica particles
tuberculosis	too-**BER**-kyu-**LOW**-sis	S/ R/	-osis *condition* tubercul- *nodule, swelling, tuberculosis*	Infectious disease that can infect any organ or tissue

EXERCISES

Case Report 8.2

You are

. . . a sleep technologist in the Sleep Disorders Clinic at Fulwood Medical Center. You are about to position the electrodes on your patient for an overnight **polysomnography** (sleep study).

You are communicating with

. . . Mr. Tye Gawlinski, a 29-year-old professional football player, and his wife. Mrs. Helen Gawlinski states that her husband snores loudly and has 40 or 50 periods in the night when he stops breathing. The snoring is so loud that she cannot sleep, even in the adjoining bedroom. Mr. Gawlinski complains of being tired all day and not having the energy he needs for his job. The sleep study is being performed to confirm a diagnosis of obstructive sleep **apnea**.

Initially, Mr. Gawlinski was instructed to sleep on his side and to use a device that, through a mask over his nose and mouth, produces a continuous positive airway pressure **(CPAP)** in his airways. He found this very uncomfortable, and it kept him awake. Instead, he chose to have the pillar procedure, in which three tiny pillars were placed in the back of his throat to support the tissues. Subsequently, Mr. Gawlinski has stopped snoring and Mrs. Gawlinski is back in the same bed.

A. After reading Case Report 8.2, *answer the following questions.*   **LO 8.7 and 8.9**

1. What are Mr. Gawlinski's symptoms? (choose all that apply)

   a. daytime sleepiness

   b. sore throat

   c. lack of energy

   d. runny nose

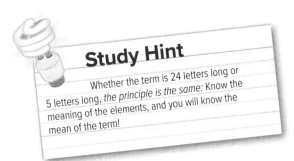

Study Hint

Whether the term is 24 letters long or 5 letters long, *the principle is the same:* Know the meaning of the elements, and you will know the mean of the term!

2. Mr. Gawlinski underwent the diagnostic procedure of:

   a. tonsillectomy

   b. endoscopy

   c. polysomnography

   d. sonogram

3. The first therapy Mr. Gawlinski used to treat his sleep apnea was:

   a. PFTs   **b.** CPAP   **c.** tonsillectomy   **d.** hypoxemia

4. Why is polysomnography done overnight?

   a. The test requires at least 8 hours of monitoring.

   b. The technicians are only hired for the night shift.

   c. Sleep apnea only occurs in the nighttime hours.

   d. The test requires monitoring of a typical night's sleep.

B. Use the medical terms *relating to the pharynx and its disorders.*   **LO 8.2 and 8.6**

1. Inflammation of the tonsils: _____ .

2. Low oxygen level in the arterial blood: _____ .

3. The medical term for a common sore throat: _____ .

4. Absence of spontaneous respiration: _____ .

5. Condition in which the body is deficient in oxygen: _____ .

C. Deconstruction: *For long or short medical terms, deconstruction into word elements is your key to solving the meaning of the term. Follow the directions and fill in the blanks.* **LO 8.1**

1. *laryngotracheobronchitis* _____ / _____ / _____ / _____

2. *epiglottitis* _____ / _____ / _____ / _____

3. *papilloma* _____ / _____ / _____ / _____

D. Apply *the language of pulmonology to answer the following questions correctly.* **LO 8.2, 8.4, and 8.6**

1. What is another term meaning *croup?* _____

2. What disorder directly affects the ability to phonate? _____

3. What is the squeaky noise on *inspiration* termed? _____

4. What is the medical term for a benign tumor of the *larynx?* _____

5. Which term means *low level of oxygen in arterial blood?* _____

E. Translate everyday language *to medical terms. Use the provided terms below to complete each sentence. Not all terms will be used. Fill in the blanks.* **LO 8.2, 8.4, 8.5, 8.6, and 8.10**

cyanotic	receiving	cyanosis	expectorate	hemoptysis	phlegm

Mrs. Algohim has arrived to the Emergency Department. Her skin appears **(1)** _____ (blue in color). She is immediately brought back to a bed. After oxygen via nasal prongs, she states that she is unable to inhale deeply. She is able to **(2)** _____ (cough up) large amounts of thick green **(3)** _____ (mucus coughed up from the respiratory tract). She denies **(4)** _____ (bloody sputum).

F. Construct terms: *Knowing just one element will enable you to build more terms with the addition of other elements. Practice building your pulmonology terms with the following root and various prefixes. Fill in the blanks.* **LO 8.1, 8.2, and 8.6**

1. The root *pnea* means _____.

Add the following prefixes to the root pnea *to form the new terms.*

tachy	brady	dys	eu	hyper

2. difficult breathing _____ / pnea

3. deeper breathing than normal _____ / pnea

4. slow breathing _____ / pnea

5. normal breathing _____ / pnea

6. rapid breathing _____ / pnea

G. Apply *the language of pulmonology to answer the following questions correctly.* **LO 8.2, 8.6, and 8.10**

1. A sticky fluid that is resistant to flow is said to be: _____

2. More than one bubble-like dilated structure: _____

3. *Hypercapnia* is excessive: _____.

4. *Hypoxia* is deficient: _____.

H. Suffixes: *Confirm your knowledge of suffixes by filling in the chart with the correct meaning for the element.* **LO 8.1, 8.2, and 8.6**

Term	Suffix	Meaning of the Suffix
pneumonitis	1.	2.
tuberculosis	3.	4.
bronchogenic	5.	6.
atelectasis	7.	8.

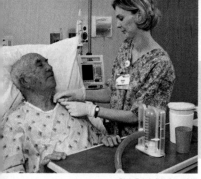

Rick Brady/McGraw-Hill

Section 8.5

Diagnostic and Therapeutic Procedures and Pharmacology

Diagnostic Procedures (LO 8.4, 8.5, and 8.7)

Specific diagnostic and therapeutic procedures, as well as a wide range of pharmacologic agents, are available to help patients with lung diseases.

Pulmonary Function Tests (PFTs) (LO 8.4, 8.5, and 8.7)

Many of the diagnostic and therapeutic procedures used in the diagnosis and treatment of respiratory disorders are performed by registered respiratory therapists (RRTs) or respiratory care practitioners under the orders of **pulmonologists** and physicians of other specialties. Pulmonary function can be measured by the following PFTs to estimate the quality of a patient's respiratory function. A **spirometer** is a device for measuring the volume of air that patients move in and out of their respiratory system. The total volume of air expired during spirometry is the patient's **forced expiratory vital capacity (FVC).** The spirometer also measures **flow rates.** For example, the **forced expiratory volume in 1 second (FEV1)** is the amount of air expired the first second of the expiratory maneuver during spirometry.

A **peak flow meter** records the greatest flow of air that can be sustained for 10 milliseconds on forced expiration, the **peak expiratory flow rate (PEFR)** which is the maximum flow rate of air that can be forcefully expired during a single blast. This test is valuable in following the course of asthma, in monitoring respiratory muscle strength, and in postoperative care to monitor the return of lung function after anesthesia.

Arterial blood gases (ABGs), the measurement of oxygen and carbon dioxide levels in the blood, are good indicators of respiratory function.

Polysomnography, also known as a sleep study, measures blood oxygen levels, heart rate and rhythm, and respiratory effort while a person sleeps to diagnose sleep disorders such as obstructive sleep apnea (OSA).

A **pulse oximeter** is a sensor placed on the finger to measure the oxygen saturation of the blood.

Auscultation (LO 8.4, 8.5, and 8.7)

The stethoscope is used to detect normal and abnormal breath sounds. Abnormal breath sounds are categorized as:

- **Wheezes (rhonchi):** musical quality; associated with bronchoconstriction found with asthma. Wheezes are characteristic of asthma.

- **Crackles** (formally known as **rales**): nonmusical, explosive sounds; attributed to the popping opening of the airways with or without the movement of air through secretions in larger airways or due to fluid in the alveoli. Crackles can be auscultated with pneumonia, pulmonary edema, and atelectasis.

- **Pleural rub:** nonmusical sound, often described as a grating or creaking sound. It is caused by the inflamed visceral and parietal pleurae rubbing together, which can occur with pleurisy.

- **Stridor:** loud, high-pitched sound with a musical quality. Associated with constriction of the airways of the upper respiratory tract such as with croup or inflamed epiglottis.

Other Diagnostic Procedures (LO 8.4, 8.5, and 8.7)

Chest X-ray (CXR) is a radiographic image of the chest taken in **anteroposterior (AP), posteroanterior (PA),** lateral, and sometimes oblique and lateral decubitus positions.

Computed tomography (CT), used for visualizing the blood vessels of the pulmonary circulation using contrast materials, **magnetic resonance angiography (MRA)** to define emboli in the pulmonary arteries, and **ultrasonography** of the pleural space, using sound waves to visualize underlying structures, are chest-imaging techniques in modern use. **Positron emission tomography (PET)** can allow the differentiation between benign and malignant lesions through the use of radioactive material.

Abbreviations

ABG	arterial blood gas
AP	anteroposterior
CT	computed tomography
CXR	chest X-ray
FEV1	forced expiratory volume in 1 second
FVC	forced vital capacity
MRA	magnetic resonance angiography
PA	posteroanterior
PEFR	peak expiratory flow rate
PET	positron emission tomography
PFTs	pulmonary function tests
RRT	registered respiratory therapist

During **auscultation** (examination by stethoscope) of the chest, the air bubbling through abnormal fluid in the alveoli and smallest airways, as in pulmonary edema, produces a noise called **crackles,** also known as rales. When air moves past fluid or secretions in the larger airways, a noise known as **rhonchi** is produced. When the bronchi are partly obstructed and air is being forced past the obstruction, a high-pitched noise known as a **wheeze** is heard.

Word Analysis and Definition

S = Suffix   P = Prefix   R = Root   R/CF = Combining Form

WORD	PRONUNCIATION		ELEMENTS	DEFINITION
auscultation	aws-kul-**TAY**-shun	S/ R/	-ation *a process* auscult- *listen to*	Diagnostic method of listening to body sounds with a stethoscope
crackle rale (syn) rales (pl)	**KRAK**-el RAHL RAHLS		*To crack* French *rattle*	Explosive popping sound due to the sudden opening of small airways or air moving through secretions
pleural rub	**PLOOR**-al RUB	S/ R/	-al *pertaining to* pleur- *pleura* rub East Frisian *to rub, scrape*	Grating sound due to pleural membranes rubbing against each other
pulmonary (adj) pulmonology pulmonologist	**PULL**-moh-**NAIR**-ee **PULL**-moh-**NOL**-oh-jee **PULL**-moh-**NOL**-oh-jist	S/ R/ S/ R/CF S/	-ary *pertaining to* pulmon- *lung* -logy *study of* pulmon/o- *lung* -logist *one who studies, specialist*	Pertaining to the lungs and their blood supply Study of the lungs, or the medical speciality of disorders of the respiratory tract Medical specialist in pulmonary disorders
rhonchus rhonchi (pl) *wheeze* (syn)	**RONG**-kuss **RONG**-key		Greek *snoring*	Wheezing sound heard on auscultation of the lungs, made by air passing through a constricted lumen
spirometer	spy-**ROM**-eh-ter	R/CF R/	spir/o- *to breathe* -meter *measure*	An instrument used to measure respiratory volumes
stridor	**STRIE**-door		Latin *a harsh, creaking sound*	High-pitched noise made when there is respiratory obstruction in the larynx or trachea
wheeze wheezes (pl)	WEEZ		Old English *action of blowing*	Musical sound of the airways associated with asthma

WORD	PRONUNCIATION	ELEMENTS		DEFINITION
aspiration	as-pih-**RAY**-shun	S/ R/	-ion *process* aspirat- *to breathe on*	Removal by suction of fluid or gas from a body cavity
bronchoscopy	brong-**KOS**-koh-pee	S/ R/CF	-scopy *to examine, view* bronch/o- *bronchus*	Examination of the interior of the tracheobronchial tree with an endoscope
bronchoscope	**BRONG**-koh-skope	S/	-scope *instrument for viewing*	Endoscope used for bronchoscopy
endotracheal	en-doh-**TRAY**-kee-al	S/ P/ R/	-al *pertaining to* endo- *inside* -trache- *trachea*	Pertaining to being inside the trachea
laryngoscope	lah-**RING**-oh-skope	S/ R/CF	-scope *instrument for viewing* laryng/o- *larynx*	Hollow tube with a light and camera used to visualize or operate on the larynx
mediastinoscopy	**ME**-dee-ass-tih-**NOS**-koh-pee	S/ R/CF	-scopy *to examine, view* mediastin/o- *mediastinum*	Examination of the mediastinum using an endoscope
percutaneous	**PER**-kyu-**TAY**-nee-us	S/ P/ R/CF	-ous *pertaining to* per- *through* -cutane- *skin*	Passage through the skin, in this case, by needle puncture
polysomnography	**POLL**-ee-som-**NOG**-rah-fee	S/ P/ R/CF	-graphy *process of recording* poly- *many* -somn/o- *sleep*	Test to monitor brain waves, muscle tension, eye movement, and oxygen levels in the blood as the patient sleeps
spirometer	spy-**ROM**-eh-ter	S/ R/CF	-meter *measure* spir/o- *to breathe*	An instrument used to measure respiratory volumes
spirometry	spy-**ROM**-eh-tree	S/	-metry *process of measuring*	Use of a spirometer
thoracentesis (*same as* pleural tap)	**THOR**-ah-sen-**TEE**-sis	S/ R/	-centesis *to puncture* thora- *chest*	Insertion of a needle into the pleural cavity to withdraw fluid or air
thoracotomy	thor-ah-**KOT**-oh-me	S/ R/CF	-tomy *surgical incision* thorac/o- *chest*	Incision through the chest wall
tomography	toe-**MOG**-rah-fee	S/ R/CF	-graphy *process of recording* tom/o- *cut, slice, layer*	Radiographic image of a selected slice of tissue
transthoracic	tranz-thor-**ASS**-ik	S/ P/ R/	-ic *pertaining to* trans- *across* -thorac- *chest*	Going through the chest wall
ultrasonography	**UL**-trah-soh-**NOG**-rah-fee	S/ P/ R/CF	-graphy *process of recording* ultra- *beyond* -son/o- *sound*	Delineation of deep structures using sound waves

Tracheal aspiration uses a semi-rigid catheter that allows irrigation and suctioning to be performed to remove cells and secretions from the trachea and main bronchi. The catheter can be passed through a tracheostomy or **endotracheal** (windpipe) tube, or through the mouth and nose.

Percutaneous transthoracic needle aspiration is the insertion of a needle with a cutting chamber through an intercostal space (between the ribs) to take a specimen of parietal pleura for examination.

Thoracotomy is used to obtain an open biopsy of tissue from the lung, hilum, pleura, or mediastinum. It is performed through an intercostal incision under local or general anesthesia.

Bronchoscopy is a procedure where a fiber optic tube is inserted into the bronchial tubes to visually examine the tubes, take a tissue biopsy, or do a washing for secretions.

Mediastinoscopy is used to stage lung cancer and diagnose mediastinal masses. The mediastinoscope is inserted through an incision in the suprasternal notch.

Thoracentesis is the insertion of a needle through an intercostal space to remove fluid from a pleural effusion for laboratory study or to relieve pressure. The procedure is also called a pleural tap.

Therapeutic Procedures (LO 8.6 and 8.7)

Many effective therapeutic procedures are available for successfully treating pulmonary function disorders. These procedures are outlined below.

Most nose bleeds can be treated at home by pinching the soft part of the nose for 15 to 20 minutes. If this fails, medical treatment can consist of **cauterization,** or nasal packing with gauze strips.

Pulmonary rehabilitation includes education, breathing exercises and retraining, exercises for the upper and lower extremities, and psychosocial support.

Nutritional support is critical for patients who have difficulty breathing, or who need to lose or have lost a lot of weight.

Immunizations are available against influenza, COVID-19 and pneumococcal bacteria—one of the most common causes of bacterial pneumonia.

Postural drainage therapy (PDT) uses gravity (by positioning and tilting the patient) to promote the drainage of secretions from lung segments. Chest percussion (tapping) on the chest wall can help loosen, mobilize, and drain any retained secretions. These two procedures are part of chest physiotherapy (CPT).

Continuous positive airway pressure (CPAP) and **Bi-level positive airway pressure (BiPAP)** apply pressure to airways through a nasal or oral mask or nose piece. CPAP provides the one pressure during inhalation and exhalation; BiPAP provides different pressures during inhalation and exhalation.

CPAP and BiPAP are used at home for obstructive sleep apnea (OSA).

Noninvasive ventilation is the application of CPAP or BiPAP to avoid invasive mechanical ventilation in acute respiratory failure or COPD exacerbation. This application is performed by a health care professional. A mask is fitted over the patient's nose and mouth and attached to a **ventilator**.

Positive end expiratory pressure (PEEP) is a ventilation technique to keep the alveoli from collapsing in patients who are experiencing respiratory failure and being mechanically ventilated by a respirator.

An **oropharyngeal airway** is used to stabilize the tongue and maintain an open airway in the unconscious patient during bag and mask ventilation. A tube is inserted to prevent the tongue from falling back and obstructing the airway and to facilitate suctioning the airway. An **endotracheal intubation** involves the placement of a flexible tube into the trachea. This bypasses the upper airway and allows the patient to be placed on a ventilator so breathing can be controlled.

Mechanical ventilation is a process of breathing through a **ventilator (respirator)** in which gases are directed under pressure into the respiratory tract to support the movement of oxygen in and carbon dioxide out. An apparatus such as a mask, endotracheal tube, or tracheostomy must be employed to allow patient connection to the ventilator. In order to place an oral endotracheal tube, a **laryngoscope** is used to visualize various upper airway structures. Mechanical ventilation can augment or replace the patient's own ventilatory efforts.

Pulmonary resection is the surgical removal of lung tissue.

- **Wedge resection** is the removal of a small, localized area of diseased lung.

- **Segmental resection** is the removal of a segment of lung tissue.

- **Lobectomy** is the removal of a lobe of the lung.

- **Pneumonectomy** is the removal of an entire lung.

- **Tonsillectomy** is used to treat OSA when the tonsils are large and block the airway. It is also performed to treat recurrent tonsillitis.

Tracheotomy is an incision made into the trachea (windpipe) to create a temporary or permanent opening into the windpipe, called a **tracheostomy** *(Figure 8.15)*. A rigid plastic or stainless steel tube is placed into the opening to provide an airway. A tracheostomy is used to maintain an airway when the upper airway is compromised, usually causing a life-threatening obstruction.

Pulmonary Pharmacology (LO 8.7)

- **Bronchodilators** relax the smooth muscles of the bronchioles. Examples are theophylline, beta2-agonists such as albuterol and vilanterol and anticholinergics such as ipratropium bromide.

- **Anti-inflammatory** drugs, such as corticosteroids, are best given by inhalation, but can be used orally or intravenously in acute episodes of asthma or COPD.

- **Mucolytics** are agents that attempt to break up mucus so it can be cleared more effectively from the airways. Examples are guaifenesin (common in over-the-counter cough medications) and N-acetylcysteine taken via **nebulizer**.

- **Antibiotics** are used when a bacterial infection is present. Penicillin, erythromycin, cefotaxime, and amoxicillin are frequently used.

- **Decongestants** decrease the swelling of tissue in the nasal cavity and sinuses. They are frequently used to treat sinusitis.

- **Oxygen** is used in hypoxemia and can be given by nasal **cannula** or mask or through an artificial airway such as with tracheostomy or intubation. Patients with severe, chronic COPD are sometimes attached to a portable oxygen cylinder.

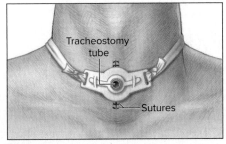

① Tracheotomy incision is made superior to the sternal notch.

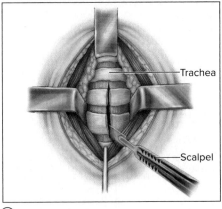

② Retractors separate the tissue, and an incision is made through the third and fourth tracheal rings.

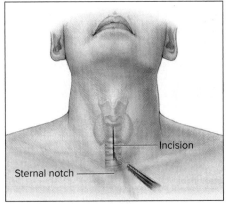

③ A tracheostomy tube is inserted, and the remaining incision is sutured closed.

▲ **FIGURE 8.15** Tracheostomy Procedure.

Word Analysis and Definition

S = Suffix   P = Prefix   R = Root   R/CF = Combining Form

WORD	PRONUNCIATION	ELEMENTS		DEFINITION
bronchodilator	**BRONG**-koh-die-**LAY**-tor	S/ R/CF R/	**-or** *one who does, that which does something* **bronch/o-** *bronchus* **-dilat-** *expand, open up*	Agent that increases the diameter of a bronchus
cannula	**KAN**-you-lah		Latin *reed*	Tube inserted into a blood vessel or cavity as a channel for fluid or gas
cautery cauterize cauterization	**KAW**-ter-ee **KAW**-ter-ize **KAW**-ter-eye-**ZAY**-shun	 S/ R/ S/	Greek *branding iron* **-ize** *action* **cauter-** *to burn* **-ation** *a process*	A device to scar, burn, or cut a tissue To apply a cautery The act of cauterizing
decongestant	dee-con-**JESS**-tant	S/ P/ R/	**-ant** *pertaining to* **de-** *take away, remove* **-congest-** *accumulation of fluid*	Agent that reduces the swelling and fluid in the nose and sinuses
immunization	im-you-nih-**ZAY**-shun	S/ R/	**-ation** *process* **immuniz-** *make immune*	Administration of an agent to provide immunity
intubation	**IN**-tyu-**BAY**-shun	S/ P/ R/	**-ation** *a process* **in-** *in* **-tub-** *tube*	Insertion of a tube into the trachea
lobectomy	low-**BECK**-toe-me	S/ R/	**-ectomy** *surgical excision* **lob-** *lobe*	Surgical removal of a lobe
mucolytic	**MYU**-koh-**LIT**-ik	S/ R/CF R/	**-ic** *pertaining to* **muc/o-** *mucus* **-lyt-** *dissolve*	Agent capable of dissolving or liquefying mucus
nebulizer	**NEB**-you-liz-er	S/ R/	**-izer** *line of action, affects in a particular way* **nebul-** *cloud*	Device used to deliver liquid medicine in a fine mist
pneumonectomy	**NEW**-moh-**NECK**-toe-me	S/ R/	**-ectomy** *surgical excision* **pneumon-** *lung, air*	Surgical removal of a lung
resection resect (verb)	ree-**SEK**-shun ree-**SEKT**	S/ P/ R/	**-ion** *action, condition* **re-** *back* **-sect-** *cut off*	Removal of a specific part of an organ or structure
respirator	**RES**-pih-**RAY**-tor	S/ P/ R/	**-ator** *person or thing that does something* **re-** *again* **-spir-** *to breathe*	Another name for mechanical ventilator
tracheostomy tracheotomy	tray-kee-**OST**-oh-me tray-kee-**OT**-oh-me	S/ R/CF S/	**-stomy** *new opening* **trache/o-** *trachea* **-tomy** *surgical incision*	Insertion of a tube into the windpipe to assist breathing Incision made into the trachea to create a tracheostomy
tonsillectomy (Note: double *"ll"*)	ton-sih-**LEK**-toh-me	S/ R/CF	**-ectomy** *surgical excision* **tonsil-** *tonsil*	Surgical removal of the tonsils
ventilation ventilator	ven-tih-**LAY**-shun **VEN**-tih-lay-tor	S/ R/ S/	**-ation** *a process* **ventil-** *wind* **-ator** *person or thing that does something*	Movement of gases into and out of the lungs Device that breathes for the patient

EXERCISES

A. Identify the meaning *of the word elements of pulmonary diagnostic terms. Select the correct answer.*   **LO 8.1, 8.2, and 8.7**

1. The root in the term spirometer means:

   a. surgical incision   **b.** to breathe   **c.** chest   **d.** measure

2. The root in the term ultrasonography means:

   a. beyond   **b.** cut, slice, layer   **c.** sound   **d.** process of recording

3. The suffix in the term bronchoscopy means:

   a. to view   **b.** across   **c.** instrument for viewing   **d.** lung

4. The prefix in the term transthoracic means:

   a. through   **b.** across   **c.** chest   **d.** pertaining to

5. The prefix in the term endoscope means:

   a. process of recording   **b.** to view   **c.** inside   **d.** surgical incision

B. Provide the abbreviation *that each statement is describing. Fill in the blanks.* **LO 8.3 and 8.7**

1. X-ray of the chest: _____

2. A group of diagnostic tests that measures flow rates, the amount of air brought into and out of the lungs: _____

3. An X-ray that passes first through the front of the chest: _____

4. A diagnostic test that provides high-resolution images of blood vessels. This test does not use radiation to create the image: _____

C. Deconstruct: *Define the elements related to therapeutic procedures used to treat pulmonary disorders. Fill in the blanks.* **LO 8.1, 8.6, and 8.7**

Medical Term	Meaning of Root/CF	Meaning of Suffix
immunization	1.	2.
nebulizer	3.	4.
tracheostomy	5.	6.
tracheotomy	7.	8.
decongestant	9.	10.

D. Meet section and chapter objectives *by applying the language of pulmonology to answer the following questions correctly.* **LO 8.2, 8.6, and 8.9**

1. A person who has trouble expectorating thick mucus may benefit from this type of drug: _____

2. A device that breathes for the patient: _____

3. The removal of a small piece of the lung is termed a _____ resection.

4. An airway that is placed in the mouth and pharynx is termed an _____ airway.

E. Identify the medical term used to describe each of the following: **LO 8.2, 8.6, and 8.7**

1. A patient that has developed allergic rhinitis describes a "stuffy nose." You should suspect they may benefit from treatment with a _____ medication.

2. A patient who presents with massive, uncontrollable epistaxis may benefit from having a procedure known as _____ to prevent further bleeding.

F. Elements. *The elements below all appear in the language of pulmonology. Match the word element in the first column with its correct meaning in the second column.* **LO 8.1, 8.2, 8.6, and 8.7**

   _____ **1.** ectasis   **a.** listen to

   _____ **2.** capn   **b.** sticky

   _____ **3.** physema   **c.** carbon dioxide

   _____ **4.** viscos   **d.** blowing

   _____ **5.** auscult   **e.** small

   _____ **6.** ole   **f.** dilation

G. Identify the proper pronunciation of the following medical terms. Correctly spell the term. **LO 8.1, 8.2, and 8.6**

1. The correct pronunciation for the inflammation of the pleura:

   a. PLUR-ih-see

   b. PLOOR-it-is

   c. KOR-ee-zah

   d. koh-RYE-zah

   Correctly spell the term: _____

2. The correct pronunciation for the region of the pharynx below the epiglottis that includes the larynx:

   a. LAIR-ink-oh-FAIR-inks

   b. RIN-go-FAH-rinks

   c. NAY-zoh-FAIR-inks

   d. NOH-zoh-FAIR-inks

   Correctly spell the term: _____

3. The correct pronunciation for the process of breathing out:

   a. IN-spy-eh-RAY-shun

   b. in-spih-RAY-shun

   c. EKS-pie-er-AY-shun

   d. EKS-pih-RAY-shun

   Correctly spell the term: _____

4. The correct pronunciation for the explosive popping sound due to the sudden opening of small airways, alveoli, or air moving through secretions:

   a. RAILS

   b. RAHLS

   c. RONG-key

   d. RONG-kih

   Correctly spell the term: _____

5. The correct pronunciation for the agent that is capable of dissolving or liquefying mucus:

   a. MYU-koh-LIT-ik

   b. MYU-cool-IT-ik

   c. AG-on-ist

   d. AYG-on-ist

   Correctly spell the term: _____

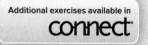
Additional exercises available in connect

Chapter Review exercises, along with additional practice items, are available in Connect!

The Digestive System

The Essentials of the Language of Gastroenterology

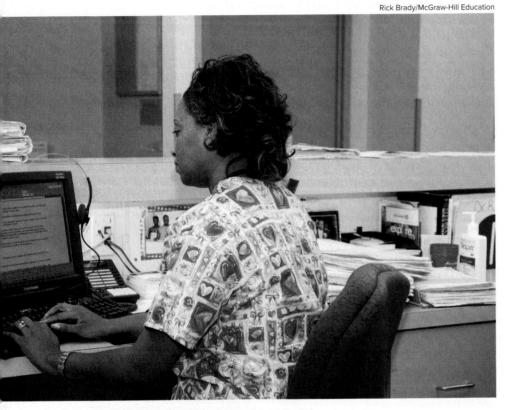

CHAPTER 9

Rick Brady/McGraw-Hill Education

In your future career, being able to communicate comfortably, accurately, and effectively with the health professionals involved in the diagnosis and treatment of problems in the **gastroenterological** system is key. You may work directly and/or indirectly with one or more of the following:

- **Gastroenterologists** are medical specialists in the field of gastroenterology.
- **Proctologists** are surgical specialists in diseases of the anus and rectum.
- **Dentists** are practitioners specially trained to diagnose and treat conditions that affect oral health.
- **Periodontists** are specialists in disorders of the tissues surrounding the teeth.
- **Nutritionists** are professionals who prevent and treat illness by promoting healthy eating habits.
- **Dietitians** are professionals who manage food services systems and promote sound eating habits.

Learning Outcomes

It may be a necessary part of your job to accurately transcribe the voice-recorded reports of physicians and any other health care professionals into readable text. To ensure that your patients receive the best possible care, you and the health care professionals directly and indirectly involved with patient care need to be able to:

LO 9.1 Use roots, combining forms, suffixes, and prefixes to construct and analyze medical terms related to the digestive system.

LO 9.2 Spell and pronounce correctly medical terms related to the digestive system to communicate them with accuracy and precision in any health care setting.

LO 9.3 Define accepted abbreviations related to the digestive system.

LO 9.4 Relate the overall anatomy of the alimentary canal to the actions and functions of digestion.

LO 9.5 Explain the anatomy and roles of the mouth, pharynx, stomach, small intestine, and large intestine in digestion.

LO 9.6 Explain the anatomy and roles of the liver, gallbladder, and pancreas in digestion.

LO 9.7 Describe diseases and disorders related to the digestive system.

LO 9.8 Describe the diagnostic procedures used for diseases and disorders of the digestive system.

LO 9.9 Describe the therapeutic procedures and pharmacologic agents used for disorders of the digestive system.

LO 9.10 Identify health care professionals involved in the care of patients with digestive diseases and disorders.

LO 9.11 Apply your knowledge of the medical terms of the digestive system to documentation, medical records, and medical reports.

LO 9.12 Translate the medical terms of the digestive system into everyday language to communicate clearly with patients and their families.

Section 9.1

The Digestive System

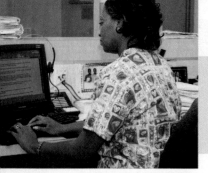

Rick Brady/McGraw-Hill Education

Keynote

- Water added in along the alimentary canal liquefies the food to make it easier to digest and absorb.

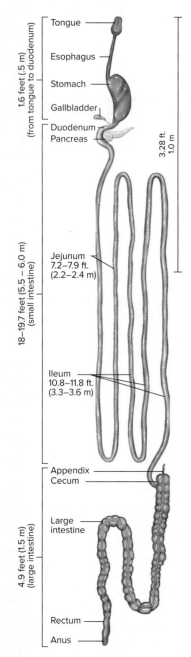

▲ **FIGURE 9.1**
Alimentary Canal.

Alimentary Canal and Accessory Organs (LO 9.4)

Every cell in your body requires a constant supply of nourishment in a form that can be absorbed across its cell membrane. The **digestive system** breaks down food into elements that can be transported to the cells via the blood and lymphatics.

The digestive system consists of the **alimentary canal,** or digestive tract, which extends from the mouth to the anus, and **accessory organs** connected to the canal to assist in digestion.

The alimentary canal *(Figure 9.1)* includes the:

- Mouth
- Stomach
- Pharynx
- Small intestine
- Esophagus
- Large intestine

The accessory organs of digestion include the:

- Teeth
- Liver
- Tongue
- Gallbladder
- Salivary glands
- Pancreas

Actions and Functions of the Digestive System (LO 9.4)

The actions and functions of your digestive system have these five components:

1. **Ingestion:** The selective intake of food into the mouth.

2. **Movement:** The mechanical movement of food from the mouth to the anus *(Figure 9.2)*. Normally, this takes 24 to 36 hours. **Deglutition** (swallowing) moves the **bolus** (mass or lump) of food from the mouth into the esophagus. **Peristalsis** (waves of contraction and relaxation) moves food material through most of the alimentary canal.

3. **Digestion:** The breakdown of foods into forms that can be transported to cells and absorbed into these cells. This process has two parts:

   a. **Mechanical digestion** breaks larger pieces of food into smaller ones without altering their chemical composition. **Mastication** (chewing) breaks down the food into smaller particles so that digestive **enzymes** have a larger surface area with which to interact.

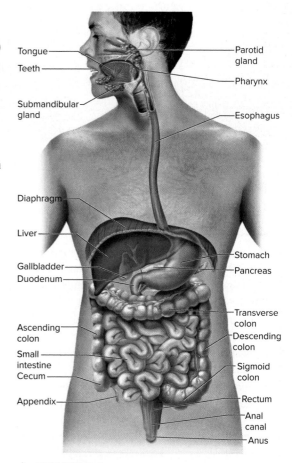

▲ **FIGURE 9.2**
The Digestive System.

b. **Chemical digestion** breaks down large molecules of food into smaller and simpler chemicals by way of digestive enzymes (made by the salivary glands, stomach, small intestine, and pancreas). The digestive enzymes have three main groups:

- **Amylases,** which digest carbohydrates
- **Lipases,** which digest fats
- **Proteases,** which digest proteins

4. **Secretion:** The addition of secretions like mucus that lubricate, liquefy, and digest food throughout the digestive tract, while also keeping the tract's lining lubricated.

5. **Absorption:** The movement of nutrient molecules out of the digestive tract, through the epithelial cells lining the tract, and into the blood or lymph for transportation to body cells.

6. **Elimination:** The process by which the body removes undigested food residue.

Word Analysis and Definition

S = Suffix   P = Prefix   R = Root   R/CF = Combining Form

WORD	PRONUNCIATION	ELEMENTS		DEFINITION
absorption	ab-**SORP**-shun	S/ R/	-ion *action, condition* absorpt- *to swallow*	Uptake of nutrients and water by cells in the GI tract
alimentary	al-ih-**MEN**-tar-ee	S/ R/	-ary *pertaining to* aliment- *nourishment, food*	Pertaining to the digestive tract
alimentary canal	kah-**NAL**		canal, Latin *a duct or channel*	Digestive tract
amylase	**AM**-ih-lase	S/ R/	-ase *enzyme* amyl- *starch*	One of a group of enzymes that breaks down starch
bolus	**BOH**-lus		Greek *lump*	A single mass of a substance
deglutition	dee-glue-**TISH**-un	S/ R/	-ion *action, condition* deglutit- *to swallow*	The act of swallowing
digestion	die-**JESS**-chun	S/ R/	-ion *action* digest- *to break down food*	Breakdown of food into elements suitable for cell metabolism
digestive (adj)	die-**JEST**-iv	S/	-ive *nature of, quality of*	Pertaining to digestion
elimination	ee-lim-ih-**NAY**-shun	S/ R/	-ation *process* elimin- *throw away*	Removal of waste material from the digestive tract
enzyme	**EN**-zime	P/ R/	en- *in* -zyme *fermenting*	Protein that induces changes in other substances
gastric (adj)	**GAS**-trik	S/ R/	-ic *pertaining to* gastr- *stomach*	Pertaining to the stomach
gastroenterology	**GAS**-troh-en-ter-**OL**-oh-gee	S/ R/CF R/CF	-logy *study of* gastr/o- *stomach* -enter/o- *intestine*	Medical specialty of the stomach and intestines
ingestion	in-**JEST**-shun	S/ R/	-ion *action* ingest- *carry in*	Intake of food or drink into the digestive tract
lipase	**LIE**-pase	S/ R/	-ase *enzyme* lip- *fat*	Enzyme that breaks down fat
masticate (verb)	**MAS**-tih-kate	S/ R/	-ate *pertaining to, composed of* mastic- *chew*	To chew
mastication (noun)	mas-tih-**KAY**-shun	S/	-ation *process*	The process of chewing
nutrient nutritive (adj)	**NYU**-tree-ent **NYU**-trih-tiv	 S/ R/	Latin *to nourish* -ive *nature of, pertaining to* nutrit- *nourishment*	A substance in food required for normal physiologic function Providing nourishment
nutrition	nyu-**TRISH**-un	S/	-ion- *action, condition*	The study of food and liquid requirements for normal function of the human body
nutritionist	nyu-**TRISH**-un-ist	S/	-ist *specialist in*	Certified professional in nutrition science
peristalsis	**PAIR**-ih-**STAL**-sis	P/ R/	peri- *around* -stalsis *constrict*	Waves of alternate contraction and relaxation of the intestinal wall to move food along the digestive tract
protease	**PRO**-tee-ase	S/ R/CF	-ase *enzyme* prot/e- *protein*	Group of enzymes that breaks down protein
secrete secretion (noun)	se-**KREET** se-**KREE**-shun		Latin *to separate*	To release or give off, as substances produced by cells Producton by a cell or gland

EXERCISES

A. Analyzing *the elements can help you determine the meaning of a medical term. Use the terms provided below to complete each sentence.*

Fill in the blanks.   **LO 9.1, 9.4, 9.7, 9.8, and 9.10**

gastric   gastroenterology   gastrointestinal   gastroenterologist   gastroscope

1. After completion of his training, the physician's assistant chose to work in the field of _____ .

2. After eating a large amount of fatty and sugary food, the patient experienced _____ upset.

3. Due to chronic pain in the digestive tract, the family practice physician referred the patient to a _____ .

4. The _____ is used to view the inside of the stomach.

5. The patient is complaining of intense burning pain in the stomach; you document this as _____ pain.

B. Match *the correct medical term in column 2 to the definition in column 1. The body process, or action, is described for you below. Fill in the blanks.*
LO 9.4 and 9.5

_____ 1. swallowing   **a.** mastication

_____ 2. intestinal muscle contractions   **b.** elimination

_____ 3. chewing   **c.** deglutition

_____ 4. removal of waste material   **d.** peristalsis

C. Read *the text to obtain answers to the following questions. Fill in the blanks.*   **LO 9.4 and 9.5**

1. What is the mechanical movement of food from mouth to anus called? _____

2. Which enzyme helps to break down protein? _____

3. What lubricates the food in the digestive tract? _____

4. Which enzyme breaks down fat? _____

5. Which enzyme breaks down starch? _____

6. What is the medical term used to describe the lump of food that is moved from the mouth to esophagus? _____

D. Build *the medical terms by filling in their missing elements. Fill in the blanks.*   **LO 9.1, 9.4, and 9.5**

1. The process of chewing: _____ / _____

2. Removal of waste material from the digestive tract: _____ / _____

3. The act of swallowing: _____ / _____

4. To chew: _____ / _____

5. Waves that move food in intestines: _____ / _____

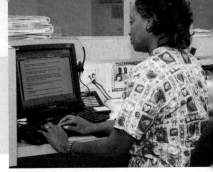

Rick Brady/McGraw-Hill Education

When you pop a piece of chicken and some vegetables into your mouth, you start a cascade of digestive tract events that will occur during the next 24 to 36 hours. In this chapter, you will follow the food as it moves through the digestive tract. The first stages in the cascade of events begins when the food is in the mouth and then swallowed.

The Mouth and Mastication (LO 9.5)

Your **mouth** (**oral** cavity)*(Figure 9.3)* is the gateway to your digestive tract. It's the first site of mechanical digestion, through **mastication** (chewing), and of chemical digestion, through an enzyme in your **saliva.**

The roof of your mouth is called the **palate,** and its anterior two-thirds is the bony hard **palate.** The posterior one-third is the muscular **soft palate.** The skeletal muscle of the soft palate has a projection or flap called the **uvula,** which partially closes off the **nasopharynx** (upper pharynx) when swallowing and produces additional saliva for lubricating the throat.

Your **tongue** moves food around your mouth and helps the cheeks, lips, and gums hold food in place while you chew it. Small, rough, raised areas on the tongue, called **papillae,** contain some 4,000 taste buds that react to the chemical nature of food to give you different taste sensations *(Figure 9.4).* A taste-bud cell lives for 7 to 10 days before it's replaced.

Adult Teeth (LO 9.5)

The average adult has 32 teeth—16 rooted in the upper jaw (maxilla) and 16 in the lower jaw (mandible) *(Figure 9.3).* The bulk of a tooth is composed of **dentin** (also spelled *dentine),* a substance like bone but harder, that is covered in **enamel.** The dentin surrounds a central **pulp** cavity, containing blood vessels, nerves, and connective tissue. The blood vessels and nerves reach this cavity from the jaw through tubular root canals. The **gingiva** is a soft pink tissue that surrounds and attaches to teeth and the jaw bones. The area around the tooth is referred to as the **periodontal** region.

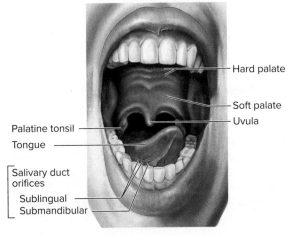

▲ **FIGURE 9.3**   Mouth.

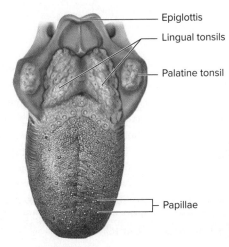

▲ **FIGURE 9.4**   Tongue.

WORD	PRONUNCIATION	ELEMENTS		DEFINITION
dentin (*also spelled* dentine)	**DEN**-tin	S/ R/	-ine *pertaining to, substance* dent- *tooth*	Dense, ivory-like substance located under the enamel in a tooth
enamel	ee-**NAM**-el		French *enamel*	Hard substance covering a tooth
gingiva gingival (adj)	**JIN**-jih-vah **JIN**-jih-val	S/ R/	Latin *gum* -al *pertaining to* gingiv- *gum*	Tissue surrounding the teeth and covering the jaw Pertaining to the gums
masticate (verb)	**MAS**-tih-kate	S/ R/	-ate *pertaining to, composed of* mastic- *chew*	To chew
mastication (noun)	mas-tih-**KAY**-shun	S/	-ation *process*	The process of chewing
mouth	MOWTH		Old English *mouth*	External opening of a cavity or canal
nasopharynx	**NAY**-zoh-**FAIR**-inks	R/CF R/	nas/o- *nose* -pharynx *throat*	Region of the pharynx at the back of the nose and above the soft palate
oral	**OR**-al	S/ R/	-al *pertaining to* or- (os) *mouth*	Pertaining to the mouth
palate	**PAL**-at		Latin *palate*	Roof of the mouth
papilla papillae (pl)	pah-**PILL**-ah pah-**PILL**-ee		Latin *small pimple*	Any small projection
parotid	pah-**ROT**-id	S/ P/ R/	-id *having a particular quality* par- *beside* -ot- *ear*	The parotid gland is the salivary gland beside the ear
periodontal	**PAIR**-ee-oh-**DON**-tal	S/ P/ R/	-al *pertaining to* peri- *around* -odont- *tooth*	Around a tooth
pulp	PULP		Latin *flesh*	Dental pulp is the connective tissue in the cavity in the center of the tooth
saliva (noun) salivary (adj)	sa-**LIE**-vah **SAL**-ih-var-ee	S/ R/	Latin *spit* -ary *pertaining to* saliv- *saliva*	Secretion in mouth from salivary glands Pertaining to saliva
sublingual	sub-**LING**-wal	S/ P/ R/	-al *pertaining to* sub- *underneath* -lingu- *tongue*	Underneath the tongue
submandibular	sub-man-**DIB**-you-lar	S/ P/ R/	-ar *pertaining to* sub- *underneath* -mandibul- *mandible*	Underneath the mandible
tongue	TUNG		Latin *tongue*	Mobile muscle mass in the mouth; bears the taste buds
uvula	**YOU**-vyu-lah		Latin *grape*	Fleshy projection of the soft palate

Salivary Glands (LO 9.5)

Salivary glands secrete saliva. The two **parotid** glands (beside the ears), the two **submandibular** glands (beneath the mandible), the two **sublingual** glands (beneath the tongue) *(Figure 9.5),* and numerous minor salivary glands scattered in the mucosa of the tongue and cheeks secrete more than a quart of saliva daily.

Saliva is 95% water, and its major functions are to begin the digestion of starch and fat and to lubricate food so it's easier to swallow. Imagine you are eating a piece of chicken and some vegetables. By mastication, the chicken has been torn and ground into small pieces by your teeth, and its fat has begun to be digested by the lipase in your saliva. The vegetables have also been ground into small pieces, and their starch has begun to be digested by the amylase in your saliva.

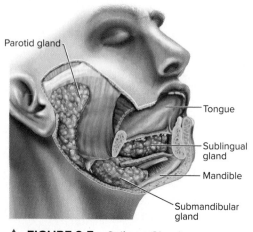

Parotid gland

Tongue

Sublingual gland

Mandible

Submandibular gland

▲ **FIGURE 9.5**   Salivary Glands.

Pharynx and Esophagus (LO 9.5)

The esophagus *(Figure 9.6)* is a tube 9 to 10 inches long. It pierces the diaphragm at the esophageal **hiatus** to go from the thoracic cavity to the abdominal cavity *(Figure 9.6)*. Under normal conditions, the esophagus remains collapsed unless filled with a food bolus.

The chicken and vegetables that you ingested earlier have now been sliced and ground into small particles by the teeth. These particles are partly digested and lubricated by saliva, and rolled into a bolus between the tongue and the hard palate—the bony roof of the mouth. The bolus is now ready to be swallowed down the oropharynx (upper part of the throat) *(Figure 9.7)* into the **esophagus.**

The bolus enters the esophagus from the lower end of the pharynx. In the esophagus, peristaltic, or wavelike, contractions of the esophageal wall muscles move it downward *(Figure 9.8)*. At the lower end of the esophagus, the lower esophageal **sphincter** (cardiac sphincter) relaxes to allow the bolus to enter the stomach.

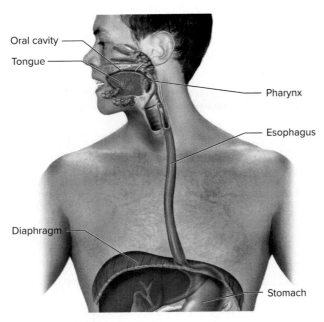

▲ FIGURE 9.6
Esophagus.

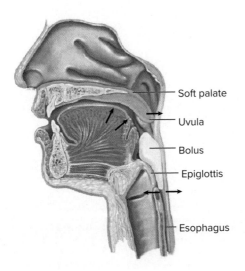

▲ FIGURE 9.7
Swallowing. The bolus of food is in the oropharynx.

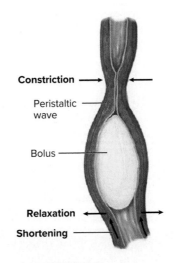

▲ FIGURE 9.8
Swallowing. The bolus of food is shown in the esophagus.

Word Analysis and Definition

S = Suffix   P = Prefix   R = Root   R/CF = Combining Form

WORD	PRONUNCIATION	ELEMENTS		DEFINITION
esophagus esophageal (adj)	ee-**SOF**-ah-gus ee-**SOF**-ah-**JEE**-al	S/ R/	Greek *gullet* -eal *pertaining to* esophag- *esophagus*	Tube linking pharynx to stomach Pertaining to the esophagus
hiatus (noun) hiatal (adj)	high-**AY**-tus high-**AY**-tal	S/ R/	Latin *an aperture* -al *pertaining to* hiat- *opening*	An opening through a structure Pertaining to a hiatus
sphincter	**SFINK**-ter		Greek *a band*	A band of muscle that encircles an opening; when it contracts, the opening squeezes closed

EXERCISES

A. Apply *your knowledge of the same elements to various terms, and increase your medical vocabulary. Focus on what is the same and what is different about the following terms. Fill in the chart.*   **LO 9.1, 9.2, and 9.5**

Medical Term	Meaning of Prefix	Meaning of Root	Meaning of Suffix
submandibular	1.	2.	3.
sublingual	4.	5.	6.
parotid	7.	8.	9.

B. Use *medical terms relating to the mouth and mastication to correctly complete each sentence. Fill in the blanks.*   **LO 9.2 and 9.5**

1. The roof of the mouth is termed the _____ .

2. During swallowing, the _____ covers the entrance to the nose from the back of the throat.

3. Taste buds are located on the sides of the tongue's _____ .

4. The _____ moves food around in the mouth during mastication.

Section 9.3

Digestion—Stomach, Small Intestine, and Large Intestine

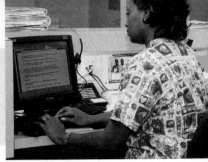

Rick Brady/McGraw-Hill Education

The bolus of food that you swallowed has now passed down your esophagus and into your stomach. The process of digestion begins to accelerate. The stomach continues the mechanical breakdown of the food particles and initiates the chemical digestion of protein and fats. The small intestine is where the greatest amount of food digestion and absorption occurs.

Digestion: The Stomach (LO 9.5)

Your stomach's peristaltic contractions mix different boluses of food together and push these contents toward the **pylorus** (the stomach opening that leads to the bowel's small intestine) *(Figure 9.9)* to produce a mixture of semi-digested food called **chyme.**

The cells of your stomach's lining secrete *(Figure 9.10):*

1. **Mucus,** which lubricates food and protects the stomach lining;

2. **Hydrochloric acid (HCl),** which breaks up the connective tissue of meat and the cell walls of vegetables (think of the chicken-and-vegetables meal you ate earlier);

3. **Pepsin** (an active enzyme), which digests chicken and vegetable proteins;

4. **Intrinsic factor,** which is essential for vitamin B_{12} absorption in the small intestine; and

5. **Gastrin** (a chemical), which stimulates HCl and **pepsinogen** production, and encourages the stomach's peristaltic contractions.

A typical meal like chicken and vegetables takes 3 to 4 hours to exit the stomach as **chyme.** Peristaltic waves squirt 2 to 3 milliliters **(ml)** of this chyme at a time through the **pyloric sphincter** into the **duodenum** (the first part of the small intestine) *(Figure 9.9).*

Abbreviations

HCl	hydrochloric acid
ml	milliliter

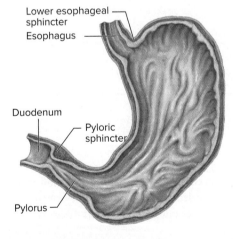

▲ **FIGURE 9.9**
Stomach.

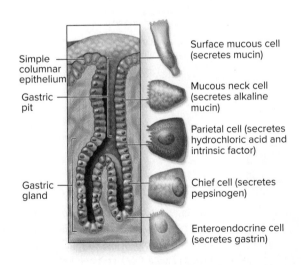

▲ **FIGURE 9.10**
Gastric Cells and Their Secretions.

S = Suffix   P = Prefix   R = Root   R/CF = Combining Form

WORD	PRONUNCIATION		ELEMENTS	DEFINITION
chyme	KYME		Greek *juice*	Semifluid, partially digested food passed from the stomach into the duodenum
cecum (noun)	SEE-kum		Latin *blind*	Blind pouch that is the first part of the large intestine
cecal (adj)	SEE-kal	S/ R/	-al *pertaining to* cec- *cecum*	Pertaining to the cecum
duodenum	du-oh-**DEE**-num	S/ R/	-um *structure* duoden- *twelve*	The first part of the small intestine; approximately 12 finger-breadths (9 to 10 inches) in length
duodenal (adj)	du-oh-**DEE**-nal	S/	-al *pertaining to*	Pertaining to the duodenum
gastrin	GAS-trin	S/ R/	-in *substance, chemical compound* gastr- *stomach*	Hormone secreted in the stomach that stimulates secretion of HCl and increases gastric motility
glycogen	GLYE-koh-jen	S/ R/CF	-gen *to produce* glyc/o- *sugar/glucose*	The body's principal carbohydrate reserve, stored in the liver and skeletal muscle
hydrochloric acid (HCl)	high-droh-**KLOR**-ik **ASS**-id	S/ R/CF R/	-ic *pertaining to* hydr/o- *water* -chlor- *green*	The acid of gastric juice
ileum	**ILL**-ee-um	S/ R/	-um *structure* ile- *ileum*	Third portion of small intestine
ileocecal	**ILL**-ee-oh-**SEE**-cal	S/ R/CF R/	-al *pertaining to* ile/o- *ileum* cec- *cecum*	Pertaining to the junction of the ileum and cecum
intrinsic factor	in-**TRIN**-sik **FAK**-tor	S/ R/ R/	-ic *pertaining to* intrins- *on the inside* factor *maker*	Makes the absorption of vitamin B_{12} happen
jejunum (noun)	je-**JEW**-num		Latin *empty*	Segment of small intestine between the duodenum and the ileum
jejunal (adj)	je-**JEW**-nal	S/ R/	-al *pertaining to* jejun- *jejunum*	Pertaining to the jejunum
mucus (noun) mucous (adj) mucin	MYU-kus MYU-kus MYU-sin		Latin *slime*	Sticky secretion of cells in mucous membranes Relating to mucus or the mucosa Protein element of mucus
pepsin pepsinogen	PEP-sin pep-**SIN**-oh-jen	S/ R/CF	Greek *to digest* -gen *produce* pepsin/o- *pepsin*	Enzyme produced by the stomach that breaks down protein Converted by HCl in the stomach to pepsin
pylorus	pie-**LOR**-us	S/ R/	-us *pertaining to* pylor- *gate, pylorus*	Exit area of the stomach
pyloric (adj)	pie-**LOR**-ik	S/	-ic *pertaining to*	Pertaining to the pylorus
portal vein	**POR**-tal **VANE**		portal, Latin *gate* vein, Latin *vein*	The vein that carries blood from the intestines to the liver
starch	STARCH		Anglo-Saxon *stiffen*	Complex carbohydrate made of multiple units of glucose attached together
villus villi (pl)	VILL-us VILL-eye		Latin *shaggy hair*	Thin, hairlike projection, particularly of a mucous membrane lining a cavity

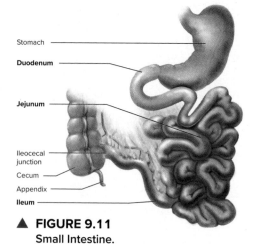

▲ FIGURE 9.11
Small Intestine.

Small Intestine (LO 9.5)

The small intestine, called *small* because of its diameter, completes the chemical digestion process. It is responsible for the **absorption** of most of the nutrients. The small intestine extends from the pylorus of the stomach to the beginning of the large intestine, and it has three segments *(Figure 9.11)*, as listed below:

1. The **duodenum** is the first 9 to 10 inches of the small intestine. It receives chyme from the stomach, together with pancreatic juices and bile;

2. The **jejunum** makes up about 40% of the small intestine's length. It is the primary region for chemical digestion and nutrient absorption; and

3. The **ileum** makes up the last 55% of the small intestine's length. It ends at the **ileocecal** valve, a **sphincter** that controls entry into the large intestine.

Digestion in the Small Intestine (LO 9.5)

After leaving the stomach as chyme, food spends 3 to 5 hours in the small intestine.

Anywhere from 4 to 6 hours after consuming the chicken and vegetables mentioned earlier, the food has passed through the small intestine and is ready to be passed into the large intestine. While in the small intestine, the protein, carbohydrates, and fats have been broken down by enzymes and absorbed into the bloodstream.

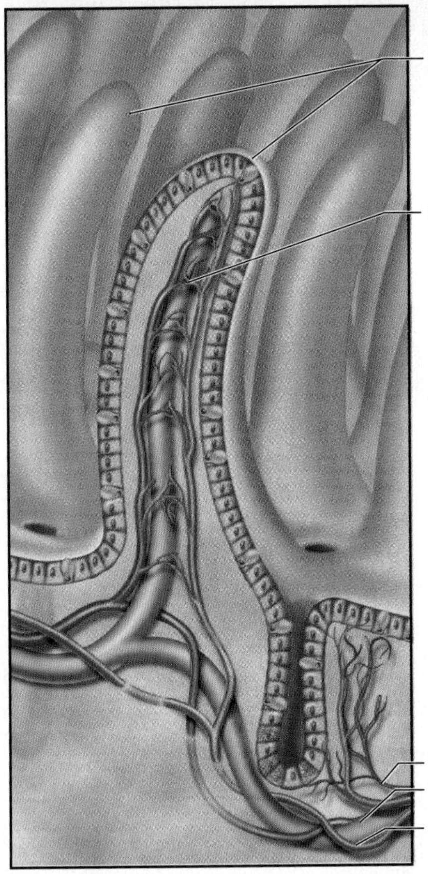

Chemical Digestion, Absorption, and Transport (LO 9.6 and 9.9)

Carbohydrates (LO 9.4, 9.5, and 9.6)

In your small intestine, carbohydrates like **starches** are broken down into simple sugars—glucose and fructose—which are absorbed by the lining cells and transferred to the capillaries of the **villi** *(Figure 9.12).* The most commonly consumed carbohydrates are bread, soft drinks, cookies, cakes, doughnuts, syrups, jams, potatoes, and rice. From the capillaries of the villi, the simple sugars are carried by the **portal vein** to the liver, where the non-glucose sugars are converted to glucose. Glucose is the major source of energy for all cells.

Glycogen, the storage form of carbohydrate, is found in the liver and skeletal muscle. Glycogen in muscles supplies glucose during high-intensity and endurance exercise.

Proteins (LO 9.5 and 9.6)

Proteins are only 10% to 20% digested when they arrive in the duodenum and small intestine. Enzymes produced by cells in the small intestine, and the pancreatic enzyme trypsin, break down the remaining proteins into **amino acids.**

The amino acids are carried away in the blood and are transported to cells all over the body to be used as building blocks for new tissue formation.

Lipids (LO 9.5 and 9.6)

Lipids (fats) enter the duodenum and small intestine as large globules. These have to be **emulsified** by the bile salts into smaller droplets so that pancreatic **lipase** (fat-reducing enzymes) can digest them into very small droplets of free **fatty acids** and monoglycerides.

These small droplets are taken up by the **lacteals** (lymphatic vessels) inside the villi and then move into the lymphatic system. The droplets now comprise a milky, fatty lymphatic fluid called **chyle,** which eventually reaches the thoracic duct and moves into the bloodstream *(see Chapter 7).* Chyle is stored in adipose tissue. The fat-soluble vitamins A, D, E, and K are absorbed with the lipids.

Water (LO 9.5 and 9.6)

Water has no caloric value and makes up approximately 60% of your body weight (about 10 gallons) as an adult. Your small intestine absorbs 92% of your body's water, which is taken into the bloodstream through the capillaries in the villi. Water-soluble vitamins, C and the B complex, are absorbed with water, except for B_{12}.

You can survive 6 to 8 weeks without food, but only a few days without water.

Minerals (LO 9.5 and 9.6)

Minerals are absorbed along the whole length of the small intestine. Iron and calcium are absorbed according to the body's needs. The other minerals are absorbed regardless of need, and the kidneys excrete the surplus.

The major minerals are sodium **(Na)**, potassium **(K)**, calcium **(Ca)**, and magnesium **(Mg).**

▲ **FIGURE 9.12**
Intestinal Villi.

Keynotes

- **Proteins are broken down into amino acids.**
- **Minerals are electrolytes.**
- **In malnutrition, the body breaks down its own tissues to meet its nutritional and metabolic needs.**
- **Milk sugar is lactose. The enzyme lactase breaks down lactose into glucose.**

Abbreviations

Ca	calcium
ED	emergency department
K	potassium
Mg	magnesium
Na	sodium

S = Suffix P = Prefix R = Root R/CF = Combining Form

WORD	PRONUNCIATION		ELEMENTS	DEFINITION
amino acid	ah-**ME**-no ASS-id	R/CF	**amin/o-** *nitrogen containing* acid, Latin *sour*	The basic building block for protein
chyle	KYLE		Greek *juice*	A milky fluid that results from the digestion and absorption of fats in the small intestine
diarrhea	die-ah-**REE**-ah	P/ R/	**dia-** *complete* **-rrhea** *flow, discharge*	Abnormally frequent and loose stools
emulsify	ee-**MUL**-sih-fye	S/ R/	**-ify** *to become* **emuls-** *suspend in a liquid*	Break up into very small droplets to suspend in a solution (emulsion)
emulsion (noun)	ee-**MUL**-shun	S/	**-ion** *condition, action*	The system that contains small droplets suspended in a liquid
lacteal	**LAK**-tee-al	S/ R/CF	**-eal** *pertaining to* **lact-** *milk*	A lymphatic vessel carrying chyle away from the intestine
lipase	**LIE**-pase	S/ R/	**-ase** *enzyme* **lip-** *fat*	Enzyme that breaks down fat
lipid	**LIP**-id		Greek *fat*	General term for all types of fatty compounds; e.g., cholesterol, triglycerides, and fatty acids
malabsorption	mal-ab-**SORP**-shun	S/ P/ R/	**-ion** *action, condition* **mal-** *bad, difficult* **-absorpt-** *swallow, take in*	Inadequate gastrointestinal absorption of nutrients
mineral	**MIN**-er-al	S/ R/	**-al** *pertaining to* **miner-** *mines*	Inorganic compound usually found in the earth's crust

Structure and Functions of the Large Intestine (LO 9.9)

Once your small intestine has digested and absorbed the nutrients, the residual materials must be prepared in your large intestine so they can be eliminated from your body.

Structure of the Large Intestine (LO 9.5)

Your **large intestine** is so named because its diameter is much greater than that of your small intestine. In your abdominal cavity, the large intestine forms a perimeter around the central mass of the small intestine.

At the junction between the small and large intestines, a ring of smooth muscle called the **ileocecal sphincter** forms a one-way valve. This allows chyme to pass into the large intestine and prevents the large intestine's contents from backing into the ileum.

The **cecum** is located at the beginning of the large intestine. It is a pouch in the abdomen's right lower quadrant. A narrow tube with a closed end (the **vermiform appendix**) projects downward from the cecum *(Figure 9.13a and b)*. The function of the appendix is not known.

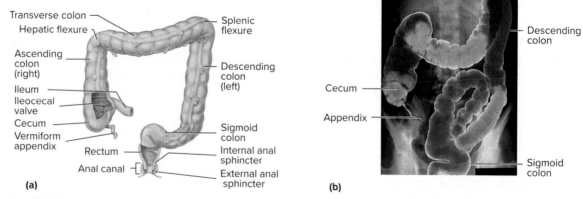

▲ **FIGURE 9.13**
Large Intestine.
(a) Surface anatomy. (b) X-ray of large intestine following barium enema.
CNRI/Science Photo Library/Science source

The ascending **colon** begins at the cecum and extends upward to underneath the liver. Here, it makes a sharp turn at the hepatic **flexure** and becomes the transverse colon. At the left side of the abdomen, near the spleen at the splenic flexure, the transverse colon turns downward to form the descending colon. At the pelvic brim, the descending colon forms an S-shaped curve called the **sigmoid** colon. This descends in the pelvis to become the rectum and then the **anal canal.**

The **rectum** has three transverse folds—rectal valves that enable it to retain **feces** while passing gas (flatus).

The anal canal *(Figure 9.14)* is the last 1 to 2 inches of the large intestine, opening to the outside as the **anus.** An internal anal sphincter, composed of smooth muscle from the intestinal wall, and an external anal sphincter, composed of skeletal muscle that can be controlled voluntarily, guard the exit of the anus.

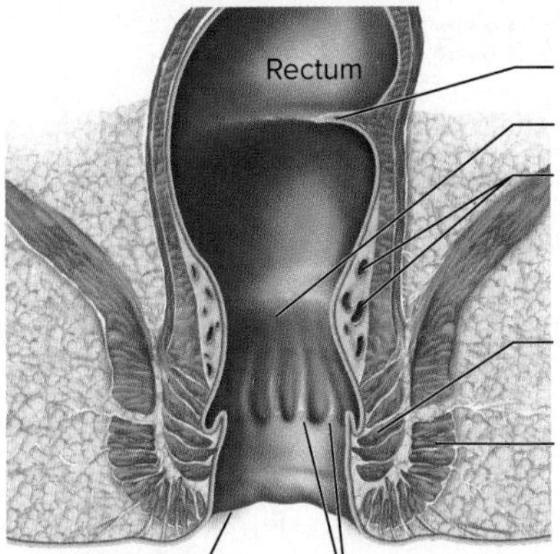

▲ **FIGURE 9.14**
Anal Canal.

Functions of the Large Intestine (LO 9.5)

Your large intestine has the following key functions:

- Absorption of water and electrolytes. The large intestine receives more than 1 liter (1,000 ml) of chyme each day from the small intestine. It reabsorbs water and electrolytes to reduce the volume of chyme to 100 to 150 ml of feces, which are eliminated by **defecation;**

- **Secretion** of mucus that protects the intestinal wall and holds particles of fecal matter together;

- **Digestion** (by the bacteria that inhabit the large intestine) of any food remnants that have escaped the small intestine's digestive enzymes;

- **Peristalsis** happens a few times a day in the large intestine to produce mass movements toward the rectum; and

- **Elimination** of materials that were not digested or absorbed.

Word Analysis and Definition

S = Suffix   P = Prefix   R = Root   R/CF = Combining Form

WORD	PRONUNCIATION		ELEMENTS	DEFINITION
anus	A-nus		Latin *ring*	Terminal opening of the digestive tract through which feces are discharged
anal (adj)	A-nal	S/ R/	-al *pertaining to* an- *anus*	Pertaining to the anus
appendix	ah-**PEN**-dicks		Latin *appendage*	Small blind projection from the pouch of the cecum
cecum	**SEE**-kum		Latin *blind*	Blind pouch that is the first part of the large intestine
colon	**KOH**-lon		Greek *colon*	The large intestine, extending from the cecum to the rectum
colic (adj)	**KOL**-ik	S/ R/	-ic *pertaining to* col- *colon*	Spasmodic, crampy pains in the abdomen
feces	**FEE**-seez		Latin *dregs*	Undigested, waste material discharged from the bowel
fecal (adj)	**FEE**-kal	S/ R/	-al *pertaining to* fec- *feces*	Pertaining to feces
defecation	def-eh-**KAY**-shun	S/ P/	-ation *process* de- *removal*	Evacuation of feces from rectum and anus
flatus	**FLAY**-tus		Latin *blowing*	Gas or air expelled through the anus
flatulence	**FLAT**-you-lents	S/	-ence *forming*	Excessive amount of gas in the stomach and intestines
flatulent (adj)	**FLAT**-you-lent	R/	flatul- *excessive gas*	Relating to or suffering from flatulence
flexure	**FLEK**-shur		Latin *bend*	A bend in a structure
ileocecal sphincter	**ILL**-ee-oh-**SEE**-cal **SFINK**-ter	S/ R/CF R/	-al *pertaining to* ile/o- *ileum* -cec- *cecum* sphincter, Greek *band*	Band of muscle that encircles the junction of ileum and cecum
rectum	**RECK**-tum		Latin *straight*	Terminal part of the colon from the sigmoid to the anal canal
rectal (adj)	**RECK**-tal	S/ R/	-al *pertaining to* rect- *rectum*	Pertaining to the rectum
sigmoid	**SIG**-moyd		Greek *letter "S"*	Sigmoid colon is shaped like an "S"
vermiform	**VER**-mih-form		Latin *wormlike*	Worm shaped; used as a descriptor for the appendix

EXERCISES

A. Define the actions of the secretions of the stomach. *Match the secretion in the first column with its function listed in the second column. Fill in the blanks.* **LO 9.5**

_____ **1.** intrinsic factor   **a.** protects the lining of the stomach

_____ **2.** pepsin   **b.** breaks up cell walls of plants

_____ **3.** mucus   **c.** allows for absorption of vitamin B_{12}

_____ **4.** hydrochloric acid   **d.** enzyme that breaks down protein

B. Identify *the meaning of word elements. Select the correct answer that completes each statement.* **LO 9.1**

1. The suffix that is used to form the names of enzymes is

    a. -ic

    b. -al

    c. -ase

    d. -ous

    e. -ion

2. The medical term that has an element that means **milk:**

    a. lipid

    b. chyme

    c. protease

    d. chyle

    e. lacteal

3. The medical term that has an element that means **mines:**

    a. chyle

    b. fats

    c. lipids

    d. minerals

    e. emulsify

4. The root **enter** means:

    a. blood

    b. to begin

    c. water

    d. small intestine

    e. bile

C. Apply *the language of the digestive system and answer the following questions. Fill in the blanks.* **LO 9.2, 9.5, 9.6, 9.8, and 9.11**

1. What part of the digestive system contains both an internal and external sphincter? _____

2. What body part is thought to have no known use or function? _____

3. What is a ring of smooth muscle that forms a one-way valve called? _____

4. What is the name of the area of the colon that is shaped like an "S"? _____

5. What is the name of the procedure where the appendix is removed? _____

6. The *hepatic flexure* is near what major body organ? _____

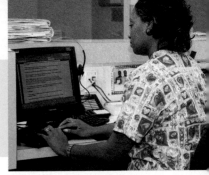

Rick Brady/McGraw-Hill Education

Section 9.4

Digestion—Liver, Gallbladder, and Pancreas

Your liver and pancreas secrete enzymes that are responsible for the majority of digestion occurring in the small intestine.

The Liver (LO 9.6)

Your **liver** is your largest internal organ. It is a complex structure located under your right ribs just below your diaphragm *(Figure 9.15)*.

As a complex organ, your liver's multiple functions include:

- Manufacturing and excreting **bile;**
- Removing **bilirubin** (a rust-colored pigment) from the bloodstream;
- Storing excess sugar as **glycogen;** and
- Manufacturing blood proteins, including those needed for clotting *(see Chapter 7).*
- Filters and purifies blood from the small intestine and lower portion of the body just before the venous blood flows into the heart

Keynotes

- Only the production of bile relates the liver to digestion.
- Vaccines are available to prevent hepatitis A and B.

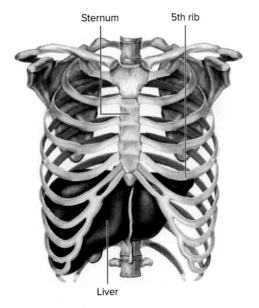

Sternum   5th rib

Liver

▲ **FIGURE 9.15**
Location of Liver.

Word Analysis and Definition

S = Suffix   P = Prefix   R = Root   R/CF = Combining Form

WORD	PRONUNCIATION		ELEMENTS	DEFINITION
bile bile acids biliary (adj)	BILE **BILE AH**-sids **BILL**-ee-air-ee	S/ R/CF	Latin *bile* -ary *pertaining to* bil/i- *bile*	Fluid secreted by the liver into the duodenum Steroids synthesized from cholesterol Pertaining to bile or the biliary tract
bilirubin	bill-ee-**RU**-bin	S/ R/CF	-rubin *rust colored* bil/i- *bile*	Bile pigment formed in the liver from hemoglobin
glycogen	**GLYE**-koh-gen	S/ R/CF	-gen *produce, create* glyc/o- *sugar, glycogen*	The body's principal carbohydrate reserve, stored in the liver and skeletal muscle
hepatic	hep-**AT**-ik	S/ R/	-ic *pertaining to* hepat- *liver*	Pertaining to the liver
liver	**LIV**-er		Old English *liver*	Body's largest organ, located in the right upper quadrant of the abdomen

- Between meals, the gallbladder absorbs water and electrolytes from the bile and concentrates it 10 to 20 times.
- Jaundice is caused by deposits of bilirubin in the tissues.
- The pancreas is the only organ that is both an endocrine and an exocrine gland.

Abbreviation

GB   gallbladder

Gallbladder, Biliary Tract, and Pancreas (LO 9.7)

Gallbladder and Biliary Tract (LO 9.6)

On the underside of your liver is your **gallbladder (GB),** which stores and concentrates the bile produced by the liver. The **cystic duct** from the gallbladder joins with the **hepatic duct** to form the **common bile duct.** This duct system, which moves the bile from the liver to the duodenum, is called the **biliary tract** *(Figure 9.16a and b).*

The Pancreas (LO 9.6)

Your **pancreas** is a spongy, exocrine gland. **Exocrine** glands secrete fluids. In fact, many of the glands in your body are exocrine glands, including your sweat glands, mammary glands, and other digestive enzyme-releasing glands. The majority of the pancreas secretes digestive juices, but smaller areas of pancreatic islet cells secrete the hormones **insulin** and **glucagon** *(see Chapter 12).*

The pancreas produces pancreatic digestive juices that are excreted through the pancreatic duct. This duct joins the common bile duct shortly before it opens into the duodenum *(Figure 9.16b),* which encircles the top or head of the pancreas *(Figure 9.16b).* Pancreatic and bile juices then enter the duodenum.

Other pancreatic cells secrete insulin and glucagon, which go directly into the bloodstream. This part of the pancreas is an **endocrine** (hormone-secreting) gland.

Pancreatic juices contain alkaline electrolytes, which help neutralize the acid chyme as it comes from the stomach, and enzymes, which break down starches, fats, and proteins into simpler elements.

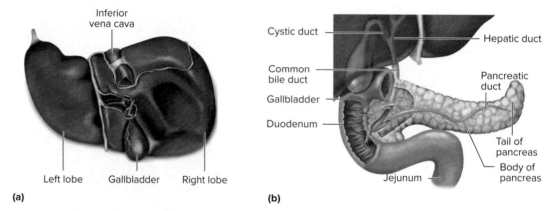

(a)

(b)

▲ **FIGURE 9.16**
(a) Underside of liver. (b) Anatomy of gallbladder, pancreas, and biliary tract.

S = Suffix   P = Prefix   R = Root   R/CF = Combining Form

WORD	PRONUNCIATION		ELEMENTS	DEFINITION
cyst cystic (adj)	SIST SIS-tik	 S/	Greek sac, *bladder* -ic *pertaining to*	Abnormal fluid-filled sac surrounded by a membrane Pertaining to a cyst
duct	DUKT		Latin *to lead*	Tube or channel that carries a substance
endocrine exocrine	EN-doh-krin EK-soh-krin	P/ R/ P/	endo- *within, inside* -crine *secrete* exo- *outward, outside*	A gland that produces an internal or hormonal substance and secretes it into the bloodstream A gland that secretes substances outwardly through excretory ducts
gallbladder	GAWL-blad-er		bladder, Old English *receptacle*	Receptacle on the inferior surface of the liver for storing bile
glucagon	GLU-kah-gon	R/ R/	gluc- *glucose, sugar* -agon *to fight*	Hormone that mobilizes glucose from body storage
insulin	IN-syu-lin	S/ R/	-in *chemical compound* insul- *island*	Pancreatic hormone that suppresses blood glucose levels and transports glucose into cells
pancreas pancreatic (adj)	PAN-kree-as pan-kree-AT-ik	 S/ R/	Greek *sweetbread* -ic *pertaining to* pancreat- *pancreas*	Lobulated gland, the head of which is tucked into the curve of the duodenum Pertaining to the pancreas

EXERCISES

A. Elements: *Select the answer that correctly completes each statement.*   **LO 9.1 and 9.7**

1. In the term *hepatic,* the root means:

   a. pancreas   **b.** stomach   **c.** liver

2. The suffix in *cirrhosis* indicates this is:

   a. a condition   **b.** surgical excision   **c.** a structure

3. *Bilirubin* is the color of:

   a. coal   **b.** milk   **c.** rust

4. The root in *cirrhosis* indicates a:

   a. color   **b.** size   **c.** location

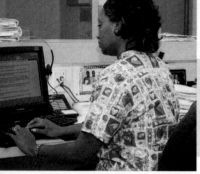

Section 9.5

Disorders of the Digestive System

Overall Digestive System Disorders (LO 9.7)

Many disorders produce symptoms from the gastrointestinal tract but have no specific lesions discoverable in any part of the tract. These disorders include:

- **Food intolerance** has gastrointestinal symptoms such as bloating, cramps, gas, heartburn, diarrhea, and general nonspecific symptoms such as irritability and headache.

- **Food allergies** occur when the immune system (*see Chapter 7*) overreacts to a food **antigen,** identifying it as a danger, and triggering a protective response. Gastrointestinal symptoms involve vomiting, stomach cramps, and difficulty swallowing. Eight types of food account for 90% of all allergic food reactions: eggs, milk, peanuts, tree nuts, fish, shellfish, wheat, and soy.

- **Irritable bowel syndrome (IBS)** is a symptom-based diagnosis with chronic abdominal pain, abdominal discomfort, bloating, and either diarrhea or constipation. There is no known organic cause and routine testing shows no abnormality. Dietary adjustments involving fiber intake and psychological interventions can help.

- **Inflammatory bowel disease (IBD)** involves chronic inflammation of all or part of the digestive tract, but primarily includes ulcerative colitis and Crohn's disease.

- **Aging** has less effect on the digestive system than on other organ systems. In the small intestine, **lactase** levels decrease, leading to intolerance of dairy products **(lactose intolerance).**

Keynotes

- There is a very definite difference between being intolerant to a food and having a food allergy.
- Intolerance can be due to enzyme deficiencies or sensitivity to food additives.
- A food allergy involves the immune system and can be serious or life threatening.

Disorders of the Mouth (LO 9.7)

The human mouth is the entrance to the digestive system. Since so many elements pass through it, the human mouth is prone to tooth disorders and a host of other conditions.

A buildup of **dental plaque** (a collection of oral microorganisms and their products), or **tartar** (calcified deposits on the surface of teeth), is a precursor to invasion by dental disease–causing bacteria.

Dental caries, which describe tooth decay and cavity formation, are erosions of the tooth surface caused by bacteria *(Figure 9.17)*. If untreated, it can lead to an abscess at the root of the tooth. **Gingivitis** is an infection of the gums. **Periodontal disease** occurs when the gums and the jawbone are involved in a disease process. In **periodontitis,** infection causes the gums to pull away from the teeth, forming pockets that become sources of infection that can spread to underlying bone. Infection of the gums with a purulent or pus-like discharge is called **pyorrhea.**

Keynotes

- Cleft palate is a congenital fissure in the median line of the palate, often associated with a cleft lip.
- Periodontal disease is thought to be associated with coronary artery disease, but no causal relationship has been established.

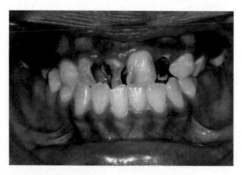

▲ **FIGURE 9.17**   Dental Caries.

WORD	PRONUNCIATION	ELEMENTS		DEFINITION
aphthous	**AF**-thus		Greek *ulcer*	Painful small oral ulcers (canker sores)
canker	**KANG**-ker		Latin *crab*	Nonmedical term for aphthous ulcer
caries	**KARE**-eez		Latin *dry rot*	Bacterial destruction of teeth
dental	**DEN**-tal		Latin *tooth*	Pertaining to the teeth
gingivitis	jin-jih-**VI**-tis	S/ R/	-itis *inflammation* gingiv- *gum*	Inflammation of the gums
glossodynia	gloss-oh-**DIN**-ee-ah	S/ R/CF	-dynia *pain* gloss/o- *tongue*	Painful, burning tongue
halitosis	hal-ih-**TOE**-sis	S/ R/	-osis *condition* halit- *breath*	Bad odor of the breath
periodontitis	**PAIR**-ee-oh-don-**TIE**-tis	P/ R/ S/	peri- *around* -odont- *tooth* -itis *inflammation*	Inflammation of the tissues around a tooth
plaque	PLAK		French *plate*	Patch of abnormal tissue
pyorrhea	pie-oh-**REE**-ah	R/ R/CF	-rrhea *flow* py/o- *pus*	Purulent discharge
stomatitis	**STOH**-mah-**TI**-tis	S/ R/CF	-itis *inflammation* stomat/i- *oral cavity, mouth*	Inflammation of the mucous membrane in the mouth
tartar	**TAR**-tar		Latin *crust on wine casks*	Calcified deposit at the gingival margin of the teeth
thrush	THRUSH		Root unknown	Infection with *Candida albicans*

The term **stomatitis** is used for any infection of the mouth, including:

- **Mouth ulcers,** also called **canker** sores, are erosions of the mucous membrane lining the mouth. **Aphthous** ulcers are the most common and occur in clusters of small ulcers that last for 3 or 4 days. These are usually stress- or illness-related but can also be caused by trauma.

- **Cold sores,** or fever blisters *(Figure 9.18),* are recurrent blisters on the lips, lining of the mouth, and gums due to infection with the virus **herpes simplex type 1 (HSV-1).** These blisters usually clear up spontaneously.

- **Thrush** *(Figure 9.19)* is an infection occurring anywhere in the mouth that is caused by the fungus *Candida albicans.* This fungus is normally found in the mouth, but it can multiply out of control as a result of prolonged antibiotic or steroid treatment, cancer chemotherapy, or diabetes. Newborn babies can acquire oral thrush from the mother's vaginal yeast infection during the birth process. Treatment with antifungal agents is usually successful.

- **Oral cancer** occurs most often on the lip, but it can also occur on the tongue. Eighty percent of oral cancers are associated with smoking or chewing tobacco. Metastasis occurs to lymph nodes, bones, lungs, and liver.

  Halitosis is the medical term for bad breath, which occurs in association with any of the above mouth disorders.

- **Glossodynia** is a painful, burning sensation of the tongue that occurs in postmenopausal women. Its etiology is unknown and there is no successful treatment.

Abbreviation

HSV-1   Herpes simplex
virus, type 1

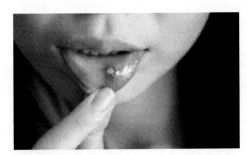

▲ **FIGURE 9.18**
Cold Sores on the Inside of the Lower Lip.

C.PIPAT/Shutterstock

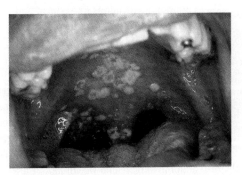

▲ **FIGURE 9.19**   Oral Thrush.

Dr. Sol Silverman, Jr., DDS/CDC

WORD	PRONUNCIATION	ELEMENTS		DEFINITION
asymptomatic	A-simp-toe-**MAT**-ik	S/ P/	-ic *pertaining to* a- *without*	Without any symptoms or abnormalities experienced by the patient
symptomatic (*with symptoms*)	simp-toe-**MAT**-ik	R/	symptomat- *symptom*	Pertaining to the symptoms of a disease
dysphagia	dis-**FAY**-jee-ah	P/ R/	dys- *difficulty* -phagia *swallowing*	Difficulty in swallowing
esophagitis	ee-**SOF**-ah-**JI**-tis	S/ R/	-itis *inflammation* espohag- *esophagus*	Inflammation of the lining of the esophagus
hernia	**HER**-nee-ah		Latin *rupture*	Protrusion of a structure through the tissue that normally contains it
reflux	**REE**-fluks	P/ R/	re- *back* -flux *flow*	Backward flow
varix varices (pl) varicose (adj)	**VAIR**-iks **VAIR**-ih-seez **VAIR**-ih-kose	 S/ R/	Latin *dilated vein* -ose *full of* varic- *varicosity; dilated, tortuous vein*	Dilated, tortuous vein Characterized by or affected with varices

Abbreviations

GERD	Gastroesophageal reflux disease
NSAID	Nonsteroidal anti-inflammatory drug

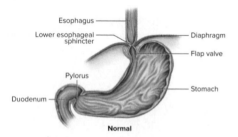

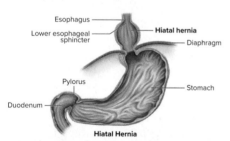

▲ **FIGURE 9.20**   Hiatal Hernia.

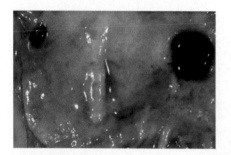

▲ **FIGURE 9.21**   Bleeding Peptic Ulcer.

Jose Luis Calvo/Shutterstock

Disorders of the Esophagus (LO 9.7)

Just like the mouth, the esophagus, too, can be prone to illness. **Esophagitis** is an inflammation of the lining of the esophagus, producing a burning chest pain **(heartburn)** after eating, pain on swallowing. The most common cause is **reflux** of the stomach's acid contents into the esophagus, also known as **gastroesophageal reflux disease (GERD).**

Hiatal hernia occurs when a portion of the stomach protrudes through the diaphragm alongside the esophagus at the esophageal hiatus *(Figure 9.20)*.

Esophageal varices are varicose veins of the esophagus. They are **asymptomatic** until they rupture, causing massive bleeding and hematemesis. They are a common finding with cirrhosis of the liver *(see later in this chapter)*.

Cancer of the esophagus arises from the tube's lining. Symptoms are **dysphagia** (difficulty swallowing), a burning sensation in the chest, and weight loss. Risk factors include cigarette smoking, alcohol abuse, obesity, and esophageal reflux. The cancer can metastasize to the liver, bones, and lungs.

Disorders of the Stomach (LO 9.7)

Gastroesophageal reflux disease (GERD) refers to the regurgitation of stomach contents back into the esophagus. The acidity of regurgitated food can irritate and ulcerate the esophageal lining and cause bleeding. Scar tissue can cause an esophageal **stricture** and **dysphagia.**

Emesis (vomiting) can result from overexpansion or irritation of any part of the digestive tract. The muscles of the diaphragm and abdominal wall forcefully contract and expel the stomach contents upward into the esophagus and mouth.

Gastritis is an inflammation of the stomach lining, producing symptoms of epigastric pain, feeling of fullness, nausea, and occasional bleeding. It can be acute or chronic, and is caused by common medications like aspirin and **NSAIDs,** by radiotherapy and chemotherapy, and by alcohol and smoking. Treatment involves removing the factors causing the gastritis, acid neutralization, and suppression of gastric acid.

Peptic ulcers occur in the stomach and duodenum when the mucosal lining breaks down *(Figure 9.21)*. Most peptic ulcers are caused by the bacterium *Helicobacter pylori (H. pylori)*, which produces enzymes that weaken the protective mucus. These ulcers usually respond to antibiotics. **Dyspepsia** (epigastric pain with bloating and nausea) is the most common symptom.

Gastric ulcers are peptic ulcers that occur in the stomach. If a blood vessel erodes, bleeding may also be present. If untreated, the ulcer can eat into the entire wall, causing a **perforation.**

Gastric cancer can be asymptomatic for a long period and then cause **indigestion, anorexia,** abdominal pain, and weight loss. It affects men twice as often as women. It metastasizes to the lymph nodes, liver, peritoneum, chest, and brain. It is usually treated with surgery and chemotherapy.

WORD	PRONUNCIATION	ELEMENTS		DEFINITION
anorexia	an-oh-**RECK**-see-ah	S/ P/ R/	-ia *condition* an- *without* -orex- *appetite*	Without an appetite; or an aversion to food
dyspepsia	dis-**PEP**-see-ah	S/ P/ R/	-ia *condition* dys- *difficult, bad* -peps- *digestion*	"Upset stomach," epigastric pain, nausea, and gas
gastritis	gas-**TRY**-tis	S/ R/	-itis *inflammation* gastr- *stomach*	Inflammation of the lining of the stomach
gastroesophageal	**GAS**-troh-ee-sof-ah-**JEE**-al	S/ R/CF R/CF	-al *pertaining to* gastr/o- *stomach* -esophag/e- *esophagus*	Pertaining to the stomach and esophagus
gastroscope gastroscopy	**GAS**-troh-skope gas-**TROS**-koh-pee	S/ R/CF S/	-scope *instrument for viewing* gastr/o- *stomach* -scopy *to examine, to view*	Endoscope for examining the inside of the stomach Endoscopic examination of the stomach
indigestion	in-dih-**JESS**-chun	S/ P/ R/	-ion *action, condition* in- *in, not* -digest- *to break down*	Symptoms resulting from difficulty in digesting food
intestine intestinal (adj)	in-**TESS**-tin in-**TESS**-tin-al	S/ R/	Latin *intestine, gut* -al *pertaining to* intestin- *gut, intestine*	The digestive tube from stomach to anus Pertaining to the intestines
peptic	**PEP**-tik	S/ R/	-ic *pertaining to* pept- *digest*	Relating to the stomach and duodenum
perforation	per-foh-**RAY**-shun	S/ R/	-ion *action, condition* perforat- *bore through*	A hole through the wall of a structure
stricture	**STRICK**-shur		Latin *draw tight*	Narrowing of a tube
ulcer ulceration ulcerative	**ULL**-sir ull-cer-**A**-shun **UL**-sir-ah-tiv	 S/ R/ S/	Latin *sore* -ation *a process* ulcer- *a sore* -ative *quality of*	Erosion of an area of skin or mucosa Formation of an ulcer Marked by an ulcer or ulcers

Disorders of the Small Intestine (LO 9.7)

The absorption of nutrients occurs primarily through the small intestine. Impairment of absorption, including Crohn's disease and lactose intolerance, is covered in *Section 9.5.*

- **Gastroenteritis,** or inflammation of the stomach and small intestine, can result in acute vomiting and diarrhea. It can be caused by a variety of viruses and bacteria and, occasionally, the parasite *Giardia lamblia* each of which is usually initiated by contact with contaminated food (food poisoning) and water.

- **Bleeding** from the small intestine is usually caused by a duodenal ulcer.

- **Celiac disease** is an autoimmune disease which causes an immune reaction to eating **gluten,** a protein contained in wheat, rye, barley, and other grains. Celiac disease *(Figure 9.22)* damages the lining of the small intestine and can cause abdominal swelling, gas, pain, weight loss, fatigue, and weakness. Treatment is a strict gluten-free diet.

- An **intussusception** *(Figure 9.23)* occurs when a part of the small intestine slides into a neighboring portion of the small intestine—much like the way that parts of a collapsible telescope slide into each other. Eighty percent of intussusceptions can be cured with an enema; the remaining 20% require surgical intervention.

- **Ileus,** also known as **paralytic ileus,** is a disruption of the normal peristaltic ability of the small intestine. It can be caused by a bowel obstruction or by intestinal paralysis. Risk factors for ileus include GI surgery, diabetic ketoacidosis *(see Chapter 12),* peritonitis, and medications, such as opiates.

- **Cancer** of the small intestine occurs infrequently compared with tumors in other parts of the GI tract. An **adenocarcinoma** is the most common malignant tumor of the small bowel.

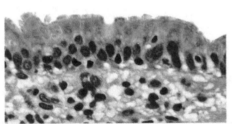
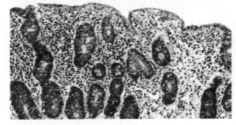

◀ **FIGURE 9.22**
Photomicrograph of Celiac Disease Showing Atrophy of Duodenal Villi.

Biophoto Associates/Science Source

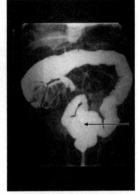

▲ **FIGURE 9.23**
Abdominal X-ray Showing Intussusception of the Intestines.

CNRI/Science Source

Disorders of Absorption (LO 9.7)

The term **malabsorption syndromes** refers to a group of diseases in which intestinal absorption of nutrients is impaired.

Malnutrition can arise from malabsorption, but can also result from a lack of food, as with famine and poverty. Malnutrition can also result from a loss of appetite in people with cancer or a terminal illness.

Lactose intolerance occurs when the small intestine is not producing enough of the enzyme **lactase** to break down the milk sugar lactose. The result is diarrhea and cramps. Lactase can be taken in pill form before eating dairy products, and milk products can be avoided.

Diarrhea is caused by irritation of the intestinal lining that causes feces to pass through the intestine too quickly for adequate amounts of water to be reabsorbed.

Crohn's disease (or **regional enteritis**) is an inflammation of the small intestine, frequently in the ileum and occasionally also in the large intestine. The symptoms are abdominal pain, diarrhea, fatigue, and weight loss. There is no cure.

Constipation occurs when fecal movement through the large intestine is slow and thus too much water is reabsorbed by the large intestine. The feces become hardened. Constipation can be caused by lack of dietary fiber, lack of exercise, dehydration and emotional upset.

Gastroenteritis (stomach "flu") is an infection of the stomach and intestine that can be caused by a large number of bacteria and viruses. It causes vomiting, diarrhea, and fever. An outbreak of gastroenteritis can sometimes be traced to contaminated food or water.

Dysentery is a severe form of bacterial gastroenteritis with blood and mucus in frequent, watery stools.

Malnutrition, malabsorption, and severe forms of diarrhea and vomiting can cause **dehydration** and an electrolyte imbalance, possibly leading to coma and death.

Word Analysis and Definition

S = Suffix   P = Prefix   R = Root   R/CF = Combining Form

WORD	PRONUNCIATION	ELEMENTS		DEFINITION
adenocarcinoma	ADD-eh-noh-kar-sih-NOH-mah	S/ R/CF R/	-oma *tumor* aden/o- *gland* -carcin- *cancer*	A cancer arising from glandular epithelial cells
celiac	SEE-lee-ack	S/ R/	-ac *pertaining to* celi- *abdomen*	Relating to the abdominal cavity
celiac disease	SEE-lee-ack diz-EEZ	P/ R/	dis- *apart* -ease *normal function*	Disease caused by a sensitivity to gluten
gastroenteritis	GAS-troh-en-ter-I-tis	S/ R/CF R/	-itis *inflammation* gastr/o- *stomach* -enter- *intestine*	Inflammation of the stomach and intestines
Giardia	jee-AR-dee-ah		Alfred Giard, 1846–1908 French biologist	Parasite that can affect the small intestine
gluten	GLU-ten		Latin *glue*	Insoluble protein found in wheat, barley, and rye
ileus	ILL-ee-us		Greek *intestinal colic*	Dynamic or mechanical obstruction of the small intestine
intussusception	IN-tuss-sus-SEP-shun	S/ P/ R/	-ion *action* intus- *within* -suscept- *to take up*	The slippage of one part of the bowel inside another, causing obstruction

WORD	PRONUNCIATION		ELEMENTS	DEFINITION
allergy	AL-er-jee	P/ R/ R/	all- *other* -ergy *process of working* -erg *work*	An acquired sensitivity to certain proteins
allergen allergic (adj)	AL-er-jen ah-LER-jic	R/ S/	-gen *to produce* -ic *pertaining to*	The substance that incites an allergic reaction Relating to any response to an allergen
Crohn's disease	KRONE diz-EEZ		Burrill Crohn, New York gastroenterologist 1884–1983	Narrowing and thickening of terminal small intestine
constipation	kon-stih-PAY-shun	S/ R	-ation *process* constip- *press together*	Hard, infrequent bowel movements
dehydration	dee-high-DRAY-shun	S/ P/ R/	-ation *a process* de- *without* -hydr- *water*	Process of losing body water
diarrhea	die-ah-REE-ah	P/ S/	dia- *complete, through* -rrhea *flow, discharge*	Abnormally frequent and loose stools
dysentery	DISS-en-tare-ee	P/ R/	dys- *bad, difficult* -entery *condition of the small intestine*	Disease with diarrhea, bowel spasms, fever, and dehydration
intolerance	in-TOL-er-ance		Latin *unable to cope with*	Inability of the small intestine to digest and dipose of a particular dietary constituent
lactose lactase	LAK-toes LAK-tase	S/ R/	Latin *milk sugar* -ase *enzyme* lact- *milk*	The disaccharide in cow's milk Enzyme that breaks down lactose to glucose
malabsorption	mal-ab-SORP-shun	S/ P/ R/	-ion *action, condition* mal- *bad* -absorpt- *to swallow*	Inadequate gastrointestinal absorption of nutrients
malnutrition	mal-nyu-TRISH-un	S/ P/ R/	-ion *action, condition* mal- *bad* nutri- *nourish*	Inadequate nutrition from poor diet or inadequate absorption of nutrients

Disorders of the Liver (LO 9.7)

Hepatitis is an inflammation of the liver, often causing **jaundice,** where the skin and sometimes the eyes have a yellowish hue. Viral hepatitis is the most common cause of hepatitis and is related to three major types of virus:

1. **Hepatitis A virus (HAV)** is highly contagious and causes a mild to severe infection. It is transmitted by contaminated food.
2. **Hepatitis B virus (HBV),** or serum hepatitis, is transmitted through contact with blood, semen, vaginal secretions, or saliva, as well as by a needle prick and the sharing of contaminated needles. Vaccines are available to prevent hepatitis A and B.
3. **Hepatitis C virus (HCV)** is the most common blood-borne infection in the United States, occurring mostly through injections given with contaminated syringes and needles. The disease can vary in severity from a mild illness lasting a few weeks to a serious, lifelong condition that can lead to cirrhosis of the liver or liver cancer. More than 3 million Americans are chronically infected with hepatitis C virus. Combination antiviral drugs are used, and new therapeutic agents are being licensed. There is no vaccine yet available.

In addition, **hepatitis D,** although considered rare, can occur in association with hepatitis B, making the infection worse. **Hepatitis E** is similar to hepatitis A and occurs mostly in under developed countries.

Chronic hepatitis occurs when the acute hepatitis does not subside after 6 months. It progresses slowly, can last for years, and is difficult to treat.

Cirrhosis of the liver is a chronic irreversible disease, replacing normal liver cells with hard, fibrous scar tissue. Its most common causes are alcoholism, prolonged hepatitis, and non-alcoholic fatty liver disease. There is no known cure.

Cancer of the liver as a primary cancer usually arises in patients with chronic liver disease, often from hepatitis B infection.

Word Analysis and Definition

S = Suffix   P = Prefix   R = Root   R/CF = Combining Form

WORD	PRONUNCIATION	ELEMENTS		DEFINITION
cholecystitis	KOH-leh-sis-TIE-tis	S/ R/CF R/	-itis *inflammation* chol/e- *bile* -cyst- *bladder*	Inflammation of the gallbladder
choledocholithiasis	koh-**LED**-oh-koh-lih-**THIGH**-ah-sis	S/ R/CF R/	-iasis *condition* choledoch/o- *common bile duct* -lith- *stone*	Presence of a gallstone in the common bile duct
cholelithiasis	KOH-leh-lih-THIGH-ah-sis	S/ R/CF R/CF	-iasis *condition* chol/e- *bile* -lith/o- *stone*	Condition of having bile stones (gallstones)
cirrhosis	sir-**ROE**-sis	S/ R/	-osis *condition* cirrh- *yellow*	Extensive fibrotic liver disease
gallstone	GAWL-stone	R/ R/	gall- *bitter* -stone *pebble*	Hard mass of cholesterol, calcium, and bilirubin that can be formed in the gallbladder and bile duct
hepatitis	hep-ah-**TIE**-tis	S/ R/	-itis *inflammation* hepat- *liver*	Inflammation of the liver
jaundice	JAWN-dis		French *yellow*	Yellow staining of tissues with bile pigments, including bilirubin
pedal	PEED-al	S/ R/	-al *pertaining to* ped- *foot*	Pertaining to the foot
provisional diagnosis (*also called* **preliminary** diagnosis)	pro-**VIZH**-un-al die-ag-**NO**-sis	S/ R/ P/ R/	-al *pertaining to* provision- *provide* dia- *complete* -gnosis *knowledge of an abnormal condition*	A temporary diagnosis pending further examination or testing The determination of the cause of a disease
pancreatitis	PAN-kree-ah-**TIE**-tis	S/ R/	-itis *inflammation* pancreat- *pancreas*	Inflammation of the pancreas

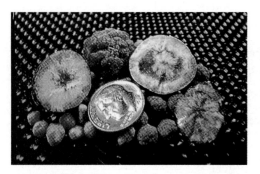

▲ **FIGURE 9.24**   Gallstones. The dime is included to illustrate the relative size of the gallstones.

Southern Illinois University/Science Source

Abbreviation

CF   cystic fibrosis

Disorders of the Gallbladder (LO 9.7)

Gallstones (cholelithiasis) can form in the gallbladder from excess cholesterol, bile salts, and bile pigment (*Figure 9.24*). The stones can vary in size and number. Risk factors are obesity, high-cholesterol diets, rapid weight loss, and in certain cases, prolonged improper emptying of the gallbladder.

Choledocholithiasis occurs when small stones become impacted in the common bile duct. This can cause biliary colic and jaundice (*see below*).

Cholecystitis is an acute or chronic inflammation of the gallbladder, usually associated with cholelithiasis and obstruction of the cystic duct with a stone.

Jaundice (icterus) is a symptom of many different diseases in the biliary tract and liver. It is a yellow discoloration of the skin and sclera of the eyes caused by deposits of bilirubin just below the skin's outer layers.

Disorders of the Pancreas (LO 9.7)

Pancreatitis is an inflammation of the pancreas. This acute condition ranges from a mild, self-limiting episode to an acute life-threatening emergency. In the chronic form, there is a progressive destruction of pancreatic tissue leading to malabsorption and diabetes.

Pancreatic cancer is the fourth leading cause of cancer-related death. Early diagnosis is difficult because the presenting symptoms are very vague. Treatment is surgical resection of the cancer. The prognosis is poor.

Cystic fibrosis (CF) is an inherited disease that becomes apparent in infancy or childhood. With CF, the pancreas, liver, intestines, sweat glands, and lungs all produce abnormally thick mucous secretions. The malabsorption of fat and protein leads to large, bulky, foul-smelling stools. Problems with thick mucous secretions in the lungs lead to chronic lung disease.

WORD	PRONUNCIATION	ELEMENTS		DEFINITION
bowel	**BOUGH**-el		Latin *sausage*	Another name for intestine
emesis hematemesis	**EM**-eh-sis he-mah-**TEM**-eh-sis	R/ R/	Greek *to vomit* **hemat**- *blood* **-emesis** *to vomit*	Vomiting Vomiting of red blood
hematochezia	he-mat-oh-**KEY**-zee-ah	S/ R/CF	**-chezia** *pass a stool* **hemat/o**- *blood*	The passage of red, bloody stools
melena	mel-**LEE**-nah		Greek *black*	The passage of black, tarry stools
occult blood	oh-**KULT BLUD**		occult, Latin *to hide*	Blood that cannot be seen in the stool but is positive on a fecal occult blood test

Gastrointestinal (GI) Bleeding (LO 9.7)

GI tract bleeding can have a variety of causes, which are not always easy to recognize. Sometimes, the bleeding can be internal and painless. It can present in different ways, however, to provide a clue as to the site of bleeding:

- **Hematemesis** is the vomiting of bright red blood, which indicates an upper GI source of bleeding (esophagus, stomach, duodenum) that is brisk.
- **Vomiting of "coffee grounds"** occurs when bleeding from an upper GI source has slowed or stopped.
- **Melena,** the passage of black, tarry stools, usually indicates upper GI bleeding.
- **Occult blood** cannot be seen in the stool the source of the bleeding can be anywhere in the GI tract.
- **Hematochezia** is the passage of bright red bloody stools, which usually indicates lower GI bowel bleeding from the sigmoid colon, rectum, or anus.

Disorders of the Large Intestine and Anal Canal (LO 9.7)

Disorders of the Large Intestine (LO 9.9)

Appendicitis is the most common cause of acute abdominal pain in the right lower quadrant. If neglected, the inflamed appendix can rupture, leading to **peritonitis.**

Diverticulosis is the presence of small pouches (**diverticula**) bulging outward through weak spots in the large intestine's lining *(Figure 9.25)*. The pouches are asymptomatic until they become infected and inflamed, a condition called **diverticulitis.** The most likely cause of **diverticular disease** (diverticulosis and diverticulitis) is a low-fiber diet.

Ulcerative colitis is an extensive inflammation and ulceration of the large intestine's lining. It produces bouts of bloody diarrhea, crampy pain, weight loss, and an electrolyte imbalance.

Irritable bowel syndrome (IBS) is an increasingly common large-bowel disorder presenting with crampy pain, gas, and changes in bowel habits to either constipation or diarrhea. There are no anatomical changes seen in the bowel. The cause is unknown.

Polyps, which vary in size and shape, are masses of tissue arising from the large intestine's wall and protruding into the bowel lumen. Most polyps are benign.

Colon and rectal cancers are the second cause of cancer deaths after lung cancer. The majority of these cancers occur in the rectum and sigmoid colon. They can spread through the bowel wall, extend down the lumen, and metastasize to regional lymph nodes and to liver, lungs, bones, and brain through the bloodstream.

Obstruction of the large bowel can be caused by cancers, large polyps, or diverticulitis.

Proctitis is an inflammation of the rectum's lining, often associated with ulcerative colitis, Crohn's disease, or radiation therapy.

Disorders of the Anal Canal (LO 9.7)

Hemorrhoids are dilated veins in the submucosa (connective tissue layer) of the anal canal, often associated with pregnancy, chronic constipation, diarrhea, or aging. They protrude into the anal canal **(internal)** or bulge out along the edge of the anus **(external)** *(Figure 9.26),* producing pain and bright red blood from the anus. A thrombosed hemorrhoid, in which blood has clotted, is very painful.

Anal fissures are tears in the anal canal's lining, perhaps from difficult bowel movements **(BMs).** **Anal fistulas** occur following abscesses in the anal glands and are an abnormal passage (fistula) between the anal canal and the skin outside the anus.

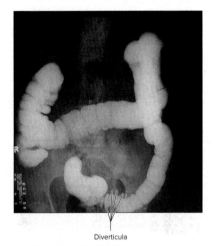

Diverticula

▲ **FIGURE 9.25**   Barium Enema Showing Diverticulosis.

Susan Leavine/Science Source

Abbreviations

BM	bowel movement
IBS	irritable bowel syndrome

Keynotes

- A proctologist is a surgical specialist in diseases of the anus and rectum.
- Fissures are tears; fistulas are abnormal passages.
- Consuming black licorice, Pepto-Bismol, or blueberries can non-disease related produce black stools.

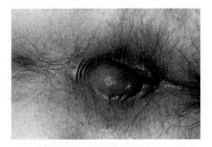

▲ **FIGURE 9.26**
External Hemorrhoid.

Dr. P. Marazzi/Science Source

Word Analysis and Definition

S = Suffix   P = Prefix   R = Root   R/CF = Combining Form

WORD	PRONUNCIATION		ELEMENTS	DEFINITION
appendicitis	ah-pen-dih-**SIGH**-tis	S/ R/	-itis *inflammation* **appendic-** *appendix*	Inflammation of the appendix
colitis	koh-**LIE**-tis	S/ R/	-itis *inflammation* **col-** *colon*	Inflammation of the colon
diverticulum diverticula (pl) diverticulosis diverticulitis	die-ver-**TICK**-you-lum di-ver-**TICK**-you-lah DIE-ver-tick-you-**LOW**-sis DIE-ver-tick-you-**LIE**-tis	S/ R/ S/ S/	-um *tissue, structure* **diverticul-** *byroad* -osis *condition* -itis *inflammation*	A pouchlike opening or sac from a tubular structure (e.g., intestine) Presence of a number of small pouches in the wall of the large intestine Inflammation of the diverticula
fissure	**FISH**-ur		Latin *slit*	Deep furrow or cleft
fistula	**FIS**-tyu-lah		Latin *pipe, tube*	Abnormal passage
hemorrhoid hemorrhoids (pl)	**HEM**-oh-royd	S/ R/CF	-rrhoid *flow* **hem/o-** *blood*	Dilated rectal vein producing painful anal swelling
peritoneum peritoneal (adj) peritonitis	**PAIR**-ih-toe-**NEE**-um **PAIR**-ih-toe-**NEE**-al **PAIR**-ih-toe-**NIE**-tis	S/ R/CF S/ S/	-um *tissue* **periton/e-** *stretch over* -al *pertaining to* -itis *inflammation*	Membrane that lines the abdominal cavity Pertaining to the peritoneum Inflammation of the peritoneum
polyp polyposis	**POL**-ip pol-ih-**POH**-sis	 S/ R/	Latin *foot* -osis *condition* **polyp-** *polyp*	Mass of tissue that projects into the lumen of the bowel Presence of several polyps
proctitis	prok-**TIE**-tis	S/ R/	-itis *inflammation* **proct-** *anus, rectum*	Inflammation of the lining of the rectum

EXERCISES

Case Report 9.1

You are

. . . a medical interpreter working in Fulwood Medical Center.

You are communicating with

. . . Mr. Xavier Ramirez, a 45-year-old farm worker, who has come to Dr. Susan Lee's primary care clinic. Mr. Ramirez complains of persistent, burning epigastric pain for several months. He has been a chain-smoker since the age of 14. His pain is eased by antacids but quickly returns. He has been taking aspirin because of joint pain in his fingers while he works. Dr. Lee has decided to refer him to a gastroenterologist for a gastroscopy. Your role is to explain the procedure to Mr. Ramirez and ensure that he keeps his appointments.

A **gastroscopy** on Mr. Ramirez reveals a gastric ulcer.

A. Use Case Report 9.1 *to answer the following questions. Select the correct answer that completes each statement.*   **LO 9.7, 9.8, and 9.10**

1. Mr. Ramirez complains of pain:

   a. in his abdomen   **c.** above his stomach

   b. in his mouth   **d.** of his tongue

2. The doctor that he has been referred to is a specialist in the treatment of:

   a. stomach and intestines   **c.** blood and cancer

   b. heart and blood vessels   **d.** ear, nose, and throat

3. Mr. Ramirez takes antacids to treat his:

   a. cough   **c.** joint pain

   b. stomach pain   **d.** nausea

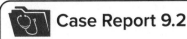

Case Report 9.2

You are

. . . a medical coder in the Health Information Management department at Fulwood Medical Center.

You are communicating with

. . . Dr. Susan Lee and you are questioning the documentation of Mrs. Sandra Jacobs's care. Mrs. Jacobs, a 46-year-old mother of four, presented in Dr. Lee's primary care clinic with episodes of cramping pain in her upper abdomen associated with nausea and vomiting. A physical examination reveals an obese, white woman with tenderness over her gallbladder. Her BP is 170/90 and she has slight **pedal** edema. A **provisional diagnosis** of gallstones has been made. She has been referred for an ultrasound examination and an appointment has been made to see Dr. Walsh in the surgery department.

Mrs. Jacobs presented with the classic gallstone symptoms of severe waves of right upper quadrant pain (biliary colic), nausea, and vomiting.

B. Refer *to Case Report 9.2. Then select the choice that correctly completes each statement or answers each question.*   **LO 9.7, 9.8, 9.9, and 9.11**

1. A provisional diagnosis means that the diagnosis is:
   a. confirmed
   b. unsupported
   c. temporary

2. Aside from pain in her abdomen, Mrs. Jacobs also has:
   a. swelling in her feet
   b. pain in her calf
   c. yellow-colored skin
   d. low blood pressure

3. The pain in Mrs. Jacobs' abdomen is thought to be due to:
   a. viral infection of digestive tract
   b. gallstones
   c. cancer in the liver
   d. inflammation of the pancreas

4. What additional diagnostic procedure is she scheduled for?
   a. sigmoidoscopy
   b. cholecystectomy
   c. barium enema
   d. ultrasound

Case Report 9.3

You are

. . . a dietitian working at Fulwood Medical Center.

You are communicating with

. . . Mrs. Jan Stark, a 36-year-old pottery maker, and her husband, Mr. Tom Stark. From her medical record, you see that Mrs. Stark has been referred to you by Dr. Cameron Grabowski, a gastroenterologist.

For the past 10 years, Mrs. Stark has had spasmodic episodes of **diarrhea** and **flatulence** associated with severe headaches and fatigue. During those episodes, her stools were greasy and pale. She has seen several physicians who have recommended low-fat, high-carbohydrate diets, but she has had no relief. Dr. Grabowski has performed an intestinal biopsy through an oral **endoscopy** and diagnosed **celiac disease.** This condition is a sensitivity to the protein **gluten** that is found in wheat, rye, barley, and oats. Dr. Grabowski has asked you to ensure that Mrs. Stark accepts a diet free of gluten-containing foods like breads, cereals, cookies, and beer.

C. Read *Case Report 9.3. Select the correct answer to complete each statement.*   **LO 9.7, 9.10, and 9.11**

1. The endoscope was inserted through Mrs. Stark's:
   a. mouth
   b. rectum
   c. abdominal incision

2. Mrs. Stark's discomfort is due to:

   a. smoking

   b. diet

   c. drinking alcohol

   d. lack of exercise

3. Dr. Grabowski is a specialist in the treatment of disorders of the:

   a. mouth

   b. stomach and intestines

   c. stomach only

   d. liver

Study Hint

Endoscope is a generic (general) term that means any instrument *(scope)* used to examine the inside *(endo)* of a tubular or hollow organ. The instrument obtains its specific name from the organ it is used to examine. Thus, an instrument used to view a stomach is a gastroscope specifically, but it is also an endoscope in general.

D. Suffixes: *Find the correct suffix to complete the medical terms. Fill in the blanks.* **LO 9.1, 9.7, and 9.8**

-ist   -itis   -ectomy   -rrhea   -osis   -al   -ics

1. inflammation of the gums   gingiv/ _____

2. specialized branch of dentistry   periodont/ _____

3. around a tooth   periodont/ _____

4. bad breath   halit/ _____

5. surgical removal of diseased gum tissue   gingiv/ _____

6. specialist in periodontics   periodont/ _____

7. purulent discharge   pyo/ _____

E. Identify *the following medical terms that have their origin in Greek, Latin, or French. Fill in the blanks.* **LO 9.2 and 9.7**

1. patch of abnormal tissue _____

2. canker sores _____

3. pertaining to the gums _____

4. nonmedical term for a mouth ulcer _____

5. bacterial destruction of teeth _____

F. Define *the elements chol/e- and choledoch/o-. Fill in the blanks.* **LO 9.2 and 9.6**

1. The element chol/e- means _____.

2. The element choledoch/o- means _____.

G. Knowledge *of elements is your best tool for increasing your medical vocabulary. Each of the following terms has an element in bold. Identify that element and give its meaning. Fill in the chart.* **LO 9.1 and 9.7**

Medical Term	Identity of Element (P, R, CF, or S)	Meaning of Element
*re*flux	1.	2.
dys*phagia*	3.	4.
hernio*rrhaphy*	5.	6.
hemat*emesis*	7.	8.
*a*symptomatic	9.	10.

H. Apply *the language of gastroenterology and fill in the blanks.* **LO 9.2 and 9.7**

1. What is another term for *varicose veins* of the esophagus? _____

2. What is the medical term for inflammation of the lining of the esophagus? _____

3. What structure does the esophagus travel through from the *thoracic cavity* to the abdominal cavity? _____

4. What is burning chest pain called? _____

5. What are you vomiting in *hematemesis?* _____

I. The definitions *of the elements will help you understand the meaning of the term. Select the correct answer that completes each statement.*   **LO 9.1 and 9.7**

1. The meaning of the prefix in the medical term **dyspepsia** is:

   a. digestion   **c.** difficult

   b. condition   **d.** stomach

2. The meaning of the root in the medical term **peptic** is:

   a. pump   **c.** ulcer

   b. digest   **d.** tear

3. The meaning of the suffix in the medical term **perforation** is:

   a. structure   **c.** pertaining to

   b. condition   **d.** inflammation

4. The meaning of the root in the medical term **anorexia** is:

   a. digestion   **c.** without

   b. stomach   **d.** appetite

J. Fill in the blanks *with the medical term being described.*   **LO 9.2, 9.3, and 9.7**

1. This condition can be caused by *Helicobacter pylori:* _____ ulcer

2. Inflammation of the lining of the stomach: _____

3. Regurgitation of the stomach contents back into the esophagus (provide the abbreviation): _____

K. Match *the disorder of the small intestine with the correct description.*   **LO 9.3 and 9.7**

_____ **1.** ileus   **a.** Parasite that causes gastroenteritis

_____ **2.** IBS   **b.** Part of the small intestine slides into a neighboring part

_____ **3.** celiac disease   **c.** Disruption of the normal peristalsis of the small intestine

_____ **4.** *Giardia lamblia*   **d.** Treatment is difficult and often unsuccessful

_____ **5.** intussusception   **e.** Allergy to gluten

L. Use your knowledge *of the small intestine and answer the questions. Select T if the statement is true. Select F if the statement is false.*   **LO 9.3, 9.5, and 9.7**

1. The absorption of nutrients occurs primarily through the small intestine.   T   F

2. Gastroenteritis can result in acute vomiting and diarrhea.   T   F

3. Bleeding from the small intestine is usually from an infection.   T   F

4. Chronic abdominal pain, bloating, and either diarrhea or constipation can be signs of IBS.   T   F

5. Risk factors for paralytic ileus include GI surgery, diabetic ketoacidosis, and medicines such as opiates.   T   F

M. Provide *the correct terms being described below. Fill in the blanks.*   **LO 9.2, 9.7, and 9.11**

1. Lymphatic vessel that carries chyle away from the intestine: _____

2. Inorganic compounds found in the earth's crust: _____

3. Condition of hardened fecal matter: _____

4. Condition caused by severe bacterial infection resulting in frequent watery stools containing blood and mucus: _____

5. Crohn's disease is also known as: _____

N. Deconstruct: *Break down these terms into their elements to define the word. Know the meaning of the elements = know the meaning of the term. If a term does not have a particular word element, insert N/A. Fill in the chart.*   **LO 9.1, 9.7, and 9.11**

Medical Term	Meaning of Prefix	Meaning of Root/CF	Meaning of Suffix
colitis	1.	2.	3.
defecation	4.	5.	6.
appendicitis	7.	8.	9.
junction	10.	11.	12.

O. Suffixes: *Insert the correct suffix to complete the term. There are more suffixes than you need. Fill in the blanks.*   **LO 9.1, 9.7, and 9.8**

-osis   -ectomy   -um   -itis   -al   -ion

1. excision or removal of a polyp   polyp/ _____

2. inflammation of the diverticula   diverticul/ _____

3. membranous structure lining the abdominal cavity   peritone/ _____

4. condition of having multiple polyps   polyp/ _____

5. pertaining to the peritoneum   peritone/ _____

P. Singular and plural terms. *Insert the correct medical terms in the blanks; watch for spelling. Fill in the blanks.*   **LO 9.2, 9.7, and 9.8**

diverticulitis   diverticulum   diverticulosis   diverticula

1. What starts out as a single _____ can be followed by many other _____. The condition of having a number of these small pouches in the wall of the intestine is known as _____. Should these pouches become inflamed, _____ will result.

polypectomy   polyps   polyposis   polyp

2. The first _____ was found on sigmoidoscopy. A follow-up colonoscopy 6 months later found several more _____ in the large intestine. Diagnosis is _____. Proposed treatment is _____.

peritoneum   peritonitis   peritoneal

3. The _____ laceration sliced completely through the _____. Because of an infection in the wound, the patient developed _____.

Q. Construct *terms related to the gallbladder. Use this group of elements, in addition to* chol/e *and* choledoch/o *to form the medical terms that are defined. Some elements you will use more than once; some elements you will not use at all. Fill in the blanks.*   **LO 9.1, 9.7, and 9.8**

lith-   -iasis   chole-   -ectomy   -osis   cyst-   -tomy   cyst/o-   -itis   choledoch/o-

1. condition of gallstones: _____ / _____ / _____

2. surgical removal of gallbladder: _____ / _____ / _____

3. gallstone in the common bile duct: _____ / _____ / _____

4. surgical incision into gallbladder to remove gallstones: _____ / _____ / _____

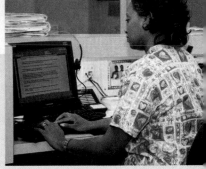

Rick Brady/McGraw-Hill Education

Diagnostic Procedures (LO 9.8)

Many diagnostic procedures rely on video cameras to display the inside of the alimentary tract. Visualizing this area assists the health care professionals to identify sections that may develop into problems and those that are presently causing problems.

An **intraoral** camera allows a **dentist** to view oral structures, such as the teeth, for caries, and the tongue, sublingual areas, and cheeks for cancerous growths.

Endoscopes are long, flexible devices with a light and tiny camera at the tip. They are connected to an endoscopic system consisting of a computer and a screen to display and record the inside of the GI tract. The size and shape of the endoscope changes based on the structure of the organs it is meant to visualize.

Enteroscopy uses an endoscope to view upper GI structures for signs of cancer, polyps, bleeding, or ulcers.

- **Gastroscopy** limits the view to the stomach.

- **Panendoscopy** views all upper GI structures.

- **Ileoscopy** views the ileum (last part of the small intestine) by inserting an endoscope through an ileostomy.

- **Double balloon endoscopy** uses two balloons at the tip of the endoscope, which are inflated sequentially to move the endoscope farther into the small intestine than what can be done with a usual endoscope.

Endoscopic ultrasound (EUS) is a type of endoscopic examination that enables detailed imaging and analysis of the pancreas. A thin tube tipped with an ultrasound probe is inserted through the mouth down into the stomach and the first part of the small intestine. The probe emits sound waves that bounce off surrounding structures, and these sound waves are recaptured by the probe and converted to black and white images that can be interpreted by the physician. EUS is of great value in assessing pancreatic tumors and cysts and acute and chronic pancreatitis.

Colonoscopy uses a **colonoscope** to view the entire colon (large intestine). Specialized scopes exist to view specific areas of the colon. A **proctologist,** also called a **colorectal** surgeon, specializes in theses procedures.

- **Anoscopy** views the tissue of the anus for signs of trauma or disorders such as anal fissures or fistulas.

- **Proctoscopy** uses a **proctoscope** to view the anal cavity and rectum for the presence of polyps or hemorrhoids. A proctoscope, also known as a **rectoscope,** is a short, rigid, hollow tube with a light at the end of it.

- **Sigmoidoscopy** uses a **sigmoidoscope** to view the rectum up through the sigmoid colon. The sigmoidoscope can either be a form of the flexible endoscope or a rigid device.

Capsule endoscopy enables examination of the entire small intestine by ingesting a pill-sized video capsule with its own camera and light source that sends images to a data recorder worn on the patient's belt.

Angiography uses injected dye to highlight blood vessels and is used to detect the site of bleeding in the GI tract.

In a **digital rectal examination** the physician palpates the rectum and prostate gland with a gloved, lubricated index finger to determine the presence of lesions.

Fecal occult blood test (Hemoccult) is used to detect the presence of blood in the stool not visible to the naked eye. It is a good first screening test for cancer of the large intestine.

In a **barium swallow,** the patient ingests barium sulfate, a contrast material, to show details of the pharynx and esophagus on X-rays.

Upper GI tract barium X-rays (barium swallow) use barium sulfate, a contrast material, to study the distal esophagus, the stomach, and duodenum. They are less accurate than enteroscopy at identifying bleeding lesions.

In a **barium meal,** barium sulfate is consumed and used to study the distal esophagus, stomach, and duodenum on X-rays *(Figure 9.27).*

Barium enema uses the contrast material barium sulfate, which is injected into the large intestine as an enema and X-ray films are taken *(Figure 9.28).*

Abbreviation

EUS   endoscopic ultrasound

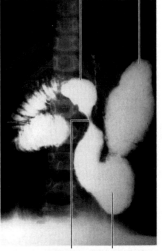

Jejunum   Pylorus of stomach

Pyloric   Duodenum
sphincter

▲ **FIGURE 9.27**   Barium Meal Showing Pylorus and Duodenum.

Medicimage/UIG/Shutterstock

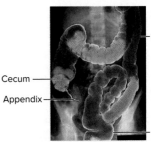

Descending colon

Cecum

Appendix

Sigmoid colon

▲ **FIGURE 9.28**   Barium Enema of the Large Intestine.

CNRI/Science Photo Library/Science source

WORD	PRONUNCIATION	ELEMENTS		DEFINITION
angiography	an-jee-**OG**-rah-fee	S/ R/CF	-graphy *process of recording* angio- *blood vessel*	Process of recording the image of blood vessels after injection of contrast material
anoscopy	**A**-nos-koh-pee	S/ R/CF	-scopy *to examine* an/o- *anus*	Endoscopic examination of the anus
colonoscope colonoscopy	koh-**LON**-oh-skope koh-lon-**OSS**-koh-pee	S/ S/ R/CF	-scope *instrument for viewing* -scopy *to examine* colon/o- *colon*	Instrument to examine the inside of the colon Endoscopic examination of the colon
dentist	**DEN**-tist	S/ R/	-ist *specialist* dent- *tooth*	A qualified practitioner specially trained to diagnose and treat conditions that affect oral health
digital	**DIJ**-ih-tal	S/ R/	-al *pertaining to* digit- *finger or toe*	Pertaining to a finger or toe
endoscope endoscopic (adj) endoscopy panendoscopy	**EN**-doh-skope **EN**-doh-**SKOP**-ik en-**DOSS**-koh-pee pan-en-**DOS**-koh-pee	P/ R/ S/ S/ P/	endo- *within, inside* -scope *instrument for viewing* -ic *pertaining to* -scopy *to examine* pan- *all*	Instrument to examine the inside of a tubular or hollow organ Pertaining to the use of an endoscope The use of an endoscope Endoscopic examination of the esophagus, stomach, and duodenum
enema	**EN**-eh-mah		Greek *injection*	An injection of fluid into the rectum
enteroscopy	en-ter-**OSS**-koh-pee	S/ R/CF	-scopy *to examine, to view* enter/o- *intestine*	The examination of the lining of the digestive tract
gastroscope gastroscopy	**GAS**-troh-skope gas-**TROS**-koh-pee	S/ R/CF S/	-scope *instrument for viewing* gastr/o- *stomach* -scopy *to examine*	Instrument to view the inside of the stomach Endoscopic examination of the stomach
ileoscopy ileostomy	**ILL**-ee-**OS**-koh-pee **ILL**-ee-**OS**-toh-mee	R/CF S/	ile/o- *ileum* -stomy *new opening*	Endoscopic examination of the ileum Artificial opening from the ileum to the outside of the body
intraoral	**IN**-trah-**OR**-al	P/ R/	intra- *inside* -oral *mouth*	Pertaining to inside the mouth
laparoscope laparoscopic (adj) laparoscopy	**LAP**-ah-roh-skope **LAP**-ah-roh-**SKOP**-ik lap-ah-**ROS**-koh-pee	S/ R/CF S/ S/	-scope *instrument for viewing* lapar/o- *abdomen in general* -ic *pertaining to* -scopy *to view, to examine*	Instrument (endoscope) used for viewing abdominal contents Pertaining to laparoscopy Examination of contents of abdomen using an endoscope
occult Hemoccult test	oh-**KULT** **HEEM**-o-kult **TEST**		Latin *to hide*	Not visible on the surface Trade name for a fecal occult blood test
proctology proctologist proctoscope proctoscopy	prok-**TOL**-oh-jee prok-**TOL**-oh-jist **PROK**-toh-skope prok-**TOSS**-koh-pee	S/ R/CF S/ S/ S/	-logy *study of* proct/o- *anus and rectum* -logist *one who studies, specialist* -scope *instrument for viewing* -scopy *to examine*	Medical specialty of the anus and rectum Medical specialist in proctology Instrument to view the inside of the anus and rectum Examination of the inside of the anus and the rectum by proctoscope or rectoscope
sigmoidoscopy	**SIG**-moi-**DOS**-koh-pee	S/ R/CF	-scopy *to examine* sigmoid/o- *sigmoid colon*	Endoscopic examination of the sigmoid colon
ultrasound	**UL**-trah-sownd	P/ R/	ultra- *higher* -sound *noise*	Very-high-frequency sound waves

Therapeutic Procedures (LO 9.9)

Abbreviation

PEG — percutaneous endoscopic gastrostomy

Many of the diagnostic procedures in the previous section can also be used as therapeutic procedures. For example, endoscopy can be used to remove polyps (**polypectomy**), biopsy suspicious lesions, stop bleeding, and be used as screening procedures for cancer.

When patients have an inability to feed normally or when certain portions of the alimentary canal are diseased or damaged, artificial devices can be employed to allow feeding and digestion to continue. Food can be inserted directly into the stomach via a **nasogastric** or stomach tube, when medically indicated. A more invasive procedure, the placement of a **percutaneous endoscopic gastrostomy (PEG) tube** involves the insertion of a feeding tube into the stomach across the skin into the stomach wall.

Laparoscopy uses a thin, lighted tube inserted through an **incision** in the abdominal wall to examine abdominal and pelvic organs. Biopsy samples can be taken through the **laparoscope,** and in many cases surgery can be performed instead of using a much larger incision. Laparoscopy is done to check for and remove abnormal tumors; repair **hiatal** and **inguinal hernias** via **herniorrhaphy;** and perform several procedures on the organs of the digestive system. An **appendectomy** completely removes the appendix. This procedure is performed on patients with acute appendicitis.

A **fistulotomy** involves an incision the length of the fistula to lay it open to drain pus and other fluids. The fistula is cleaned and sutured closed if necessary. A **fistulectomy** is an **excision** of the fistula and surrounding tissue after a fistulotomy.

Hemorrhoidectomy is the removal of hemorrhoids, either internal or external. Methods include rubber band ligation, removal with scalpel or laser, and stapling.

Intestinal resections surgically remove diseased portions of the intestine. The remaining portions of the intestine can be joined back together through an **anastomosis** *(Figure 9.29a).* If there is insufficient bowel remaining for an anastomosis, an **ostomy** *(Figure 9.29b)* can be performed, where the end of the bowel opens onto the skin at a **stoma.** Ileostomy and **colostomy** are two such procedures. GI tract cancer can be treated this way, along with radiation therapy, targeted therapy, and chemotherapy *(see Gastrointestinal Drugs section).*

Bariatric surgeries are used to help patients lose weight by surgically separating the stomach into a smaller section which decreases the amount of food it takes for a patient to feel full.

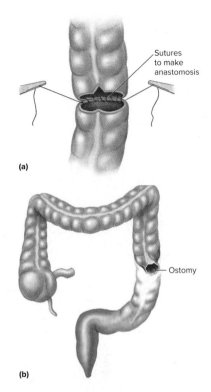

(a) Sutures to make anastomosis

(b) Ostomy

▲ **FIGURE 9.29**
Intestinal Resections.

Word Analysis and Definition

S = Suffix   P = Prefix   R = Root   R/CF = Combining Form

WORD	PRONUNCIATION	ELEMENTS		DEFINITION
anastomosis anastomoses (pl)	ah-**NAS**-to-**MOH**-sis ah-**NAS**-to-**MOH**-seez	S/ R/	-osis *condition* anastom- *join together*	A surgically made union between two tubular structures
appendectomy (**Note:** *elimination of "ic" prior to "ec" of* -ectomy)	ah-pen-**DEK**-toh-mee	S/ R/	-ectomy *surgical excision* append- *appendix*	Surgical removal of the appendix
aspiration	**AS**-pih-**RAY**-shun	S/ R/CF	-ion *process* aspirat- *to breathe on*	Removal by suction of fluid or gas from a body cavity
bariatric	bar-ee-**AT**-rik	S/ R/	-atric *treatment* bari- *weight*	Treatment of obesity
fistulectomy	**FIS**-tyu-**LEK**-toh-mee	S/ R/	-ectomy *surgical excision* fistul- *fistula*	Surgical removal of a fistula
fistulotomy	**FIS**-tyu-**LOT**-toh-mee	S/	-tomy *surgical incision*	Incision of a fistula
hernia	**HER**-nee-ah		Latin *rupture*	Protrusion of a structure through the tissue that normally contains it
herniorrhaphy	**HER**-nee-**OR**-ah-fee	S/ R/CF	-rrhaphy *suture* herni/o- *hernia*	Repair of a hernia
hemorrhoidectomy (**Note:** *This term has two suffixes.*)	**HEM**-oh-royd-**EK**-toh-me	S/ R/CF S/	-ectomy *surgical excision* hem/o- *blood* -rrhoid *flow*	Surgical removal of hemorrhoids
inguinal	**IN**-gwin-al	S/ R/	-al *pertaining to* inguin- *groin*	Pertaining to the groin
lavage	lah-**VAHZH**		Latin *to wash*	Washing out of a hollow cavity, tube, or organ
nasogastric	**NAY**-zoh-**GAS**-trik	S/ R/CF R/	-ic *pertaining to* ndas/o- *nose* -gastr- *stomach*	Pertaining to the nose and stomach
percutaneous	**PER**-kyu-**TAY**-nee-us	S/ P/ R/	-ous *pertaining to* per- *through* -cutane- *skin*	Passage through the skin, in this case, by needle puncture
polypectomy	pol-ip-**ECK**-toh-mee	S/ R/	-ectomy *surgical excision* polyp- *polyp*	Excision or removal of a polyp
resect (verb) resection	ree-**SEKT** ree-SEK-shurn	S/ P/ R/	Latin *to cut off* -ion *action, condition* re- *back* -sect- *cut off*	To remove a part
stoma ostomy (**Note:** *an "s" is removed for the purpose of spelling*)	**STOH**-mah **OS**-toh-mee	S/ R/	Greek *mouth* -stomy *new opening* -os- *mouth*	Artificial opening Surgery to create an artificial opening into a tubuar structure.
colostomy	ko-**LOS**-toh-mee	R/CF	col/o- *colon*	Artificial opening from the colon to the outside of the body
gastrostomy	gas-**TROS**-toh-mee	R/CF	gastr/o- *stomach*	Artificial opening from the stomach to the outside of the body
ileostomy	**LL**-ee-**OS**-toh-mee	R/CF	ile- *ileum*	Artificial opening from the ileum to the outside of the body

Abbreviation

ERCP   endoscopic retrograde cholangiopancreatography

Accessory Organs

Gingivectomy is the removal of gingiva to decrease the pocket depths of patients with periodontitis , gingival enlargement, or for cosmetic reasons. The procedure is carried out by a dentist or **periodontist** via scalpel or laser.

A **cholelithotomy** is the operative removal of one or more gallstones. A **cholecystectomy** completely removes the gallbladder to treat complications of the gallbladder such as cholelithiasis and choledocholithiasis.

Endoscopic retrograde cholangiopancreatography (ERCP) is used to diagnose and treat problems in the biliary ductal system. Through an endoscope, the physician can see the inside of the duodenum and inject radiographic contrast dye into the biliary tract ducts. Gallstones and cancer can be treated with this technique.

Nasogastric aspiration and lavage are used to detect upper GI bleeding. The presence of bright red blood in the lavage material indicates active upper GI bleeding; "coffee grounds" indicate the bleeding has slowed or stopped.

WORD	PRONUNCIATION	ELEMENTS		DEFINITION
cholangiography	KOH-lan-jee-OG-rah-fee	S/ R/ R/CF	-graphy *process of recording* chol- *bile* -angi/o- *blood vessel,*	X-ray of the bile ducts after injection or ingestion of a contrast medium
cholangiopancreatography	KOH-lan-jee-oh-PAN-kree	R/CF	-pancreat/o- *pancreas*	X-ray of the bile ducts and pancreatic ducts after injection or ingestion of a contrast medium
cholecystectomy	KOH-leh-sis-TEK-toh-mee	S/ R/CF R/	-ectomy *surgical excision* chol/e- *bile* -cyst- *bladder*	Surgical removal of the gallbladder
cholelithotomy	KOH-leh-lih-THOT-oh-mee	S/ R/	-otomy *surgical incision* -lith- *stone*	Surgical incision to remove a gallstone(s)
gingivectomy	jin-jih-VEC-toe-me	S/ R/	-ectomy *surgical excision* ginviv- *gum*	Surgical removal of diseased gum tissue
periodontics	PAIR-ee-oh-DON-tiks	S/ P/ R/	-ics *knowledge of* peri- *around* -odont- *tooth*	Branch of dentistry specializing in disorders of tissues around the teeth
periodontist	PAIR-ee-oh-DON-tist	S/	-ist *specialist*	Specialist in periodontics
retrograde	RET-roh-grade	P/ R/	retro- *backward* -grade *going*	Reversal of a normal flow

Gastrointestinal Drugs (LO 9.9)

Abbreviations

H₂-blocker — histamine-2 receptor antagonist

PPI — proton pump inhibitor

Drugs to Treat Excess Gastric Acid

Antacids, which are taken orally, neutralize gastric acid and relieve heartburn and acid indigestion. Examples of antacids include:

- aluminum hydroxide and magnesium hydroxide (*Maalox, Mylanta*)
- magnesium hydroxide (*Milk of Magnesia*)
- calcium carbonate (*Tums, Rolaids*)

Histamine-2 receptor antagonists (H₂-blockers) block signals that tell the stomach cells to produce acid. They are used to treat gastroesophageal reflux (GERD) and esophagitis (*see Lesson 9.2*). Examples include:

- cimetidine (*Tagamet*)
- famotidine (*Pepcid*)
- ranitidine (*Zantac*)
- nizatidine (*Axid*)

Less potent OTC variants of these drugs are also available.

Proton pump inhibitors (PPIs) suppress gastric acid secretion in the lining of the stomach by blocking the secretion of gastric acid from the cells into the lumen of the stomach. Examples include:

- omeprazole (*Prilosec*)
- lansoprazole (*Prevacid*)
- pantoprazole (*Protonix*)
- esomeprazole (*Nexium*)

Misoprostol (*Cytotec*) inhibits the secretion of gastric acid and is approved for the prevention of **nonsteroidal anti-inflammatory drug (NSAID)**–induced gastric acid.

Sucralfate (*Carafate*) reacts with gastric acid (hydrogen chloride [**HCl**]) to form a paste that binds to stomach mucosal cells and inhibits the **diffusion** of acid into the stomach lumen. It also forms a protective barrier on the surface of an ulcer. Its main use is in the **prophylaxis** of stress ulcers.

Anti-*H. pylori* therapy for the treatment of peptic ulcer and chronic gastritis is given with a combination of two antibiotics (for example, amoxicillin [generic] and clarithromycin [generic]) and a proton pump inhibitor.

Drugs to Treat Nausea and Vomiting

Antiemetics, drugs that are effective against vomiting and nausea, are used to treat motion sickness and the side effects of opioid analgesics, general anesthetics, and chemotherapy. The types of antiemetics include:

- **Serotonin antagonists,** which block serotonin receptors in the CNS and GI tract. They are used to treat postoperative and chemotherapy nausea and vomiting. Examples include dolasetron (*Anzemet*), granisetron (*Kytril*), and ondansetron (*Zofran*).

- **Dopamine antagonists,** which act in the brain. They are inexpensive but have an extensive side-effect profile and have been replaced by serotonin antagonists. Examples include chlorpromazine (*Thorazine*) and prochlorperazine (*Compazine*).

- **Antihistamines,** which are used to treat motion sickness, morning sickness in pregnancy, and opioid nausea. Examples include diphenhydramine (*Benadryl*) and promethazine (*Phenergan*).

- **Cannabinoids,** which are used in patients with **cachexia** or who are unresponsive to other antiemetics. Examples include cannabis (medical marijuana) and dronabinol (*Marinol*).

- **Antimuscarinics,** which block the effects of acetylcholine on the central nervous system. An example is scopolamine *(Scopace)* which also comes in transdermal patch form.

Drugs to Treat Constipation

Laxative drugs are used to treat chronic constipation:

- If increased water and fiber are unsuccessful, OTC forms of magnesium hydroxide are the first-line agents to be used.

- Bisacodyl *(Dulcolax)* and senna *(Docusate)* are both stimulant-category laxatives, acting on the intestinal wall to increase smooth muscle contractions.

- Lubiprostone (*Resolor*) acts on the epithelial cells of the GI tract to produce a chloride-rich fluid that softens the **stool** and increases bowel **motility**.

Drugs to Treat Diarrhea

Antidiarrheal drugs are widely available OTC. Examples include loperamide (*Imodium A-D, Maalox*), which reduces bowel motility; bismuth subsalicylate (*Pepto-Bismol*), which decreases the secretion of fluid into the intestine; and attapulgite (*Kaopectate*), which pulls fluid and electrolytes away from the GI tract; as well as enzymes and nutrients. A combination of diphenyloxylate and atropine (*Lomotil*), a Schedule V drug, reduces bowel motility.

WORD	PRONUNCIATION	ELEMENTS		DEFINITION
antidiarrheal	**AN**-tee-die-ah-**REE**-al	S/ P/ P/ R/	-al *pertaining to* anti- *against* -dia- *complete, through* -rrhea *flow, discharge*	Drug that prevents abnormally frequent and loose stools
antiemetic	**AN**-tee-eh-**MEH**-tik	P/ R/	anti- *against* -emetic *causing vomiting*	Agent that prevents vomiting
antihistamine	an-tee-**HISS**-tah-meen	P/ R/ R/CF	anti- *against* -hist- *tissue* -amine *nitrogen compound*	Drug that can be used to treat allergic symptoms or prevent vomiting
antimuscarinic	**AN**-tee-**MUS**-ka-**RIN**-ik	S/ P/ R/	-ic *pertaining to* anti- *against* -muscarin- *muscarine*	Blocking the muscarinic acetylcholine receptors
cachexia	kah-**KEK**-see-ah	P/ R/	cach- *bad* -exia *condition of body*	A general weight loss and wasting of the body
cannabinoid	can-**AH**-bi-noyd	S/ R/	-oid *resembling* cannabin- *hemp*	A group of chemical compounds, some of which increase appetite and others treat nausea and vomiting
laxative	**LAK**-sah-tiv	S/ R/CF	-tive *pertaining to* lax/a- *looseness*	An oral agent that promotes the expulsion of feces
motility	moh-**TILL**-ih-tee	S/ R/	-ility *condition, state of* mot- *to move*	The ability for spontaneous movement
proton pump inhibitor (PPI)	**PROH**-ton PUMP in-**HIB**-ih-tor	R/ R/ S/ R/	proton *first* pump *pump* -or *a doer* inhibit- *repress*	Agent that blocks production of gastric acid
stool	STOOL		Old English *a seat*	The matter discharged in one movement of the bowels

Exercises

 Case Report 9.4

You are

. . . a medical transcriptionist at Fulwood Medical Center.

You are communicating with

. . . one of Fulwood's physicians, Dr. Stewart Walsh, who has dictated this letter to request authorization for a surgical procedure:

In Mrs. Jones's case, the **gastric** bypass procedure reduced the size of her stomach from 2 quarts to 2 ounces. The bypass was taken to the mid-ileum (middle part of the small intestine). This resulted in her being able to eat less and to absorb less. She had no complications from the **laparoscopic** procedure and lost 35 pounds in the 2 months that followed.

Fulwood Medical Center
3333 Medical Parkway, Fulwood, MI 01234
555-247-6100

Center for Bariatric Surgery

Charles Leavenworth, MD
Medical Director
Lombard Insurance Company
One Lombard Place
Haverson, MI 01233

10/07/2024
Request for authorization of surgery
Mrs. Martha Jones   Subscriber ID: 056437

Dear Doctor Leavenworth,

Mrs. Jones is a 52-year-old former waitress, recently divorced. She is 5 feet 4 inches tall and weighs 275 pounds. She has type 2 diabetes with frequent episodes of hypoglycemia and also ketoacidosis, requiring three different hospitalizations. She now has diabetic retinopathy and peripheral vasculitis. Complicating this are hypertension (185/110), coronary artery disease, and pulmonary edema. In spite of monthly meetings with our nutritionist, she has gained 25 pounds in the past six months.

To reduce and control her weight, I am proposing to perform a gastric bypass using a laparoscopic approach. We will need to admit her two days prior to surgery to control her blood sugar and cardiovascular problems, and we anticipate that she will remain in the hospital for two days after surgery, barring any complications. She is also very aware of the necessary follow-up to the procedure and the counseling required for a new lifestyle.

We believe not only that this is an essential procedure medically but that it will reduce in the long term the financial burden of her multiple therapies and improve the quality of the patient's life. Enclosed is supportive documentation of her current history and medical problems.

Your company has designated our hospital as a Center of Excellence for bariatric surgery, and I look forward to your prompt agreement with this approach for this patient.

Sincerely,

Stewart Walsh, MD, FACS
Chief of Surgery

A. Read *Case Report 9.4. Then provide the correct term that answers each question. Fill in the blanks.*   **LO 9.2, 9.4, 9.7, 9.8, 9.10, and 9.11**

1. What is the term for the type of surgery being proposed for Mrs. Jones? _____

2. What method of surgery will be used to perform the procedure?_____

3. What disease has previously caused Mrs. Jones to be hospitalized?_____

4. What type of specialist has worked with Dr. Walsh to explain the procedure to Ms. Jones?_____

5. What type of specialist attempted to help Ms. Jone with her diet?_____

B. Use *the correct terms for patient documentation. Using the terms provided below, fill in the blanks with the correct term. Not all terms will be used. Fill in the blanks.*   **LO 9.2, 9.7, and 9.8**

endoscopy   proctoscopy   colonoscopy   enema   gastroenterologist   sigmoidoscopy   barium   angiography

A patient is complaining of blood in his stool. The physician requested that you schedule a **(1)**_____ **(2)**_____ with the radiology department. One week later, the test results came back inconclusive.
The physician decided that further tests were needed, and therefore wished to view the inside of the large intestines. Because the physician believed the source of the bleeding was in the large intestine, she ordered a **(3)**_____. The medical assistant called the hospital's **(4)**_____ department to schedule the procedure.

C. Use *word elements to build medical terms. Given the definition of the procedure, provide the correct word element to create the medical term. Fill in the blanks.*   **LO 9.1 and 9.9**

1. Surgical incision to remove a gallstone: cholelitho/ _____

2. Surgical removal of the appendix: _____ /ectomy

3. Surgery to create an opening from a tubular structure to the outside: _____ /tomy

4. Surgical removal of the gallbladder: chole/ _____ /ectomy

5. Artificial opening from the ileum to the outside of the body: ile/ _____ /tomy

D. Deconstruct *medical terms to determine their meanings. Select the correct answer for each question.*   **LO 9.1, 9.3, and 9.9**

1. In the procedure ERCP, the "E" stands for
   a. enteric   **b.** echo   **c.** endoscopic   **d.** electrical

2. In the procedure of inserting a nasogastric tube, the practitioner first inserts the tube through the
   a. nose   **b.** mouth   **c.** stomach   **d.** rectum

3. In the procedure ERCP, the "C" tells you that the structure being treated is the
   a. stomach   **b.** pancreas   **c.** biliary ducts   **d.** duodenum

4. In an anastomosis, the root means
   a. removal   **b.** creation of an opening   **c.** join together   **d.** incision

E. Match *the definition in the first column with the correct medication it is describing in the second column.*   **LO 9.9**

_____   1. inhibits proton pumps in the stomach   **a.** Maalox

_____   2. treats motion sickness   **b.** Imodium

_____   3. neutralizes gastric acid and relieves heartburn   **c.** Tagamet

_____   4. used for treatment of chemotherapy nausea   **d.** Nexium

_____   5. antidiarrheal drug   **e.** Benadryl

_____   6. histamine blocker used to treat GERD   **f.** Zofran

F. Construct *the correct medical term to match the definitions. If a term does not have a particular element, insert N/A. Fill in the blanks.* **LO 9.1, 9.7, and 9.8**

1. inadequate gastrointestinal absorption of nutrients

   _____ / _____ / _____
   P   R/CF   S

2. abnormally frequent and loose stools

   _____ / _____ / _____
   P   R/CF   S

3. examination of a hollow structure with a special instrument

   _____ / _____ / _____
   P   R/CF   S

4. excessive amount of gas in stomach and intestines

   _____ / _____ / _____
   P   R/CF   S

5. the instrument used for endoscopy

   _____ / _____ / _____
   P   R/CF   S

G. Correct pronunciation is key when communicating to other health care providers, patients, and their families. Choose the correct pronunciation for each medical term. **LO 9.1 and 9.2**

1. The first portion of the root in the term ileum sounds like:
   a. ill
   b. eye
   c. uhl
   d. iee

2. The first syllable in the term sphincter rhymes with:
   a. rank
   b. bike
   c. rink
   d. beak

3. Identify the proper pronunciation of dysentery:
   a. **DIS**-en-tare-ee
   b. **DIS**-en-tar-eh
   c. dice-en-tar-**EE**
   d. di-**YICE**-en-**TARE**-ee

4. The correct pronunciation for the term that means an examination of the inside of the anus and rectum:
   a. pan-en-**DOS**-koh-pee
   b. **EN**-te-oss-**KOH**-pee
   c. prok-**TOSS**-koh-pee
   d. koh-**LON**-oss-**KOH**-pee

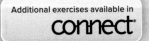
Additional exercises available in
connect

Chapter Review exercises, along with additional practice items, are available in Connect!

The Nervous System and Mental Health

The Essentials of the Languages of Neurology and Psychiatry

Learning Outcomes

Your roles are to perform electroneurodiagnostic evaluations, communicate with patients and family members communicate with other health professionals, and maintain and document history and care for patients with nervous system or mental health issues. To perform these roles, you must be able to:

LO 10.1 Use roots, combining forms, **suffixes,** and **prefixes** to construct and analyze (deconstruct) medical terms related to the nervous system and mental health.

LO 10.2 Spell and pronounce correctly medical terms related to the nervous system and mental health to communicate them with accuracy and precision in any health care setting.

LO 10.3 Define accepted abbreviations related to the nervous system and mental health.

LO 10.4 Relate the structures of the brain, cranial nerves, spinal cord, peripheral nerves, and meninges to their functions.

LO 10.5 Identify and describe disorders of the brain, cranial nerves, spinal cord, and meninges, and in the management of pain.

LO 10.6 Identify and describe common mental health disorders.

LO 10.7 Describe the diagnostic procedures, therapeutic methods, and pharmacologic agents used in treating disorders of the nervous system and mental health.

LO 10.8 Identify health professionals involved in the care of patients with nervous system diseases and disorders.

LO 10.9 Identify health professionals involved in the care of patients with mental health diseases and disorders.

LO 10.10 Apply your knowledge of medical terms relating to the nervous system and mental health to documentation, medical records, and medical reports.

LO 10.11 Translate the medical terms relating to the nervous system and mental health into everyday language in order to communicate clearly with patients and their families.

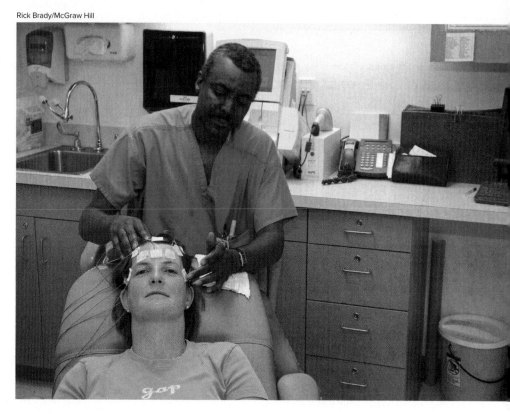
Rick Brady/McGraw Hill

The health professionals involved in the diagnosis and treatment of problems with the neurological system and mental health include the following:

- **Neurologists** are medical doctors who specialize in disorders of the nervous system.
- **Neurosurgeons** are medical doctors who perform surgical procedures on the nervous system.
- **Psychiatrists** are medical doctors who are licensed in the diagnosis and treatment of mental disorders.
- **Anesthesiologists** are medical doctors who are certified to administer anesthetics and can also be responsible for pain management.
- **Psychologists** are professionals who are licensed in the science concerned with the behavior of the human mind.
- **Licensed Professional Counselors (LPC)** are professionals who treat individuals with mental, behavioral, and emotional problems and disorders.
- **Neuropsychologists** are licensed professionals who evaluate the patient's memory, language, and cognitive functions, and develop appropriate treatment plans.
- **Electroneurodiagnostic technologists (END)** (also called EEG technicians) are professionals who operate specialized equipment that measures the electrical activity of the brain, peripheral nervous system, and spinal cord.

Structure and Function of the Nervous System

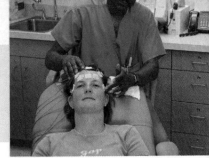

Rick Brady/McGraw Hill

The trillions of cells in your body must communicate and work together for you to function effectively. This communication is done through your **nervous system**, so it is essential that you understand how this system operates.

Structure of the Nervous System (LO 10.2 and 10.4)

The nervous system *(Figure 10.1)* has two major anatomical subdivisions.

1. The **central nervous system (CNS)**, consisting of the brain and spinal cord *(Figure 10.2)*; and
2. The **peripheral nervous system (PNS)**, consisting of all the **neurons** and **nerves** outside the central nervous system. It includes 12 pairs of cranial nerves originating from the brain and 31 pairs of spinal nerves originating from the spinal cord.

The peripheral nervous system is further subdivided into:

i. The **sensory division,** in which sensory nerves (**afferent** nerves) carry messages toward the spinal cord and brain from sense organs; and

ii. The **motor division,** in which motor nerves (**efferent** nerves) carry messages away from the brain and spinal cord to muscles and organs.

  a. The **visceral motor division** is called the **autonomic nervous system (ANS).** It carries signals to glands and to cardiac and smooth muscles. It operates at a subconscious level outside your voluntary control and has two subdivisions:

  • The **sympathetic division** arouses the body for action by increasing the heart and respiratory rates to increase oxygen supply to the brain and muscles.

  • The **parasympathetic division** calms the body, slowing down the heart and respiratory rates but stimulating digestion.

  b. The **somatic motor division** carries signals to the skeletal muscles and is within your voluntary control.

Abbreviations

ANS	autonomic nervous system
CNS	central nervous system
PNS	peripheral nervous system

▼ **FIGURE 10.1**
Components of the Nervous System.

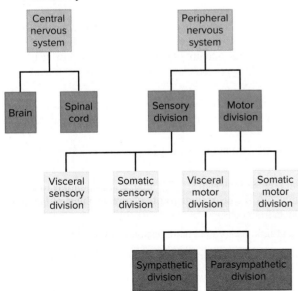

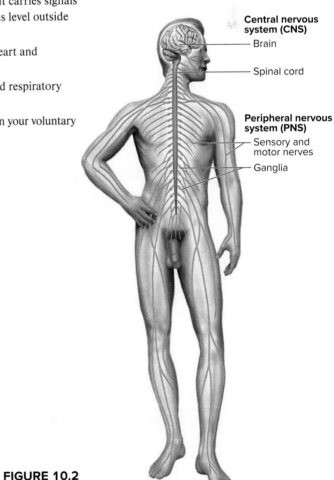

Central nervous system (CNS)
— Brain
— Spinal cord

Peripheral nervous system (PNS)
— Sensory and motor nerves
— Ganglia

▶ **FIGURE 10.2**
The Nervous System.

WORD	PRONUNCIATION	ELEMENTS		DEFINITION
afferent (Note: *Also called sensory; opposite of efferent*)	**AFF**-eh-rent		Latin *to bring to*	Moving toward a center; for example, nerve fibers conducting *impulses to the spinal cord and brain*
efferent (Note: *Also called motor; opposite of afferent*)	**EFF**-eh-rent		Latin *to bring away from*	Moving away from a center; for example, conducting nerve impulses away *from the brain or spinal cord*
autonomic	awe-toh-**NOM**-ik	S/ P/ R/	-ic *pertaining to* auto- *self* -nom- *law*	Self-governing visceral motor division of the peripheral nervous system
motor	**MOH**-tor		Latin *to move*	Structures of the nervous system that send impulses out to cause muscles to contract or glands to secrete
nerve	NERV		Latin *nerve*	A cord of nerve fibers bound together by connective tissue
nervous system	**NER**-vus **SIS**-tem	S/ R/	-ous *pertaining to* nerv- *nerve* system, Greek *an organized whole*	The whole, integrated nerve apparatus
neuron	**NYUR**-on		Greek *nerve*	Technical term for a nerve cell; consists of cell body with its dendrites and axons
parasympathetic (Note: *This term contains two prefixes.*)	pair-ah-sim-pah-**THET**-ik	S/ P/ P/ R/	-ic *pertaining to* para- *beside* -sym- *together* -pathet- *suffering*	Division of the autonomic nervous system; has opposite effects to the sympathetic division
sensory	**SEN**-soh-ree	S/ R/	-ory *having the function of* sens- *feel*	Pertaining to sensation; structures of the nervous system that carry impulses to the brain
somatic	soh-**MAT**-ik	S/ R/	-ic *pertaining to* somat- *body*	A division of the peripheral nervous system serving the skeletal muscles OR relating to the body in general
sympathetic	sim-pah-**THET**-ik	S/ P/ R/	-ic *pertaining to* sym- *together* -pathet- *suffering*	Division of the autonomic nervous system operating at an unconscious level
visceral (adj)	**VISS**-er-al	S/ R/	-al *pertaining to* viscer- **internal organs**	Pertaining to the internal organs
viscus viscera (pl)	**VISS**-kus **VISS**-er-ah		Latin *an internal organ*	Any single internal organ

Functions of the Nervous System (LO 10.2 and 10.4)

Optimal communication between your nervous system and all the cells in your body requires that the following five functions are always working smoothly:

1. **Sensory input** to the brain comes from receptors all over your body at both the conscious and subconscious levels. You are conscious of external stimuli that you receive from your body as it interacts with your environment. Inside your body, internal stimuli concerning the amount of oxygen and carbon dioxide in your blood, and other homeostatic variables like your body temperature, are being processed continually at the subconscious level.

2. **Motor output** from your brain stimulates the skeletal muscles to contract, which enables you to move. Your nervous system controls the production of sweat, saliva, and digestive enzymes without active input from you (involuntary).

3. **Evaluation and integration** occur in your brain and spinal cord to process the **sensory** input, initiate a response, and store the event in memory.

4. **Homeostasis** is maintained by your nervous system taking in internal sensory input and responding to it. For example, the nervous system responds by stimulating the heart to deliver the correct volume of blood to ensure oxygenation of and removal of waste products from cells.

5. **Mental activity** occurs in your brain so that you can think, feel, understand, respond, and remember.

Cells of the Nervous System (LO 10.2 and 10.4)

Neurons (nerve cells) receive stimuli and transmit impulses to other neurons or to organ receptors. Each neuron consists of a cell body and two types of processes or extensions, called **axons** and **dendrites** *(Figure 10.3)*.

Dendrites are short, multiple, highly branched extensions of the neuron's cell body. They direct impulses toward the cell body. A single axon, or nerve fiber, arises from the cell body, is covered in a fatty **myelin** sheath, and carries the impulse away from the cell body. Each axon measures a few millimeters to a meter in length.

Bundles of axons appear white in color and create the **white matter** of the brain and spinal cord. Neuron cell bodies, dendrites, and synapses appear gray and create the **gray matter**.

The axon terminates in a network of small branches that ends at a **synapse** (junction) with a dendrite from another neuron, or with a receptor on a muscle cell or gland cell *(Figure 10.4)*. **Neurotransmitters** cross the synapse to stimulate or inhibit another neuron or the cell of a muscle or gland. Examples of neurotransmitters are norepinephrine, serotonin, and **dopamine**.

Groups of cell bodies cluster together to form ganglia, and groups of cell bodies and axons collect together to form nerves.

The trillion neurons in the nervous system are outnumbered 50 to 1 by the supportive **glial** cells (**neuroglia**).

The blood-brain barrier is a physical barrier—composed of glial cells and the capillary blood vessel walls—that prevents foreign substances, toxins, and infections from leaving the bloodstream and affecting the brain cells.

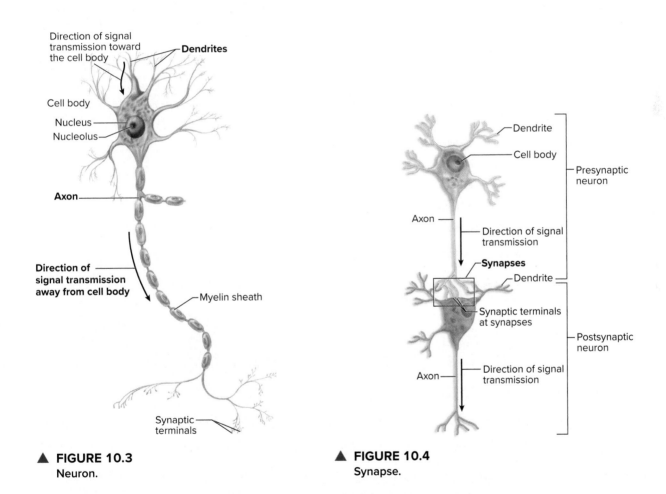

▲ **FIGURE 10.3**
Neuron.

▲ **FIGURE 10.4**
Synapse.

P = Prefix   S = Suffix   R = Root   R/CF = Combining Form

WORD	PRONUNCIATION		ELEMENTS	DEFINITION
axon	ACK-son		Greek *axis*	Single process of a nerve cell carrying nervous impulses away from the cell body
dendrite	DEN-dright		Greek *looking like a tree*	Branched extension of the nerve cell body that receives nervous stimuli
dopamine	DOH-pah-meen		Precursor of norepinephrine	Neurotransmitter in some specific small areas of the brain
glia glial (adj) neuroglia	GLEE-ah GLEE-al nyu-ROG-lee-ah	S/ R/ R/CF	Greek *glue* -al *pertaining to* -glia *glue* neur/o- *nerve*	Connective tissue that holds a structure together Pertaining to glia or neuroglia Connective tissue holding nervous tissue together
myelin	MY-eh-lin	S/ R/	-in *substance, chemical compound* myel- *spinal cord*	Material of the sheath around the axon of a nerve
neurotransmitter (Note: Transmit *is a word itself, so the prefix trans is in the middle of the overall word.)*	NYUR-oh-trans-MIT-er	S/ R/CF P/ R/	-er *agent* neur/o- *nerve* -trans- *across* -mitt- *send*	Chemical agent that relays messages from one nerve cell to the next
synapse	SIN-aps	P/ R/	syn- *together* -apse *clasp*	Junction between two nerve cells, or a nerve fiber and its target cell, where electrical impulses are transmitted between the cells

EXERCISES

A. Elements: *Solid knowledge of elements is the key to learning medical terminology. Match each element in first column with its correct meaning in second column.*   **LO 10.1**

_____ **1.** -ic

_____ **2.** syn-

_____ **3.** viscer-

_____ **4.** auto-

_____ **5.** myel-

_____ **6.** -glia-

a. self

b. pertaining to

c. spinal cord

d. together

e. internal organ

f. glue

B. Deconstruct *the following terms into their elements.*   **LO 10.1**

1. neurotransmitter _____ / _____ / _____ / _____

2. neuroglia _____ / _____ / _____ / _____

3. autonomic _____ / _____ / _____ / _____

4. synapse _____ / _____ / _____ / _____

The Brain and Cranial Nerves

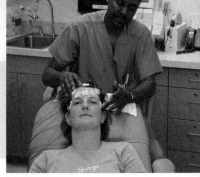

Rick Brady/McGraw Hill

The sensations of smelling the roses, seeing them, and touching them are recognized and interpreted in your brain, as are all sensations. The actions of kneeling down, cutting the rose stem, walking into the house, and placing it in a vase originate in your brain, as do all your voluntary actions.

The Brain (LO 10.2 and 10.4)

Your adult brain weighs about 3 pounds. Its size and weight are proportional to your body size, not your intelligence. Your brain is divided into three major regions: the **cerebrum**, the **brain stem**, and the **cerebellum**.

Cerebrum (LO 10.2 and 10.4)

The cerebrum makes up about 80% of your brain. It consists of two **cerebral** hemispheres, right and left which are mirror images of each other. These hemispheres are separated by a deep longitudinal fissure, and at the bottom of this, they are connected by a bridge of nerve fibers (the **corpus callosum**).

On the surface of the cerebrum, numerous ridges, **gyri,** are separated by fissures called **sulci** *(Figure 10.5).* The cerebral hemispheres are covered by a thin layer of gray matter (nerve cells and dendrites) called the cerebral **cortex**. It is folded into the gyri, and sulci, and contains 70% of all the neurons in the nervous system. Below the cerebral cortex is a mass of white matter, in which bundles of myelinated nerve fibers connect the neurons of the cortex to the rest of the nervous system.

Functional Cerebral Regions (LO 10.2 and 10.4)

Each cerebral hemisphere is divided into four lobes:

1. The **frontal lobe,** located behind the forehead, forms the anterior part of the hemisphere. This lobe is responsible for intellect, planning, problem solving, behavior, emotions and the voluntary motor control of muscles.
2. The **parietal lobe** is posterior to the frontal lobe. This lobe receives and interprets sensory information, like taste, hearing, touch, sight, and smell.
3. The **temporal lobe** is below the frontal and parietal lobes. This lobe interprets sensory experiences such as understanding language and processing emotions and information relayed by your senses.
4. The **occipital lobe** forms the posterior part of the hemisphere. This lobe interprets visual images and written words.

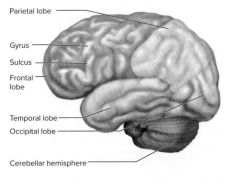

Parietal lobe

Gyrus

Sulcus

Frontal lobe

Temporal lobe

Occipital lobe

Cerebellar hemisphere

(a)

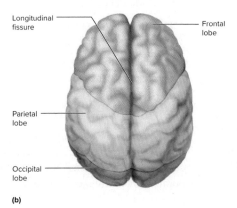

Longitudinal fissure

Frontal lobe

Parietal lobe

Occipital lobe

(b)

▲ **FIGURE 10.5** Brain.
(a) View from the left side.
(b) View from above.

Word Analysis and Definition

S = Suffix   P = Prefix   R = Root   R/CF = Combining Form

WORD	PRONUNCIATION		ELEMENTS	DEFINITION
brainstem	BRAYN-stem		brain Old English *brain* stem Old English *support*	Region of the brain that includes the thalamus, pineal gland, pons, fourth ventricle, and medulla oblongata
cerebellum	ser-eh-**BELL**-um	S/ R/	-um *structure* cerebell- *little brain*	The most posterior area of the brain located between the midbrain and the cerebral hemispheres
cerebrospinal (adj) cerebrospinal fluid (CSF)	**SER**-ee-broh-**SPY**-nal	S/ R/CF R/	-al *pertaining to* cerebr/o- *brain* -spin- *spinal cord*	Pertaining to the brain and spinal cord Fluid formed in the ventricles of the brain; surrounds the brain and spinal cord
cerebrum cerebral (adj)	**SER**-ee-brum **SER**-ee-bral	S/ R/	Latin *brain* -al *pertaining to* cerebr- *cerebrum*	Cerebral hemispheres Pertaining to the cerebral hemispheres of the brain
corpus callosum	**KOR**-pus kah-**LOW**-sum	R/ S/ R/	corpus *body* -um *structure* callos- *thickening*	Bridge of nerve fibers connecting the two cerebral hemispheres
cortex cortical (adj)	**KOR**-teks **KOR**-tih-kal		Latin *shell*	Gray covering of cerebral hemispheres
frontal lobe	**FRUNT**-al LOBE	S/ R/	-al *pertaining to* front- *front of*	Front area of the cerebral hemisphere
gyrus gyri (pl)	**JI**-rus **JI**-ree		Greek *circle*	Rounded elevation on the surface of the cerebral hemispheres
hypothalamus hypothalamic (adj)	high-poh-**THAL**-ah-muss high-poh-thah-**LAM**-ik	P/ S/ S/ R/	hypo- *below* -us *pertaining to* -ic *pertaining to* -thalam- *thalamus*	An endocrine gland in the floor and wall of the third ventricle of the brain Pertaining to the hypothalamus
occipital lobe	ock-**SIP**-it-al LOBE	S/ R/	-al *pertaining to* occipit- *back of head*	Posterior area of the cerebral hemisphere
parietal lobe	pah-**RYE**-eh-tal LOBE	S/ R/	-al *pertaining to* pariet- *wall*	Area of the brain under the parietal bone
sulcus sulci (pl)	**SUL**-cuss **SUL**-sigh		Latin *furrow, ditch*	Groove on the surface of the cerebral hemispheres that separates gyri
temporal lobe	**TEM**-pore-al LOBE	S/ R/	-al *pertaining to* tempor- *time, temple*	Posterior two-thirds of the cerebral hemispheres
thalamus	**THAL**-ah-mus		Greek *inner room*	Mass of gray matter under the ventricle in each cerebral hemisphere

Abbreviation

CSF   cerebrospinal fluid

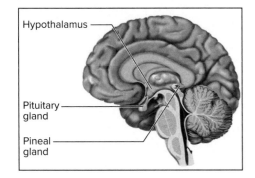

▲ FIGURE 10.6
Hypothalamus, Pituitary Gland, and Pineal Gland.

Deep inside each cerebral hemisphere are spaces called ventricles, which contain watery **cerebrospinal fluid (CSF)**. CSF circulates through the ventricles and around the brain and spinal cord. It helps to protect, cushion, and provide nutrition for the brain and spinal cord.

Located beneath the cerebral hemispheres and ventricles are the:

- **Thalamus**, which receives all sensory impulses and channels them to the appropriate region of the cortex for interpretation; and
- **Hypothalamus**, *Figure 10.6* which regulates blood pressure, body temperature, water, and electrolyte balance.

Brainstem and Cerebellum (LO 10.2 and 10.4)

The **brainstem** relays sensory impulses from peripheral nerves to higher brain centers. It also controls vital cardiovascular and respiratory activities.

The **cerebellum**, a smaller portion of the brain located between the cerebrum and brainstem, coordinates skeletal muscle activity to maintain the body's posture and balance.

Cranial Nerves, Spinal Cord, and Meninges (LO 10.4)

Cranial Nerves (LO 10.4)

Your brain communicates with the rest of your body through the cranial nerves and spinal cord. The cranial nerves are part of the peripheral nervous system. They originate on the lower or inferior surface of the brain and are identified by names and numbers, the latter written in Roman numerals *(Figure 10.7)*.

The cranial nerves provide sensory and motor functions for your head and neck areas except for the vagus nerve, which supplies your thorax and abdomen.

Spinal Cord (LO 10.2 and 10.4)

Your spinal cord lies within, and is protected by, the vertebral canal of the spinal column. It has 31 segments, each of which gives rise to a pair of spinal nerves *(Figure 10.8)*. These are the major link between the brain and the peripheral nervous system, and are the pathway for sensory and motor impulses.

Your spinal cord is divided into four regions *(Figure 10.8)*:

1. The **cervical** region is continuous with the brain stem (lower part of the brain). It contains the motor neurons that supply the neck, shoulders, and upper limbs through 8 pairs of cervical spinal nerves (C1–C8);

2. The **thoracic** region contains the motor neurons that supply the thoracic cage, rib movement, vertebral column movement, and postural back muscles through 12 pairs of thoracic spinal nerves (T1–T12);

3. The **lumbar** region supplies the hips and the front of the lower limbs through 5 pairs of lumbar nerves (L1–L5); and

4. The **sacral** region supplies the buttocks, genitalia, and backs of the lower limbs through 5 sacral nerves (S1–S5) and 1 coccygeal nerve, relative to the small bone at the base of the spine.

Meninges (LO 10.2 and 10.4)

Your brain and spinal cord are protected by the cranium and the vertebrae, cushioned by the CSF, and covered by the **meninges** *(Figure 10.9)*. The meninges have three layers:

1. The **dura mater** is the outermost layer of tough connective tissue attached to the cranium's inner surface. Within the vertebral canal the dura mater splits into two sheets, separated by the **epidural space**.

2. The **arachnoid mater** is a thin web over the brain and spinal cord. The CSF is contained in the **subarachnoid space** between the arachnoid and pia mater.

3. The **pia mater** is the innermost layer of the meninges, attached to the surface of the brain and spinal cord. It supplies nerves and blood vessels that nourish the outer cells of the brain and spinal cord.

Oh	(olfactory-I)
once	(optic-II)
one	(oculomotor-III)
takes	(trochlear-IV)
the	(trigeminal-V)
anatomy	(abducens-VI)
final	(facial-VII)
very	(vestibulocochlear-VIII)
good	(glossopharyngeal-IX)
vacations	(vagus-X)
are	(accessory-XI)
heavenly!	(hypoglossal-XII)

▲ **FIGURE 10.7** Cranial Nerves.
This mnemonic device will help you remember the cranial nerves. Use the sentence in column one (read down) to help you remember the correct order and names of the cranial nerves.

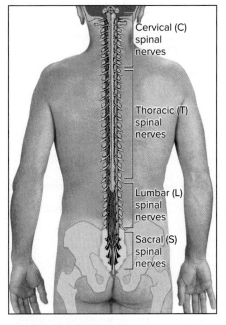

▲ **FIGURE 10.8**
Spinal Cord Regions.

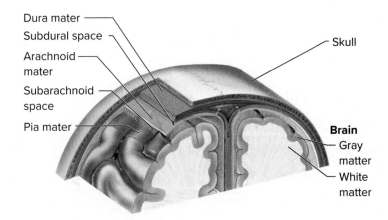

▲ **FIGURE 10.9** Meninges of Brain.

WORD	PRONUNCIATION	ELEMENTS		DEFINITION
arachnoid mater	ah-**RACK**-noyd **MAY**-ter	S/ R/ R/	-oid *resembling* arachn- *cobweb, spider* mater *mother*	Weblike middle layer of the three meninges
cervical (**Note:** Cervical also is used to refer to a region of the uterus.)	**SER**-vih-kal	S/ R/	-al *pertaining to* cervic- *neck*	Pertaining to the neck region
dura mater (**Note:** Both terms are stand-alone roots.)	**DYU**-rah **MAY**-ter	R/ R/	dura *hard* mater *mother*	Hard, fibrous outer layer of the meninges
epidural	ep-ih-**DYU**-ral	S/ P/ R/	-al *pertaining to* epi- *above* -dur- *dura*	Above the dura
epidural space				Space between the dura mater and the wall of the vertebral canal
lumbar	**LUM**-bar		Latin *loins*	Pertaining to the region in the back and sides between the ribs and pelvis
meninges	meh-**NIN**-jeez		Greek *membrane*	Three-layered covering of the brain and spinal cord
pia mater (stand-alone roots)	**PEE**-ah **MAY**-ter	R/ R/	pia *delicate* mater *mother*	Delicate inner layer of the meninges
subarachnoid space	sub-ah-**RACK**-noyd **SPASE**	S/ P/ R/	-oid *resembling* sub- *under* -arachn- *cobweb, spider*	Space between the pia mater and the arachnoid membrane
thoracic	thor-**ASS**-ik	S/ R/	-ic *pertaining to* thorac- *chest*	Pertaining to the chest (thorax)

EXERCISES

A. Roots. *The lobes of the cerebral hemispheres share a common suffix -al, meaning pertaining to. It is the root that describes the exact location of the lobe in the cerebral hemispheres. Use your knowledge of roots to understand the anatomical location of the lobes. Fill in the blanks.*   **LO 10.1, 10.2, and 10.4**

1. The cerebral lobe located above the ear: _____/al. The root means _____.

    2. The cerebral lobe located behind the forehead: _____/al. The root means _____.

3. The most posterior cerebral lobe: _____/al. The root means: _____.

B. Describe the structure of the cerebrum. *Identify the cerebral structures being described. Fill in the blanks.*   **LO 10.1 and 10.2**

1. Elevation or "ridge" of the cerebrum:

    singular form _____.

    plural form _____.

2. Gray covering of the cerebrum: _____.

3. Shallow indention of the cerebrum:

    singular form _____.

    plural form _____.

C. Construct the following *medical terms by filling in the missing elements. Fill in the blanks.*   **LO 10.1, 10.4, and 10.5**

1. under the arachnoid mater: _____/arachn/oid

2. weblike middle layer of meninges: _____/ _____/oid mater

3. pertaining to above the dura: _____/dur/al

4. hard, fibrous outer layer of meninges: _____ _____

D. Place the meninges in order from superficial to deep. *Place a "1" in the blank for the most superficial layer and "3" for the deepest layer. Fill in the blanks.* **LO 10.4**

_____ arachnoid mater

_____ pia mater

_____ dura mater

E. Deconstruct the terms into their basic elements. *Select the correct answer that completes each sentence.* **LO 10.1 and 10.4**

1. The term that has an element that means below:

    a. epidural

    b. analgesia

    c. subarachnoid

    d. meningitis

2. The term that has an element that means cobwebb or spider:

    a. epidural

    b. arachnoid

    c. pia mater

    d. meningitis

3. The term that has an element that means hard:

    a. dura mater

    b. analgesia

    c. subarachnoid

    d. pia mater

4. The term that has an element that means delicate:

    a. dura mater

    b. analgesia

    c. subarachnoid

    d. pia mater

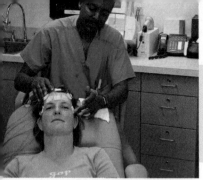

Section 10.3

Disorders of the Brain, Cranial Nerves, and Meninges

Rick Brady/McGraw Hill

AMS   altered mental status
FTD   frontotemporal dementia

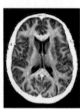

(a)

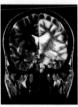

(b)

▲ **FIGURE 10.10**
Brain Sections.
(a) MRI scan of normal brain.
(b) MRI scan of Alzheimer disease showing cerebral atrophy (yellow).

Science History Images/aAamy Stock Photo

Disorders of the Brain (LO 10.2 and 10.5)

Dementia (LO 10.2 and 10.5)

The symptoms of dementia include an irreversible short-term memory loss, the inability to solve problems, and confusion. Inappropriate behavior, like wandering away, and impaired intellectual function that interferes with normal activities and relationships are also key signs of dementia.

- **Senile dementia** is not a normal part of aging and is not a specific disease. It is a term used for a collection of symptoms that can be caused by a number of disorders affecting the brain.

- **Alzheimer disease** *(Figure 10.10)*—the most common form of dementia—affects about 10% of the population over 65, and up to 50% of the population over 85. Nerve cells in the areas of the brain associated with memory and **cognition** are replaced by abnormal protein clumps and tangles.

- **Vascular dementia**—the second most common form of dementia—can come on gradually when arteries supplying the brain become arteriosclerotic (narrowed or blocked), depriving the brain of oxygen. It can also occur suddenly after a stroke *(see later in this chapter).*

- **Frontotemporal dementia (FTD)** is caused by progressive cell degeneration in the brain's frontal and temporal lobes, which control planning and judgment, emotions, speaking and understanding speech, and certain types of movement. It accounts for 10% to 15% of all dementias, but it is more common in those younger than 65.

Other conditions causing dementia include reactions to medications, like sedatives and antiarthritics; depression in the elderly; and infections, such as AIDS or encephalitis.

Confusion is used to describe people who cannot process information normally. They cannot answer questions appropriately, understand where they are, or remember important facts, like their name and address.

Delirium is an altered mental state, also known as altered mental status **(AMS),** characterized by the sudden onset of disorientation, an inability to think clearly or pay attention. The level of consciousness varies from increased wakefulness to drowsiness. It is not a disease, is reversible, and can be part of dementia or a stroke.

Word Analysis and Definition

S = Suffix   P = Prefix   R = Root   R/CF = Combining Form

WORD	PRONUNCIATION		ELEMENTS	DEFINITION
Alzheimer disease	**AWLZ**-high-mer diz-**EEZ**		Dr. Alois Alzheimer, German physician, 1864–1915	Common form of dementia
cognition	kog-**NIH**-shun		Latin *knowledge*	Process of acquiring knowledge through thinking, learning, and memory
confusion	kon-**FEW**-zhun	S/ R/	-ion *condition, action* confus- *bewildered*	Mental state in which environmental stimuli are not processed appropriately
delirium	de-**LIR**-ee-um	S/ R/	-um *structure* deliri- *disorientation, confusion*	Acute altered state of consciousness with agitation and disorientation
dementia	dee-**MEN**-she-ah	S/ P/ R/	-ia *condition* de- *removal, without* -ment- *mind*	Chronic, progressive, irreversible loss of the mind's cognitive, and intellectual functions
senile	**SEE**-nile	S/ R/	-ile *pertaining to* sen- *old age*	Characteristic of old age
vascular	**VAS**-kyu-lar	S/ R/	-ar *pertaining to* vascul- *blood vessel*	Pertaining to a blood vessel

Epilepsy (LO 10.5)

Epilepsy is a chronic disorder in which clusters of neurons (nerve cells) discharge their electrical signals in an abnormal rhythm. This disturbed electrical activity (a **seizure** or a **convulsion**) can cause strange sensations and behavior, convulsions, and loss of consciousness. The causes of epilepsy are numerous, from abnormal brain development to brain damage.

In 2017, the **International League Against Epilepsy** revised its classification system for seizures based on the onset of the seizure. The three categories are focal, generalized, and unknown, and within each are the subcategories of motor and nonmotor. Focal seizures also have the subcategory of retained or impaired awareness.

Focal seizures, previously termed partial seizures, occur when the epileptic activity is in one localized area of the brain only, causing, for example, involuntary jerking movements of a single limb.

1. **Generalized onset seizures** occur in both sides of the brain and are categorized as motor onset or nonmotor onset.

   a. Nonmotor (**Absence) seizures,** previously known as "**petit mal,**" which begin between ages 4 and 14. The child stares vacantly for a few seconds and may be accused of daydreaming.

   b. Motor (**Tonic-clonic) seizures,** previously called "**grand mal,**" which are dramatic. The person experiences a **loss of consciousness (LOC),** breathing stops, the eyes roll up, and the jaw is clenched. This "tonic" phase lasts for 30 to 60 seconds. It is followed by the "clonic" phase, in which the whole body shakes with a series of violent, rhythmic jerkings of the limbs. The seizures last for a couple of minutes, and then consciousness returns.

2. **Focal onset seizures** can also be categorized as either motor onset or nonmotor onset. For either category of focal onset seizures, the description is relatively the same except motor onset can result in epileptic spasms and tonic-clonic seizures.

3. **Unknown onset seizures** can also be categorized as either motor onset or nonmotor onset. With the motor type of unknown onset seizure, tonic-clonic or epileptic spasms are present, whereas with nonmotor unknown onset seizure, behavior arrest is the most common observation.

   Febrile seizures, which are triggered by a fever in infants and toddlers aged 6 months to 5 years. Very few of these children go on to develop epilepsy.

   Status epilepticus is considered to be a medical emergency. It is defined as having one continuous seizure or recurrent seizures without regaining consciousness for 30 minutes or more.

Any seizure may be followed by a period of diminished function in the area of the brain surrounding the seizure's main origin. This temporary neurologic deficit is called a **postictal** state.

Seizures may be followed by a **postictal state** period of diminished function in the area of the brain surrounding the seizure focus.

Syncope and cataplexy are symptoms of other conditions that resemble symptoms of epilepsy.

- **Syncope** (fainting or passing out) is a temporary loss of consciousness and posture. It is usually due to hypotension and the associated deficient oxygen supply (hypoxia) to the brain.

- **Cataplexy** is the sudden loss of voluntary muscle tone with brief episodes of total paralysis associated with **narcolepsy.** Sleep-paralysis, excessive daytime sleepiness, and hallucinations are also symptoms of narcolepsy.

Keynotes

- Epilepsy affects 1 in 200 people, and 50% of cases develop before age 10.

- Status epilepticus is a medical emergency and requires maintenance of the airway, breathing, and circulation and intravenous administration of anticonvulsant drugs.

- The first-aid treatment during a seizure is to place the person in a reclining position, cushion the head, and turn the person on his or her side. Do not try to hold down the person's arms or legs or restrain the tongue.

- There is no cure for tic disorders, but they can be treated pharmacologically with haloperidol or clonidine.

Abbreviations

ILEA	International League Against Epilepsy
LOC	loss of consciousness

Word Analysis and Definition

S = Suffix P = Prefix R = Root R/CF = Combining Form

WORD	PRONUNCIATION		ELEMENTS	DEFINITION
epilepsy	EP-ih-LEP-see		Greek *seizure*	Chronic brain disorder due to paroxysmal excessive neuronal discharges
epileptic (adj) (**Note:** *An epileptic episode is called a* seizure.)	EP-ih-LEP-tik SEE-zhur	S/ R/	-ic *pertaining to* epilept- *seizure*	Pertaining to or suffering from epilepsy
febrile	FEB-ril or FEB-rile or FEE-bril		Latin *febris*	Pertaining to or having a fever
grand mal	GRAHN MAL	R/ R/	grand *big* mal *bad*	Previous name for generalized motor (tonic-clonic) seizure
narcolepsy	NAR-koh-lep-see	S/ R/CF	-lepsy *seizure* narc/o- *stupor*	Involuntary falling asleep
petit mal	peh-TEE MAL	R/ R/	petit *small* mal *bad*	Previous name for nonmotor (absence) seizures
postictal (adj)	post-IK-tal	S/ P/ R/	-al *pertaining to* post- *after* -ict- *seizure*	Transient neurologic deficit after a seizure
ictal (adj)	IK-tal	S/	-al *pertaining to*	Pertaining to, or a condition caused by, a stroke or epilepsy
tic	TIK		French *tic*	Sudden, involuntary, repeated contraction of muscles
tonic	TON-ik	S/ R/	-ic *pertaining to* ton- *pressure, tension*	State of muscular contraction
tonic-clonic seizure	TON-ik-KLON-ik SEE-zhur	R/ S/ R/	clon- *tumult* -ure *process* seiz- *to grab*	The body alternates between excessive muscular rigidity (tonic) and jerking muscular contractions (clonic)

- Risk factors for ischemic strokes are hypertension, diabetes mellitus, high cholesterol levels, smoking, and obesity.
- Risk factors for hemorrhagic strokes are hypertension, cerebral arteriovenous malformations, and cerebral aneurysms.
- More than 10% of people who have a TIA will have a stroke within 3 months.

Cerebrovascular Accidents (CVAs) or Strokes (LO 10.3 and 10.5)

A **stroke** (also known as a **cerebrovascular accident** or **CVA**) occurs when the blood supply to a part of the brain is suddenly interrupted, depriving the brain cells of oxygen. Some cells die; others are badly damaged. With timely treatment, the damaged cells can be saved. There are two types of stroke:

1. **Ischemic strokes** account for about 90% of all strokes and are caused by:

   a. **Atherosclerosis**: Plaque in the wall of a cerebral artery *(Figure 10.11a);* or

   b. **Embolism:** A blood clot in a cerebral artery originating from elsewhere in the body *(Figure 10.11b).*

2. **Hemorrhagic strokes (intracranial hemorrhages)** occur when a blood vessel in the brain bursts or when a cerebral **aneurysm** ruptures.

Symptoms of Strokes (LO 10.3 and 10.5)

The symptoms of a stroke can include the sudden onset of numbness or weakness, especially on one side of the body; difficulty in walking, balance, or coordination; trouble speaking or understanding speech; trouble seeing in one or both eyes; dizziness; confusion; and severe headache. A method to remember common warning signs of stroke is to use the acronym FAST:

Face—Ask the person to smile. Does one side of the Face droop?

Arms—Ask the person to raise both arms. Does one Arm drift downward?

Speech—Ask the person to repeat a simple phrase. Is his or her Speech slurred or strange?

Time—If any of the previous signs is present, Time to call 911 immediately.

Although stroke is a disease of the brain, it can affect the whole body. A common residual disability is complete paralysis of one side of the body, called **hemiplegia.** If one side of the body is weak rather than paralyzed, the disability is **hemiparesis.**

Transient Ischemic Attack (TIA) (LO 10.3 and 10.5)

Transient ischemic attacks (TIAs) are small, short-term strokes with symptoms lasting for less than 24 hours. If neurologic symptoms persist for more than 24 hours, the condition is considered a full-blown stroke (CVA) with resulting brain cell damage and cell death.

The most frequent cause of TIAs is a small embolus that occludes (blocks) a small artery in the brain. Often, the embolus arises from a clot in the atrium in atrial fibrillation or from an atherosclerotic plaque in a carotid artery. Treatment is directed at the underlying cause. A **carotid endarterectomy** (CEA) may be necessary if a carotid artery is significantly blocked with plaque.

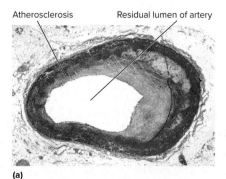

Atherosclerosis   Residual lumen of artery

(a)

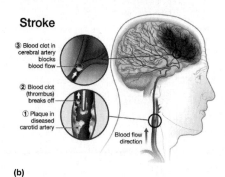

Stroke

③ Blood clot in cerebral artery blocks blood flow

② Blood clot (thrombus) breaks off

① Plaque in diseased carotid artery

Blood flow direction

(b)

◀ **FIGURE 10.11**
Causes of Ischemic Strokes.
(a) Atherosclerosis in a cerebral artery, leaving a small, residual lumen.
(b) Embolus blocking an artery. Healthy tissue is on the left (tan); blood-starved tissue is on the right (gray).

Kateryna Kon/Shutterstock

WORD	PRONUNCIATION		ELEMENTS	DEFINITION
aneurysm aneurysm (adj)	AN-yur-izm		Greek *dilation*	Circumscribed dilation of an artery or cardiac chamber
atherosclerosis	ATH-er-oh-skler-OH-sis	S/ R/CF R/CF	-sis *abnormal condition* ather/o- *porridge, gruel* -scler/o- *hardness*	Atheroma in arteries
cerebrovascular accident (**Note:** also known as a stroke)	SER-eh-broh-VAS-cyoo-lar AK-si-dent STROHK	S/ R/CF R/	-ar *pertaining to* cerebr/o- *brain* -vascul- *blood vessel* French *accident, what comes by chance*	Acute clinical event caused by an impaired cerebral circulation
embolus emboli (pl)	EM-boh-lus		Greek *plug, stopped*	Detached piece of thrombus, a mass of bacteria, quantity of air, or foreign body that blocks a blood vessel
hemiparesis	HEM-ee-pah-REE-sis	P/ R/	hemi- *half* -paresis *weakness*	Weakness of one side of the body
hemiplegia hemiplegic (adj)	hem-ee-PLEE-jee-ah hem-ee-PLEE-jik	S/ P/ R/ S/	-ia *condition* hemi- *half* -pleg- *paralysis* -ic *pertaining to*	Paralysis of one side of the body Pertaining to or suffering from hemiplegia
hemorrhage hemorrhagic	HEM-oh-raj HEM-oh-raj-ik	S/ R/ S/	-rrhage *to flow profusely* hem/o- *blood* -ic *pertaining to*	To bleed profusely Pertaining to a hemorrhage
ischemia ischemic (adj)	is-KEE-mee-ah is-KEE-mik	S/ R/ S/	-emia *blood condition* isch- *to keep back* -emic *in the blood*	Lack of blood supply to a tissue Pertaining to or affected by ischemia
transient ischemic attack (TIA)	TRAN-see-ent is-KEE-mik a-TACK	S/ R/	Latin *to pass* -emic *in the blood* isch- *to keep back* Italian *to attack*	Temporary blockage of a cerebral blood vessel resulting in stroke—like symptoms lasting less than 24 hours

Movement Disorders (LO 10.3 and 10.5)

Parkinson disease is caused by the degeneration of neurons in the basal ganglia that produce a neurotransmitter called dopamine. Motor symptoms of abnormal movements, **tremor** of the hands, rigidity, a shuffling gait, and weak voice appear and gradually become more and more severe. There is no cure.

Tourette syndrome and other **tic** disorders are characterized by episodes of involuntary, rapid, repetitive, fixed movements of individual muscle groups in the face or the limbs. They are associated with meaningless vocal sounds or meaningful words and phrases. The tics may be genetic.

Huntington disease (also known as **Huntington chorea**) is a hereditary disorder starting with mild personality changes between the ages of 30 and 50. Involuntary, irregular, jerky (**choreic**) movements and muscle weakness follow, and dementia occurs in the later stages. There is no known cure.

Neoplasm (LO 10.3 and 10.5)

Brain tumors are most often secondary tumors that have metastasized from cancers in the lung, breast, skin, or kidney. **Primary brain tumors** arise from any of the glial cells and are called **gliomas.**

Headache (LO 10.3 and 10.5)

Migraine produces an intense throbbing, pulsating pain in one area of the head, often with nausea and vomiting. It can be preceded by an **aura,** visual disturbances like flashing lights, or temporary loss of vision. Prevention is difficult.

Infections of the Brain (LO 10.3 and 10.5)

Creutzfeldt-Jakob disease (CJD) produces a rapid deterioration of mental function with difficulty in coordination of muscle movement. The agent that caused the 1996 outbreak of **mad cow disease (bovine spongiform encephalopathy, or BSE)** in the United Kingdom is the same agent causing an outbreak of **Variant Creutzfeldt-Jakob disease (vCJD)** in humans.

Brain abscess is usually a direct spread of infection from sinusitis, otitis media (middle ear infection), or mastoiditis (an infection in the skull bone behind the ear). It can also result from blood-borne pathogens arising from lung or dental infections.

Encephalitis is inflammation of the parenchyma of the brain. It is usually caused by a virus such as human immunodeficiency virus (HIV), West Nile virus, herpes simplex, or the childhood diseases of measles, mumps, chickenpox, and rubella.

Abbreviations

BSE	bovine spongiform encephalopathy
CJD	Creutzfeldt-Jakob disease
vCJD	Variant Creutzfeldt-Jakob disease

WORD	PRONUNCIATION		ELEMENTS	DEFINITION
abscess	AB-sess		Latin *a going away*	A collection of pus
aneurysm	AN-yur-izm		Greek *dilation*	Small, circumscribed dilation of an artery or cardiac chamber
aura	AWE-rah		Greek *breath of air*	Sensory experience preceding an epileptic seizure or a migraine headache
bovine spongiform encephalopathy (BSE)	BO-vine SPON-jee-form en-sef-ah-LOP-ah-thee	S/ R/ S/ R/CF S/ R/CF	-ine *pertaining to* bov- *cattle* -form *appearance of* spong/i- *sponge* -pathy *disease* encephal/o- *brain*	Disease of cattle ("mad cow disease") that can be transmitted to humans, causing Creutzfeldt-Jakob disease
Creutzfeldt-Jakob disease (CJD)	KROITS-felt YAK-op DIZ-eez		Hans Creutzfeldt, 1885–1964, and Alfons Jakob, 1884–1931, German psychiatrists	Progressive, incurable, neurologic disease caused by infectious prions
encephalitis	en-SEF-ah-LIE-tis	S/ R/	-itis *inflammation* encephal- *brain*	Inflammation of brain cells and tissues
glioma	glie-OH-mah	S/ R/	-oma *tumor, mass* gli- *glue*	Tumor arising in a glial cell
Huntington disease Huntington chorea (syn)	HUN-ting-ton diz-EEZ kor-EE-ah		George Huntington, U.S. physician, 1851–1916 chorea Greek *dance*	Progressive inherited, degenerative, incurable neurologic disease
migraine	MY-grain	P/ R/	mi- *derived from hemi, half* -graine *head pain*	Paroxysmal severe headache confined to one side of the head
Parkinson's disease	PAR-kin-sons diz-EEZ		James Parkinson, British physician, 1755–1824	Disease of muscular rigidity, tremors, and a masklike facial expression
prion	PREE-on		acronym for **pr**oteinaceous **in**fectious particles	Small, infectious proteinaceous particle
stroke (same as **cerebrovascular accident, CVA**)	STROHK		Old English *to strike*	Acute clinical event caused by impaired cerebral circulation
syncope	SIN-koh-pee		Greek *cutting short*	Temporary loss of consciousness and postural tone due to diminished cerebral blood flow
tremor	TREM-or		Latin *to shake*	Small, shaking, involuntary, repetitive movements of hands, extremities, neck, or jaw
Tourette syndrome	tur-ET SIN-drome		Gilles de la Tourette, French neurologist, 1857–1904	Disorder of multiple motor and vocal tics

Keynote

- About 5.3 million Americans (2% of the population) are living with disabilities from TBI.

Abbreviations

ADL   activity of daily living
TBI   traumatic brain injury

Traumatic Brain Injury (TBI) (LO 10.3 and 10.5)

Traumatic brain injury (TBI) results from any one of many types of injuries to the head, from a fall on to a hard surface to a car accident to war injuries. Every year, physicians treat over 1 million patients who have experienced TBI; as many as 10% of these have long-term damage affecting their normal **activities of daily living (ADLs)**.

Imagine driving your car along the highway at 50 miles per hour. Suddenly, you are hit head-on by another driver. Your brain goes from 50 miles per hour to zero—instantly. Your soft brain is propelled forward and compacted against the front of your hard skull (**coup**). Next, you rebound backward, and your brain slams against the back of your skull (**contrecoup**). Your brain now has a bruise or **contusion**, if not worse damage, such as an active bleed.

A mild head injury (**concussion**) may leave you feeling dazed, confused, or unable to recall the event that caused your concussion. Repeated concussions, like those experienced by famous boxer Muhammad Ali, have a cumulative effect, leading to a reduced mental ability and reaction time, and/or trauma-induced Parkinson's disease.

A severe injury may include torn blood vessels that bleed into the brain. The brain may also tear, or swell within the hard, inflexible skull, cutting off important signals and connections.

Shaken baby syndrome (SBS) is a type of TBI produced when a baby is violently shaken. A baby has weak neck muscles and a heavy head. Shaking makes the brain bounce back and forth in the skull, leading to severe brain damage.

Posttraumatic stress disorder is associated with TBI and discussed later in this chapter.

Disorders of the Meninges (LO 10.5)

Meningitis is an inflammation of the membranes (meninges) covering the brain and spinal cord. Viral meningitis—the most common form—can occur at any age. Bacterial meningitis predominantly affects the very young or very old. **Meningococcal** meningitis is contagious, transmitted through a simple cough or sneeze. It is most commonly passed among people who live in close quarters—such as students in college dormitories.

A **subdural hematoma** is bleeding into the subdural space (below the dura mater), frequently associated with closed-head injuries and bleeding from broken veins caused by violent head rotations.

An **epidural hematoma** is a pooling of blood in the epidural space between the skull and the dura mater, often associated with a fractured skull and bleeding from an artery within the meninges.

Disorders of the Cranial Nerves (LO 10.5)

Bell palsy is a facial nerve (7th cranial nerve) disorder characterized by a sudden weakness or paralysis of muscles on one side of the face. The inability to smile or whistle, the uncontrollable drooping of the mouth and drooling of saliva, and an inability to close the eye *(Figure 10.12)* are common symptoms. The use of steroids in the early stages can prevent the paralysis from becoming permanent.

Trigeminal neuralgia (TN), **tic douloureux**, is an extremely painful chronic disorder of the trigeminal nerve (5th cranial nerve) caused by nerve injury or compression of the nerve by a blood vessel. The facial pain can be constant or sporadic and is very intense. The anticonvulsant carbamazepine *(Tegretol)* is the first-line treatment, and opiates can be prescribed for pain. There is limited evidence that surgical treatment options are effective.

An **acoustic neuroma** is a benign, slow-growing tumor on the vestibulocochlear nerve (8th cranial nerve) that causes hearing loss, tinnitus, and dizziness. Treatment is with surgery and/or radiation.

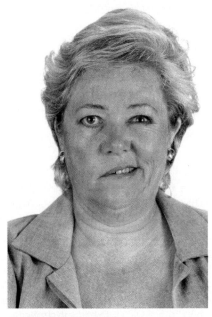

▲ **FIGURE 10.12**
Bell Palsy of Left Side of Face.

Jo Ann Snover/Shutterstock

Word Analysis and Definition

S = Suffix   P = Prefix   R = Root   R/CF = Combining Form

WORD	PRONUNCIATION		ELEMENTS	DEFINITION
acoustic	ah-**KYU**-stik		Greek *hearing*	Pertaining to hearing
Bell palsy	BELL **PAWL**-zee		Charles Bell, Scottish -surgeon, 1774–1842	Paresis, or paralysis, of one side of the face
concussion	kon-**KUSH**-un	S/ R/	**-ion** *action, condition* **concuss-** *shake or jar violently*	Mild brain injury
contrecoup	**KON**-treh-koo		French *counterblow*	Injury to the brain at a point directly opposite the point of contact
contusion	kon-**TOO**-zhun	S/ R/	**-ion** *action, condition* **contus-** *bruise*	Hemorrhage into a tissue (bruising), including the brain
coup	KOO		French *a blow*	Injury to the brain directly under the skull at the point of contact
meningitis	men-in-**JIE**-tis	S/ R/	**-itis** *inflammation* **mening-** *meninges*	Inflammation of the meninges
meningococcal	meh-nin-goh-**KOK**-al	S/ R/CF R/	**-al** *pertaining to* **mening/o-** *meninges* **-cocc-** *round bacterium*	Pertaining to the meningococcus bacterium
neuroma	nyu-**ROH**-mah	S/ R/	**-oma** *tumor* **neur-** *nerve*	Any tumor arising from cells in the nervous system
subdural space	sub-**DYU**-ral SPASE	S/ P/ R/	**-al** *pertaining to* **sub-** *below* **-dur-** *dura, hard*	Space between the arachnoid and dura mater layers of the meninges
trauma traumatic (adj)	**TRAW**-mah traw-**MAT**-ik	S/ R/	Greek *wound* **-tic** *pertaining to* **trauma-** *injury*	A physical or mental injury Pertaining to or caused by trauma
trigeminal neuralgia	try-**GEM**-in-al	S/ P/ R/	**-al** *pertaining to* **tri-** *three* **-gemin-** *double*	Fifth (v) cranial nerve with three branches supplying the face
	nyu-**RAL**-jee-ah	S/ R/	**-algia** *pain* **neur-** *nerve*	Trigeminal neuralgia; painful facial muscles supplied by the trigeminal nerve
tic douloureux (syn)	TIK duh-luh-**RUE**		douloureux French *painful tic*	

EXERCISES

 Case Report 10.1

You are

. . . a medical assistant working with Dr. Raul Cardenas, a neurologist at Fulwood Medical Center.

You are communicating with

. . . Mr. Lester Rood, a 75-year-old man who was diagnosed with **dementia** a year ago. He lives with his daughter, Judy, and she is with him today.

Patient Interview:

Mr. Rood: "How am I feeling? Scared stiff. Sometimes I don't know where I am. I get so messed up. I can't cook anymore. I forget what I'm doing, can't get things straight. I find myself in the street and don't know how I got there. Judy has to help me shower and remind me to go to the bathroom. And it's only going to get worse. I don't want to be a burden. I used to have 100 people working for me. It's so frustrating, so frightening."

A. Disorders of the brain. *Match each disorder in the first column with its correct description in the second column. Fill in the blanks.*   **LO 10.5**

_____ **1.** delirium

_____ **2.** Alzheimer disease

_____ **3.** confusion

_____ **4.** vascular dementia

a. common form of dementia due to protein clumps and tangles

b. dementia due to decreased blood flow to the brain

c. altered state of consciousness with agitation and disorientation

d. condition in which a person cannot properly process information

B. Identify *the elements in each medical term, and unlock the meaning of the word. Fill in the chart.*   **LO 10.1, 10.5, and 10.11**

Medical Term	Meaning of Prefix	Meaning of Root/CF	Meaning of Suffix
dementia	**1.**	**2.**	**3.**
sympathy	**4.**	**5.**	**6.**
delirium	**7.**	**8.**	**9.**
confusion	**10.**	**11.**	**12.**
empathy	**13.**	**14.**	**15.**
sedation	**16.**	**17.**	**18.**

 ## Case Report 10.2

You are

. . . an **electroneurodiagnostic** technologist (END) working with Gregory Solis, MD, a **neurosurgeon** at Fulwood Medical Center.

You are communicating with

. . . Ms. Roberta Gaston, a 39-year-old woman, who has been referred by Raul Cardenas, MD, a **neurologist**, for evaluation for possible **neurosurgery**. Ms. Gaston has had **epileptic** seizures since the age of 16. She also has daily minor spells in which she stops interacting and blinks rhythmically for about 20 seconds, after which she returns to normal. She is unable to work and is cared for by her parents. Her **neurologic** examination is normal. Her **electroencephalogram (EEG)** shows diffuse epileptic discharges in the left frontal region. Her CT scan is normal. An MRI shows a 20-mm-diameter mass adjacent to her left ventricle.

For Ms. Roberta Gaston, who was seen in Dr. Solis's neurosurgery clinic, the EEG did not pinpoint an epileptic source. In order to further investigate the source, Dr. Solis inserted deep brain electrodes into the region of the suspicious mass that showed on the MRI. Seizures were recorded arising in the mass itself. Dr. Solis performed a surgical resection of the mass, which was a **glioma**. Ms Gaston has been seizure-free since the surgery a year ago.

Ms. Gaston suffered from both **absence** and **tonic-clonic** seizures.

C. Documentation: *Fill in the following paragraph with the appropriate language of neurology. Review Case Report 10.2 to assist you in completing this exercise. Fill in the blanks.*   **LO 10.2, 10.3, 10.7, 10.10, and 10.11**

electroencephalography	electroneurodiagnostic	epilepsy	electroencephalograph
neurologist	electroencephalogram	neurosurgeon	

Roberta Gaston and her parents were sent to this office by her (1) _____.

Dr. Solis has ordered some (2) _____ because of her (3) _____.

The particular type of test is an (4) _____, which will produce an EEG on the (device) (5) _____.

After the results of the (6) _____, if Ms. Gaston needs surgery, it will be performed by a(n) (7) _____.

D. Refer to Case Report 10.2 *to correctly complete each statement and answer the question. Fill in the blanks.*   **LO 10.2, 10.3, 10.5, and 10.7**

1. Provide the medical term (not the abbreviation) for the diagnostic test that can determine the electrical activity of the brain: _____

2. Provide the medical term (not the abbreviation) for the diagnostic test that provided an image of the mass: _____

3. The cause of Ms. Gaston's seizures is a(n): _____

4. Provide the therapeutic procedure written in the Case Report that Dr. Solis performed: _____

5. Did the therapeutic procedure correct Ms. Gaston's neurological disorder? (yes or no) _____

E. In practice, *you will find that some people will use the new terms for seizures, and some will use the older traditional terms. It is important that you know both. Fill in the blanks with the correct term.* **LO 10.2 and 10.5**

1. A tonic-clonic seizure is traditionally known as a _____ mal seizure.

2. An absence seizure is traditionally known as a _____ mal seizure.

F. Signs of brain disorders. *Match the sign of the brain disorder in the first column with its corresponding condition in the second column. Fill in the blanks.* **LO 10.5**

_____	1. multiple seizures for 30 minutes without regaining consciousness	**a.** absence seizure
_____	2. infant with high fever	**b.** narcolepsy
_____	3. child appears to be daydreaming	**c.** febrile seizure
_____	4. transient neurologic deficit after a seizure	**d.** Tourette syndrome
_____	5. person suddenly falls asleep	**e.** status epilepticus
_____	6. a tic disorder	**f.** postictal state

G. Diagnosis: *Patient documentation is given to you below. Select the correct language of neurology for the diagnosis.* **LO 10.5 and 10.7**

1. Patient is experiencing shaking, involuntary movements of her extremities.
   Diagnosis: **a.** *syncope*   **b.** *prion*   **c.** *tremor*

2. Radiologic studies show a small, circumscribed dilation of the cerebral artery.
   Diagnosis: **a.** *Parkinson disease*   **b.** *aneurysm*   **c.** *migraine*

3. The patient's paroxysmal headache is confined to the left temporal region.
   Diagnosis: **a.** *syncope*   **b.** *tremor*   **c.** *migraine*

4. Tests and studies have confirmed inflammation of the brain cells and tissues to make this diagnosis.
   Diagnosis: **a.** *meningitis*   **b.** *fasciitis*   **c.** *encephalitis*

5. This patient has experienced loss of consciousness due to diminished cerebral blood flow.
   Diagnosis: **a.** *syncope*   **b.** *tremor*   **c.** *migraine*

H. Provide the abbreviation *for the described condition. Fill in the blanks.* **LO 10.3 and 10.5**

1. Short episodes of low oxygen delivery to the brain usually due to an embolus: _____

2. An embolus in a cerebral artery that is stopping the delivery of oxygen to an area of the brain: _____

3. Rapid deterioration of mental function, some of which are caused by bovine spongiform encephalopathy: _____

4. General term that describes a condition that has a range of developmental disorders including physical repetitive movements: _____

I. Diseases and disorders. *Are you familiar enough with their terminology and symptoms to match the correct disease or disorder with the appropriate statement for each patient? Select the correct answer that completes each sentence.* **LO 10.5**

1. The patient has a slow-growing tumor on the vestibulocochlear nerve:
   a. acoustic neuroma   **b.** tic douloureux   **c.** intracranial hemorrhage

2. Patient has inflammation of the coverings of the brain:
   a. meningitis   **b.** encephalitis   **c.** vasculitis

3. Brain injury occurred after the patient was hit head-on while driving his truck:
   a. acoustic neuroma   **b.** Bell palsy   **c.** contusion

4. Patient complains of intermittent, shooting pain in the area of the face and head:
   a. trigeminal neuralgia   **b.** peripheral neuropathy   **c.** neuritis

Section 10.4

Disorders of the Spinal Cord and Peripheral Nerves

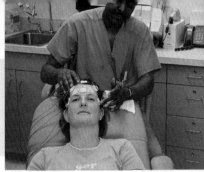

Rick Brady/McGraw Hill

Disorders of the Myelin Sheath of Nerve Fibers (LO 10.3 and 10.5)

Many disorders of the nervous system can affect the spinal cord and the peripheral nerves without affecting the brain. When the myelin sheath surrounding nerve fibers is damaged, nerves do not conduct impulses normally. In newborns, many of their nerves have immature myelin sheaths, which is why some of their movements are jerky and uncoordinated.

Demyelination, the destruction of an area of the myelin sheath, can occur in the **PNS** and be caused by inflammation, vitamin B_{12} deficiency, poisons, and some medications.

Multiple sclerosis (MS), a chronic, progressive, autoimmune disorder, is the most common condition in which demyelination of nerve fibers in the brain, spinal cord, and optic nerves can occur *(Figure 10.13)*. **Intermittent** myelin damage and scarring slow nerve impulses. This leads to muscle weakness, pain, abnormal sensations (**paresthesias**), numbness, and vision loss. Because different nerve fibers are affected at different times, MS symptoms often worsen (**exacerbations**) or show partial or complete reduction (**remissions**).

Abbreviations

MS	multiple sclerosis
PNS	peripheral nervous system

Keynote

- MS is most common in women, has an average age of onset between 20 and 40 years, and its cause is unknown.

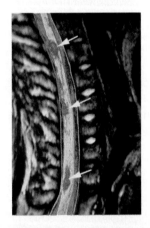

◀ **FIGURE 10.13**
Multiple Sclerosis of the Spinal Cord. Areas of demyelination are arrowed and shown in red.

Source: CAVALLINI JAMES/BSIP/age fotostock

Word Analysis and Definition

S = Suffix   P = Prefix   R = Root   R/CF = Combining Form

WORD	PRONUNCIATION	ELEMENTS		DEFINITION
demyelination	dee-**MY**-eh-lin-**A**-shun	S/ P/ R/	-ation *process* de- *without* -myelin- *myelin*	Process of losing the myelin sheath of a nerve fiber
exacerbation (contrast **remission**)	ek-zas-er-**BAY**-shun	S/ R/	-ion *condition, action* exacerbat- *increase, aggravate*	Period when there is an increase in the severity of a disease
intermittent	**IN**-ter-**MIT**-ent	S/ P/ R/	-ent *end result* inter- *between* -mitt- *send*	Alternately ceasing and beginning again
paresthesia paresthesias (pl) (**Note:** the "a" following the "r" in *para* is dropped for ease of pronunciation.)	pair-es-**THEE**-ze-ah	S/ P/ R/	-ia *condition* par(a)- *abnormal* -esthes- *sensation*	Abnormal sensation; e.g., tingling, burning, and pricking
remission (contrast **exacerbation**)	ree-**MISH**-un	S/ P/ R/	-ion *condition, action* re- *back* -miss- *send*	Period when there is a lessening or absence of the symptoms of a disease
sclerosis	skleh-**ROH**-sis	S/ R/CF	-sis *abnormal condition* scler/o- *hardness*	Thickening and hardening of a tissue; in the nervous system, hardening of nervous tissue by fibrous and glial connective tissue

Abbreviations

SCI	spinal cord injury
PPS	Postpolio syndrome
ALS	Amyotrophic lateral sclerosis
POLIO	Poliomyelitis

Disorders of the Spinal Cord (LO 10.5)

Trauma (LO 10.5)

The spinal cord can be injured in three ways:

1. **Severed,** by a fractured vertebra *(Figure 10.14a);*
2. **Contused,** as in a sudden, violent jolt to the spine; and
3. **Compressed,** by a dislocated vertebra, bleeding, or swelling *(Figure 10.14b).*

Because of its anatomy—with nerve fibers and tracts going up and down, to and from the brain—a spinal cord injury results in a loss of function below the injury site. For example, if the cord is injured in the thoracic region, the arms function normally but the legs may become **paralyzed.** Both muscle control and sensation are lost. **Paresis** is partial paralysis.

If the spinal cord is severed, the loss of function is permanent. Contusions can cause temporary loss of function and movement, lasting days, weeks, or months.

Compression of the cord can also occur from a tumor in the cord or spine or from a **herniated disc.** The intervertebral disc *(see Section 4.2 of Chapter 4)* can move out of place (herniate, slip) or break open (rupture) from injury or strain. This causes pressure on the spinal nerves, leading to pain, numbness, and/or weakness. Cancer or osteoporosis can cause a vertebra to collapse and also compress the cord.

Severed spinal cord

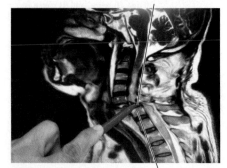

(a)   Fracture-dislocation of vertebra

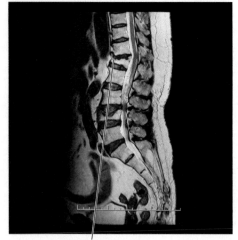

(b)   Fractured vertebra

▲ FIGURE 10.14

Spinal Cord Injuries.
(a) Severed spinal cord from fracture-dislocation of vertebra.
(b) Compressed spinal cord with vertebral fracture.

10.14a: Richman Photo/Shutterstock
10.14b: Suttha Burawonk/Shutterstock

Other Disorders of the Spinal Cord (LO 10.3 and 10.5)

Acute transverse myelitis is a localized spinal cord disorder that blocks the transmission of impulses up and down the spinal cord.

Subacute combined degeneration of the spinal cord is due to a deficiency of vitamin B_{12}. The spinal cord's sensory nerve fibers degenerate, producing weakness, clumsiness, tingling, and a sensory loss as to the position of the limbs.

In **syringomyelia,** fluid-filled cavities form in the spinal cord and compress nerves that detect pain and temperature.

Poliomyelitis (POLIO) is an acute infectious disease, occurring mostly in children, due to the poliovirus. The virus destroys motor neurons.

Postpolio syndrome (PPS) is when people develop tired, painful, and weak muscles many years after recovery from polio.

Amyotrophic lateral sclerosis (ALS), or "Lou Gehrig's disease," occurs when motor nerves in the spinal cord progressively deteriorate.

Disorders of Peripheral Nerves (LO 10.5)

Peripheral neuropathy is used here as any disorder affecting one or more peripheral nerves.

Mononeuropathy is damage to a single peripheral nerve. Examples are:

- **Carpal tunnel syndrome,** in which the median nerve at the wrist is compressed between the wrist bones and a strong overlying ligament.

- **Ulnar nerve palsy,** which results from nerve damage as the forearm's ulnar nerve crosses close to the surface over the humerus at the back of the elbow.

- **Peroneal nerve palsy,** which arises from nerve damage as the peroneal or lower leg bone nerve passes close to the surface near the back of the knee. Compression of this nerve occurs in people who are bedridden or strapped in a wheelchair.

Polyneuropathy is damage to, and the simultaneous malfunction of, many motor and/or sensory peripheral nerves throughout the body. There are many causes of peripheral polyneuropathy; diabetes is a common cause. Symptoms include numbness, pain, tingling sensations, and weakness. Treatment is aimed at the underlying problem and pain reduction.

Herpes zoster, or **shingles,** is an infection of peripheral nerves arising from a reactivation of the dormant childhood chickenpox (varicella) virus.

Neuralgia will often accompany neuropathy.

WORD	PRONUNCIATION	ELEMENTS		DEFINITION
amyotrophic	a-my-oh-**TROH**-fik	S/ P/ R/CF R/	-ic *pertaining to* a- *without* -my/o- *muscle* -troph- *nourishment, development*	Pertaining to muscular atrophy
compression	kom-**PRESH**-un	S/ P/ R/	-ion *action, condition* com- *together* -press- *squeeze*	Squeeze together to increase density and/or decrease a dimension of a structure
herniation hernia (noun) herniate (verb)	her-nee-**AY**-shun **HER**-nee-ah **HER**-nee-ate	S/ R/ S/	-ation *process* herni- *rupture* -ate *composed of*	Protrusion of an anatomical structure from its normal location Protrusion of a structure through the tissue that normally contains it
myelitis	**MY**-eh-**LIE**-tis	S/ R/	-itis *inflammation* myel- *spinal cord*	Inflammation of the spinal cord

neuropathy
 	
   mononeuropathy
   polyneuropathy
	nyu-**ROP**-ah-thee
	
	MON-oh-nyu-**ROP**-ah-thee
	POL-ee-nyu-**ROP**-ah-thee
		S/
		R/CF
		P/
		P/
			-pathy *disease*
			neur/o- *nerve*
			mono- *one*
			poly- *many*
				Any disorder of the nervous system
				
				Disorder affecting a single nerve
				Disorder affecting many nerves

paralyze (verb) paralysis (noun) paralytic (adj)	**PAIR**-ah-lyze pah-**RAL**-ih-sis pair-ah-**LYT**-ik	P/ R/ R/ S/ R/	para- *beside, abnormal* -lyze *destroy* -lysis *destruction* -ic *pertaining to* -lyt- *destroy*	To make incapable of movement Loss of voluntary movement Suffering from paralysis
paresis hemiparesis	par-**EE**-sis **HEM**-ee-pah-**REE**-sis	 P/ R/	Greek *weakness* hemi- *half* -paresis *weakness*	Partial paralysis (weakness) Weakness of one side of the body
poliomyelitis (Note: abbreviated as polio) postpolio syndrome (PPS)	**POE**-lee-oh-**MY**-eh-lie-tis post-**POE**-lee-oh **SIN**-drome	S/ R/ R/ P/ R/ P/ R/	-itis *inflammation* polio- *gray matter* -myel- *spinal cord* post- *after* -polio *gray matter* syn- *together* -drome *running*	Inflammation of the gray matter of the spinal cord, leading to paralysis of the limbs and muscles of respiration Progressive muscle weakness in a person previously affected by polio
syringomyelia	sih-**RING**-oh-my-**EE**-lee-ah	S R/CF R/	-ia *condition* syring/o- *tube, pipe* -myel- *spinal cord*	Abnormal longitudinal cavities in the spinal cord that cause paresthesias and muscle weakness
trauma traumatic (adj)	**TRAW**-mah traw-**MAT**-ik	 S/ R/	Greek *wound* -tic *pertaining to* trauma- *injury*	A physical or mental injury Pertaining to or caused by trauma

Congenital Anomalies of the Nervous System (LO 10.3 and 10.5)

Some of the most devastating congenital neurologic abnormalities develop in the first 8 to 10 weeks of pregnancy, when the nervous system is in its early stages of formation. These malformations can be detected using ultrasonography and amniocentesis *(see Chapter 15)*. Many of these can be prevented by the mother taking 400 mcg/day of folic acid before conception and during early pregnancy.

A **teratogen** is an agent that can cause **anomalies** of an embryo or fetus *(see Chapter 15)*. It can be a chemical, a virus, or radiation. Some teratogens found in the workplace include textile dyes, photographic chemicals, semiconductor materials, and the metals lead, mercury, and cadmium.

Anencephaly is the absence of the cerebral hemispheres and is incompatible with life. **Microcephaly**, decreased head size, is associated with small cerebral hemispheres and moderate to severe motor and intellectual disability.

Hydrocephalus *(Figure 10.15)* is ventricular enlargement in the cerebral hemispheres with excessive CSF; it is usually due to a blockage that prevents the CSF from exiting the ventricles to circulate around the spinal cord. Treatment involves placing a tube (shunt) into the ventricle to divert the excess fluid into the abdominal cavity or a neck vein.

Spina bifida (neural tube defect) occurs mostly in the lumbar and sacral regions. It is variable in its presentation and symptoms. **Spina bifida occulta** has a small partial defect in the vertebral arch. The spinal cord or meninges do not protrude. Often the only sign is a tuft of hair on the skin overlying the defect.

In **spina bifida cystica** there is no vertebral arch formed. The spinal cord and meninges protrude through the opening and may or may not be covered with a thin layer of skin *(Figure 10.16a and b)*. Protrusion of only the meninges is called a **meningocele**. Protrusion of the meninges and spinal cord is called a **meningomyelocele** (myelomeningomyelocele). The lower limbs may be paralyzed.

Fetal alcohol syndrome (FAS) can occur when a pregnant woman drinks alcohol. A child born with FAS has a small head, narrow eyes, and a flat face and nose. Intellect and growth are impaired. FAS is the third most common cause of intellectual disabilities in newborns.

Cerebral Palsy (LO 10.3 and 10.5)

Cerebral palsy (CP) is the term used to describe the motor impairment resulting from brain damage in an infant or young child. It is not hereditary. In congenital CP, the cause is often unknown but can be a brain malformation from maternal use of cigarettes, drugs, and alcohol. CP developed at birth or in the neonatal period is usually related to an incident causing hypoxia (low oxygen) of the brain.

CP causes delay in the development of normal milestones in infancy and childhood.

The affected limbs can be **spastic** (muscles are tight and resistant to stretch) and may show **athetoid** movements, where the limbs involuntarily writhe and constantly move. A poor sense of balance and coordination may also be present, leading to **ataxia**.

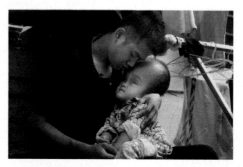

▲ **FIGURE 10.15**
Infant with Hydrocephalus.

Imaginechina Limited/Alamy Stock Photo

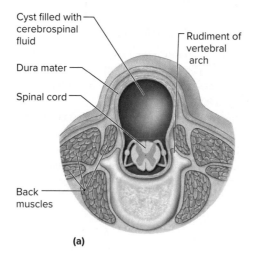

Cyst filled with cerebrospinal fluid
Rudiment of vertebral arch
Dura mater
Spinal cord
Back muscles

(a)

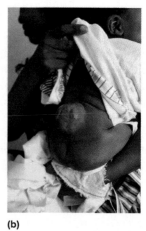

(b)

▲ **FIGURE 10.16**
Spina Bifida Cystica.
(a) Cross section of a spinal meningocele. (b) Child with spina bifida cystica.

Photo By BSIP/UIG Via Getty Images

S = Suffix   P = Prefix   R = Root   R/CF = Combining Form

WORD	PRONUNCIATION	ELEMENTS		DEFINITION
anomaly	ah-**NOM**-ah-lee		Greek *abnormality*	A structural abnormality
anencephaly	**AN**-en-**SEF**-ah-lee	S/ P/ R/	-aly *condition* an- *without* -enceph- *brain*	Born without cerebral hemispheres
microcephaly	**MY**-kroh-**SEF**-ah-lee	P/ R/	micro- *small* -ceph- *head*	An abnormally small head
ataxia	a-**TAK**-see-ah	S/ P/ R/	-ia *condition* a- *without* -tax- *coordination*	Inability to coordinate muscle activity, leading to jerky movements
ataxic (adj)	a-**TAK**-sik	S/	-ic *pertaining to*	Pertaining to or suffering from ataxia
athetosis	ath-eh-**TOE**-sis	S/ R/	-osis *condition* athet- *without position, uncontrolled*	Slow, writhing involuntary movements
athetoid (adj)	**ATH**-eh-toyd	S/	-oid *resembling*	Resembling or suffering from athetosis
hemiplegia	hem-ee-**PLEE**-jee-ah	S/ P/ R/	-ia *condition* hemi- *half* -pleg- *paralysis*	Paralysis of one side of the body
hemiplegic (adj) hemiparesis	hem-ee-**PLEE**-jik **HEM**-ee-pah-**REE**-sis	S/ R/	-ic *pertaining to* -paresis *weakness*	Pertaining to or suffering from hemiplegia Weakness of one side of the body
hydrocephalus	**HIGH**-droh-**SEF**-ah-lus	S/ R/CF R/	-us *pertaining to* hydr/o- *water* -cephal- *head*	Enlarged head due to excess CSF in the cerebral ventricles
meningocele	meh-**NIN**-goh-seal	S/ R/CF	-cele *hernia* mening/o- *meninges*	Protrusion of the meninges from the spinal cord or brain through a defect in the vertebral column or cranium
meningomyelocele	meh-nin-goh-**MY**-el-oh-seal	S/ R/CF	-cele *hernia* -myel/o- *spinal cord*	Protrusion of the spinal cord and meninges through a defect in the vertebral arch of one or more vertebrae
monoplegia	**MON**-oh-**PLEE**-jee-ah	S/ P/ R/	-ia *condition* mono- *one* -pleg- *paralysis*	Paralysis of one limb
monoplegic (adj)	**MON**-oh-**PLEE**-jik	S/	-ic *pertaining to*	Pertaining to or suffering from monoplegia
palsy	**PAWL**-zee		Latin *paralysis*	Paralysis or paresis from brain damage
paraplegia	pair-ah-**PLEE**-jee-ah	S/ P/ R/	-ia *condition* para- *abnormal* -pleg- *paralysis*	Paralysis of both lower extremities
paraplegic (adj)	pair-ah-**PLEE**-jik	S/	-ic *pertaining to*	Pertaining to or suffering from paraplegia
quadriplegia	kwad-rih-**PLEE**-jee-ah	S/ P/ R/	-ia *condition* quadri- *four* -pleg- *paralysis*	Paralysis of all four limbs
quadriplegic (adj)	kwad-rih-**PLEE**-jik	S/	-ic *pertaining to*	Pertaining to or suffering from quadriplegia
spina bifida	**SPY**-nah **BIH**-fih-dah	R/CF P/ R/	spin/a *spine* bi- *two* -fida *split*	Failure of one or more vertebral arches to close during fetal development
spina bifida cystica	**SIS**-tik-ah	S/ R/	-ica *pertaining to* cyst- *cyst*	Meninges and spinal cord protruding through the absent vertebral arch and having the appearance of a cyst
spina bifida occulta	**OH**-kul-tah	R/CF	occult/a *hidden*	The deformity of the vertebral arch is not apparent from the surface
teratogen	**TER**-ah-toe-gen	S/ R/CF	-gen *create, produce* terat/o- *monster, malformed fetus*	Agent that produces fetal deformities

EXERCISES

 Case Report 10.3

You are

. . . Tanisha Colis, an electroneurodiagnostic technologist working for Raul Cardenas, MD, a neurologist at Fulwood Medical Center.

You are communicating with

. . . Mrs. Suzanne Kalish, a 42-year-old social worker employed by the medical center. Mrs. Kalish has recently had an exacerbation of her symptoms due to **multiple sclerosis (MS).** She is going to have a visual evoked potential **(VEP)** test, followed by an MRI of her brain and spinal cord.

Patient Interview:

Tanisha: "Good morning, Mrs. Kalish. I'm Tanisha Colis, the technologist who'll be performing your visual evoked potential test. How are you feeling?"

Mrs. Kalish: "I've been doing OK for the last 4 or 5 years. Then, a few weeks ago, I started dragging my right foot and just couldn't make it work. I've got to hang onto the walls to stay vertical. I'm tired out, can't come to work. It's a struggle to walk the few yards just to pick up the mail."

Tanisha: "The MRI you are going to have today will give us a lot of information about what's going on."

Mrs. Kalish: "My mind is going 'wheelchair, wheelchair, wheelchair.' Especially since in the last couple of days the vision in my right eye has gotten all blurred."

Tanisha: "That's the reason you are having the visual evoked potential test."

Mrs. Kalish: "I hate this disease. It's just so frustrating not to be able to control or fix my body. This just seems to be getting worse, you know."

Tanisha: "Let me help you up, and we'll go get this test done."

Mrs. Kalish: "I can manage, thank you."

A. Read Case Report 10.3. *Select the answer that answers the question or completes the statement.* **LO 10.3, 10.5, 10.7, and 10.8**

1. Why did Dr. Cardenas order the VEP for Mrs. Kalish?

   a. she has trouble standing

   b. she has blurred vision

   c. her energy level has decreased

2. Mrs. Kalish states that her condition ". . . just seems to be getting worse." The medical term for her statement is:

   a. exacerbation

   b. acute

   c. remission

3. Which disorder does Mrs. Kalish have?

   a. peripheral neuritis

   b. fibromyalgia

   c. multiple sclerosis

4. The focus of Dr. Cardenas, speciality is to:

   a. treat autoimmune diseases

   b. surgically treat neurological disorders

   c. medically treat neurological disorders

   d. counsel patients on psychological disorders

B. Test yourself *on the elements and terms related to neurologic disorders. Select the correct answer.* **LO 10.1 and 10.5**

1. The term *intermittent* contains:

    a. prefix, root, and suffix

    b. prefix and root

    c. combining form and suffix

2. *Remission* is the opposite of:

    a. intermittent

    b. exacerbation

    c. demyelination

3. In the term *demyelination* the prefix means:

    a. without

    b. in front of

    c. half

C. Abbreviations *are common in medical documentation. Provide the abbreviation each statement is describing. Fill in the blanks.* **LO 10.3 and 10.5**

1. The muscle weakness the occurs after having poliomyelitis: _____

2. Injury to the spinal cord: _____

3. Another name for Lou Gehrig's disease: _____

4. Inflammation of the gray matter of the spinal cord due to virus: _____

D. Identify the element *and give its meaning. Fill in the chart.* **LO 10.1, 10.5, 10.7, and 10.11**

Element	Element Identity (P, R, CF, or S)	Meaning of Element
myo-	1.	2.
herni-	3.	4.
-pathy	5.	6.
syringo-	7.	8.

E. Search and find *the correct term for the element you are given. Select the correct answer.* **LO 10.1 and 10.5**

1. Find the term with the prefix meaning *without*:

    a. hydrocephalus

    b. anencephaly

    c. bifida

2. Find the term with the suffix meaning *hernia*:

    a. meningocele

    b. cystica

    c. teratogen

3. Find the term with the root meaning *hidden*:

    a. spina bifida

    b. spina bifida cystica

    c. spina bifida occulta

4. Find the term with the root meaning *coordination*:

    a. monoplegia

    b. athetosis

    c. ataxia

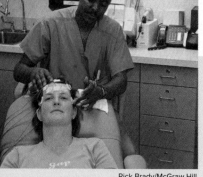
Rick Brady/McGraw Hill

Section 10.5

Diagnostic and Therapeutic Procedures and Pharmacology of the Nervous System

Abbreviations

CT	computed tomography
EEG	Electroencephalography
EMG	electromyography
LP	lumbar puncture
MRI	magnetic resonance imaging
PET	positron emission tomography
VEP	visual evoked potential

Diagnostic Procedures in Neurology (LO 10.5 and 10.7)

To obtain a specimen of CSF, a **lumbar puncture (LP)** or **spinal tap** is performed *(Figure 10.17)*. A needle is inserted through the skin, back muscles, spinal ligaments of an intervertebral space, epidural space, dura mater, and arachnoid mater into the subarachnoid space. The CSF is then aspirated. Laboratory examination of the CSF that shows white blood cells suggests meningitis. High protein levels indicate meningitis or damage to the brain or spinal cord. Blood suggests a brain hemorrhage or a traumatic tap.

Electroencephalography (EEG) records the brain's electrical activity and helps identify seizure disorders, sleep disturbances, degenerative brain disorders, and brain damage.

Electroneurodiagnostic technologists monitor and record electrical activity in the brain and the electrical activity of muscles and nerves.

Tests measuring the electrical activity of the brain:

Evoked responses are a procedure in which stimuli for vision, sound, and touch are used to activate specific areas of the brain and their responses are measured with EEG or PET scans. The **Visual Evoked Response (VEP)** etects damage to the optic nerve, a condition associated with MS.

Electromyography (EMG) involves placing small needles into a muscle to record its electrical activity at rest and during contraction. It is used to provide information in disorders of muscles, peripheral nerves, and the **neuromuscular** junction.

Nerve conduction studies measure the speed at which motor or sensory nerves conduct impulses. The studies exclude disorders of the brain, spinal cord, and muscles and focus on the peripheral nerves.

Computed tomography (CT), a computer-enhanced X-ray technique, generates images of slices of the brain and spinal cord to detect a wide range of disorders, including tumors, areas of dead brain tissue due to stroke, and birth defects.

Magnetic resonance imaging (MRI) produces highly detailed anatomical images of most neurologic disorders, including strokes, brain tumors, and myelin sheath damage.

Magnetic resonance angiography uses an injection of a radiopaque dye to produce images of blood vessels of the head and neck during MRI.

Cerebral angiography is an invasive procedure in which a radiopaque dye is injected into the blood vessels of the neck and brain. It can detect blood vessels that are partially or completely blocked, aneurysms, or arteriovenous malformations.

Cerebral arteriography can determine the site of bleeding in hemorrhagic strokes.

Color Doppler ultrasonography uses high-frequency sound (ultrasound) waves to show different rates of blood flow through the arteries of the neck or the base of the brain. This evaluates TIAs and the risk of a full-blown stroke.

Echoencephalography uses ultrasound waves to produce an image of the brain in children under age 2 because their skulls are thin enough for the waves to pass through them.

Positron emission tomography (PET) involves attaching radioactive molecules onto a substance necessary for brain function (for example, the sugar glucose). As the molecules circulate in the brain, the radioactive labels give off positively charged signals that can be recorded *(Figure 10.18)*.

Myelography is the use of X-rays of the spinal cord that are taken after a radiopaque dye has been injected into the CSF by spinal tap. It has been replaced by MRI when that is available.

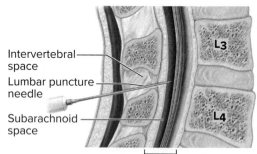

Intervertebral space
Lumbar puncture needle
Subarachnoid space
L3
L4
Vertebral canal

▲ **FIGURE 10.17**
Lumbar Puncture (spinal tap).

Primary motor cortex

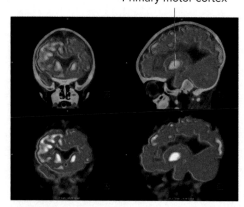

▲ **FIGURE 10.18**
PET Scan of the Brain Showing the Motor Cortex.

wenht/Getty Images

WORD	PRONUNCIATION		ELEMENTS	DEFINITION
angiography	an-jee-**OG**-rah-fee	S/	-graphy *process of recording*	Process of recording the image of blood vessels after injection of contrast material
		R/CF	angi/o- *blood vessel*	
arteriography	ar-teer-ee-**OG**-rah-fee	S/	-graphy *process of recording*	X-ray visualization of an artery after injection of contrast material
		R/CF	arteri/o- *artery*	
Doppler	**DOP**-ler		Johann Christian Doppler, 1803–1853, Austrian mathematician and physicist	Diagnostic instrument that sends an ultrasonic beam into the body
Doppler ultrasonography	**DOP**-ler **UL**-trah-soh-**NOG**-rah-fee	S/	-graphy *process of recording*	Imaging that detects direction, velocity, and turbulence of blood flow; used in workup of stroke patients
		P/	ultra- *beyond*	
		R/CF	-son/o- *sound*	
color Doppler ultrasonography				Computer-generated color image to show directions of blood flow
echoencephalography	**EK**-oh-en-sef-ah-**LOG**-rah-fee	S/	-graphy *process of recording*	Use of ultrasound in the diagnosis of intracranial lesions
		R/CF	ech/o- *sound wave*	
		R/CF	-encephal/o- *brain*	
electroencephalogram (EEG)	ee-**LEK**-troh-en-**SEF**-ah-loh-gram	S/	-gram *recording*	Record of the electrical activity of the brain
		R/CF	electr/o- *electricity*	
		R/CF	-encephal/o- *brain*	Device used to record the electrical activity of the brain
electroencephalograph	ee-**LEK**-troh-en-**SEF**-ah-loh-graf	S/	-graph *to write, record*	
electroencephalography	ee-**LEK**-troh-en-**SEF**-ah-**LOG**-rah-fee	S/	-graphy *process of recording*	The process of recording the electrical activity of the brain
electromyogram	ee-**LECK**-troh-**MY**-oh-gram	S/	-gram *record, recording*	Record of the electrical activity of a muscle
electromyography	ee-**LEK**-troh-my-**OG**-rah-fee	S/	-graphy *process of recording*	Recording of electrical activity in muscle
		R/CF	electr/o- *electricity*	
		R/CF	-my/o- *muscle*	
electroneurodiagnostic (adj)	ee-**LEK**-troh-**NYUR**-oh-die-ag-**NOS**-tik	S/	-ic *pertaining to*	Pertaining to the use of electricity in the diagnosis of a neurologic disorder
		R/CF	electr/o- *electricity*	
		R/CF	-neur/o- *nerve*	
		R/	-diagnost- *decision*	
myelography	my-eh-**LOG**-rah-fee	S/	-graphy *process of recording*	Radiography of the spinal cord and nerve roots after injection of contrast medium into the subarachnoid space
		R/CF	myel/o- *spinal cord*	
nerve conduction study	NERV kon-**DUK**-shun **STUD**-ee	R/	nerve *nerve*	Procedure to measure the speed at which an electrical impulse travels along a nerve
		S/	-ion *action*	
		P/	con- *with, together*	
		R/	-duct- *lead*	
		R/	study *inquiry*	

Therapeutic Procedures (LO 10.5 and 10.7)

Surgical Procedures (LO 10.5 and 10.7)

Neurosurgeons diagnose and surgically treat conditions of the central and peripheral nervous systems.

Craniotomy is the surgical removal of part of a skull bone (the bone flap) to expose the brain for surgery. A craniotomy is used to remove subdural and epidural hematomas if they do not resolve on their own.

Cranioplasty is the repair of a bone defect in the skull, often the result of craniotomy.

Deep brain stimulation is the surgical placement of electrodes deep into specific areas of the brain to deliver electrical stimulations to treat the tremors of Parkinson disease, essential tremor, or multiple sclerosis.

Endoscopic pituitary surgery utilizes an approach through the inside of the nose to remove pituitary tumors.

Endovascular coiling, also known as endovascular embolization, blocks the blood flow to an aneurysm.

Flow diversion uses **stents** placed via a catheter to maintain blood flow through a blood vessel where blockage or an aneurysm has occurred.

• Surgical procedures for many
conditions are often used after
medication and rehabilitation
therapy fail.

Treatment for TIA is directed at the underlying cause. **Carotid endarterectomy** may be necessary if a carotid artery is significantly occluded with plaque.

Treatment of many acute ischemic strokes is by thrombolysis using medications known asclot busters. Thes include such as **tissue plasminogen activator (tPA)** within 4½ hours of the stroke, with supportive measures followed by rehabilitation.

Treatment of gliomas is a combination of surgery, radiotherapy, and chemotherapy. The combination is necessary because even if you remove 99% of a tumor, there will be up to 1 billion cells remaining. A more recent therapy, **brachytherapy,** implants small radioactive pellets directly into the tumor. The radiation is released over time.

A **shunt** is used in hydrocephalus to drain the excess CSF from the ventricles to either the peritoneal cavity or an atrium of the heart.

Spina bifida—correction of defect by removing the sac and closing the opening with skin within 24–48 hours after birth to reduce the chance of infection.

Microvascular decompression (MVD)—an endoscopic surgery that wraps a sponge around the compressed nerve, preventing the blood vessel from touching and further irritating the nerve. Treats trigeminal neuralgia and other cranial nerve neuralgias.

Treatment of Cerebral Palsy (LO 10.5 and 10.7)

A multidisciplinary team of health professionals is required to develop an individualized treatment plan and to involve the patients, families, teachers, and caregivers in decision making and planning.

Physical therapy is designed to prevent muscles from becoming weak or rigidly fixed with contractures, to improve motor development, and to facilitate independence. Speech therapy and psychotherapy complement physical therapy.

A variety of devices and mechanical aids ranging from muscle braces to motorized wheelchairs offer support for mobility.

Word Analysis and Definition

S = Suffix   P = Prefix   R = Root   R/CF = Combining Form

WORD	PRONUNCIATION		ELEMENTS	DEFINITION
brachytherapy	brah-kee-**THAIR**-ah-pee	P/ R/	**brachy-** *short* **-therapy** *medical treatment*	Radiation therapy in which the source of irradiation is implanted in the tissue to be treated
carotid endarterectomy (CEA)	kah-**ROT**-id **END**-ar-ter-**EK**-toe-me	S/ P/ R/	carotid, Greek *large neck artery* **-ectomy** *surgical excision* **end-** *inside* **-arter-** *artery*	Surgical removal of diseased lining from the carotid artery to leave a smooth lining and restore blood flow
cranium cranioplasty craniotomy	KRAY-nee-um KRAY-nee-oh-**PLASTEE** KRAY-nee-**OT**-oh-mee	S/ R/CF S/	Greek *skull* **-plasty** *surgical repair* **crani/o-** *skull* **-tomy** *surgical incision*	The bony container of the brain, excluding the face Repair of a bone defect in the skull Surgical removal of part of a skull bone to expose the brain for surgery
endovascular	**END**-oh-**VAS**-kyu-lar	S/ P/ R/	**-ar** *pertaining to* **endo-** *inside* **-vascul-** *blood vessel*	Relating to the inside of a blood vessel
microvascular decompression	**MY**-kroh-vas-kyu-lar **DEE**-kom-**PRESH**-un	S/ P/ R/CF S/ P/ R/	**-ar** *pertaining to* **micro-** *small* **-vascul-** *blood vessel* **-ion** *action* **de-** *removal* **-compress-** *press together*	Endoscopic procedure that places a sponge between the offending blood vessel and the affected nerve
neurology neurologist neurologic (adj) neurosurgeon neurosurgery	nyu-**ROL**-oh-jee nyu-**ROL**-oh-jist NYU-roh-**LOJ**-ik NYU-roh-**SUR**-jun NYU-roh-**SUR**-jer-ee	S/ R/CF S/ S/ R/ S/ R/ S/	**-logy** *study of* **neur/o-** *nerve* **-logist** *one who studies, specialist* **-ic** *pertaining to* **-log-** *to study* **-eon** *one who does* **-surg-** *operate* **-ery** *process of*	Medical specialty of disorders of the nervous system Medical specialist in disorders of the nervous system Pertaining to the nervous system One who performs surgery on the nervous system Operating surgically on the nervous system
shunt	SHUNT		**Middle English** *divert*	A bypass or diversion of fluid

Botulinum toxin *(Botox)* can also used to treat spasticity in certain patients, although this treatment is not a permanent solution and must be renewed about every 3 to 6 months.

Pain Management (LO 10.5 and 10.7)

Pain persisting longer than 3 months is said to be **chronic.** It can be caused by cancer, arthritis, fibromyalgia, low-back or neck problems, headache, or injuries that have not healed. Normal activities can be restricted or be impossible.

In 2016, the cost of chronic pain was estimated to be $560 billion due to medical costs, lost work productivity, and disability programs. In modern health care, chronic pain management has become essential and often uses a multidisciplinary approach. Pain management is now a board-certified subspecialty for **anesthesiologists.**

Medications are the cornerstone of pain management, and the following can be used depending on the severity of the pain:

- **Analgesics** (such as acetaminophen) and nonsteroidal anti-inflammatory drugs (NSAIDs) for mild pain;
- **Opioids** hydrocodone/acetaminophen *(Vicodin),* oxycodone/acetaminophen *(Percocet),* and oxycodone/aspirin *(Percodan).* These opiate medications are addictive and are frequently abused and sold on the street.
- Higher doses of opiates for severe pain. These are often used on their own, and include **morphine** and fentanyl.
- **Buprenorphine** is an opioid that has recently been recommended for treatment in chronic pain. It provides analgesia with less risk for abuse and addiction. There are strict federal regulations on the qualifications of physicians allowed to prescribe it.
- **Epidural anesthesia** is used for pain management during surgery and childbirth.

Pharmacology of the Nervous System (LO 10.3 and 10.7)

The transmission of impulses from one neuron to another and from a neuron to a cell is achieved by neurotransmitters at synaptic connections. Drugs that affect the nervous system, called *psychoactive drugs,* target this synaptic mechanism *(Table 10.1).*

Medications Treating Neurology Disorders (LO 10.3 and 10.7)

Neurologists treat neurologic conditions with drugs to prevent the transmission of nerve impulses.

Migraines

Migraines can be treated for acute episodes or preventively. Acute episode medications are NSAIDs, caffeine, and triptans such as rizatriptan *(Maxalt)* and sumatriptan *(Imitrex).* Preventive medications such as **botulinum toxins,** galcanezumab-gnlm *(Emgality),* and ubrogepant *(Ubrelvy)* have proven effective.

Medications for Dementia

There are no medications to treat senile dementia.

- Alzheimer disease—donepezil *(Aricept)* and rivastigmine *(Exelon)* prolong the amount of time neurons communicate with each other and **memantine** *(Namenda),* which works similarly to donepezil and rivastigmine.
- **Frontotemporal dementia**—no cure, treat symptoms. Antidepressants, antipsychotics, and memantine *(Namenda).*
- **Vascular dementia**—exploring use of medications to treat Alzheimer disease, however, treating vascular disease *(see Chapter 6).*

Infections

- **Antibiotics**—treat bacterial infections seen in brain abscess and bacterial encephalitis.
- **Vaccinations**—prevent most types of meningococcal meningitis and viral infections: shingles (Shingrix) and poliomyelitis.

Table 10.1 Psychoactive Drugs

Type/Mode of Action	Name	Common Effects	Effects of Abuse
Stimulants ("uppers") Speed up activity in the CNS	Caffeine	Wakefulness, shorter reaction time, alertness	Restlessness, insomnia, heartbeat irregularities
	Nicotine	Varies from alertness to calmness, appetite for carbohydrates decreases	Heart disease; high blood pressure; vasoconstriction; bronchitis; emphysema; lung, throat, mouth cancer
	Amphetamines	Wakefulness, alertness, increased metabolism, decreased appetite	Nervousness, high blood pressure, delusions, psychosis, convulsions, death
	Cocaine	**Euphoria,** high energy, illusions of power	Excitability, paranoia, anxiety, panic, depression, heart failure, death
Depressants ("downers") Slow down activity in the CNS	Alcohol	1–2 drinks—reduced inhibitions and anxiety Many drinks—slow reaction time, poor coordination and memory	Blackouts, mental and neurologic impairment, psychosis, cirrhosis of liver, death
	Barbiturates and **tranquilizers**	Reduced anxiety and tension, sedation	Impaired motor and sensory functions, amnesia, loss of consciousness, death
Narcotics Mimic the actions of natural **endorphins**	Codeine, opium, morphine, heroin	Euphoria, pleasure, relief of pain	High tolerance of pain, nausea, vomiting, constipation, convulsions, coma, death
Psychedelics Disrupt normal thought processes	Marijuana	Relaxation, euphoria, increased appetite, pain relief	Sensory distortion, hallucinations, paranoia, throat and lung damage
	LSD, mescaline, MDMA (Ecstasy)	Exhilaration, euphoria, hallucinations, insightful experiences	Panic, extreme delusions, bad trips, paranoia, psychosis
Antidepressants Affect the neurotransmitters serotonin, norepinephrine, and dopamine	Selective serotonin reuptake inhibitors (SSRIs)—Prozac, Paxil, Zoloft	Enhanced mental clarity, improved sleep, diminished depression	Anxiety, decreased sex drive, insomnia, restlessness, fatigue, headaches
	Serotonin and norepinphrine reuptake inhibitors (SNRIs)—Effexor XR, Pristiq, Cymbalta	Diminished depression, pain relief	Raised blood pressure, liver and kidney failure, fatal outcome with overdose
	Tricyclic antidepressants (TCAs)—amitriptyline, Tofranil	Effective relief of depression but numerous side effects	Decreased sex drive and outcomes, difficulty urinating, sedation, weight gain, dry mouth, fatal outcome with overdose
Anxiolytics (anti-anxiety) Affect inhibitory neurotransmitters and their synaptic receptors	Benzodiazepines—Librium, Valium, Xanax	Relief of anxiety and panic disorder in the short term with rapid action	Habit forming, addiction tendencies, drowsiness, dizziness, worsen the effects of alcohol
	Selective serotonin reuptake inhibitors (SSRIs) (see above)	Used because they are not addictive	Fatigue, nausea, depression, insomnia
	Azaspirones—BuSpar	Effective in mild to moderate anxiety—takes 2–4 weeks to have effect; not addictive	Overdose leads to unconsciousness
	Beta blockers—Inderal, Tenormin *(see Chapter 6)*	Greatly reduce certain anxiety symptoms, such as shaking, palpitations, and sweating	Nausea, diarrhea, bronchospasm, bradycardia, insomnia, erectile dysfunction
Antiepileptic drugs (AEDs) (anticonvulsants) Do not cure epilepsy, but suppress seizures while medications are in the body	Broad-spectrum AEDs—Depakote, Lamictal, Topamax, Keppra	Effective for a wide range of all types of seizures	Weight gain, tremor, hair loss, osteoporosis, low blood count, memory problems
	Narrow-spectrum AEDs—Phenobarbital, Dilantin, Tegretol, Lyrica	Effective for specific types of seizures	GI upset, weight gain, blurred vision, low blood counts, fatigue

WORD	PRONUNCIATION	ELEMENTS		DEFINITION
addict	**AD**-ikt	P/ R/	ad- *to* -dict *consent, surrender*	Person with a psychologic or physical dependence on a substance or practice
addiction	ah-**DIK**-shun	S/	-ion *condition, action*	Habitual psychologic and physiologic dependence on a substance or practice
addictive	ah-**DIK**-tiv	S/	-ive *quality of, pertaining to*	Pertaining to or causing addiction
analgesia	an-al-**JEE**-zee-ah	S/ P/ R/	-ia *condition* an- *without* -alges- *sensation of pain*	State in which pain is reduced
analgesic (adj)	an-al-**JEE**-zik	S/	-ic *pertaining to*	Substance that produces analgesia
anesthesia	an-es-**THEE**-zee-ah	P/ R/CF	an- *without* -esthesi/a- *feeling*	Complete loss of sensation
anesthesiologist	**AN**-es-thee-zee-**OL**-oh-jist	S/ P/ R/CF	-logist *one who studies, specialist* an- *without* -esthesi/o- *feeling, sensation*	Medical specialist in anesthesia
anesthesiology	**AN**-es-thee-zee-**OL**-oh-jee	S/	-logy *study of*	Medical speciality of anesthesia
anesthetic	an-es-**THET**-ik	S/ P/ R/	-ic *pertaining to* an- *without, lack of* -esthet- *sensation, perception*	Agent that causes absence of feeling sensation
antagonism	an-**TAG**-oh-nizm	S/ P/ R/	-ism *process, action* ant- *against* -agon- *contest against*	Situation of opposing
antagonist	an-**TAG**-oh-nist	S/	-ist *agent*	An opposing structure, agent, disease, or process
antiepileptic	**AN**-tee-eh-pih-**LEP**-tik	S/ P/ R/	-tic *pertaining to* anti- *against* -epilep- *seizure*	A pharmacologic agent capable of preventing or arresting epilepsy
anxiolytic	**ANG**-zee-oh-**LIT**-ik	S/ R/CF	-lytic *soluble* anxi/o- *anxiety*	An agent that reduces the symptoms of anxiety
Botox	**BOH**-tox		Botulinum toxin	Neurotoxin injected into muscles to prevent the muscles from contracting
dependence	dee-**PEN**-dense		Latin *to hang from*	State of needing someone or something
depressant	dee-**PRESS**-ant	S/ R/	-ant *agent* depress- *press down*	Substance that diminishes activity, sensation, or tone
antidepressant	**AN**-tih-dee-**PRESS**-ant	P/	anti- *against*	An agent to suppress the symptoms of depression
endorphin	en-**DOR**-fin	P/ R/	end- *within* -orphin *morphine*	Natural substance in the brain that has the same effect as opium
euphoria	yoo-**FOR**-ee-ah	S/ P/ R/	-ia *condition* eu- *normal* -phor- *bear, carry*	Exaggerated feeling of well-being
narcotic	nar-**KOT**-ik	S/ R/CF	-tic *pertaining to* narc/o- *sleep, stupor*	Drug derived from opium or a synthetic drug with similar effects
opium opioid	**O**-pee-um **O**-pee-oid	 S/	Latin *opium* -oid *resembling*	A narcotic drug derived from the poppy plant. A natural or synthetic narcotic
psychedelic	sigh-keh-**DEL**-ik	S/ R/CF R/	-ic *pertaining to* psych/e- *mind, soul* -del- *visible*	Agent that intensifies sensory perception
psychoactive	sigh-koh-**AK**-tiv	S/ R/CF R/	ive *quality of, pertaining to* psych/o- *mind, soul* -act- *to do*	Able to alter mood, behavior, and/or cognition
sedative	**SED**-ah-tiv	S/ R/	-ive *quality of, pertaining to* sedat- *to calm*	Agent that calms nervous excitement
sedation	seh-**DAY**-shun	S/	-ion *condition, action*	State of being calmed
stimulant stimulate (verb) stimulation	**STIM**-you-lant **STIM**-you-late stim-you-**LAY**-shun	S/ R/ S/	-ant *forming* stimul- *excite, strengthen* -ation *process*	Agent that excites or strengthens functional activity Arousal to increased functional activity
tolerance	**TOL**-er-ants	S/ R/	-ance *state of, condition* toler- *endure*	The capacity to become accustomed to a stimulus or drug

EXERCISE

A. Construct medical terms common to diagnostic procedures in neurology. *Given the definition, complete the medical term it is defining using word elements related to diagnostic terms in neurology. Fill in the blanks.* **LO 10.1, 10.2, 10.5, 10.6, and 10.7**

1. The machine that creates the record of the electrical activity of the brain. electro/encephalo/_____

2. The process of recording arteries. arterio/_____

3. The use of high-frequency sound waves to view blood flow. Doppler ultra/_____/graphy

4. Process of recording the spinal cord. _____/graphy

5. Process of recording the electrical activity of the muscle. electr/o/_____/graphy

B. Demonstrate understanding of word elements in medical terms. *This will make short work of answer questions in this course and interpreting patient medical records in clinical practice. This exercise uses layman's terms and asks you to replace those words the medical term they are describing. Fill in the blanks.* **LO 10.1, 10.2, 10.5, 10.7, 10.8, 10.10, and 10.11**

A 27-year-old male is brought to the emergency department by paramedics. The male is unconscious. The paramedics report that he was involved in an altercation at a bar when he was struck in the head with a barstool. After a CT confirmed intracranial bleeding, he was immediately brought to the operating room where the (1) *surgical expert in the treatment of neurological conditions* performed a (2) *procedure in which part of the skull was removed.* A large clot was removed from the subdural space. The wound was closed and the patient was admitted to the surgical ICU. The injury to skull shattered several areas of the (3) *bones that cover the brain,* and therefore the patient will require a (4) *repair of defect of the skull* at a later date when he becomes medically stable.

1. The medical term that replaces the italicized words: _____

2. The medical term that replaces the italicized words: _____

3. The medical term that replaces the italicized words: _____

4. The medical term that replaces the italicized words: _____

C. Deconstruct this *language of neurology* into its basic elements to help understand the meaning of the term. *Write the elements between the slashes. The first one is done for you. Every term does not need every element, so you will have some blanks.* **LO 10.1 and 10.7**

1. antagonist _____ ant _____ / _____ agon _____ / _____ ist _____

2. addict _____ / _____ / _____

3. tranquilizer _____ / _____ / _____

4. stimulant _____ / _____ / _____

5. psychedelic _____ / _____ / _____

6. tolerance _____ / _____ / _____

7. psychoactive _____ / _____ / _____

D. Deconstruct *each medical term into its basic elements to better understand the meaning of the term. If the term does not have a particular element, leave it blank. Fill in the blanks.* **LO 10.1, 10.6, and 10.7**

1. euphoria _____/_____/_____
         P   R, R/CF   S

2. antidepressant _____/_____/_____
             P   R, R/CF   S

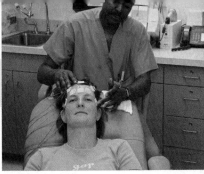
Rick Brady/McGraw Hill

Mental Health Definitions (LO 10.6 and 10.9)

- **Mental health** is defined by the World Health Organization (**WHO**) as "a state of wellbeing in which the individual realizes his or her own abilities, can cope with the normal stresses of life, can work productively and fruitfully, and is able to make a contribution to the community."

- **Psychology** is the scientific study of behavior—talking, reading, sleeping, interacting with others—and mental processes—thinking, feeling, remembering, and dreaming.

- **Psychiatry** is the medical specialty concerned with the origin, diagnosis, prevention, and treatment of mental, emotional, and behavioral disorders.

- **Mental health disorders** are of different types and will be considered in this chapter under the headings Psychosis and Schizophrenia, Mood Disorders, Anxiety Disorders, Personality Disorders, and Substance Abuse and Chemical Dependence.

Psychosis and Schizophrenia (LO 10.6)

Psychosis is an abnormal mental state in which the individual has a loss of contact with reality. People suffering from psychosis are described as **psychotic**.

Schizophrenia is a form of psychosis. People with schizophrenia do *not* have a "split personality," but their perceptions are separated from reality, their words are separated from their meanings, and their behaviors are separated from their thought processes. They perceive things without stimulation (**hallucinations**). They suffer from mistaken beliefs that are contrary to facts (**delusions**). The delusions can be **paranoid**, with pervasive distrust and suspicion of others. Their speech is disorganized and can be incoherent, and they may refuse or be unable to speak (**mute**) *(Figure 10.19)*.

Keynotes

- A specialist in psychiatry is a physician called a psychiatrist, who is licensed to prescribe medications.

- A specialist in psychology is a psychologist, who is a doctoral level healthcare provider but not licensed to prescribe medications.

- Insanity is a legal term for a severe mental illness that impairs a defendant's ability to understand the moral wrong of the act he/she committed. It is not a medical diagnosis.

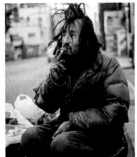

▲ **FIGURE 10.19**
A Man with Schizophrenia Living on the Streets.

RichLegg/Getty Images

Word Analysis and Definition

S = Suffix   P = Prefix   R = Root   R/CF = Combining Form

WORD	PRONUNCIATION		ELEMENTS	DEFINITION
delusion	dee-**LOO**-zhun	S/ R/	-ion *condition* delus- *deceive*	Fixed, unyielding false belief despite strong evidence to the contrary
hallucination	hah-loo-sih-**NAY**-shun	S/ R/	-ation *condition* hallucin- *imagination*	Perception of an object or event when there is no such thing present
mute	MYUT		Latin *silent*	Unable or unwilling to speak
paranoia	pair-ah-**NOY**-ah	P/ R/	para- *abnormal* -noia *to think*	Presence of persecutory delusions
paranoid	**PAIR**-ah-noyd	S/	-oid *resembling*	Having persecutory delusions
psychiatry	sigh-**KIGH**-ah-tree	S/ R/	-iatry *treatment* psych- *mind*	Diagnosis and treatment of mental disorders
psychiatrist	sigh-**KIGH**-ah-trist	S/	-iatrist *one who treats*	Licensed medical specialist in psychiatry
psychology	sigh-**KOL**-oh-jee	S/ R/CF	-logy *study of* psych/o- *mind*	Science concerned with the behavior of the human mind
psychologist	sigh-**KOL**-oh-jist	S/	-logist *one who treats*	Licensed specialist in psychology
psychosis	sigh-**KOH**-sis	S/ R/	-osis *condition* psych- *mind*	Disorder with loss of contact with reality
psychotic (adj)	sigh-**KOT**-ik	S/ R/CF	-tic *pertaining to* psych/o- *mind*	Affected by psychosis
schizophrenia	skitz-oh-**FREE**-nee-ah	S/ R/CF R/	-ia *condition* schiz/o- *to split* -phren- *mind*	Disorder of perception and behavior with loss of reality
schizophrenic (adj)	skitz-oh-**FREN**-ik	S/	-ic *pertaining to*	Suffering from schizophrenia

GAD	generalized anxiety disorder
OCD	obsessive-compulsive disorder
PTSD	posttraumatic stress disorder
SAD	seasonal affective disorder
SSD	somatic symptom disorder

Mood Disorders (LO 10.2, 10.3, and 10.6)

Mood involves a subjective emotional state that persists for a period of time. A person's mood is **congruent** when the symptoms of psychosis matches their mood state.

Major depression, also called **unipolar disorder,** occurs when a person is deeply sad, despairing, and hopeless for at least 2 weeks; sees nothing but sorrow and despair in the future; and may have thoughts of suicide.

- **Bipolar disorder,** which used to be called **manic-depressive disorder,** is the alternation of major episodes of depression with periods of excessive overexcitement, impulsive behavior, **insomnia,** and lack of fatigue, called **mania.** Untreated mixed (manic and depressive) episodes usually last around 4 to 5 months.

- **Dysphoric mania** combines the frenetic energy of mania with dark thoughts and paranoid delusions. It may be the cause of some mass shootings.

- **Seasonal affective disorder (SAD)** entails episodes of depression that occur in the fall and winter months. It appears to be related to a lack of sunshine causing increased melatonin production by the pineal gland (*see Chapter 12*).

Anxiety Disorders (LO 10.2, 10.3, and 10.6)

Anxiety disorders are the most common category of mental disorder found in the United States. They are characterized by an unreasonable anxiety and fear so intense and persistent that it disrupts the person's life. There are five categories of anxiety disorders:

1. **Generalized anxiety disorder (GAD)** consists of uncontrollable anxiety not focused on one situation or event that has lasted for 6 months or more. People with the disorder develop physical fear reactions, including palpitations, insomnia, difficulty concentrating, and irritability.

2. **Posttraumatic stress disorder (PTSD)** affects about 7.7 million American adults. It arises after significant trauma, such as a life-threatening incident, loss of a loved one, abuse, torture or combat in war, or a high level of stress in daily life. Symptoms include flashbacks of the traumatic event, nightmares, intense physical reactions to reminders of the event, feeling emotionally numb, irritability, outbursts of anger, and difficulty concentrating. Alcohol and drug abuse are common.

3. **Panic disorder** is characterized by sudden, brief attacks of intense fear that cause physical symptoms, occur often for no reason, and peak in 10 minutes or less.

4. **Phobias** differ from panic attacks in that a *specific* situation or event brings on a strong fear response. There are two categories of phobias:

   - **Situational phobias** involve a fear of specific situations. Examples are **acrophobia** (fear of heights), **agoraphobia** (fear of crowded places), and **claustrophobia** (fear of confined spaces).

   - **Social phobias** involve a fear of being embarrassed in social situations. The most common are fear of public speaking and fear of eating in public.

5. In **obsessive-compulsive disorder (OCD),** most patients have both **obsessions** and **compulsions.** Obsessions are recurrent thoughts, fears, doubts, images, or impulses. Compulsions are recurrent, irresistible impulses to perform actions such as counting, hand washing, checking, and systematically arranging things.

Psychosomatic disorder is a real physical illness in which anxiety and stress play a causative role. Examples are tension headaches and low back pain.

The DSM-V replaced hypochondriasis with two new disorders.

Somatic symptom disorder (SSD) is a condition in which the patient has distressing physical (somatic) symptoms together with abnormal thoughts, feelings, and behaviors in response to these symptoms.

Illness anxiety disorder is an intense anxiety of having an undiagnosed illness.

S = Suffix   P = Prefix   R = Root   R/CF = Combining Form

WORD	PRONUNCIATION		ELEMENTS	DEFINITION
acrophobia	ak-roh-**FOH**-be-ah	S/ R/CF	-phobia *fear* acr/o- *peak, highest point*	Pathologic fear of heights
affect affective (adj)	**AF**-fekt af-**FEK**-tiv	S/ R/	Latin *state of mind* -ive *pertaining to* affect- *mood*	External display of feelings, thoughts, and emotions Expressing emotion
agoraphobia	ah-gor-ah-**FOH**-be-ah	S/ R/CF	-phobia *fear* agor/a- *marketplace*	Pathologic fear of being trapped in a public place
anxiety	ang-**ZI**-eh-tee		Greek *distress, anxiety*	Distress caused by fear
biofeedback (Note: *This term has no prefix or suffix.*)	bi-oh-**FEED**-back	R/CF R/ R/	bi/o- *life* -feed- *to give food, nourish* -back *back, return*	Training techniques to achieve voluntary control of responses to stimuli
bipolar disorder	bi-**POH**-lar dis-**OR**-der	S/ P/ R/	-ar *pertaining to* bi- *two* -pol- *pole*	A mood disorder with alternating episodes of depression and mania
claustrophobia	klaw-stroh-**FOH**-be-ah	S/ R/CF	-phobia *fear* claustr/o- *confined space*	Pathologic fear of being trapped in a confined space
congruent	**KON**-gru-ent	S/ P/ R/	-ent *end result* con- *with* -gru- *to move*	Coinciding or agreeing with
cognitive	**KOG**-nih-tiv	S/ R/	-ive *quality of* cognit- *thinking*	Pertaining to the mental activities of thinking and learning
compulsion	kom-**PULL**-shun	S/ R/	-ion *action, condition* compuls- *drive, compel*	Uncontrollable impulses to perform an act repetitively
compulsive (adj)	kom-**PULL**-siv	S/	-ive *nature of, quality of*	Possessing uncontrollable impulses to perform an act repetitively
depression	de-**PRESH**-un	S/ R/	-ion *condition, process* depress- *press down*	Mental disorder with feelings of deep sadness and despair
dysphoria	dis-**FOR**-ee-ah	S/ P/ R/	-ia *condition* dys- *bad, difficult* -phor- *carry, bear*	A condition of severe depression, agitation, and paranoid delusions
dysphoric (adj)	dis-**FOR**-ick	S/	-ic *pertaining to*	Pertaining to dysphoria
insomnia	in-**SOM**-nee-ah	S/ P/ R/	-ia *condition* in- *not* -somn- *sleep*	Inability to sleep
mania manic (adj)	**MAY**-nee-ah **MAN**-ik	S/ R/	Greek *frenzy* -ic *pertaining to* man- *mania*	Mood disorder with hyperactivity, irritability, and rapid speech Pertaining to or characterized by mania
manic-depressive disorder	**MAN**-ik-de-**PRESS**-iv dis-**OR**-der	S/ R/	-ive *quality of* depress- *press down*	An outdated name for bipolar disorder
obsession	ob-**SESH**-un	S/ R/	-ion *action, condition* obsess- *besieged by thoughts*	Persistent, recurrent, uncontrollable thoughts or impulses
obsessive (adj)	ob-**SES**-iv	S/	-ive *nature of, quality of*	Possessing persistent, recurrent, uncontrollable thoughts or impulses
phobia	**FOH**-be-ah	S/	Greek *fear* -ic *pertaining to*	Pathologic fear or dread
posttraumatic	post-traw-**MAT**-ik	P/ R/	post- *after* -traumat- *wound*	Occurring after and caused by trauma
psychosomatic	sigh-koh-soh-**MAT**-ik	S/ R/CF R/	-tic *pertaining to* psych/o- *mind* -soma- *body*	Pertaining to disorders of the body usually resulting from disturbances of the mind
somatic symptom disorder	soh-**MAT**-ik **SIMP**-tum dis-**OR**-der	S/ R/ P/ R/	-ic *pertaining to* somat- *body* symptom *Greek sign* dis- *apart, away from* -order *arrange*	Distressing physical symptoms occur, causing abnormal thoughts, feelings, and behaviors
unipolar disorder	you-nih-**POLE**-ar dis-**OR**-der	S/ P/ R/	-ar *pertaining to* uni- *one* -pol- *pole (at the pole of depression)*	Depression

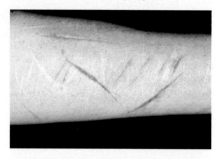

Personality Disorders (LO 10.3 and 10.6)

Personality is defined as an individual's unique and stable patterns of thoughts, feelings, and behaviors. When these patterns become rigid and inflexible in response to different situations, they can cause impairment of the individual's ability to deal with other people (i.e., to function socially).

- **Borderline personality disorder (BPD)** is a frequent diagnosis in people who are impulsive, unstable in mood, and manipulative. They can be exciting, charming, and friendly one moment and angry, irritable, and sarcastic the next. Their identity is fragile and insecure, their self-worth is low. They can be promiscuous and self-destructive; for example, with **self-mutilation (self-injury)** *(Figure 10.20)* or **suicide.**

- People with **narcissistic personality disorder** have an exaggerated sense of self-importance and seek constant attention, and lack **empathy**.

- **Antisocial personality disorder,** used interchangeably with the terms **sociopath** and **psychopath**, describes people who lie, cheat, steal, and have no sense of responsibility and no anxiety or guilt about their behavior. Psychopaths have these characteristics but tend to be more violent and anger easily.

- **Schizoid** and **paranoid personality disorders** describe people who are absorbed with themselves, untrusting, and fearful of closeness with others.

Dissociative Disorders (LO 10.3 and 10.7)

Dissociative disorders involve a disassociation (splitting apart) of past experiences from present memory or consciousness. The development of distinctly separate personalities is called **dissociative identity disorder (DID).** It was formerly called **multiple personality disorder (MPD).** Two or more distinct personalities, each with its own memories and behaviors, inhabit the same person at the same time *(Figure 10.21)*. The basic origin of all these disorders is the need to escape, usually from extreme trauma, and most often from sexual, emotional, or physical abuse in childhood. Treatment is with psychotherapy.

Impulse Control Disorders (LO 10.3 and 10.6)

Impulse control disorders involve an inability to resist an impulse to perform an action that is harmful to the individual or to others. These disorders include:

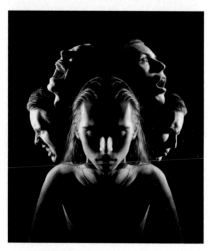

▲ **FIGURE 10.21**
Dissociative Identity Disorder
(Multiple Personality Disorder).

Stepan Kapl/Shutterstock

- **Kleptomania,** which is characterized by stealing—not for gain but to satisfy an irresistible urge to steal. Behavior therapy can help, and SSRIs appear to be of value.

- **Trichotillomania (TTM),** which is characterized by the repeated urge to pull out one's own scalp, beard, pubic, and other body hair.

- **Pyromania**, which is repeated fire setting with no motive other than a fascination with fire and fire engines. Some pyromaniacs end up as volunteer firefighters.

Abbreviations

BPD	borderline personality disorder
DID	dissociative identity disorder
MPD	multiple personality disorder
TTM	trichotillomania

Keynotes

- Empathy is understanding another person's feelings.
- Sympathy is to feel sorry about a person's problem.

Substance Abuse and Chemical Dependence (LO 10.3 and 10.6)

Substance abuse involves a person's continued use of psychoactive drugs, including alcohol and illicit drugs, despite having significant problems or distress related to their use. This continued use can lead to a **dependence** syndrome, which includes the strong need to take the drug, persistence in its use despite harmful consequences to the user and others, daily priority given to drug use, and increased tolerance.

- **Addiction** includes dependence syndrome, but it refers to not only psychoactive drugs but also such entities as exercise addiction, food addiction, computer addiction, and gambling. The patterns of behavior and habits of use associated with an addiction are characterized by immediate gratification coupled with the long-term harmful effects, which include changes in the structure and function of the brain.

- **Abused substances** include tobacco, alcohol, marijuana, cocaine, heroin, methamphetamines, Ecstasy, LSD, and PCP. In addition, prescription drug abuse is increasing dramatically. The three classes of prescription drugs being abused are:

  1. **Opioids,** which include oxycodone (Oxycontin), hydrocodone (Vicodin), meperidine (Demerol), hydromorphone (Dilaudid), and fentanyl (Duragesic and others).

  2. **CNS depressants** such as the **benzodiazepines** Xanax and Valium.

  3. **CNS stimulants** such as Adderall and Ritalin.

  Abuse of prescription drugs now ranks second to marijuana among illicit drug users, and the number of fatal poisonings from prescription opioid analgesics outnumbers total deaths from heroin and cocaine.

WORD	PRONUNCIATION		ELEMENTS	DEFINITION
addict addiction	ADD-ikt ah-DIK-shun	P/ R/ S/	ad- *toward* -dict *surrender* -ion *condition, action*	Person with a psychologic or physical dependence on a substance or practice Habitual psychologic and physiologic dependence on a substance or practice
antisocial personality disorder	AN-tee-SOH-shal per-son-AL-ih-tee dis-OR-der	S/ P/ R/ S/ S/ R/	-al *pertaining to* anti- *against* -soci- *partner, ally, community* -ity *condition, state* -al- *pertaining to* person- *person*	Disorder in which affected persons experience no empathy or remorse and engage in harmful and manipulative behavior toward others.
dissociative identity disorder	di-SO-see-ah-tiv eye-DEN-tih-tee dis-OR-der	S/ P/ R/	-ative *quality of* dis- *apart, away from* -soci- *partner, ally, community*	Mental disorder in which part of an individual's personality is separated from the rest, leading to multiple personalities
empathy sympathy	EM-pah-thee SIM-pah-thee	P/ R/ P/ R/	em- *into* -pathy *emotion, disease* sym- *together* -pathy *emotion, disease*	Ability to place yourself into the feelings, emotions, and reactions of another person Appreciation and concern for another person's mental and emotional state
kleptomania	klep-toe-MAY-nee-ah	S/ R/CF	-mania *frenzy* klept/o- *to steal*	Uncontrollable need to steal
narcissism	NAR-sih-sizm		Greek mythical character, Narcissus, who was in love with his own reflection in water	Disorder in which affected persons experience no empathy, remorse, or emotional connection with others. They believe themselves to be superior and require excessive praise.
narcissistic (adj)	NAR-sih-SIS-tik	S/ S/ R/	-ism *a process* -istic *pertaining to* narciss- *self-love*	Relating everything to oneself
psychopath	SIGH-koh-path	S/ R/CF	-path *disease* psych/o- *mind*	Person with antisocial personality disorder
pyromania	pie-roh-MAY-nee-ah	S/ R/CF	-mania *frenzy* pyr/o- *fire*	Morbid impulse to set fires
schizoid	SKITZ-oyd	S/ R/	-oid *resemble* schiz- *split*	Characteristic of being withdrawn, separated, and uninterested in social contact
self-mutilation	self-myu-tih-LAY-shun	S/ R/ R/	-ation *process* self- *own individual* -mutil- *to maim*	Injury or disfigurement made to one's own body
sociopath	SO-see-oh-path	S/ R/CF	-path *disease* soci/o- *partner, ally, community*	Person with antisocial personality disorder
suicide suicidal (adj)	SOO-ih-side SOO-ih-SIGH-dal	R/CF R/CF S/	su/i- *self* -cid/e *kill* -al *pertaining to*	The act of killing oneself Wanting to kill oneself

EXERCISES

 ## Case Report 10.4

You are

. . . a **psychiatric technician** employed in the Psychiatric Department of Fulwood Medical Center. Your patient has been referred from the Emergency Department, where he was seen earlier this morning.

You are communicating with

. . . Mr. Dante Costello, a 21-year-old homeless man, brought in by the police after he was found sitting immobile in the middle of a main street (**catatonia**).

Mr. Costello's explanation is "the voices told me to do it." He has heard voices (**hallucinations**) telling him to do things for the past year. The voices often comment on his behavior. He has isolated himself from other people because "they are not who they say they are, and they are trying to get me" (**delusions**). He is taking no drugs or medications, and he denies any **suicidal** or **homicidal** intent.

Mr. Costello appears dirty and disheveled, with poor hygiene. He can give no home or family address. His **affect** is **congruent,** though expressionless. His speech is slow, and his thoughts are disorganized and confused.

The most probable diagnosis is **schizophrenia**. He needs to be admitted to the hospital because he is a potential danger to himself and other people.

A. **After reading Case Report 10.4,** *select the correct answer to complete each statement.*   **LO 10.6**

1. The term that means wanting to kill oneself:

   a. homicidal   b. schizophrenic   c. suicidal   d. psychotic

2. Mr. Costello's inappropriate behavior is due to:

   a. homicidal thoughts   b. poor hygiene   c. hearing voices   d. homelessness

3. In the statement "His affect is congruent, though expressionless," the term **congruent** means:

   a. the behavior matches his appearance   c. he believes people are out to get him

   b. he is not speaking   d. his behavior points to hurting other people

4. His behavior of sitting in the street for long periods of time describes which condition?

   a. paranoia   b. mutism   c. homicidal   d. catatonia

B. **Reinforce** *your learning of the languages of psychology and psychiatry by providing the term that is being defined. Fill in the blanks.*   **LO 10.2, 10.7, and 10.9**

1. A medical doctor who specializes in the origin, diagnosis, prevention, and treatment of mental, emotional, and behavioral disorders: _____

2. A front-line worker who directly cares for those with mental illnesses and/or developmental disabilities: _____ technician.

3. The general term for a licensed specialist in psychology: _____

C. **Match** *the term in the first column to its correct definition in the second column. Pay close attention to the word elements to assist you in choosing the correct definition for each term.*   **LO 10.6 and 10.11**

_____	1. psychosomatic	a. fear of being trapped in a public space
_____	2. acrophobia	b. fear of heights
_____	3. obsessive	c. inability to sleep
_____	4. insomnia	d. disorder of body due to disturbance of the mind
_____	5. agoraphobia	e. uncontrollable impulses to perform acts repetitively
_____	6. compulsion	f. persistent, recurrent, uncontrollable thoughts

D. **Use the correct abbreviation** *for personality disorders. Read the description of the personality disorder and give the correct abbreviation or term/s for which it is describing. Fill in the blanks.*   **LO 10.2, 10.3, and 10.6**

1. A person who repeatedly pulls the hairs from the eyebrows and eyelids: _____

2. The current title for a condition in which a person states that he or she has two separate and distinct personalities: _____

3. The older abbreviation for a person with two separate and distinct personalities: _____

4. A person that consistently cannot resist a sudden urge to do a particular act may be considered to have a: _____

Diagnostic and Therapeutic Procedures and Pharmacology for Mental Health Disorders

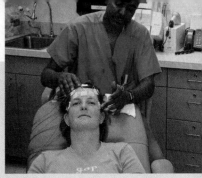

Rick Brady/McGraw Hill

Diagnostic Methods for Mental Disorders

While mental illness is common (about one in five adults has a mental illness in any given year) and is a leading cause of disability, diagnostic tests and treatment procedures are limited, and medications do not cure the illness but can significantly improve symptoms. At this time, there are no tests (examination of blood or body fluids) for mental illnesses as is the case with a physical health condition, though research to identify markers for schizophrenia and depression is ongoing. To define a mental health diagnosis, the following steps can be taken:

- A **physical examination** by a primary care physician to rule out physical problems that could be causing the symptoms.

- **Lab tests** to rule out physical causes of the symptoms; for example, tests of thyroid function and screening for alcohol and drugs.

- A **psychological evaluation** by a psychiatrist or psychologist to determine the patient's symptoms, thoughts, feelings, mood **congruence,** and behavior patterns by talking to the patient and using questionnaires. The defining symptoms of each mental illness are detailed in the ***Diagnostic and Statistical Manual of Mental Disorders,*** fifth edition (DSM-5), compiled by the American Psychiatric Association, which is used by mental health providers to make the diagnosis of mental health disorders and by insurance companies to set reimbursements for treatment.

Therapeutic Methods for Mental Disorders

Mental disorders are characterized by changes in mood, thought, and/or behavior that interfere with the daily activities of living and impair the ability to work and interact with family and the community.

Bright light therapy stimulates the pineal gland to treat seasonal affective disorder. This is one of the few mental health disorders that has a treatment outside of psychotherapy. **Psychotherapy,** also called talk therapy, explores with a trained mental health professional thoughts, feelings, and behaviors on the assumption that the cure for a person's suffering lies within that person. The therapist's roles are to generate emotional awareness and insight to help the person identify the source of the problems and consider alternatives for dealing with them. There are six types of psychotherapy:

1. **Supportive psychotherapy,** in which the expression of feelings is encouraged and the therapist provides help with problem solving.

2. **Psychoanalysis,** which is the oldest form of psychotherapy, developed by Sigmund Freud in the early 20th century. It encourages the person to say whatever comes to mind and helps the person develop an understanding of how the past affects the present, enabling the person to develop new and more adaptive ways of functioning.

3. **Psychodynamic psychotherapy,** which is similar to psychoanalysis and focuses on identifying unconscious patterns in current thoughts, feelings, and behaviors.

4. **Cognitive therapy,** which helps people identify distortions in interpreting experiences and learn to think in different ways about the experiences, which leads to an improvement in behavior and feelings.

5. **Behavioral therapy,** which is similar to cognitive therapy. A combination of the two—**cognitive behavioral therapy (CBT)**—is often used. Behavioral therapy believes that abnormal behaviors are due to faulty learning, and these maladaptive behaviors can be unlearned and corrected.

6. **Interpersonal therapy** involves treatment for depression and focuses on unresolved grief and conflicts that arise when people have to fill roles that differ from their expectations both at work and in the family.

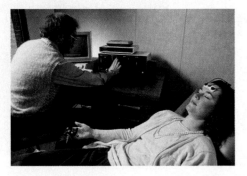

FIGURE 10.22
Patient Receiving Biofeedback Therapy.

Phototherapy, also called bright light therapy, uses bright fluorescent lights to stimulate the pineal gland to treat seasonal affective disorder.

Biofeedback *(Figure 10.22),* and relaxation techniques can be helpful in reducing the tension and spasm associated with psychosomatic disorders.

Brain stimulation treatment, in the form of **electroconvulsive therapy (ECT),** is an effective treatment for severe depression that is unresponsive to other treatments. Electrodes are attached to the head and a series of electrical shocks are delivered to the brain to induce a brief seizure. The effect of this on the brain cells is not fully understood.

The treatment of **posttraumatic stress disorder is multimodal,** involving **psychotherapy,** social interventions, and family and patient education.

Forms of psychotherapy are **cognitive behavioral therapy (CBT)** and **cognitive processing therapy (CPT),** in which thoughts and beliefs generated by the trauma are reframed.

Word Analysis and Definition

S = Suffix   P = Prefix   R = Root   R/CF = Combining Form

WORD	PRONUNCIATION	ELEMENTS		DEFINITION
biofeedback (**Note:** This term has no prefix or suffix.)	bye-oh-**FEED**-back	S/ R/ R/	-**back** *back, return* **bio-** *life* -**feed-** *to nourish*	Training techniques to achieve voluntary control of responses to stimuli
cognitive behavioral therapy (**Note:** Behavioral has two suffixes.)	KOG-nih-tiv be-**HAYV**-yur-al **THAIR**-ah-pee	S/ R/ S/ S/ R/	-**ive** *quality of* **cognit-** *thinking* -**al** *pertaining to* -**ior-** *pertaining to* **behav-** *mental activity* **therapy** Greek *medical treatment*	Psychotherapy that emphasizes thoughts and attitudes in one's behavior
cognitive processing therapy	KOG-nih-tiv **PROSS**-es-ing **THAIR**-ah-pee	S/ R/ S/ P/ R/	-**ive** *quality of* **cognit-** *thinking* -**ing** *doing* **pro-** *before* -**cess-** *going forward* **therapy** Greek *medical treatment*	Psychotherapy to build skills to deal with the effects of trauma in other areas of life
electroconvulsive	ee-**LEK**-troh-**KON-VUL**-siv	S/ R/CF P/ R/	-**ive** *quality of* **electr/o-** *electricity* -**con-** *with* -**vuls-** *tear, pull*	Use of electrical current to produce convulsions
psychoanalysis	sigh-koh-ah-**NAL**-ih-sis	R/CF R/	**psych/o-** *mind* -**analysis** *process to define*	Method of psychotherapy

Pharmacologic Agents Used for Mental Disorders

Psychiatric medications do not cure mental disorders, but they can significantly improve symptoms and help to make other treatments such as psychotherapy more effective. Commonly used classes of prescription medications are discussed below. Two examples of psychiatric medications and their effect on anxiety disorder are listed in *Table 10.2.*

- **Selective serotonin reuptake inhibitors (SSRIs),** with generic and brand names fluoxetine (*Prozac*), fluoxamine (*Luvox*), paroxeline (*Paxil*), and sertraline (*Zoloft*); depression, bipolar disorder, anxiety disorders.

- **Serotonin and norepinephrine reuptake inhibitors (SNRIs),** with generic and brand names venlafaxine (*Effexor*), milnacipran (*Dalcipran*), and duloxetine (*Cymbalta*); depression, bipolar disorder.

- **Affect mainly dopamine and norepinephrine**—bupropion (*Wellbutrin*); depression.

- **Novel serotonergic drugs** such as vortioxetine (*Trintellix*—formerly called *Brintellix*) or vilazodone.

- **Mood stabilizers** to control manic or hypomanic episodes are lithium (*Lithobid*), valproic acid (*Depakene*), divalproex (*Depakote*), carbamazepine (*Tegretol*), and lamotrigine (*Lamictal*); bipolar disorder.

- **Antipsychotics** to help persistent symptoms of depression or mania are the newer, second generation aripiprazole psychotics olanzapine *(Zyprexa)*, risperidone *(Risperdal)*, quetiapine *(Seroquel)*, and aripiprazole *(Abilify)*. These medications are also used to treat schizophrenia, often in combination with **benzodiazepine.**

- **Antidepressant-psychotic**—the medication *Symbyax* is a combination of the antidepressant fluoxetine and the antipsychotic olanzapine and is approved for the treatment of depressive disorders in bipolar disorder.

- **Benzodiazepines** such as diazepam *(Valium)*, alprazolam *(Xanax)*, clonazepam *(Klonopin)*, and lorazepam *(Ativan);* anxiety disorders.

- **Stimulants** such as dextroamphetamine *(Adderal, Dexedrene)* and methylphenidate *(Ritalin, Metylin)* are used to treat attention-deficit/hyperactivity disorder (ADHD) and are also available in longacting formats.

- **Hypnotics** such as zolpidem *(Ambien)*, zaleplon *(Sonata)*, and eszopiclone *(Lunesta)* also are used to treat insomnia.

- **Tranquilizers** such as chlorpromazine *(Thorazine)*, haloperidol *(Aloperidin)*, and the benzodiazepines calm like sedatives but without a sleep-inducing effect.

Table 10.2 Pharmacotherapy of Panic Disorder

Type of Drug	Effect
Benzodiazepines:	Effective prophylaxis
alprazolam *(Xanax)*	Reduce anticipatory anxiety
clonazepam *(Klonopin)*	Rapid onset of action
lorazepam *(Ativan)*	
diazepam *(Valium)*	
Selective Serotonin Reuptake Inhibitors (SSRIs):	Reduce frequency of attacks
sertraline *(Zoloft)*	Reduce intensity of panic
paroxetine *(Paxil)*	Take 2 weeks to produce effect
fluvoxamine *(Luvox)*	

WORD	PRONUNCIATION	ELEMENTS		DEFINITION
antidepressant	AN-tih-dee-**PRESS**-ant	S/ P/ R/	-ant *agent* anti- *against* -depress- *press down*	An agent to suppress the symptoms of depression
antipsychotic	AN-tih-sigh-**KOT**-ik	S/ P/ R/CF	-tic *pertaining to* anti- *against* -psych/o- *mind*	An agent helpful in the treatment of psychosis
barbiturate	bar-**BIT**-chu-rat	S/ R/	-urate *salt of uric acid* barbit- *barbituric acid*	Central nervous system depressant used as a hypnotic, anxiolytic, or anticonvulsant
benzodiazepine	ben-zoh-die-**AZ**-ah-peen	S/ P/ R/CF	-pine *pine* -diaze- *organic compound* benz/o- *benzene*	Central nervous system depressant used as a hypnotic, anxiolytic, or anticonvulsant, or to produce amnesia
hypnotic	hip-**NOT**-ik	S/ R/CF	-tic *pertaining to* hypn/o- *sleep*	An agent that promotes sleep
stabilizer	**STAY**-bill-ize-er	S/ S/ R/	-er *agent* -ize *action* stabil- *fixed, steady*	Agent that helps create a steady state
tranquilizer	**TRANG**-kwih-lie-zer	S/ R/	-izer *affects in a particular way* tranquil- *calm, serene*	Agent that calms without sedating or depressing

EXERCISES

A. Elements remain your best clue to the meaning of a medical term. *Match the element in the left column with its correct meaning in the right column.*   **LO 10.2**

_____ **1.** *electr/o*

_____ **2.** *cognit*

_____ **3.** *bio*

_____ **4.** *pro-*

_____ **5.** *vuls*

_____ **6.** *behav*

_____ **7.** *con-*

_____ **8.** *-ior*

_____ **9.** *-ive*

_____ **10.** *feed*

    a. mental activity

    b. before

    c. nourish

    d. pertaining to

    e. tear

    f. life

    g. quality of

    h. electricity

    i. with

    j. thinking

B. Apply the elements of the language of medical terminology to answer the following questions. *Fill in the blanks.*   **LO 10.7**

1. What are the differences between behavioral, processing, and feedback therapies?

    a. Behavioral therapy _____

    _____

    b. Processing therapy _____

    _____

    c. Biofeedback therapy _____

    _____

C. Define the types of medications used to treat mental disorders. *Choose the correct definition for the given medication.*   **LO 10.7**

1. The action of a **sedative** is to:

    a. suppress the symptoms of depression

    b. calm without depressing

    c. promote wakefulness

    d. calm nervous excitement

2. A reason why a physician would prescribe a benzodiazepine would be due to its ability to induce:

    a. seizures

    b. muscle spasms

    c. memory loss

    d. insomnia

D. Pronunciation is important whether you are saying the word or listening to a word from a coworker. Identify the proper pronunciation of the following medical terms.   **LO 10.1, 10.2, 10.5, and 10.7**

1. The correct pronunciation for an agent that causes an absence of feeling:

    a. **ANAL**-jeh-zik

    b. an-al-**JEE**-zik

    c. **AN**-eh-thet-ik

    d. an-es-**THET**-ik

Correctly spell the term: _____

2. The correct pronunciation for the failure of one or more vertebral arches to close during fetal development:

    a. **SPY**-na **BYE**-fih-day

    b. **SPY**-nah **BIH**-fih-dah

    c. **MAY**-nin-go-sell

    d. meh-**NING**-oh-seal

Correctly spell the term: _____

3. The correct pronunciation for a pharmacologic agent capable of preventing or arresting epilepsy:

    a. sed-**AY**-tiv

    b. **SED**-ah-tiv

    c. **AN**-tee-eh-pih-**LEP**-tik

    d. **AN**-tee-**PIE**-lep-**TIK**

Correctly spell the term: _____

4. The correct pronunciation for the disorder described as the presence of persecutory delusions:

    a. pair-ah-**NOY**-ah

    b. par-uh-nyu-**OH**-yuh

    c. **NEE**-ralj-**EE**-ah

    d. nyu-**RAL**-jee-ah

Correctly spell the term: _____

5. The correct pronunciation for the time occurring after a seizure:

    a. post-**IK**-tal

    b. pah-**STICK**-tal

    c. **TON**-ik

    d. tone-**IK**

Correctly spell the term: _____

Additional exercises available in **connect**

Chapter Review exercises, along with additional practice items, are available in Connect!

Special Senses of the Eye and Ear

The Essentials of the Languages of Ophthalmology and Otology

Rick Brady/McGraw Hill

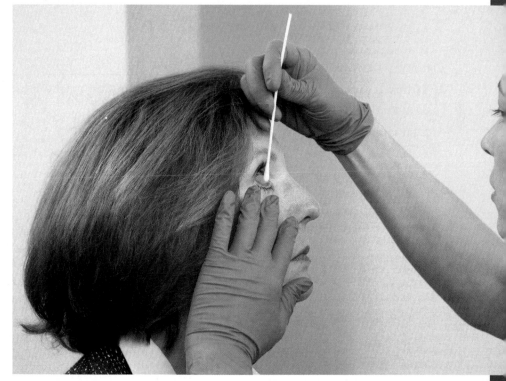

Learning Outcomes

In order to make correct decisions in situations where you are caring for patients with eye and ear issues, to communicate with other health care team members about the patient, to participate in patient education, and to document the patient's care, you need to be able to:

LO 11.1 Use roots, combining forms, suffixes, and prefixes to construct and analyze (deconstruct) medical terms related to the eye and ear.

LO 11.2 Spell and pronounce correctly medical terms related to the eye and ear to communicate them with accuracy and precision in any health care setting.

LO 11.3 Define accepted abbreviations related to the eye and ear.

LO 11.4 Relate the structures of the eyes and ears to their functions.

LO 11.5 Identify and describe disorders and pathological conditions related to the eyes and ears.

LO 11.6 Identify the diagnostic and therapeutic procedures and pharmacologic agents used for diseases and disorders of the eyes and ears.

LO 11.7 Identify health professionals involved in the care of patients with eye and ear diseases and disorders.

LO 11.8 Apply your knowledge of the medical terms of the eyes and ears to documentation, medical records, and medical reports.

LO 11.9 Translate the medical terms of the eyes and ears into everyday language to communicate clearly with patients and their families.

NOTE: The sense of smell is discussed as an integral part of the respiratory system; the sense of taste, as an integral part of the digestive system; and the sense of touch, as an integral part of the nervous system.

In your future career, you may work directly and/or indirectly with one or more of the following:

- **Ophthalmologists** are medical doctors who specialize in the diagnosis and treatment of diseases of the eye.
- **Optometrists** are doctors of optometry, skilled in the measurement of vision, and maintaining eye health.

The health professionals listed below perform specific assigned procedures and support ophthalmologists according to the depth of their training:

- **Certified ophthalmic medical technicians**
- **Certified ophthalmic assistants**
- **Certified ophthalmic technicians**
- **Certified ophthalmic technologists**
- **Registered ophthalmic ultrasound biometrists**
- **Diagnostic ophthalmic sonographers**

In your future career, being able to communicate comfortably, accurately, and effectively with the health professionals involved in the diagnosis and treatment of problems of the ear is key. You may work directly and/or indirectly with one or more of the following:

- **Otologists** are physician medical specialists in diseases of the ear.
- **Otorhinolaryngologists**, also known as ENTs, are physician medical specialists in diseases of the ear, nose, and throat.
- **Audiologists** are specialists in the evaluation of hearing function.

Section 11.1

Structure and Function of the Accessory Structures of the Eye

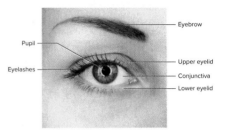

Rick Brady/McGraw Hill

Accessory Structures, Extrinsic Muscles and Their Functions (LO 11.2 and 11.4)

Accessory Structures (LO 11.2 and 11.4)

A beam of light travels to the eye at 186,000 miles per second, or 671 million miles per hour. Before it can reach the eyeball, it passes through the external **periorbital accessory** structures, which have important functions that support and protect the exposed front surface of the eye.

- **Eyebrows** *(Figure 11.1)* keep sweat from running into the eyes and function in nonverbal communication to show how you're feeling in response to certain stimuli.

- **Eyelids** protect the eyes from foreign objects. They blink to move tears across the eyes' surface and sweep debris away. They close during sleep to keep out visual stimuli and prevent the eye from drying out. They are the body's thinnest layer of skin.

- **Eyelashes** are strong hairs that help keep debris out of the eyes. They arise from hair follicles with their sebaceous glands on the edge of the lids.

The **conjunctiva** is a transparent mucous membrane that lines the inside of both eyelids. It moves freely over the eyeball and covers the front of the eye but not the central portion (the cornea). In the conjunctiva, numerous goblet cells secrete a thin film of mucin (a complex protein) that keeps the eyeball moist. It has numerous small blood vessels and is richly supplied with nerve endings that make it very sensitive and easily irritated.

The **lacrimal apparatus** *(Figure 11.2)* consists of the **lacrimal (tear) gland** located in the superolateral corner of the orbit. This gland secretes tears, and short ducts carry the tears to the conjunctiva's surface. After washing across the conjunctiva, the tears leave the eye at its medial corner by draining into the **lacrimal sac.** They then flow into the **nasolacrimal duct**, which carries the tears into the nose, from where they are eventually swallowed.

The functions of tears are to:

- **Clean and lubricate** the surface of the eyes;

- **Deliver** nutrients and oxygen to the conjunctiva; and

- **Prevent infection** through bactericidal (bacteria-killing) enzymes.

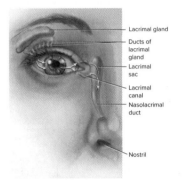

▲ **FIGURE 11.1**
External Anatomy of the Eye.

Africa Studio/Shutterstock

▲ **FIGURE 11.2**
Lacrimal Apparatus.

Word Analysis and Definition

S = Suffix   P = Prefix   R = Root   R/CF = Combining Form

WORD	PRONUNCIATION		ELEMENTS	DEFINITION
accessory	ak-**SESS**-oh-ree		Latin *to move toward*	A muscle, nerve, or other structure that is supplemental to a more major
alignment	a-**LINE**-ment		French *arrange in a straight line*	Having structures in its correct position relative to other structures
conjunctiva conjunctival (adj)	kon-junk-**TIE**-vah kon-junk-**TIE**-val	S/ R/	Latin *inner lining of eyelids* -al *pertaining to* conjunctiv- *conjunctiva*	Inner lining of eyelids Pertaining to the conjunctiva
extrinsic	eks-**TRIN**-sik		Latin *on the outer side*	Any muscle located entirely on the outside of the structure under consideration; e.g., the eye
intrinsic	in-**TRIN**-sik		Latin *on the inner side*	Any muscle located entirely within (inside) the structure under consideration; e.g., the eye
lacrimal	**LAK**-rim-al	S/ R/	-al *pertaining to* lacrim- *tear*	Pertaining to tears and the tear apparatus
nasolacrimal duct	**NAY**-zoh-**LAK**-rim-al DUKT	R/CF R/	nas/o- *nose* duct *to lead*	Passage from the lacrimal sac to the nose
orbit orbital (adj)	**OR**-bit **OR**-bit-al	S/ R/	Latin *circle* -al *pertaining to* orbit- *orbit*	The bony socket that holds the eyeball Pertaining to the orbit
periorbital (adj)	pair-ee-**OR**-bit-al	P/	peri- *around*	Pertaining to tissues around the orbit
stereopsis	stair-ee-**OP**-sis	S/ R/	-opsis *vision* stere- *three-dimensional*	Three-dimensional vision

- The cornea protects the eye and, by changing shape, provides about 60% of the eye's focusing power.
- The iris controls the amount of light entering the eye.
- The lens changes its shape to focus rays of light on to the retina.

Extrinsic Muscles of the Eye (LO 11.2 and 11.4)

The position of the eyes on the human face allows them to work closely together, giving us very good three-dimensional perception (**stereopsis**) and hand-eye coordination. Stereopsis depends on an accurate **alignment** of the two eyes.

Six coordinated **extrinsic** eye muscles in each eye—attached to the inner wall of the orbit and outer surface of the eyeball—keep the eyes properly aligned, and move the eyes in all directions.

The Eyeball (Globe) (LO 11.2 and 11.4)

Although your eyeball may appear to be solid, it's actually a hollow sphere that measures around 1 inch in diameter.

The functions of the eyeball are to continuously:

1. **Adjust** the amount of light it lets in to reach the retina;
2. **Focus** on near and distant objects; and
3. **Produce** images of those objects and instantly transmit them to the brain.

There are three layers of the eyeball:

1. outer fibrous layer
   a. **sclera**—white; protects inner eye structures
   b. **cornea**—transparent; bends light rays
2. middle vascular layer, also known as the **uvea,**
   a. **iris**—colored part of the eye; controls size of the pupil
   b. **ciliary body**—bends the lens; focuses light rays
   c. **choroid**—vascular layer of the eye; absorbs light
3. inner layer
   a. **retina**—neural layer of the eye; absorbs light

As shown earlier in this chapter, the front of the eyeball is covered by the conjunctiva. This thin layer of tissue lines the inside of the eyelids and curves over the eyeball to meet the **sclera** *(Figure 11.3),* the tough, white outer layer of the eye.

At the center of the front of the eye is the **cornea**, a transparent, dome-shaped membrane. The cornea has no blood supply and obtains its nutrients from tears and from fluid in the anterior chamber behind it.

When light rays strike the eye, they pass through the cornea. Because of its dome curvature, those rays striking the edge of the cornea are bent toward its center. The light rays then go through the **pupil**, the black opening in the center of the colored area (the **iris**) in the front of the eye.

The iris controls the amount of light entering the eye. For example, when you are in the dark outside at night, the iris opens (**dilates**) to allow more light into the eye. When you are in bright sunlight or in a well-lit room, the iris closes (**constricts**) to allow less light into the eye.

After traveling through the pupil, the light rays pass through the transparent **lens**. This lens can become thicker and thinner, enabling it to bend light rays and focus them on the **retina** at the back of the eye. **Accommodation** is the process of changing focus, and **refraction** is the process of bending light rays.

The eyeball is divided into two fluid-filled segments, the anterior cavity and the posterior cavity. These cavities are separated by the lens and ciliary muscle *(Figure 11.3 a).* **Aqueous humor** fills the anterior cavity and **vitreous humor** fills the posterior cavity.

The lens does not contain blood vessels (**avascular**) or nerves, and with increasing age, it loses its elasticity.

◄ FIGURE 11.3
(a) Anatomy of the Eyeball.
(b) Eye Layers.

Africa Studio/Shutterstock

Word Analysis and Definition

S = Suffix   P = Prefix   R = Root   R/CF = Combining Form

WORD	PRONUNCIATION	ELEMENTS		DEFINITION
accommodation (noun)	ah-kom-oh-**DAY**-shun	S/ P/ R/	-ion *action* ac- *toward* -commodat- *adjust*	The act of adjusting something to make it fit the needs; in this case, the lens of the eye adjusts itself
accommodate (verb)	ah-**KOM**-oh-date	S/	-ate *pertaining to, composed of*	To adapt to meet a need
accommodative (adj)	ah-kom-oh-**DAY**-tiv	S/	-ive *pertaining to*	Pertaining to accommodation
aqueous humor	**AYK**-wee-us **HEW**-mor	S/ R/CF	-ous *pertaining to* aqu/e- *watery* humor *Greek liquid*	Watery liquid in the anterior and posterior chambers of the eye
avascular	a-**VAS**-cue-lar	S/ P/ R/	-ar *pertaining to* a- *without* -vascul- *blood vessel*	Without a blood supply
constrict (verb)	kon-**STRIKT**	P/ R/	con- *with, together* -strict *narrow*	Become or make narrow
constriction (noun)	kon-**STRIK**-shun	S/	-ion *action, condition*	A narrowed portion of a structure
cornea	**KOR**-nee-ah		Latin *web, tunic*	The central, transparent part of the outer coat of the eye covering the iris and pupil
corneal (adj)	**KOR**-nee-al	S/ R/	-al *pertaining to* corne- *cornea*	Pertaining to the cornea
dilate (verb) dilation (noun)	**DIE**-late die-**LAY**-shun	S/ R/	Latin *dilate* -ion *action, condition* dilat- *dilate*	To perform or undergo dilation Stretching or enlarging an opening or a structure
iris	**EYE**-ris		Greek *diaphragm of the eye*	Colored portion of the eye with the pupil in its center
lens	**LENZ**		Latin *lentil shape*	Transparent refractive structure behind the iris
pupil	**PYU**-pill		Latin *pupil*	The opening in the center of the iris that allows light to reach the lens
pupillary (adj) (**Note:** *Change to ll.*)	**PYU**-pih-**LAIR**-ee	S/ R/	-ary *pertaining to* pupill- *pupil*	Pertaining to the pupil
refract (verb) refraction (noun)	ree-**FRAKT** ree-**FRAKT**-shun	S/ R/	Latin *break up* -ion *condition* refract- *bend*	Bend or change direction of a ray of light The bending of light
retina retinal (adj)	**RET**-ih-nah **RET**-ih-nal	S/ R/	Latin *net* -al *pertaining to* retin- *retina*	Light-sensitive innermost layer of the eyeball Pertaining to the retina
sclera	**SKLAIR**-ah		Greek *hard*	Fibrous outer covering of the eyeball and the white of the eye
scleral (adj)	**SKLAIR**-al	S/ R/	-al *pertaining to* scler- *hardness, white of eye*	Pertaining to the sclera
vitreous humor	**VIT**-ree-us **HEW**-mor	S/ R/	-ous *pertaining to* vitre- *glassy* humor *Greek liquid*	A gelatinous liquid in the posterior cavity of the eyeball with the appearance of glass
uvea	**YOU**-vee-ah		Latin *vascular layer*	Middle coat of the eyeball; includes the iris, ciliary body, and choroid

The Retina (LO 11.2 and 11.4)

The retina is the size of a postage stamp and has ten layers of cells. Located at the back of the eye *(Figure 11.4a)*, it is the final destination for light rays. The retina has 130 million **rods** *(Figure 11.4b)*, which perceive only light, not color, and function mostly in dim lighting. The retina has 6.5 million light- and color-activated **cones** *(Figure 11.4b)*, which allow precise **visual acuity** (sharpness). Three different cone types respond individually to either red, green, or blue light. The perception of color is based on the intensity of various color mixtures from the three cone types.

Some people have a hereditary lack of response by one or more of the three cone types and show color blindness. The most common form of this is red-green color blindness. Here, red-green colors and related shades cannot be distinguished from each other.

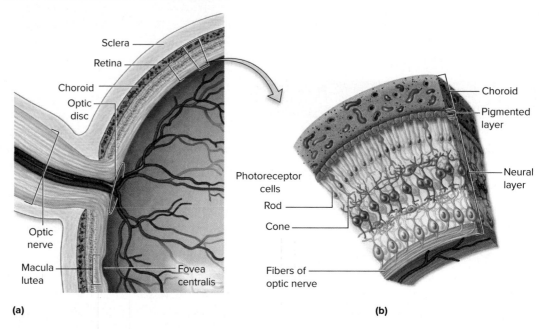

(a)

(b)

▲ **FIGURE 11.4** Structure of the Retina.
(a) Retina. (b) Rods and cones.

The rods and cones convert the light rays' energy into electrical impulses. The **optic nerve**—a bundle of more than a million nerve fibers—transmits these impulses to the visual cortex at the back of the brain. The area where the optic nerve and retina connect is called the **optic disc.** Because it has no rods and cones, the optic disc cannot form images; as a result, this area is called the "blind spot."

Just lateral to the optic disc at the back of the retina is a circular, yellowish region called the **macula lutea** *(Figure 11.4a)*. In the center of the macula is a small pit called the **fovea centralis**, which has 4,000 tiny cones but no rods. Each cone has its own nerve fiber, and this gives the fovea area the sharpest vision. As you read this text, the words are precisely focused on your fovea centralis.

Behind the light-sensitive **photoreceptor** layer of the retina is a vascular layer called the **choroid**.

Refraction (LO 11.4)

Light travels at 186,000 miles per second, and even when it hits the eye, this speed remains the same. Light rays that hit the center of the cornea pass straight through the eye, while rays that hit away from the center then bend toward the center. These light rays then hit the lens and bend again, and in normal vision, the image is focused sharply on the retina, **emmetropia** *(Figure 11.5)*.

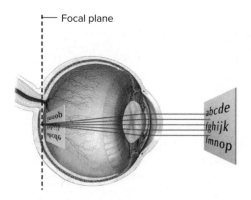

▲ **FIGURE 11.5** Normal Vision.

S = Suffix   P = Prefix   R = Root   R/CF = Combining Form

WORD	PRONUNCIATION	ELEMENTS		DEFINITION
choroid	**KOR**-oid		Greek *membrane*	Region of the retina and uvea
emmetropia	em-eh-**TROH**-pee-ah	P/ R/	emmetr- *measure* -opia *sight*	Normal refractive condition of the eye
fovea centralis	**FOH**-vee-ah sen-**TRAH**-lis	S/ R/	fovea Latin *a pit* -is *pertaining to* central- *center*	Small pit in the center of the macula that has the highest visual acuity
macula lutea	**MACK**-you-lah **LOO**-tee-ah		macula Latin *small spot* lutea Latin *yellow*	Yellowish spot on the back of the retina; contains the fovea
optic optical (adj)	**OP**-tik **OP**-tih-kal	S/ R/	Greek *eye* -al *pertaining to* optic- *eye*	Pertaining to the eye or vision Pertaining to the eye or vision
optic disc	**OP**-tik DISK		Greek *eye* Latin *disc*	Area in the back of the eye where the optic nerve and retina connect; the "blind spot"
photoreceptor	foh-toh-ree-**SEP**-tor	S/ R/CF	-or *that which does something* phot/o- *light* -recept- *receive*	A photoreceptor cell receives light and converts it into electrical impulses
visual acuity	**VIH**-zhoo-wal ah-**KYU**-ih-tee	S/ R/	-al *pertaining to* visu- *sight* acuity Latin *sharpen*	Sharpness and clearness of vision

EXERCISES

A. Build *your medical vocabulary. If the term does not have an element, insert N/A. The first one has been done for you. Fill in the chart.*   **LO 11.1**

Medical Term	Prefix	Meaning of Prefix	Root(s)/CF(s)	Meaning of R/CF	Suffix	Meaning of Suffix
corneal	1. N/A	2. N/A	3. corne-	4. cornea	5. -al	6. pertaining to
conjunctivitis	7.	8.	9.	10.	11.	12.
periorbital	13.	14.	15.	16.	17.	18.

B. Define *the statements in the first column using the language of ophthalmology in the second column. Fill in the blanks.*   **LO 11.4 and 11.5**

_____ 1. colored portion of the eye   a. lens

_____ 2. bend a ray of light   b. retina

_____ 3. opening in the iris   c. avascular

_____ 4. transparent, refractive structure   d. pupil

_____ 5. innermost layer of the eyeball   e. refract

_____ 6. fibrous, outer covering of the eye   f. iris

_____ 7. without a blood supply   g. sclera

C. Define *the meaning of the following word elements. Fill in the blanks.*   **LO 11.1 and 11.8**

1. -itis _____

2. -strict _____

3. a- _____

4. retin- _____

5. -al _____

6. dilat- _____

D. The language of ophthalmology *will be your answers in this exercise. Select the best answer.*   **LO 11.1 and 11.4**

1. Sharpness and clearness of vision is called:

    a. optical

    b. acuity

    c. vascular

    d. sclera

    e. choroid

2. Because it has no rods and cones, the optic disc cannot form images and thus is called the:

    a. fovea

    b. blind spot

    c. uvea

    d. visual cortex

    e. optic nerve

3. The term *photoreceptor* has:

    a. two combining forms and a suffix

    b. a prefix, a root, and a suffix

    c. a combining form, a root, and a suffix

    d. two roots and a suffix

    e. a suffix and a root

4. The area of sharpest vision is the:

    a. cornea

    b. rods

    c. macula lutea

    d. fovea centralis

    e. cones

E. Deconstruct *terms related to retina. Fill in the blanks.*   **LO 11.1 and 11.4**

1. centralis: _____/_____
                                R   S

2. photoreceptor: _____/_____/_____
                                    R/CF   R   S

3. optical: _____/_____
                                R   S

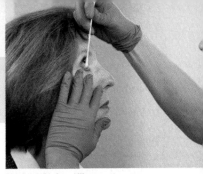

Many eye disorders can threaten a patient's vision, but if detected early, the majority of these conditions can be cured or treated to slow or prevent the progression of vision loss.

Rick Brady/McGraw Hill

Disorders of the Accessory Structures and Extrinsic Eye Muscles (LO 11.5)

The accessory glands of the eyes can be affected by a number of different disorders, most of which cause noticeable discomfort.

Conjunctivitis (pink eye) has several causes *(Figure 11.6)* but can also be considered nonspecific. Some of the most common forms of conjunctivitis are listed below:

Viral and bacterial conjunctivitis are contagious and can be spread by a person touching their eyes after coming into contact with a **contaminated** object and an infected person's eye secretions or tears.

- **Viral** is contagious and commonly caused by viruses that cause the common cold.

- **Bacterial** is contagious and frequently due to staphylococcal or streptococcal bacteria; often referred to as "pink eye."

- **Allergic conjunctivitis,** which can be part of seasonal hay fever or produced by year-round allergens like animal dander and dust mites *(Chapter 8);*

- **Irritant conjunctivitis,** which can be caused by air **pollutants** (smoke and fumes), chemicals like chlorine, and some ingredients found in soaps and cosmetics; and

- **Neonatal conjunctivitis (ophthalmia neonatorum),** which is specific to babies and can be caused by a blocked tear duct, by the antibiotic eye drops given routinely at birth, or by sexually transmitted bacteria from an infected mother's birth canal.

Eyelid edema, a generalized swelling of the eyelids, is often produced by an allergic reaction *(see Chapter 8)* from cosmetics, pollen in the air, or insect stings and bites.

A **stye** or **hordeolum** is an infection of an eyelash follicle that produces an abscess *(Figure 11.7),* with localized pain, swelling, redness, and pus at the edge of the eyelid.

Blepharitis occurs when multiple eyelash follicles become infected. The eyelid's margin shows persistent redness and crusting and may become **ulcerated** *(Figure 11.8).*

Ptosis, in which the upper eyelid is constantly drooped over the eye, is due to **paresis** of the muscle that raises the upper lid *(Figure 11.9).* The term **blepharoptosis** defines the sagging of the eyelids from excess skin.

Dry eye disease (dysfunctional tear syndrome) is due to decreased tear production by the lacrimal glands. It leads to ocular discomfort and potential damage to the conjunctiva and cornea. Dry eye is more common in females and the elderly, and in people who wear contact lenses.

Sjögren's syndrome is an autoimmune process attacking the lacrimal and salivary glands. Symptoms include dry mouth and eyes.

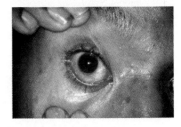

▲ **FIGURE 11.6**
Conjunctivitis.

Centers for Disease Control and Prevention

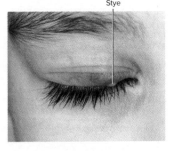

▲ **FIGURE 11.7**
Stye Showing
Pus-Filled Cyst.

ElRoi/Shutterstock

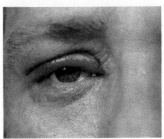

▲ **FIGURE 11.8**
Blepharitis of
the Upper Lid.

Images By Kenny/Alamy Stock Photo

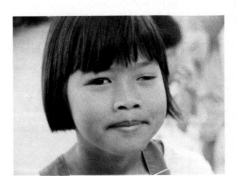

▲ **FIGURE 11.9**   Ptosis of Left Eyelid.

Richman Photo/Shutterstock

WORD	PRONUNCIATION	ELEMENTS		DEFINITION
blepharitis	blef-ah-**RYE**-tis	S/ R/	-itis *inflammation* **blephar-** *eyelid*	Inflammation of the eyelid
blepharoptosis	**BLEF**-ah-**ROP**-toh-sis	S/ R/CF	-ptosis *drooping* **blephar/o-** *eyelid*	Drooping of the upper eyelid
conjunctivitis "pink eye"	kon-junk-tih-**VI**-tis	R/CF	**conjunctiv-** *conjunctiva* Lay term for conjunctivitis	Inflammation of the conjunctiva Conjunctivitis
contagious	kon-**TAY**-jus		Latin *touch closely*	Infection can be transmitted from person to person or from a person to a surface to a person
contaminate (verb)	kon-**TAM**-in-ate	S/ P/ R/	-ate *composed of, pertaining to* con- *together* **-tamin-** *touch*	To cause the presence of an infectious agent to be on any surface
contamination (noun)	**KON**-tam-ih-**NAY**-shun	S/	-ation *process*	The presence of an infectious agent on any surface
hordeolum (*also called* stye)	hor-**DEE**-oh-lum		Latin *stye in the eye*	Abscess in an eyelash follicle
keratoconjunctivitis	**KAIR**-ah-toh-kon-**JUNK**-tih-**VI**-tis	S/ R/	-itis *inflammation* **-conjunctiv-** *conjunctiva*	Combined inflammation of the cornea and conjunctiva
ophthalmia neonatorum	off-**THAL**-me-ah ne-oh-nay-**TOR**-um	S/ R/ S/ P/ R/	-ia *condition* **ophthalm-** *eye* -orum *function of* neo- *new* **-nat-** *born*	Conjunctivitis of the newborn
paresis (can also be used as a *suffix*)	par-**EE**-sis		Greek *paralysis*	Partial paralysis
pollution	poh-**LOO**-shun		Latin *to defile*	Condition that is unclean, impure, and a danger to health
pollutant	poh-**LOO**-tant	S/ R/	-ant *pertaining to* **pollut-** *unclean*	Substance that makes an environment unclean or impure
ptosis (**Notes:** *When a word begins with two consonants, the first is silent.* **Ptosis** *can also be used as a suffix.*)	**TOH**-sis		Greek *drooping*	Drooping down of the upper eyelid or an organ
purulent	**PURE**-you-lent	S/ R/	-ulent *abounding in* **pur-** *pus*	Showing or containing a lot of pus
Sjögren's syndrome	**SHOW**-gren **SIN**-drome		Henrik Sjögren, 1889–1986, Swedish ophthalmologist	Autoimmune disease that attacks the glands that produce saliva and tears
ulcer ulceration	**ULL**-sir ull-sir-**A**-shun	S/ R/	-ation *a process* **ulcer-** *a sore*	Erosion of an area of skin or mucosa Formation of an ulcer

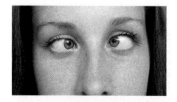

▲ FIGURE 11.10
Strabismus.

sruilk/Shutterstock

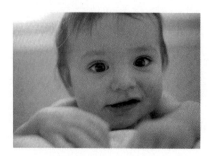

◄ FIGURE 11.11
Congenital Esotropia (both eyes are affected).

Matt Harris Photography/Alamy Stock Photo

Disorders of Extrinsic Eye Muscles (LO 11.5)

When there is a muscle imbalance in one eye, the alignment breaks down and **strabismus** (*Figure 11.10*), also known as a "cross-eyed" condition, results.

Esotropia is a condition where the eye is turned in toward the nose. In congenital or infantile esotropia, both eyes look in toward the nose—the right eye looks to the left and the left eye looks to the right (*Figure 11.11*).

Accomodative esotropia is an inward eye turn, usually noticed around age 2 in 1% to 2% of children.

Exotropia, an outward eye turn, is noticed in children around ages 2 to 4.

Amblyopia, or "lazy eye," occurs in children when vision in one eye has not developed as well as vision in the other. It occurs because the eye and the brain do not cooperate for the affected eye.

Nystagmus is a term to describe fast, uncontrollable movements of the eye that may be side to side (horizontal nystagmus), up and down (vertical nystagmus), or **rotary** (rotary nystagmus). The condition can be congenital or acquired from head injury, inner ear disorders (*see the section on the Ear in this chapter*), stroke, or drugs, such as excess alcohol, sedatives, or anti-epilepsy drugs (*see Chapter 10*).

Disorders of the Anterior Eyeball (LO 11.5)

Keratoconjunctivitis, also known as toxic conjunctivitis, is a combined inflammation of the cornea and conjunctiva. It can be viral, bacterial, or allergic in origin.

Corneal abrasions are caused by foreign bodies, by direct trauma (like being scratched by a fingernail), or by ill-fitting contact lenses. An abrasion can grow into an ulcer.

Scleritis is an inflammation of the sclera (the white outer covering of the eyeball) that can affect one or both eyes.

Anisocoria describes the presence of unequal pupils as either a normal finding in 20% of individuals or an indication of brain injury.

Uveitis, inflammation of the iris, ciliary body, and choroid, produces pain, blurred vision, and constriction of the pupil.

Glaucoma results if fluid from inside the eyeball cannot escape from the eye into the bloodstream. The fluid continues to be produced and pressure builds up inside the eye. This pressure interferes with the blood supply to the retina, causing retinal cells to die and damage to occur within the optic nerve fibers. Glaucoma is a major cause of blindness *(Figure 11.12)*.

A **cataract** is a cloudy or opaque area in the lens *(Figure 11.3)*. It is caused by aging and may be associated with diabetes and cigarette smoking. Symptoms include blurred vision *(Figure 11.4)* and **photosensitivity** and is another major cause of blindness.

Congenital (present at birth) cataracts occur in less than 0.5% of newborns and can be unilateral (present in one eye) or bilateral (present in both eyes). They are treated in the same way as any other cataract.

Photosensitivity is discomfort or pain associated with the amount of light most people tolerate. Examples of eye-related conditions that can cause photosensitivity are cataracts, damage to cornea such as abrasions and ulcers, and inflammatory conditions such as conjunctivitis, keratitis, iritis, and uveitis. Neurologic conditions causing photosensitivity include migraines, post-concussion syndrome, and other traumatic brain injuries.

Photophobia is a behavior where a person avoids light because it hurts their eyes. It is recommended that health professionals investigate the causes of a person's photophobia, one of which could be photosensitivity. The terms photosensitivity and photophobia are often used interchangeably.

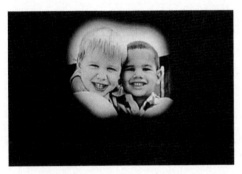

▲ **FIGURE 11.12** Vision with Glaucoma.

National Eye Institute

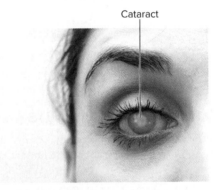

Cataract

▲ **FIGURE 11.13** Cataract.

sruilk/Shutterstock

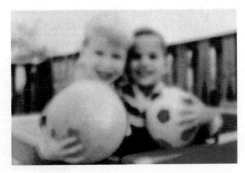

▲ **FIGURE 11.14** Vision with Cataract.

National Eye Institute

WORD	PRONUNCIATION		ELEMENTS	DEFINITION
amblyopia	am-blee-**OH**-pee-ah	P/ R/	**ambly-** *dull* **-opia** *sight*	Failure or incomplete development of the pathways of vision to the brain
abrasion	ah-**BRAY**-shun	S/ R/	**-ion** *action, condition, process* **abras-** *scrape off*	Area of skin or mucous membrane that has been scraped off
anisocoria (Note: Two prefixes)	an-**EYE**-soh-**KOR**-ee-ah	S/ P/ P/ S/ R/	**-ia** *condition* **an-** *not, lack of, without* **-iso-** *equal* **-ia** *condition* **-cor-** *pupil*	Unequal pupil size
cataract	**KAT**-ah-ract		Latin *to break down*	Complete or partial opacity of the lens
esotropia	es-oh-**TROH**-pee-ah	S/ P/ R/	**-ia** *condition* **eso-** *inward* **-trop-** *turn*	Turning the eye inward toward the nose
exotropia	ek-soh-**TROH**-pee-ah	P/	**exo-** *outward*	Turning the eye outward away from the nose
glaucoma	glau-**KOH**-mah	S/ R/	**-oma** *mass, tumor* **glauc-** *lens opacity*	Loss of vision due to increased intraocular pressure
nystagmus	nis-**TAG**-muss		Greek *nodding*	Fast, uncontrollable movements of the eyeballs
photophobia	foh-toh-**FOH**-bee-ah	S/ R/CF R/	**-ia** *condition* **phot/o-** *light* **-phob-** *fear*	Fear of the light because it hurts the eyes.
photophobic (adj)	foh-toh-**FOH**-bik	S/	**-ic** *pertaining to*	Pertaining to or suffering from photophobia
photosensitivity	**FOH**-toh-sen-sih-**TIV**-ih-tee	S/ R/CF R/	**-ity** *condition* **phot/o-** *light* **-sensitiv-** *feeling*	When light produces pain in the eye
photosensitive (adj)	foh-toh-**SEN**-sih-tiv			Having a reaction to light
rotary	**ROW**-tah-ree		Latin *to revolve*	Circular movement
scleritis	sklair-**EYE**-tis	S/ R/	**-itis** *inflammation* **scler-** *hardness, white of eye*	Inflammation of the sclera
strabismus	strah-**BIZ**-mus	S/ R/	**-ismus** *take action* **strab-** *squint*	Turning of an eye away from its normal position
uveitis	you-vee-**EYE**-tis	S/ R/	**-itis** *inflammation* **uve-** *uvea*	Inflammation of the uvea

Disorders of the Retina (LO 11.4)

An impaired retina affects your ability to see in the same way that an injured leg affects your ability to walk. In either case, your level of functioning in normal, daily life is limited.

Macular Degeneration (LO 11.4)

Degeneration of the central macula results in a loss of visual acuity or sharpness, with a dark blurry area of vision loss in the center of the visual field *(Figure 11.15)*. Photoreceptor cell loss and bleeding with capillary proliferation and scar formation *(Figure 11.16)* also occur. Macular degeneration can progress to blindness. Most cases occur in people over 55.

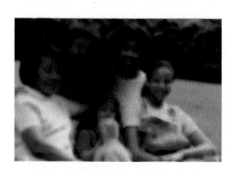

◀ **FIGURE 11.15**
Vision with Macular Degeneration.

Steve Mason/Getty Images

▶ **FIGURE 11.16**   **Ophthalmoscopic View of Macular Degeneration.**

memorisz/Shutterstock

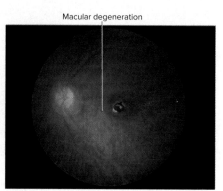

Macular degeneration

Retinal Detachment (LO 11.4)

In retinal detachment, the retina may separate partially or completely from its underlying choroid layer, creating a retinal tear or hole. This can happen suddenly, without pain, but is considered a surgical emergency. The patient sees a dark shadow invading his or her peripheral vision.

Diabetic Retinopathy (LO 11.4)

Some 50% of diabetics have **retinopathy**. Patients may experience hemorrhages (bleeding), which can lead to the destruction of the photoreceptor cells (rods and cones) and visual difficulties (*Figures 11.17 and 11.18*).

Papilledema

Papilledema is swelling of the optic disc due to increased **intracranial** pressure. It is not a diagnosis; it is a sign of some underlying pathology. It is seen on ophthalmoscopic examination.

Cancer of the Eye (LO 11.4)

Tumors of the skin of the eyelids include the **squamous cell** and basal cell carcinomas and melanoma described in Chapter 3.

Retinoblastoma is the most common eye cancer in children and is diagnosed most frequently around 18 months of age. Of those children affected, 20% have the cancer in both eyes. This condition can be hereditary. With early detection and aggressive chemotherapy and laser surgery treatment, about 90% of these cases can be cured.

In adults, the most common eye cancers are metastases to the eye from lung cancer in men and breast cancer in women.

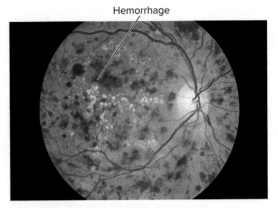

▲ **FIGURE 11.17** Ophthalmoscopic View of Diabetic Retinopathy Showing Areas of Hemorrhage.

BSIP/UIG/Getty Images

Night Blindness (LO 11.4)

Night blindness is the inability to see in poor light. It is a symptom of an underlying problem that can be:

- Uncorrected nearsightedness
- Cataracts
- Retinitis pigmentosa
- Vitamin A deficiency
- Glaucoma medications (such as pilocarpine) that constrict the pupil

Disorders of Refraction (LO 11.5)

Farsighted people are said to have **hyperopia** *(Figure 11.19)*. Because the eyeball is shortened, objects close to the eye are focused behind the retina and vision is blurred.

Nearsighted people are said to have **myopia** *(Figure 11.20)*. Because the eyeball is elongated, faraway objects are focused in front of the retina. Vision is blurred.

In **presbyopia** the lens loses its flexibility, making it difficult to focus for near vision. This usually occurs when you reach your forties.

In **astigmatism**, curvatures of the cornea cause difficulty focusing and blurred images.

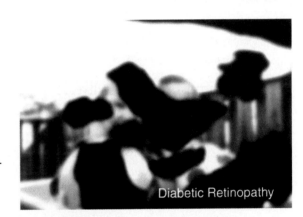

▲ **FIGURE 11.18** Vision with Diabetic Retinopathy.

National Institutes of Health/National Eye Institute

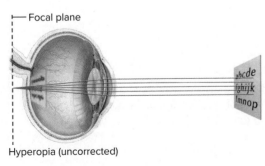

Hyperopia (uncorrected)

▲ **FIGURE 11.19** Hyperopia (farsightedness).

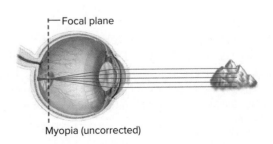

Myopia (uncorrected)

▲ **FIGURE 11.20** Myopia (nearsightedness).

Word Analysis and Definition

WORD	PRONUNCIATION	ELEMENTS		DEFINITION
astigmatism	ah-**STIG**-maht-izm	S/ P/ R/	-ism *process* a- *without* -stigmat- *focus*	Inability to focus light rays that enter the eye in different planes
hyperopia	high-per-**OH**-pee-ah	P/ R/	hyper- *beyond* -opia *sight*	Able to see distant objects but unable to see close objects
intracranial	in-trah-**KRAY**-nee-al	S/ P/ R/	-al *pertaining to* intra- *within* -crani- *skull, cranium*	Within the cranium (skull)
myopia (Note: *One "op" is removed to allow the term to flow.*)	my-**OH**-pee-ah	R/ S/	myop- *to blink* -opia *sight*	Able to see close objects but unable to see distant objects
papilledema	pah-pill-eh-**DEE**-mah	R/ S/	papill- *pimple* -edema *swelling*	Swelling of the optic disc in the retina
presbyopia	prez-bee-**OH**-pee-ah	R/ S/	presby- *old person* -opia *sight*	Difficulty in nearsighted vision occurring in middle and old age in both sexes
retinoblastoma	**RET**-in-oh-blas-**TOH**-mah	S/ R/CF R/	-oma *tumor, mass* retin/o- *retina* -blast- *immature cell*	Malignant neoplasm of primitive retinal cells
retinopathy	ret-ih-**NOP**-ah-thee	S/	-pathy *disease*	Degenerative disease of the retina

EXERCISES

Case Report 11.1

You are...

...an **ophthalmic** technician (OT) working in the office of **ophthalmologist** Angela Chun, MD, a member of the Fulwood Medical Group.

You are communicating with...

...Mrs. Jenny Hughes, a 30-year-old computer software consultant. She walked into the office with painful, red, swollen eyelids and a sticky, **purulent** discharge from both eyes. The administrative medical assistant did not hold her in the reception area but brought her directly to you. Mrs. Hughes complains of headache and **photophobia**, and says her eyelids were stuck together when she woke up this morning. She tells you that a couple of days earlier, she had gone into a small business office to install software at the firm's 10 workstations. One of the employees was absent with **pink eye**. Mrs. Hughes wants to know if she could have contracted the condition from that employee's keyboard, and how to prevent her husband and two children from getting it. In your hand, you have a pen and clipboard with the office Notice of Privacy Practices and sign-in sheet for her to sign. How do you proceed?

Mrs. Hughes' pink eye is called acute **contagious** conjunctivitis. It responds well to **antibiotic** eyedrops. Her hands were **contaminated** from the keyboard of the employee who had left work and gone home with pink eye. She transmitted the infection to her eye by touching it with her contaminated fingers.

Your documentation of Mrs. Hughes' office visit could read:

Progress Note: 04/10/23

Mrs. Jenny Hughes was brought directly into the clinical area at 1030 hrs with what appeared to be conjunctivitis. Both eyelids were red and swollen with a **purulent discharge.** She complained of headache and **photophobia.** Dr. Chun prescribed two drops q4h of Ciprofloxacin eyedrops and sent a swab of the discharge to the laboratory. I instructed and watched Mrs. Hughes wash her hands and use an alcohol-based hand gel. I then had her sign in and sign our Notice of Privacy Practices. I instructed her in the use of the eyedrops and emphasized home care and hand care measures to prevent the infection from spreading to her family. She was given a return appointment in 1 week and told to call the office if the eyedrops do not help.

—Daphne Butras, OT, 1055 hrs.

A. Read Case Report 11.1 *and content related to accessory structures of the eye to correctly complete each statement. Select the correct answer to complete each statement.* **LO 11.4, 11.5, and 11.7**

1. What words could Jenny Hughes likely use to describe her condition of **photophobia**:

    a. "It hurts to blink my eye."   **c.** "My eyelids are painful."

    b. "My eye is dry and scratchy."   **d.** "The light hurts my eye."

2. The medical term that is used to document the condition of **pink eye** is:

    a. conjunctivitis   **b.** corneal abrasion   **c.** blepharitis   **d.** ptosis

3. Dr. Chun's specialty is described as a:

    a. specialist in the measurements of vision   **c.** specialist in the diagnosis and treatment of eye disorders.

    b. technician who fits patients with prescription eyeware   **d.** technician who assists optometrists with a treatment

B. Disorders: The accessory structures of the eye have their own disorders. *The patient conditions are described in the first column; match the condition with the correct medical term in the second column from this lesson.* **LO 11.5**

_____	**1.** inflammation of the conjunctiva	**a.**	paresis
_____	**2.** drooping of upper eyelid	**b.**	hordeolum
_____	**3.** partial paralysis	**c.**	blepharoptosis
_____	**4.** red, crusted, and ulcerated eyelid	**d.**	blepharitis
_____	**5.** abscess in an eyelash follicle	**e.**	conjunctivitis

C. There are three medical terms below that need to be translated *for Mrs. Hughes so she can understand her condition and treatment. Select the answer that will correctly complete each statement.* **LO 11.4, 11.5, and 11.6**

Mrs. Hughes has **conjunctivitis (1)** of both eyes. It is important that she wash her hands before touching things, because this condition is **contagious (2)**. Instruct her to instill two drops of **antibiotic (3)** eye drops into the eyes four times per day.

1. Mrs. Hughes, you have a(n)

    a. inflammation of the inner lining of the eyelid.   **c.** partial paralysis of the eyelid.

    b. infection of the tear duct.   **d.** abscess in an eyelash follicle.

2. This condition

    a. can cause a fever.   **c.** can lead to paralysis.

    b. is a contagious infection.   **d.** remains in your body for up to one year.

3. The medication in the eye drops

    a. relieves your dry eyes.   **b.** fights off allergens.   **c.** dilates your pupils.   **d.** kills the bacterial infection.

D. Recognize *the definitions of disorders of the extrinsic muscles of the eye. Insert the disorder of the eye that is being described. Fill in the blanks.* **LO 11.2 and 11.5**

1. a turning of the eye outward away from the nose: _____

2. failure or incomplete development of the pathways of vision to the brain: _____

3. turning of the eye inward toward the nose: _____

4. a turning of an eye away from its normal position: _____

5. three-dimensional vision: _____

6. the adjustment of the lens by itself: _____

E. Deconstruct *the following medical terms into their elements. Complete the chart. If a term does not have an element, insert N/A. The first one has been done for you.* **LO 11.1**

Medical Term	Prefix	Root(s)/Combining Form(s)	Suffix
exotropia	1. exo-	2. -trop-	3. -ia
esotropia	4.	5.	6.
amblyopia	7.	8.	9.
stereopsis	10.	11.	12.

F. Construct *the correct medical term to match the meaning given in the first column 1. Write each element in the correct column to form the complete term. Fill in the chart.* **LO 11.1 and 11.5**

Meaning of Medical Term	Prefix	Root(s)/Combining Form(s)	Suffix
inability to focus light rays	1.	2.	3.
able to see distant objects but not close ones	4.	5.	6.
able to see close objects but not distant ones	7.	8.	9.

G. *Use the terms below to complete the following sentences. You may use a term only one time, but you will not use every term. Fill in the blanks.* **LO 11.2, 11.5, and 11.8**

abrasion   cataract   fluorescein   glaucoma   photosensitive   photosensitivity   pollutants   pollution

1. Loss of peripheral vision can be caused by _____.

2. Smoke and perfume are _____.

3. Scratching your eye with a tree branch can produce a(n) _____.

4. A clouding of the lens associated with aging is termed _____.

5. A person who states that light hurts theirs eyes is complaining of _____.

H. Deconstruct *the following medical terms into their elements.* **LO 11.1**

1. abrasion: _____ / _____
                        R   S

2. glaucoma: _____ / _____
                        R   S

3. ophthalmia: _____ / _____
                        R   S

4. photosensitivity: _____ / _____ / _____
                        R/CF   R   S

5. neonatorum: _____ / _____ / _____
                        P   R   S

6. uveitis: _____ / _____
                        R   S

I. Identify *the eye disorder being described. Fill in the blanks.* **LO 11.2 and 11.5**

1. This is a cancer of the eye and the most common form of eye cancer occurring in children: _____.

2. Inability to see in poor light: _____.

3. This condition can occur in diabetics and can lead to blindness, a condition known as diabetic _____.

4. A loss of central vision due to the degeneration of the retina lateral to the optic disc: _____ degeneration.

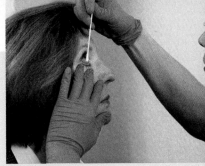

Rick Brady/McGraw Hill

Routine eye exams are important for early detection and prevention, and are recommended at different times throughout life. Diagnostic and therapeutic procedures and the application of medications to the external eye are performed by many different health professionals including **ophthalmologists, optometrists,** and **opthalmologic technicians** and **technologists.**

Abbreviation

PERRLA   pupils equal, round,
          reactive to light and
          accommodation

Ophthalmic Diagnostic Procedures (LO 11.2, 11.3, 11.4, and 11.6)

Examination of the eye includes evaluation of pupillary reaction. Medical shorthand for this quick normal eye examination can be **PERRLA,** which means *p*upils *e*qual, *r*ound, *r*eactive to *l*ight and *a*ccommodation.

Visual acuity, the sharpness and clearness of vision, is tested for each eye with the opposite eye covered with a solid object. For **distance vision,** patients look at a **Snellen letter chart** *(Figure 11.21a)* 20 feet away and vision is recorded as the smallest line in which the patient can read half of the letters. For **near vision,** the patient reads a standard **Jaeger reading card** *(Figure 11.21b)* at a distance of 14 inches.

Color vision is tested using the **Ishihara color system**. In the example shown in *Figure 11.22,* people with red-green color blindness would not be able to detect the number 74 among the colored dots.

Refractive error, the nature and degree to which light is bent by the eye, is measured with a **refractometer.**

Visual fields can be impaired by lesions anywhere in the neural visual pathway and in glaucoma, and can be assessed grossly by **direct confrontation.** The patient maintains a fixed gaze at the examiner's nose and a small object or finger is brought into the patient's visual periphery (**peripheral vision**) in each of the four visual quadrants. The patient indicates when the object is first seen. Each eye is tested separately.

Corneal examination uses **fluorescein** *(Figure 11.23)* staining to reveal abrasions and ulcers.

Pupillary reaction to light is tested in each eye with a penlight as the patient looks into the distance.

Extrinsic muscles of the eyeball are tested by guiding the patient to look in eight directions (up, up and right, right, down and right, down, down and left, left, and left and up) with a moving finger or penlight.

Fundoscopy using an **ophthalmoscope** can detect lens opacities, retinal changes, and retinal vascular changes. The vascular changes can be areas of hemorrhage or changes in the retinal arteries indicating hypertension or arteriosclerosis. The retinal changes can show age-related macular degeneration, retinoblastoma, retinal

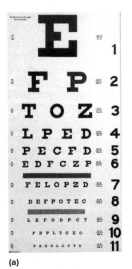

(a)   (b)

▲ **FIGURE 11.21**   Visual Acuity Tests.
(a) Snellen letter chart for distance vision. (b) Jaeger reading card.

Fig 11.21a: Rick Brady/McGraw Hill Fig 11.21b: Courtesy of Good-Lite Company

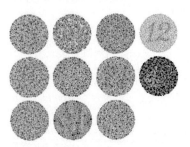

Complete Ishihara color test plates

◀ **FIGURE 11.22**   Test for Color Blindness. Reproduced with permission from *Ishihara's Tests for Color Deficiency,* published by Kanehara Trading Inc., Tokyo, Japan. Tests for color deficiency cannot be conducted with this figure. For accurate testing, the original plates should be used.

Alexander Kaludov/Alamy Stock Photo

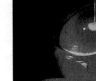

Ulcer

▶ **FIGURE 11.23**
Fluorescein-Stained Corneal Ulcer.

ARZTSAMUI/Shutterstock

detachment, signs of diabetes, signs of glaucoma, or signs of raised intracranial pressure (papilledema). Greater detail of the vessels of the eye can be seen with fluorescein **angiography**. Fluorescein is injected into the vein and pictures are taken as the dye passes through the retina revealing more details.

Slit-lamp examination focuses the height and width of a beam of light to give a **stereoscopic** view of the interior structures of the eyeball. It is used for identifying corneal foreign bodies and abrasions, and identifying retinal diseases.

Intraocular pressure is measured with a **tonometer**, which determines the eyeball's resistance to tension or indentation. There are several methods of **tonometry**, which include pneumatonometry and Goldmann tonometry.

Word Analysis and Definition

S = Suffix   P = Prefix   R = Root   R/CF = Combining Form

WORD	PRONUNCIATION		ELEMENTS	DEFINITION
fluorescein	flor-**ESS**-ee-in	P/ R/	fluo- *fluorine* -rescein *resin*	Dye that produces a vivid green color under a blue light to diagnose corneal abrasions and foreign bodies
fundus fundoscopy	**FUN**-dus fun-**DOS**-koh-pee	S/ R/CF	Latin *bottom* -scopy *to examine* fund/o- *fundus*	Part farthest from the opening of a hollow organ Examination of the fundus (retina) of the eye
fundoscopic (adj)	fun-doh-**SKOP**-ik	S/	-ic *pertaining to*	As a result of fundoscopy
Ishihara color system	ish-ee-**HAR**-ah **KUH**-ler **SIS**-tem		Shinobu Ishihara, 1879–1963, Japanese ophthalmologist **color** Latin *color* **system** Greek *to combine*	Test for color vision defects
Jaeger reading cards	**YAY**-ger **REED**-ing CARDS	S/ R/	Edward Jaeger, 1818–1884, Austrian ophthalmologist -ing *quality of, doing* read- *advise, interpret, read* card Latin *leaf of papyrus*	Printed in different sizes of print for testing near vision
ocular intraocular	**OCK**-you-lar in-trah-**OCK**-you-lar	S/ P/ R/	-ar *pertaining to* intra- *within* -ocul- *eye*	Pertaining to the eye Pertaining to the inside of the eye
ophthalmology	off-thal-**MALL**-oh-jee	S/ R/CF	-logy *study of* ophthalm/o- *eye*	Diagnosis and treatment of diseases of the eye
ophthalmologist ophthalmic (adj)	off-thal-**MALL**-oh-jist off-**THAL**-mik	S/ S/ R/	-logist *one who studies, specialist* -ic *pertaining to* ophthalm- *eye*	Medical specialist in ophthalmology Pertaining to the eye
ophthalmoscope	off-**THAL**-moh-skope	S/ R/CF	-scope *instrument for viewing* ophthalm/o- *eye*	Instrument for viewing the retina
ophthalmoscopy ophthalmoscopic (adj)	**OFF**-thal-**MOS**-koh-pee **OFF**-thal-moh-**SCOP**-ik	S/ S/	-scopy *to view, examine* -ic *pertaining to*	The process of viewing the retina Pertaining to the use of an ophthalmoscope
optometrist	op-**TOM**-eh-trist	S/ R/CF	-metrist *skilled in measurement* opt/o- *vision*	Someone skilled in the measurement of vision but who cannot treat eye diseases or prescribe medication
optometry	op-**TOM**-eh-tree	S/	-metry *process of measuring*	The profession of the measurement of vision
peripheral vision	peh-**RIF**-er-al **VIZH**-un	S/ R/	-al *pertaining to* peripher- *external boundary* vision Latin *to see*	Ability to see objects as they come into the outer edges of the visual field
refractometer	ree-frak-**TAH**-meh-tur	S/ R/CF	-meter *measure, instrument to measure* refract/o- *to bend (light)*	Device that measures refractive errors of the cornea
Snellen letter chart	**SNEL**-en **LET**-er CHART		Hermann Snellen, 1834–1908, Dutch ophthalmologist **letter** Latin *letter of the alphabet* **chart** Latin *piece of papyrus, document*	Test for acuity of distance vision
stereoscopy	**STAIR**-ee-**OS**-koh-pee	S/ R/CF	-scope *to examine, to view* stere/o- *three-dimensionale*	Optic technique that blends two identical views of one object to create the perception that the object is three-dimensional
stereoscopic (adj)	**STAIR**-ee-oh-**SKOP**-ik	S/	-ic *pertaining to*	Pertaining to stereoscopy
tonometer	toh-**NOM**-eh-ter	S/ R/CF	-meter *measure, instrument to measure* ton/o- *pressure, tension*	Instrument for determining intraocular pressure
tonometry	toh-**NOM**-eh-tree	S/	-metry *process of measuring*	The measurement of intraocular pressure

Therapeutic Procedures for Diseases and Disorders of the Eye (LO 11.2, 11.5, and 11.6)

Photocoagulation therapy is used to reattach a torn or detached portion of the retina and to prevent further growth of abnormal blood vessels that can cause a detachment. A high-intensity, narrowly focused beam of light from the **argon laser** is absorbed by pigment in the retinal cells and converted into heat, which welds the edge of the retinal detachment against the underlying choroid. **Retinal cryopexy (cryotherapy)** uses intense cold to have the same effects as the heat of photocoagulation.

Photocoagulation therapy is also used to heal bleeding **microaneurysms** of small blood vessels in the early stages of **diabetic retinopathy,** and is used with **chemotherapy** in the treatment of **retinoblastoma**. It also can be used for wet age-related macular degeneration to destroy or seal off new blood vessels to prevent leakage, but the many small retinal scars it creates cause blind spots in the patient's visual field.

When a **cataract** is interfering with vision, the opaque lens is removed by **phacoemulsification** in which ultra-sonic waves fragment the cataract to make its removal much easier. The lens is then replaced with an artificial **intraocular** lens, which becomes a permanent part of the eye.

Laser corneal surgery is a procedure that uses a laser to reshape the surface of the eye to change the curvature of the cornea. The surgical procedure **radial keratotomy** is used to treat myopia. Radial cuts, like the spokes of a wheel, flatten the cornea and enable it to refract the light rays to focus on the retina. In flattening the cornea, it can correct myopia (nearsightedness) and astigmatism (uneven curvature of the cornea) and alter the outer edges of the cornea to correct hypermetropia (farsightedness). These procedures are also called **refractive surgery** and **laser-assisted in situ keratomileusis (LASIK).** An alternative to LASIK is **photorefractive keratectomy (PRK),** in which spoke-like incisions are cut into the cornea to flatten its surface and correct nearsightedness.

Glaucoma is treated with a combination of eye drops *(see next section on ocular pharmacology),* pills, laser surgery, and traditional surgery with the goal of preventing loss of vision. The most commonly used laser procedure is **trabeculoplasty,** in which the eye's drainage system is changed by the laser beam to enable the aqueous humor fluid to drain out more easily into the blood stream. **Trabeculectomy** is the most common traditional surgical procedure, in which a passage is created in the sclera to allow excess fluid to drain out of the eye. More recently, a small silicone tube has been placed from the surface of the eye into the anterior chamber to allow drainage of the excess fluid.

Keratoplasty replaces a cornea damaged by infection or trauma.

Blepharoplasty treats blepharoptosis by surgically removing excess eyelid skin and sometimes muscle and fat.

Corrective Lenses (LO 11.2, 11.5, and 11.6)

Corrective lenses correct disorders of refraction. They bend light rays before they meet the eye's lens.

Concave lens corrects myopia.

Convex lens corrects hyperopia.

Convex **bifocal** or **progressive** lens corrects presbyopia.

Cylindrical lens corrects this astigmatism.

Exotropia and esotropia treatments depend on the severity of the problem. One treatment is patching the good eye so that the affected eye is required to focus. Surgical treatment of extrinsic eye muscle is an option with large deviation or if previous management is unsuccessful.

Amblyopia treatments include patching the good eye. Treatment is necessary to strengthen the neural connections from the affected eye to the brain. Lifetime poor vision results if amblyopia is not treated.

Keynotes

- As the eye is heavily supplied with nerves, local anesthesia is required for eye surgery. *(see the next section on ocular pharmacology).*

- Sterile precautions with the use of antiseptics, sterile drapes, gowns, and gloves are used in eye surgery to prevent infection.

Abbreviation

LASIK   laser-assisted in situ keratomileusis

WORD	PRONUNCIATION		ELEMENTS	DEFINITION
argon laser	AR-gon LAY-zer		**argon** Greek *lazy* **laser** *acronym for Light Amplification by Stimulated Emission of Radiation*	Laser used for ophthalmic procedures consisting of photons in the blue and/or green spectrum
bifocal	bi-FOH-cal	S/ P/ R/	-al *pertaining to* bi- *two* -foc- *focus*	Two powers on lens
blepharoplasty	BLEF-ah-roh-PLAS-tee	S/ R/CF	-plasty *repair* blephar/o- *eyelid*	Surgical repair of the eyelid
concave convex	kon-KAVE kon-VEKS		Latin concavus *arched* Latin convexus *vaulted*	Having a hollowed surface A surface that is evenly curved outward
cryotherapy cryopexy	CRY-oh-THAIR-ah-pee CRY-oh-PEK-see	S/ R/CF S/	-therapy *treatment* cry/o- *cold* -pexy *fixation*	The use of cold in the treatment of disease Repair of a detached retina by freezing it to surrounding tissue
in situ	IN SIGH-tyu		Latin *in its original place*	In the correct place
keratectomy keratomileusis keratoplasty keratotomy	KAIR-ah-TEK-toh-mee KAIR-ah-toh-mie-LOO-sis KAIR-ah-TOT-oh-mee KAIR-ah-toh-PLAS-tee	S/ R/ R/CF R/ S/ R/ S/	-ectomy *excision* kerat- *cornea* kerat/o- *cornea* -mileusis *lathe* -plasty *repair* kerat/o- *cornea* -tomy *surgical incision*	Surgery to remove corneal tissue A surgical procedure that involves cutting and shaping the cornea Corneal transplant or graft Incision in the cornea
phacoemulsification	FAK-oh-ee-mul-sih-fih-KAY-shun	S/ R/CF R/	-ation *process* phac/o- *lens* -emulsific- *to milk out*	Technique used to fragment the center of the lens into very tiny pieces and suck them out of the eye
photocoagulation photoreactive	foh-toh-koh-ag-you-LAY-shun foh-toh-ree-AK-tiv	S/ R/CF R/ P/ R/	-ation *process* phot/o- *light* -coagul- *clot* -re- *again* -active *movement*	The use of light (laser beam) to form a clot Initiation by light of a process previously inactive
progressive	pro-GRESS-iv	S/	Latin *going forward* -ive *nature of, quality of, pertaining to*	Lens power gradually changes from point to point
trabeculectomy	trah-BEK-you-LEK-toh-mee	S/ R/	-ectomy *excision* trabecul- *eye's fluid drainage system*	Surgical creation of passage in sclera to allow fluid to drain out of the eye
trabeculoplasty	trah-BEK-you-loh-plas-tee	S/ R/CF	-plasty *surgical repair* trabecul/o- *eye's fluid drainage system*	Laser repair of eye's fluid drainage system

Ocular Pharmacology (LO 11.2, 11.5, and 11.6)

There are a wide variety and number of medications placed directly into the conjunctival sac to treat different eye disorders or to help the clinician examine the eye more thoroughly and more easily.

- **Mydriatics** are drugs that cause the pupil to dilate and are mainly used to examine the eye fundus. **Mydriacil** *(Tropicamide)* takes 15 minutes for the eye to fully dilate and can last for 3 to 6 hours with blurred vision. Other dilating drops, for example, **atropine** and **homatropine,** are long acting, lasting 7 to 10 days.

- **Miotics** are drugs that constrict the pupil (**miosis**); for example, **pilocarpine,** which can be part of a regimen for treating glaucoma.

- **Ocular topical anesthetics** temporarily block nerve conduction in the conjunctiva and cornea. They have a quick onset of 10 to 20 seconds and last for 10 to 20 minutes. They are used to assist with eye examinations and **visual acuity** testing and to help treat chemical burns, welding flash, and foreign bodies. Examples are **amethocaine,** 0.5% and 1%, and **oxybupricaine,** 0.4%.

- **Ocular diagnostic drops** stain conjunctival cells to improve diagnostic capabilities; for example, the presence of a foreign body or a corneal abrasion. Examples are **fluorescein** and **Lissamine Green.** The drops do not interfere with vision but are taken up by soft contact lenses, which should be removed prior to instillation of the drops.

Abbreviation

q4h   Every four hours.

- **Ocular lubricant drops** are used to replace tears, treat dry eyes, moisten hard contact lenses, protect the eye during eye surgical procedures, and help treat keratitis. Examples are *Visine, Refresh Optive,* and *Retaine.*

- **Anti-infective (antibiotic) eye medications,** both drops and ointments, can be **antibacterial,** for example, **glatifloxacin** (*Zymaxid*) and **sulfacetamide** (*Klaron, Ovace*); **antifungal,** such as **natamycin** (*Natacyn*); and **antiviral,** for example, **idoxuridine** (*Herplex*) and **trifluridine** (*Viroptic*).

- **Anti-inflammatory eye medications** are used in allergic disorders, to prevent scarring and visual loss in inflammation of the eye, and to decrease postoperative eye inflammation and scarring. Examples are **corticosteroids** such as **dexamethasone** (*Decadron*) and **nonsteroidal anti-inflammatory agents** such as **flurbiprofen** (*Ocufen*) and **suprofen** (*Profenal*).

- In **glaucoma,** numerous eye medications are available and are used individually, in combinations, and/or with surgery *(see the previous section on eye therapeutic procedures).* **Miotics** decrease the size of the pupil and widen the trabecular network to enable fluid to escape more easily. **Beta-adrenergic blockers** decrease production of aqueous humor; examples are **timolol maleate** (*Timoptic*) and **betaxolol** (*Betoptic*). **Carbonic anhydrase inhibitors** reduce production of aqueous humor; examples are **acetazolamide sodium** (*Diamox*) and **dichlorphenamide** (*Daranide*); **alpha-adrenergic agents** increase the outflow of aqueous humor by unknown mechanisms; examples are **epinephrine** (*Epifrin*) and **phenylephrine** (*Neo-synephrine*).

Word Analysis and Definition

S = Suffix   P = Prefix   R = Root   R/CF = Combining Form

WORD	PRONUNCIATION		ELEMENTS	DEFINITION
antibacterial	AN-teh-bak-**TEER**-ee-al	S/ P/ R/CF	-al *pertaining to* anti- *against* -bacter/i- *bacteria*	Destructive of or preventing the growth of bacteria
antibiotic	AN-tih-bye-**OT**-ik	S/ R/	-tic *pertaining to* -bi/o- *life*	Made incapable of transmitting an infection
antifungal	AN-teh-**FUN**-gal	S/ R/	-al *pertaining to* -fung- *fungus*	Destructive of or preventing the growth of fungi
anti-infective	AN-teh-in-**FEK**-tiv	S/ R/	-ive *nature of* -infect- *taint*	Made incapable of transmitting an infection
anti-inflammatory	AN-teh-in-**FLAM**-ah-toh-ree	S/ P/ R/	-ory *having the function of* in- *in* -flammat- *inflammation*	Reducing, removing, or preventing inflammation
antiviral	an-teh-**VIE**-ral	S/ R/	-al *pertaining to* -vir- *virus*	To weaken or abolish the action or replication of a virus
atropine	**AT**-roh-peen		Greek *belladonna*	Pharmacologic agent used to dilate pupils
inhibitor	in-**HIB**-ih-tor	S/ P/ R/	-or *one who does* in- *in* -hibit- *keep back*	An agent that restrains or retards physiologic, chemical, or enzymatic action
miosis miotic	my-**OH**-sis my-**OT**-ik	 S/ R/CF	Greek *lessening* -tic *pertaining to* mi/o- *less*	Contraction of the pupil An agent that causes the pupil to contract
mydriasis mydriatic	mih-**DRY**-ah-sis mid-ree-**AT**-ik	 S/ R/	Greek *dilation of the pupil* -atic *pertaining to* mydri- *dilation of the pupil*	Dilation of the pupil Pertaining to or an agent that causes dilation of the pupil

EXERCISES

 Case Report 11.2

You are ...

. . . an ophthalmic technician employed by Angela Chun, MD, an ophthalmologist at Fulwood Medical Center.

You are communicating with ...

. . . Mrs. Vijita Patel, the mother of Aadi Patel, a 2½-year-old boy, who has been referred by his pediatrician to Dr. Chun.

Mrs. Patel states that for the past couple of months, Aadi's right eye has turned in. The only visual difficulty she has noticed is that he sometimes misses a Cheerio when he tries to grab it.

You are responsible for documenting Aadi's diagnostic and therapeutic procedures and explaining their significance to his mother.

A. **Elements** *help build your knowledge of the language of ophthalmology. One element in each of the following medical terms is bolded and italicized. Identify the type of element (P, R/CF, S) in the second column, and then write the meaning of the element in the third column. Fill in the chart.* **LO 11.1, 11.4, 11.5, and 11.6**

Medical Term	P, R/CF, S	Meaning of Element
retino*blast*oma	1.	2.
ophthalmo*scope*	3.	4.
ophthalmoscop*ic*	5.	6.
*ophthalmo*scopy	7.	8.
retino*pathy*	9.	10.
ophthalm**ology**	11.	12.

B. The ophthalmic technician in Dr. Chun's office needs to be familiar with all these terms in order to communicate with Dr. Chun and her patients. *Show your understanding of the terms by selecting the correct answers.*   **LO 11.5 and 11.6**

1. The test used to measure color blindness is
    a. Snellen   **b.** Jaeger   **c.** Ishihara   **d.** visual fields   **e.** ophthalmoscope

2. Peripheral vision measures the outer edge of the
    a. anterior chamber   **b.** vitreous body   **c.** aqueous humor   **d.** posterior chamber   **e.** visual field

3. A test for near vision is the
    a. Snellen chart   **b.** ophthalmoscope   **c.** Jaeger card   **d.** Ishihara   **e.** visual fields

4. This is used to detect corneal abrasions or ulcers
    a. ophthalmoscope   **b.** refractometer   **c.** tonometer   **d.** fluorescein

C. Identify the meaning of the word elements related to ophthalmology. *Match the element in the first column with its correct meaning in the second column.*   **LO 11.1**

Word Element	Meaning
_____ **1.** *kerat-*	**a.** cold
_____ **2.** *cry/o-*	**b.** light
_____ **3.** *-ectomy*	**c.** surgical repair
_____ **4.** *-plasty*	**d.** eye's fluid drainage system
_____ **5.** *phot/o-*	**e.** cornea
_____ **6.** *trabecul-*	**f.** excision

D. Identify the medication that would treat each condition. *Match the medication on the left with its correct indicated use.*   **LO 11.5 and 11.6**

_____ **1.** antibacterial	**a.** treatment for glaucoma
_____ **2.** mydriatic	**b.** dry eyes
_____ **3.** anti-inflammatory	**c.** bacterial infection of the eye
_____ **4.** miotic	**d.** allergic disorder of the eye
_____ **5.** ocular topical anesthetic	**e.** dilate the pupil in order to view the eye fundus
_____ **6.** lubricant	**f.** chemical burn to the eyes

E. Match *the disorder of refraction in the first column with the corrective lens in the second column.*   **LO 11.5 and 11.6**

_____ **1.** astigmatism	**a.** convex only
_____ **2.** myopia	**b.** convex bifocals
_____ **3.** presbyopia	**c.** cylindrical
_____ **4.** hyperopia	**d.** concave

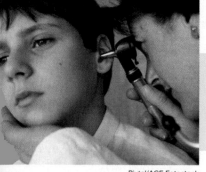

Section 11.4

Structure and Function of the Ear and Hearing

Keynotes

- The **external auditory** canal is the only skin-lined cul-de-sac in the body.
- Cerumen (earwax) is formed from a combination of secretions and combines with dead skin cells.

Your ear has three major sections *(Figure 11.24)*:

1. The external ear
2. The middle ear
3. The inner ear

External Ear (LO 11.4)

The external ear comprises several structures that keep it functioning effectively.

The **auricle** or **pinna** is a wing-shaped structure that directs sound waves into the ear canal through the external **auditory meatus**. The external auditory canal ends at the very delicate **tympanic** membrane, otherwise known as the eardrum *(Figure 11.25)*. When using an otoscope to examine the tympanic membrane, the auricle should be pulled up and out to straighten the external auditory canal.

The meatus and canal are lined with skin that contains many modified sweat glands called **ceruminous** glands, which secrete **cerumen**.

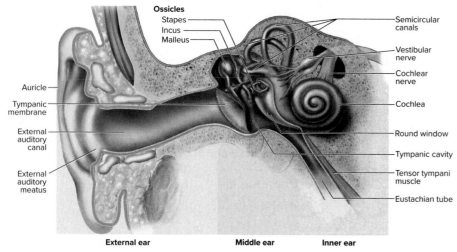

▲ **FIGURE 11.24**
Anatomical Regions of the Ear.

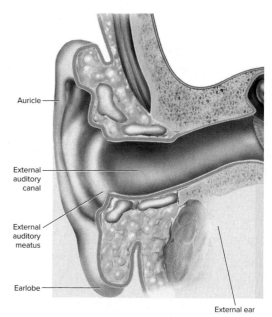

▲ **FIGURE 11.25**
External Ear.

Middle Ear (LO 11.4)

The middle ear has the following four components (*Figure 11.26*).

1. The **tympanic membrane** (eardrum) rests at the inner end of the external auditory canal. It vibrates freely as sound waves hit it. It has a good nerve supply and is very sensitive to pain. When examined through the otoscope, it is transparent and reflects light *(Figure 11.27)*.

2. The **tympanic cavity** is immediately behind the tympanic membrane. It is filled with air that enters through the eustachian tube, and the cavity is continuous with the **mastoid** air cells in the bone behind it. The cavity contains small bones called **ossicles**.

3. The three **ossicles**—the **malleus**, **incus**, and **stapes**—work to amplify sounds by vibrating one to the other, and are attached to the tympanic cavity wall by tiny ligaments. The malleus is attached to the tympanic membrane and vibrates with the membrane when sound waves hit it. The malleus is also attached to the incus, which vibrates, too, and passes the vibrations onto the stapes. The stapes is attached to the oval window, an opening that transmits the vibrations to the inner ear.

4. The **eustachian (auditory) tube** connects the middle ear with the **nasopharynx** (throat), into which it opens near the pharyngeal tonsils **(adenoids)** *(Figure 11.28)*. In children under 5 years of age, this tube is not fully developed as it is short and horizontal with undeveloped valve-like flaps in the throat that usually protect the structure.

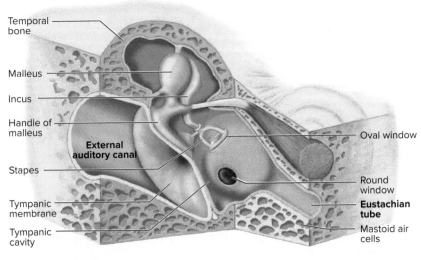

▲ **FIGURE 11.26**
Middle Ear.

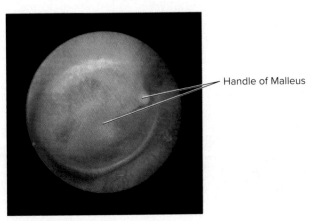

▲ **FIGURE 11.27**
Otoscopic View of Normal Tympanic Membrane.

Dr. G. Lacher/Science Source

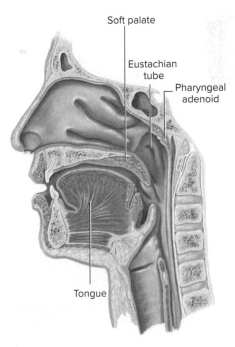

▲ **FIGURE 11.28**
Nasopharynx (throat) Showing the Eustachian Tube.

S = Suffix   P = Prefix   R = Root   R/CF = Combining Form

WORD	PRONUNCIATION	ELEMENTS		DEFINITION
adenoid	ADD-eh-noyd	S/ R/	-oid *resembling* aden- *gland*	Single mass of lymphoid tissue in the midline at the back of the throat
auditory (adj)	AW-dih-tor-ee		Latin *hearing*	Relating to hearing or the organs of hearing
auricle pinna (syn)	AW-ri-kul		Latin *ear*	The shell-like external ear
cerumen ceruminous (adj)	seh-**ROO**-men seh-**ROO**-mih-nus	S/ R/	Latin *wax* -ous *pertaining to* cerumin- *cerumen*	Waxy secretion of glands of the external ear Pertaining to cerumen
eustachian tube auditory tube (syn)	you-**STAY**-shun TYUB		Bartolomeo Eustachio, Italian anatomist, 1524–1574	Tube that connects the middle ear to the nasopharynx
incus	**IN**-cuss		Latin *anvil*	Middle one of the three ossicles in the middle ear; shaped like an anvil
malleus	**MAL**-ee-us		Latin *hammer*	Outer (lateral) one of the three ossicles in the middle ear; shaped like a hammer
mastoid	**MASS**-toyd	S/ R/	-oid *resembling* mast- *breast*	Small bony protrusion immediately behind the ear
meatus meatal (adj)	me-**AY**-tus me-**AY**-tal		Latin *go through*	Passage or channel; also the external opening of a passage
pinna pinnae (pl)	**PIN**-ah **PIN**-ee		Latin *wing*	Another name for auricle
nasopharynx nasopharyngeal (adj)	**NAY**-zoh-fair-inks **NAY**-zoh-fair-**RIN**-jee-al	R/CF R/ S/ R/	nas/o- *nose* -pharynx *throat* -eal *pertaining to* -pharyng- *pharynx*	Region of the pharynx at the back of the nose and above the soft palate Pertaining to the nasopharynx
ossicle	**OSS**-ih-kel	S/ R/CF	-cle *small* oss/i- *bone*	A small bone, particularly relating to the three bones in the middle ear
stapes	**STAY**-peez		Latin *stirrup*	Inner (medial) one of the three ossicles of the middle ear; shaped like a stirrup
tympanic	tim-**PAN**-ik	S/ R/	-ic *pertaining to* tympan- *eardrum*	Pertaining to the tympanic membrane (eardrum) or tympanic cavity

Inner Ear for Hearing (LO 11.4)

The inner ear is a **labyrinth** *(Figure 11.29)* of complex, intricate systems of passages. The passages in the **cochlea**, a part of the labyrinth, contain receptors to translate vibrations into nerve impulses so that the brain can interpret them as different sounds.

The membrane of the oval window separates the middle ear from the **vestibule** of the inner ear. From the tympanic membrane (① *in Figure 11.30*), the stapes ② moves the oval membrane to generate pressure waves in

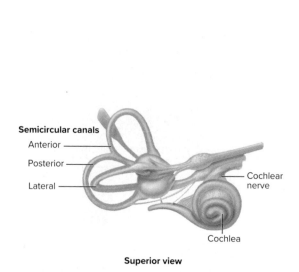

▲ **FIGURE 11.29**
Labyrinth of Inner Ear.

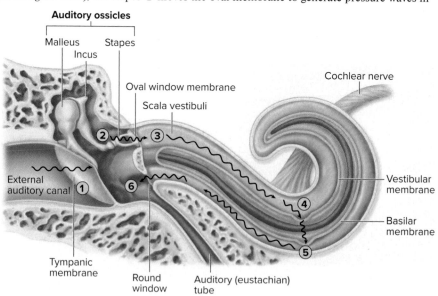

▲ **FIGURE 11.30**
Hearing Process in the Inner Ear.

the fluid inside the cochlea ③. The pressure waves cause **vestibular** and **basilar membranes** inside the cochlea to vibrate ④ and sway fine hair cells attached to the basilar membrane ⑤. The hair cells convert this motion into nerve impulses, which travel via the **cochlear nerve** to the brain. The excess pressure waves in the cochlea escape the inner ear via the round window ⑥.

Inner Ear for Equilibrium and Balance (LO 11.4)

The inner ear contains the organs in your body responsible for maintaining the true sense of balance. The vestibule and the three semicircular canals *(Figures 11.31 and 11.32)* in the inner ear maintain an individual's balance. These are the true organs of balance. Inside the fluid-filled vestibule are two raised, flat areas covered with hair cells and a jelly-like material. This gelatinous material contains calcium and protein crystals called **otoliths**. The position of the head alters the amount of pressure this gelatinous mass applies to the hair cells. The hair cells respond to horizontal and vertical changes and send impulses to the brain relating how the head is tilted.

Each of the three fluid-filled semicircular canals has a dilated end called an **ampulla**. The ampulla contains a mound of hair cells set in a gelatinous material that together are called the **crista ampullaris** *(Figure 11.32)*. This detects rotational movements of the head that distort the hair cells and lead to stimulation of connected nerve cells. The nerve impulses travel through the vestibular nerve to the brain. From the brain, nerve impulses travel to the muscles to maintain **equilibrium** and balance.

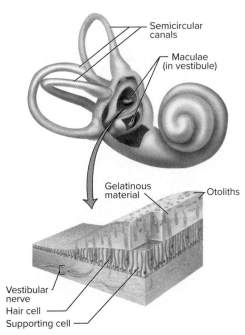

▲ **FIGURE 11.31**
Vestibule of the Inner Ear.

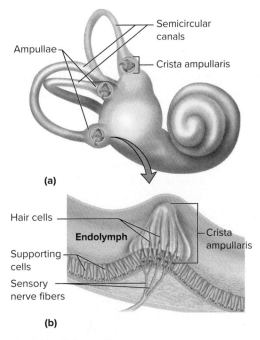

▲ **FIGURE 11.32**
Semicircular Canals.
(a) Anatomy. (b) Histology.

Word Analysis and Definition

S = Suffix   P = Prefix   R = Root   R/CF = Combining Form

WORD	PRONUNCIATION		ELEMENTS	DEFINITION
ampulla	am-**PULL**-ah		Latin *two-handled bottle*	Dilated portion of a canal or duct
basilar	**BAS**-ih-lar	S/ R/	**-ar** *pertaining to* **basil-** *base, support*	Pertaining to the base of a structure
cochlea	**KOK**-lee-ah		Latin *snail shell*	An intricate combination of passages; used to describe the part of the inner ear used in hearing
cochlear (adj)	**KOK**-lee-ar	S/ R/	**-ar** *pertaining to* **cochle-** *cochlea*	Pertaining to the cochlea
crista ampullaris	**KRIS**-tah am-**PULL**-air-is	R/ S/ R/	**crista** *crest* **-aris** *pertaining to* **ampull-** *bottle-shaped*	Mound of hair cells and gelatinous material in the ampulla of a semicircular canal
equilibrium	ee-kwi-**LIB**-ree-um	P/ R/	**equi-** *equal* **-librium** *balance*	Being evenly balanced
labyrinth	**LAB**-ih-rinth		Greek *labyrinth*	The inner ear
otolith	**OH**-toh-lith	R/CF R/	**ot/o-** *ear* **-lith** *stone*	A calcium particle in the vestibule of the inner ear
vestibule vestibular (adj)	**VES**-tih-byul ves-**TIB**-you-lar	S/ R/	Latin *entrance* **-ar** *pertaining to* **vestibul-** *vestibule of the inner ear*	Space at the entrance to a canal Pertaining to the vestibule of the inner ear

EXERCISES

A. Review *the terms. Define the meanings of the word elements that construct medical terms. Select the correct answer that completes each statement.*   **LO 11.1 and 11.4**

1. In the term *mastoid,* the suffix means:

   a. condition   **b.** resembling   **c.** inflammation

2. The element *mast* means:

   a. throat   **b.** breast   **c.** ear

3. The element *pharynx* means:

   a. throat   **b.** nose   **c.** tongue

4. The root in the term *ossicle* means:

   a. bone   **b.** small   **c.** stirrup

5. The root in the term *adenoid* means:

   a. resembling   **b.** kidney   **c.** gland

B. Employ *the language of otology and fill in the blanks with the correct term being described.*   **LO 11.2 and 11.9**

1. List the ear ossicles in order from lateral to medial: _____

2. The smallest bone in the body: _____

3. Write the synonym for *eustachian tube.* _____

4. What is the medical term for *eardrum?* _____

5. The pharyngeal tonsils are the _____

6. What is the medical term for *throat?* _____

Section 11.5

Disorders of the Ear and Hearing

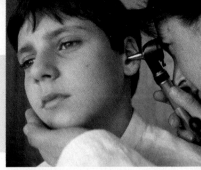

Pixtal/AGE Fotostock

Disorders of the External Ear (LO 11.5)

Some disorders of the external ear include infections and earwax buildup.

Otitis externa *(Figure 11.33)* is a bacterial or fungal infection of the external auditory canal lining. The ear canal is red and swollen, sometimes with a purulent drainage, and accompanied with pain.

Swimmer's ear is a form of otitis externa resulting from an accumulation of water that remains in the ear, commonly occuring in children after swimming. As the water persists in the ear canal, it allows bacteria to grow.

If a foreign body, like a small bead, gets into the auditory canal, or if cerumen becomes **impacted** in the canal, the result can be hearing loss.

Disorders of the Middle Ear (LO 11.5)

The middle ear can be susceptible to the disorders outlined below.

* **Acute otitis media (AOM)** is the presence of fluid in the middle ear with ear pain, **pyrexia (fever),** and redness of the tympanic membrane. AOM occurs most often in the first 2 to 4 years of age as a result of an **upper respiratory infection (URI),** also known as **coryza.** It is common that acute AOM occurs in both ears.

* **Chronic otitis media** *(Figure 11.30)* occurs when the acute infection subsides but the eustachian tube is blocked. The fluid in the middle ear caused by the infection cannot drain, and it gradually becomes stickier. This is called **chronic otitis media with effusion (OME)** and produces hearing loss because the sticky fluid prevents the ossicles from vibrating *(Figure 11.34).*

* A **perforated** tympanic membrane *(Figure 11.35)* can occur in acute otitis media **(AOM)** and chronic otitis media when fluid in the middle ear cannot escape down the eustachian tube. The fluid, usually pus, creates pressure and can cause the eardrum to rupture. Most perforations will heal spontaneously within a month, leaving a small scar. Other perforation causes include a cotton swab (Q-tip) puncture, an open-handed slap to the ear, or induced pressure as in scuba diving.

Abbreviations

AOM	acute otitis media
URI	upper respiratory infection
OME	otitis media with effusion

External auditory canal

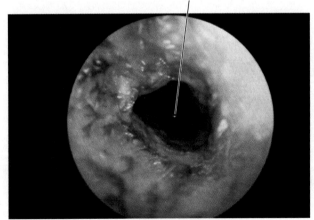

▲ **FIGURE 11.33**
Otoscopic View of Otitis Externa.

Richard Morton

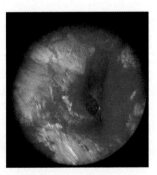

▲ **FIGURE 11.34**
Otoscopic View of Acute Otitis Media.

Mikhail V. Komarov/Shutterstock

Perforation

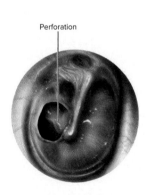

▲ **FIGURE 11.35**
Otoscopic View of Chronic Otitis Media with Perforation.

Bo Veisland/Science Source

- **Cholesteatoma** is a complication of chronic otitis media with fluid or effusion (OME). Chronically inflamed middle ear cells multiply and collect, forming a tumor. They damage the ossicles and can spread to the inner ear.
- **Otosclerosis** is a middle-ear disease that usually affects people between 18 and 35 years. It can impair one ear or both and produces a gradual hearing loss for low and soft sounds. Its etiology is unknown. Spongy bone forms around the junction of the oval window and stapes, preventing the stapes from conducting sound vibrations to the inner ear.

Disorders of the Inner Ear (LO 11.5)

Hearing Disorders of the Inner Ear (LO 11.5)

Abbreviation

BPPV   benign paroxysmal posi-
        tional vertigo

Today, the most common cause of hearing loss, aside from aging, is damage to the fine hairs in the cochlea by exposure to repeated loud noise, related either to work (e.g., jackhammers and leaf blowers) or to leisure activities (such as amplified music at concerts, personal listening devices, and motorcycles). This is a **sensorineural hearing loss**.

Disorders of the Inner Ear for Balance (LO 11.5)

Keynotes

- Repeated exposure to loud noise causes hearing loss in young people as well as in older people.
- A **conductive hearing loss** occurs when sound is not conducted efficiently through the external auditory canal to the tympanic membrane and the ossicles. Causes include
  - Middle ear pathology, such as acute otitis media, otitis media with effusion, or a perforated eardrum.
  - Impacted cerumen.
  - Infected external auditory canal.
  - Foreign body in the external canal.

The sensation of spinning or whirling that patients sometimes experience as a result of an inner ear disorder is called **vertigo**, often described by patients as dizziness. A ringing in the ears is called **tinnitus**. Both sensations arise in the inner ear. Tinnitus can also sound like hissing, buzzing, roaring, or clicking and may be associated with difficulty hearing, sleeping, or working. Treatment includes hearing aids, sound-masking devices, and learning ways to cope with the problem.

Benign paroxysmal positional vertigo (BPPV) is a common type of intermittent vertigo caused by fragments of the otoliths in the vestibule migrating into the semicircular canals. The otolith fragments brush against the hair cells, sending conflicting signals to the brain, producing vertigo.

S = Suffix   P = Prefix   R = Root   R/CF = Combining Form

WORD	PRONUNCIATION	ELEMENTS		DEFINITION
acute	ah-**KYUT**		Latin *sharp*	Disease of sudden onset
bilateral	by-**LAT**-er-al	S/ P/ R/	**-al** *pertaining to* **bi-** *two* **-later-** *side*	On two sides; e.g., in both ears
chronic	**KRON**-ik		Greek *time*	A persistent, long-term disease
cholesteatoma	**KOH**-less-**TEE**-ah-**TOH**-mah	S/ R/CF R/	**-oma** *tumor, mass* **chol/e-** *bile* **-steat-** *fat*	Yellow, waxy tumor arising in the middle ear
conductive hearing loss	kon-**DUK**-tiv **HEER**-ing LOSS	S/ R/	**conductive** Latin *to lead* **-ing** *quality of* **hear-** *to perceive sounds* **loss** Middle English *to lose*	Hearing loss caused by lesions in the outer ear or middle ear
coryza acute rhinitis (syn)	koh-**RYE**-zah		Greek *catarrh*	Viral inflammation of the mucous membrane of the nose
effusion	eh-**FYU**-shun		Latin *pouring out*	Collection of fluid that has escaped from blood vessels into a cavity or tissues
impacted	im-**PAK**-ted		Latin *driven in*	Immovably wedged, as with earwax blocking the external canal
labyrinthitis	**LAB**-ih-rin-**THIE**-tis	S/ R/	**-itis** *inflammation* **labyrinth-** *inner ear*	Inflammation of the inner ear
Ménière disease	men-ee-**AIR** diz-**EEZ**		Prosper Ménière, French physician, 1799–1862	Disorder of the inner ear with acute attacks of tinnitus, vertigo, and hearing loss
otitis externa	oh-**TIE**-tis ekz-**TER**-nah	S/ R/	**-itis** *inflammation* **ot-** *ear* Latin *from the outside*	Inflammation of the external ear
otitis media	oh-**TIE**-tis **ME**-dee-ah	S/ R/	**-itis** *inflammation* **ot-** *ear* Latin *middle*	Inflammation of the middle ear
otosclerosis	oh-toh-sklair-**OH**-sis	S/ R/CF R/CF	**-sis** *abnormal condition* **ot/o-** *ear* **-scler/o-** *hard*	Hardening at the junction of the stapes and oval window that causes loss of hearing
paroxysmal	pair-ock-**SIZ**-mal	S/ R/	**-al** *pertaining to* **paroxysm-** *sudden, sharp attack*	Occurring in sharp, spasmodic episodes
perforated perforation	**PER**-foh-ray-ted per-foh-**RAY**-shun	S/ R/	Latin *to bore through* **-ion** *action* **perforat-** *bore through*	Punctured with one or more holes A hole through the wall of a structure
pyrexia fever (syn)	pie-**REK**-see-ah **FEE**-ver	S/ R/	**-ia** *condition* **pyrex-** *fever, heat* Latin *fever*	Increased body temperature that is a physiologic response to a disease
sensorineural hearing loss	**SEN**-sor-ih-**NYUR**-al **HEER**-ing LOSS	S/ R/CF R/ S/ R/	**-al** *pertaining to* **sensor/i-** *sensory* **-neur-** *nerve* **-ing** *quality of* **hear-** *to perceive sounds* **loss** Middle English *to lose*	Hearing loss caused by lesions of the inner ear or the auditory nerve
tinnitus	**TIN**-ih-tus		Latin *jingle*	Persistent ringing, whistling, clicking, or booming noise in the ears
vertigo	**VER**-tih-go		Latin *dizziness*	Sensation of spinning or whirling

EXERCISES

Case Report 11.3

You are . . .

. . . a medical assistant working for primary care physician Susan Lee, MD, of the Fulwood Medical Group.

You are communicating with . . .

. . . Mrs. Carmen Cardenas, who has brought in her 3-year-old son, Eddie. She tells you that Eddie has had a cold for a couple of days. Early this morning, he woke up screaming, felt hot, and was tugging his ears. She gave him **acetaminophen** with some orange juice, and he threw up. She also tells you this is the third similar episode in the past year, and, since the last time, she is concerned that he is not hearing normally. You see a worried mother and a restless toddler with a green nasal discharge. His oral temperature taken with an electronic digital thermometer is 102.4°F, and his pulse is 112. You tell Mrs. Cardenas that Dr. Lee will be in to see Eddie as soon as possible.

Clinical Note. 05/10/18

Examination by Dr. Lee showed that Eddie has a bilateral **acute otitis media (AOM)** with an upper respiratory infection **(URI).** Dr. Lee is also concerned that Eddie has a **chronic** otitis media with **effusion (OME)** that is causing hearing loss. She prescribed Amoxicillin 250 mg **q.i.d.** with acetaminophen 160 **mg p.r.n.** for 10 days, when she will see Eddie again. If, after the acute infection subsides, there remains an effusion with hearing loss, Dr. Lee may need to refer Eddie to an **otologist**. I explained this to Mrs. Cardenas.

—Luis Guittierez, CMA 1115 hrs.

Eddie Cardenas's ear problems began with his eustachian tube. His cold (upper respiratory infection, **URI**, or **coryza**) inflamed the mucous membranes of his throat and eustachian tube. Because he is so young, his eustachian tube is short and horizontal, allowing the inflammation to spread easily from his throat into the middle ear, causing his acute otitis media **(AOM).** The inflammatory process produced fluid (effusion) in the middle ear. His tympanic membrane became inflamed and painful, which you could see through an otoscope *(Figure 11.30).*

A. Construct medical terms. *Insert the missing word element that correctly completes the medical term being described. Fill in the blanks.*   **LO 11.1, 11.2, 11.5, and 11.7**

1. One who specializes in the study of the ear: _____/logist

2. Pertaining to both sides: _____/later/al

3. Medical specialist in the treatment of the ear, nose, and throat: ot/o/rhino/_____ /logist

4. Infection of the middle ear: ot/_____ media

5. One who studies hearing: _____/logist

B. Match *the abbreviation in the left column with its meaning in the right column. Fill in the blanks.*   **LO 11.3, 11.5, and 11.6**

_____	1. URI	a. infection of the middle ears
_____	2. mg	b. infection in both middle ears with a fluid collection
_____	3. AOM	c. milligram
_____	4. OME	d. upper respiratory infection

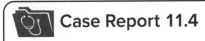

Case Report 11.4

You are...

...Sonia Ramos, a medical assistant working with Sylvia Thompson, MD, an otorhinolaryngologist at Fulwood Medical Center.

You are communicating with...

...Mr. Ernesto Santiago, a 44-year-old man who was referred to Dr. Thompson. Mr. Santiago complains of recurrent attacks of nausea, vomiting, a sense of spinning or whirling, and ringing in his ears. The attacks last about 24 hours and are getting more frequent. He has been having trouble hearing quiet speech on his left side. Your role is to document his examination, diagnosis, and care, and to act as liaison between Mr. Santiago and Dr. Thompson.

The recurrent attacks that Mr. Santiago suffered are called **Ménière disease**. The disease involves the destruction of inner-ear hair cells, but the etiology is unknown and there is no cure. Dr. Thompson prescribed medication to control Mr. Santiago's nausea and vomiting.

C. Read *Case Report 11.4. Insert the correct medical term to answer each question or complete the statement.* **LO 11.2, 11.5, 11.8, and 11.9**

1. Which medical term is used in documentation for Mr. Santiago's "ringing in his ears?" _____

2. Which medical term is used in documentation for Mr. Santiago's "spinning or whirling?" _____

3. Because the attacks come and go, they can be described as being: _____

4. Will the medication correct the disorders of the inner ear? (yes or no) _____

D. Challenge *your knowledge of the ear by filling in the correct terms for the following definitions. Fill in the blanks.* **LO 11.2, 11.5, and 11.9**

Definition	Medical Term
1. Persistent ringing in the ears	_____
2. Sensation of spinning or whirling	_____
3. Occurring in sharp, spasmodic episodes	_____
4. State of being evenly balanced	_____
5. Dilated portion of a canal or duct	_____
6. Calcium particle in the vestibule	_____
7. Mound of hair cells found in ampulla	_____

E. Test *your knowledge of the language of otology. Match the definition in the first column with its correct medical term in the second column. Fill in the blanks.* **LO 11.4 and 11.5**

_____ 1. pertaining to the eardrum   a. meatus

_____ 2. external opening of a passage   b. cerumen

_____ 3. shell-like external ear   c. tympanic

_____ 4. waxy secretion of the external ear   d. auricle

_____ 5. earwax that is wedged in the ear canal   e. impacted

F. Translate *medical terms into everyday language for your patients. Select the correct answer to each statement.* **LO 11.5, 11.6, and 11.9**

1. An otoscopic exam to look for cerumen impaction.

   a. "The doctor will look in your ear to see if there is earwax lodged in the ear canal."

   b. "The surgeon will cut a hole in the eardrum to release the fluid."

   c. "The nurse will flush the ear canal to remove ear wax."

   d. "You will need an X-ray of the skull to determine if you have a tumor in your ear."

2. Otitis externa

   a. "The eardrum has a hole in it."

   b. "Earwax in the ear canal has hardened."

   c. "Your outer ear is infected."

   d. "The inner ear is filled with thick fluid."

3. Which of the following statements describes the **external auditory meatus?**

   a. thin membrane at the end of the ear canal

   b. outer area of the ear that directs sound waves into the ear canal

   c. tube that leads to your eardrum

   d. opening between the outermost area of the ear and the ear canal

G. Build medical terms. *Fill in the blanks with the correct element to complete the terms.* **LO 11.1 and 11.5**

1. A hole through the wall of a structure: _____ /ion

2. Hardening at the junction of the stapes and oval window: oto/_____ /sis

3. Yellow, waxy tumor in the middle ear: _____ / _____ /oma

H. Choose *the correct answer to each statement.* **LO 11.1 and 11.5**

1. The root in the term **perforation** means:

   a. tumor   b. bore through   c. liquid   d. bile   e. blockage

2. In the term **cholesteatoma,** the word element that means fat is:

   a. choles-   b. -steat-   c. -oma

3. In the term **otosclerosis,** the word element oto- means:

   a. pertaining to   b. hardening   c. condition of   d. ear

I. Match *the correct element in the first column to the correct meaning in the second column below. Fill in the blanks.* **LO 11.1 and 11.5**

_____ 1. -ion   a. action

_____ 2. scler/o-   b. fat

_____ 3. -oma   c. tumor

_____ 4. steat-   d. bile

_____ 5. chol/e-   e. hard

J. Review *the material regarding the middle ear structures and their disorders; then choose the best answer.* **LO 11.1 and 11.5**

1. In the term **basilar,** *basil-* is a

   a. prefix   b. root   c. combining form

2. The **entrance to the inner ear** is the

   a. vestibule   b. labyrinth   c. cochlea   d. aqueous   e. choroid

3. **Labyrinthitis** is a(n)

   a. procedure   b. symptom   c. inflammation

4. The element *neuro-* means

   a. never   b. nerve   c. nose

5. **Hearing loss** caused by lesions of the outer ear is

   a. auditory   b. basilar   c. sensorineural   d. conductive

6. An **intricate combination of passages** in the ear is the

   a. cochlea   b. vestibule   c. labyrinth

7. The root meaning **inflammation** can be found in the word

   a. vestibule   b. labyrinthitis   c. otology

8. **Hearing loss** caused by lesions of the inner ear is called _____ hearing loss.

   a. auditory   b. basilar   c. sensorineural

9. The suffix meaning **pertaining to** is found in the term

   a. vestibular   b. labyrinthitis   c. audiometer

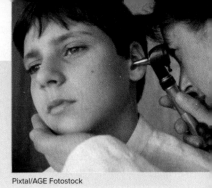
Pixtal/AGE Fotostock

Section 11.6

Diagnostic and Therapeutic Procedures and Pharmacology for Disorders of the Ear

Many of the diagnostic tests for hearing function and to determine diseases of the ear can be performed by technicians with physician overview. To communicate clearly and accurately, the terminology of these diagnostic procedures must be clearly understood by everyone involved.

Otolaryngologists are physicians specializing in the treatment, including surgical procedures, of diseases and disorders of the ear, nose, and throat. They are often referred to as **ENT** doctors.

Otology is a medical subspecialty of otolaryngology that focuses on diseases and disorders of the ear. **Otologists** are physicians who diagnose and treat ear disorders and diseases.

Audiologists are not physicians but have a doctoral degree (**AuD**). They specialize in the conditions of hearing and balance.

Diagnostic Procedures for Diseases of the Ear (LO 11.6)

Basic hearing test procedures that can be performed in an office include:

- **Whispered speech testing,** which is a simple screening method in which one ear of the patient is covered and the patient is asked to identify whispered sounds.
- **Tuning fork screening tests,** which can identify on which side a hearing loss is located (**Weber test**) and whether the hearing loss is due to loss of bone or air conduction (**Rinne test**).

    Audiometry measures hearing function and is often performed by an **audiologist,** a specialist in **audiology.**

    An **audiometer** is an electronic device that generates sounds in different frequencies and intensities and prints out a graph (**audiogram**) of the patient's responses (*Figure 11.36*).

Abbreviations	
ABR	auditory brainstem response
AD	right ear
AS	left ear
AU	both ears
AuD	doctor of audiology
CAT	computed axial tomography
ENT	ear, nose, and throat

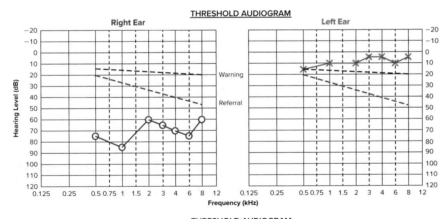

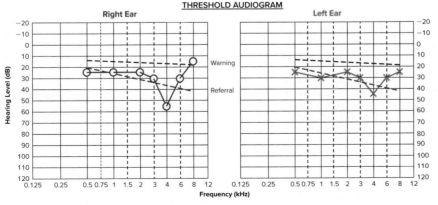

◀ **FIGURE 11.36**
Examples of Audiometry Results.

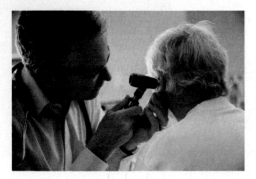

▲ FIGURE 11.37
Physician Using an Otoscope to Examine Patient's Ear.

Tympanometry helps detect problems between the tympanic membrane and the inner ear by using a small earpiece that generates pressure and sound in the ear canal to gather information (**tympanography**) about changes of pressure inside the ear.

When recording the results of hearing testing, **A** is shorthand for the right ear, **A** for the left ear, and **AU** for both ears.

The auricle pinna is examined visually and by touch. The external ear and the middle ear are examined via **otoscopy** with an **otoscope** (*Figure 11.37*). The auricle of the ear is gently manipulated in order for a health care provider to obtain an **otoscopic** view of the external and middle ear. The otoscopic view enables the tympanic membrane and the ossicles behind it to be visualized.

A **pneumatic otoscope** pushes air into the ear and enables the examiner to see if the eardrum moves freely.

Electrocochleography (ECOG) measures the response to sound by the nervous system. A soft electrode is placed deeply in the external ear canal and other electrodes are placed on the forehead to measure responses to sound.

Auditory brainstem response (ABR) test also measures the nervous system response to sound with a setup and procedure similar to ECOG.

Videonystagmography (VNG) diagnoses nystagmus. This test uses a special set of goggles with a video camera to record eye movements as a response to position changes and certain stimuli provided by a health care specialist.

Magnetic resonance imaging (MRI) of structures in the inner ear can be helpful in the diagnosis of some vestibular disorders. **Computerized axial tomography (CAT)** scan can help diagnose problems in and around the inner ear.

Word Analysis and Definition

S = Suffix   P = Prefix   R = Root   R/CF = Combining Form

WORD	PRONUNCIATION		ELEMENTS	DEFINITION
audiology	aw-dee-**OL**-oh-jee	S/ R/CF	-logy *study of* -audi/o- *hearing*	Study of hearing disorders
audiologist	aw-dee-**OL**-oh-jist	S/	-logist *specialist*	Specialist in evaluation of hearing function
audiometer	aw-dee-**OM**-eh-ter	R/CF R/	audi/o- *hearing* -meter *measure*	Instrument to measure hearing
audiometric (adj)	**AW**-dee-oh-**MET**-rik	S/ R/	-ic *pertaining to* -metr- *measure*	Pertaining to the measurement of hearing
audiometry	aw-dee-**OM**-eh-tree	S/	-metry *process of measuring*	The measurement of hearing
electrocochleography	ee-**LEK**-troh-kok-lee-**OG**-rah-fee	S/ R/CF R/CF	-graphy *process of recording* electr/o- *electric* -cochle/o- *cochlea*	Measurement of the electric potentials generated in the inner ear by sounds
otologist	oh-**TOL**-oh-jist	S/ R/CF	-logist *specialist* ot/o- *ear*	Medical specialist in diseases of the ear
otology	oh-**TOL**-oh-jee	S/	-logy *study of*	Diagnosis and treatment of disorders of the ear
otorhinolaryngologist	oh-toh-rye-no-lah-rin-**GOL**-oh-jist	R/CF R/CF	-rhin/o- *nose* -laryng/o- *larynx*	Ear, nose, and throat medical specialist
otoscope	**OH**-toh-scope	S/ R/CF	-scope *instrument for viewing* ot/o- *ear*	Instrument for examining the external and middle ears
otoscopic (adj)	oh-toh-**SKOP**-ik	S/	-ic *pertaining to*	Pertaining to examination with an otoscope
otoscopy	oh-**TOS**-koh-pee	S/	-scopy *to examine*	Examination of the ear
pneumatic	new-**MAT**-ik	S/ R/	-ic *pertaining to* pneumat- *structure filled with air*	Pertaining to a structure filled with air
Rinne test	**RIN**-eh TEST		Friedrich Rinne, 1819–1868, German otologist **test** Latin *earthen vessel*	Test for conductive hearing loss
tympanography	**TIM**-pan-**OG**-rah-fee	S/ R/CF	-graphy *process of recording* tympan/o- *eardrum, tympanic membrane*	Recording pressure changes inside the ear
tympanometry	**TIM**-pan-**OM**-eh-tree	S/	-metry *process of measuring*	Measurement of pressure changes between the middle and inner ears
video			Latin, *to see*	Media product with visual elements displayed on a computer monitor
videonystagmography		S/ R/ R/	-graphy *process of recording* video- *pertaining to visual elements* -nystagm/o- *nystagmus*	Process of recording eye movements as a response to visual stimuli and position changes
Weber test	**VAY**-ber TEST		Ernst Weber, 1794–1878, German physiologist **test** Latin *earthen vessel*	Test for sensorineural hearing loss

Therapeutic Procedures for the Ear (LO 11.6)

Hearing (LO 11.6)

Ear clearing to equalize the pressure in the middle ear with the outside air pressure by making the ear(s) "pop" can be performed by yawning, swallowing, or using a method like a **Valsalva maneuver,** in which the nose is pinched, the mouth is closed, and attempts are made to breathe out through the nose.

Ear wax blockage is removed by loosening it with warm water or oil, and then flushing, **curetting,** or suctioning out the softened wax.

Debridement is the removal of necrotic tissue and debris from the external ear canal in otitis externa using dry cotton wipes and/or suction. Mild otitis externa can then be treated with 2% acetic acid and hydrocortisone drops. Moderate infections require the addition of a **topical antibacterial suspension,** and severe infections require the insertion of an ear wick into the canal, wetted four times a day with a topical antibiotic or 5% aluminum acetate solution. Very severe infections may need systemic antibiotics.

Swimmer's ear is a form of otitis externa and can be prevented by applying a few drops of a 1:1 mixture of rubbing alcohol and vinegar immediately after swimming.

Acute otitis media responds to an antibiotic such as amoxicillin, though some infections may subside spontaneously. **Tympanocentesis** may be used for infections that do not respond to antibiotic therapy.

A chronic otitis media with effusion, when the sticky fluid persists in the middle ear. A **myringotomy** can be performed to treat small, hollow plastic tube inserted through the tympanic membrane to allow the effusion to drain out. These tubes are called **tympanostomy tubes,** or **pressure equalization tubes** (PE tubes) (*Figure 11.38*). **Mastoidectomy** is required for a cholesteatoma.

Hearing aids can help a sensorineural hearing loss and an **audiologist** will recommend the type of device for each patient. Hearing aids are becoming more sophisticated and smaller, but they do not help people with cochlear damage.

Cochlear implants can be used for a severe hearing loss. Unlike a hearing aid that amplifies sound and directs it through the ear canal, a cochlear implant compensates for damaged or nonworking elements in the cochlea. The devices pick up sound and **digitize** it, convert the digitized sound into electrical signals, and transmit those signals to electrodes embedded in the cochlea. The electrodes stimulate the cochlear nerve, sending signals to the brain.

Stapedotomy improves hearing in otosclerosis by using a laser to make a hole in the stapes footplate, removing the stapes bone, and inserting a **prosthesis** that replaces the bone.

Balance (LO 11.6)

Otolith repositioning procedures, performed by physical therapists with specialized training, are employed to return the tiny otolith granules to their correct resting place to resolve positional vertigo.

Exercises taught in a physical therapy setting can help with dizziness and vertigo to improve balance in different positions and activities.

Medications for the Ear (LO 11.6)

In the external ear canal, buildup of wax can be loosened with warm water **irrigation,** oil or with carbamide peroxide solution *(Debrox).* Otitis externa can be treated with acetic acid drops to change the pH of the external canal or with drops containing an antibiotic or an antibiotic and steroid such as ciprofloxacin and dexamethazone *(Ciprodex)* or neomycin, polymycin, and hydrocortisone *(Corticosporin).*

For infections of the middle ear, antibiotics such as penicillin, amoxicillin, and erythromycin are used.

For inner ear disorders, the antihistamine meclizine and the anti-anxiety medication diazepam *(Valium)* are used to diminish the vertigo of BPPV. The treatment of Ménière disease has been revolutionized with the use of a single transtympanic injection of a low dose of gentamycin.

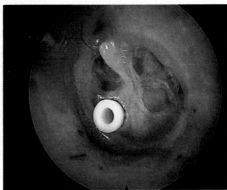

▲ **FIGURE 11.38**
Pressure Equalization (PE) Tube in Tympanic Membrane.

Professor Tony Wright, Institute of Laryngology & Otology/ Science Source

WORD	PRONUNCIATION		ELEMENTS	DEFINITION
acetaminophen	ah-seat-ah-**MIN**-oh-fen		Generic drug name	Medication that is an analgesic and antipyretic
curette	kyu-**RET**	S/ R/	-ette *little* cur- *cleanse*	Scoop-shaped instrument for scraping the interior of a cavity or removing new growths
curettage (Note: *the final "e" of curette is dropped because the suffix "–age" begins with a vowel*)	kyu-reh-**TAHZH**	S/	-age *related to*	Scraping the interior of a cavity or removing a new growth
debridement	day-**BREED**-mon	S/ P/ R/	-ment *resulting state* de- *take away* -bride- *rubbish*	The removal of necrotic or injured tissue
digitize	**DIJ**-ih-tize	S/ R/	-ize *affect in a specific way* digit- *finger, toe, number*	To change analog information into a numerical format to facilitate computer processing
implant	im-**PLANT**		French *to insert*	To insert material into tissues; or the material inserted into tissues
irrigation	ih-rih-**GAY**-shun	S/ R/	-ation *process* irrig- *to water*	Use of water; e.g., to remove wax from the external ear canal
maneuver	mah-**NYU**-ver		French *to work by hand*	A planned movement or procedure
mastoidectomy	**MASS**-toy-**DEK**-toh-me	S/ S/ R/	-etomy *surgical removal* -oid *resembling* mast- *breast*	Surgical removal of portions of the mastoid bone.
myringotomy	mir-in-**GOT**-oh-mee	S/ R/CF	-tomy *surgical incision* myring/o- *tympanic membrane*	Incision in the tympanic membrane
necrosis	neh-**KROH**-sis	S/ R/	-osis *condition* necr- *death*	Pathologic death of one or more cells
necrotic (adj)	neh-**KROT**-ik	S/ R/CF	-tic *pertaining to* necr/o- *death*	Affected by necrosis
prosthesis	**PROS**-thee-sis		Greek *addition*	Manufactured substitute for a missing or diseased part of the body
stapedotomy	**STAY**-puh-**DOT**-oh-mee	S/ R/CF	-tomy *surgical incision* staped/o- *stapes*	Microsurgical procedure for otosclerosis in which stapes prosthesis is placed in a hole in stapes footplate
topical	**TOP**-ih-kal	S/ R/	-al *pertaining to* topic- *local*	Medication applied directly to obtain a local effect
tympanocentesis	**TIM**-pah-noh-sen-**TEE**-sis	S/ R/CF	-centesis *to puncture* tympan/o- *eardrum, tympanic membrane*	Puncture of the tympanic membrane with a needle
tympanostomy	**TIM**-pan-**OS**-toh-mee	S/	-stomy *new opening*	Surgically created new opening in the tympanic membrane to allow fluid to drain from the middle ear
Valsalva	val-**SAL**-vah		Antonio Valsalva, 1666–1723, Italian physician	Any forced expiratory effort against a closed airway

EXERCISES

A. Define the different auditory diagnostic tests. *Match the test in the first column with its correct description in the second column. Fill in the blanks.*   **LO 11.6**

_____ 1. tympanometry

_____ 2. Rinne test

_____ 3. otoscopy

_____ 4. Weber test

a. used to view the external ear and tympanic membrane

b. test for conductive hearing loss

c. test for sensorineural hearing loss

d. measures pressure changes between the middle and inner ears

B. Deconstruct medical terms relating to the diagnostic tests of the ear. *Fill in the blanks* LO 11.1, 11.6, and 11.7

1. tympanometry: _____ / _____
   CF   S

2. tympanocentesis: _____ / _____
   CF   S

3. audiologist: _____ / _____
   CF   S

C. Use the following table *to list all the combining forms in the terms given and give their meaning:* LO 11.1 and LO 11.6

Terms	Combining Forms	Meaning of Combining Forms
otoscope		
electrocochleography		

D. Insert *the following terms to complete the medical documentation. Use each term only once; not all terms will be used. Fill in the blanks.* LO 11.2, 11.5, 11.6, and 11.7

otoscope   otoscopic   otoscopy   pneumatic

The patient was complaining of an earache. A(n) _____ (1) exam was necessary to quickly visualize the auditory canal and tympanic membrane. You hand Dr. Brown a(n) _____ (2) and she noticed that the membrane seemed to be abnormal. She used the _____ (3) attachment to see if the tympanic membrane moved freely.

E. Fill in the blanks *with the correct abbreviation being described.* LO 11.2 and 11.6

1. Use of goggles with a video camera to monitor eye movements as they follow different visual targets _____

2. Records images of the structures of the inner ear without the use of radiation: _____

3. Measures the nervous system's response to sound through the placement of electrodes in the ear canal and on the forehead: _____

F. Identify the therapeutic procedure indicated for each disorder. *Select the correct answer for each question.* LO 11.5 and 11.6

1. Chronic otitis media may be treated with:

   a. Valsalva maneuver   **b.** tympanostomy tubes   **c.** rubbing alcohol drops   **d.** physical therapy

2. Acute otitis media is treated with:

   a. myringotomy   **b.** tympanostomy tubes   **c.** oral antibiotics   **d.** antihistamines

3. Positional vertigo can be treated with:

   a. physical therapy   **b.** anti-anxiety medications   **c.** cochlear implants   **d.** myringotomy

4. A treatment for excessive cerumen in the auditory canal:

   a. alcohol and vinegar drops   **b.** antibiotic drops   **c.** myringotomy   **d.** curettage

5. Cholesteatoma is treated with:

   a. debridement   **b.** excision   **c.** acetic acid drops   **d.** oral antibiotics

G. Pronunciation is important whether you are saying the word or listening to a word from a coworker. Identify the proper pronunciation of the following medical terms. LO 11.1, 11.2, 11.4, and 11.5

1. The correct pronunciation for the last name of the French physician that describes an inner ear disorder that has cluster attacks of tinnitus, vertigo, and hearing loss.

   a. val-sale-VAH   **b.** val-SAL-vah   **c.** men-YEAR   **d.** man-YARE

   Correctly spell the term: _____

2. The correct pronunciation for a fungal infection in an ear

    a. ves-**TIB**-you-lar   **b.** **VES**-tih-byul-ar   **c.** **OH**-toh-migh-**KEY**-oh-sis **d.** **OH**-toh-my-**KOH**-sis

    Correctly spell the term: _____

3. The correct pronunciation for another name for auricle

    a. **PIN**-ee   **b.** **PIN**-ah   **c.** **PIN**-ay   **d.** **PIN**-ahs

    Correctly spell the term: _____

4. The correct pronunciation for pertaining to tears

    a. pair-ee-**OR**-bit-al   **b.** **PER**-ih-or-bit-al   **c.** Lak-**RIME**-al   **d.** **LAK**-rim-al

    Correctly spell the term: _____

5. The correct pronunciation for the ability to see close objects but unable to see distant objects

    a. me-**OH**-pee-ah   **b.** my-**OH**-pee-ah   **c.** em-eh-**TOH**-pee-ah   **d.** em-eh-try-**OH**-pee-ah

    Correctly spell the term: _____

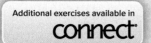

Additional exercises available in **connect**

Chapter Review exercises, along with additional practice items, are available in Connect!

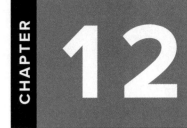

CHAPTER 12

The Endocrine System

The Essentials of the Language of Endocrinology

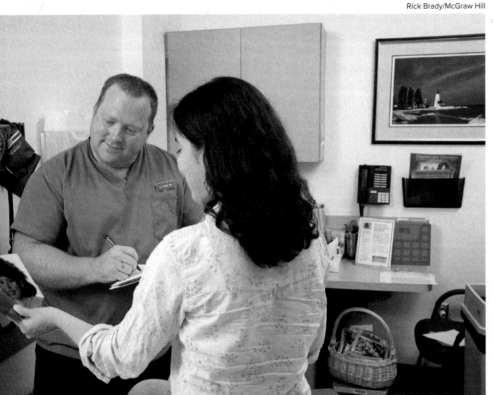

Rick Brady/McGraw Hill

Learning Outcomes

The **endocrine** system is a communication system. The *hormones* produced by this system are blood-borne messengers secreted by endocrine glands; they circulate in the bloodstream, gaining access to other body cells. They are distributed anywhere the blood travels, but only affect the target cells that have receptors for them. These hormones alter the metabolism of the target cells. The information in this chapter will enable you to:

LO 12.1 Use roots, combining forms, suffixes, and prefixes to construct and analyze (deconstruct) medical terms related to the endocrine system.

LO 12.2 Spell and pronounce correctly medical terms related to the endocrine system to communicate them with accuracy and precision in any health care setting.

LO 12.3 Define accepted abbreviations related to the endocrine system.

LO 12.4 Identify the anatomy and physiology of the organs of the endocrine system.

LO 12.5 Identify and describe disorders and pathological conditions related to the endocrine system.

LO 12.6 Identify the diagnostic and therapeutic procedures and pharmacologic agents used for disorders of the endocrine system.

LO 12.7 Identify health care professionals involved in the care of patients with endocrine diseases and disorders.

LO 12.8 Apply your knowledge of medical terms relating to the endocrine system to documentation, medical records, and medical reports.

LO 12.9 Translate the medical terms relating to the endocrine system into everyday language in order to communicate clearly with patients and their families.

The health professionals involved in the diagnosis and treatment of problems with the endocrine system include:

- **Endocrinologists,** who are medical specialists concerned with the production and effects of hormones.
- **Internal medicine physicians,** also called **internists,** are medical doctors specializing in internal medicine, who diagnose and treat chronic conditions of internal organs.
- **Endocrine physician assistants,** who are advanced practice providers who work with endocrinologists to provide care and education to endocrine and diabetes patients.
- **Endocrine nurse practitioners,** who are registered nurses with at least a Master's degree with specialized training in endocrinology.
- **Certified diabetic educators,** who are certified professionals with specialized knowledge in diabetes self-management education and monitoring.

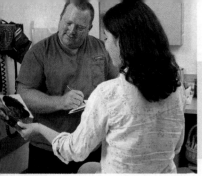

Section 12.1

Endocrine System, Hypothalamus, and Pituitary and Pineal Glands

Rick Brady/McGraw Hill

Your endocrine system is a network of ductless glands whose cells secrete **hormones** directly into your bloodstream.

The Endocrine System (LO 12.4)

The endocrine system comprises several major organs *(Figures 12.1 and 12.2)*. These organs work together to ensure that this system operates smoothly:

- **Pituitary gland** and the nearby **hypothalamus**
- **Pineal gland**
- **Thyroid gland**
- **Parathyroid glands**
- **Thymus gland**
- **Adrenal glands**
- **Pancreas**
- **Gonads: testes in the male;** ovaries **in the female** (The male gonads are discussed in *Chapter 14* and the female gonads in *Chapter 15.*)

In addition, endocrine cells found in tissues throughout the body secrete particular hormones. For example:

- **Cells in the upper GI tract** secrete gastrin, which stimulates gastric secretions.
- **Cells in the kidney** secrete **erythropoietin,** which stimulates erythrocyte (red blood cell) production in the bone marrow.
- **Fat cells** secrete **leptin,** which helps suppress appetite. Lack of leptin can lead to overeating and obesity.
- **Cells in tissues throughout the body** secrete **prostaglandins**, which act locally to dilate blood vessels, relax airways, stimulate uterine contractions in menstrual cramps or labor, and lower acid secretion in the stomach. When tissues are injured, prostaglandins promote an inflammatory response.

Keynotes

- A hormone is secreted by an endocrine gland or cell and carried by the bloodstream to act at distant target sites.
- The medical specialty concerned with the hormonal secretions of the endocrine glands is called **endocrinology**.

Abbreviation

ADH   antidiuretic hormone

▲ **FIGURE 12.1**
Hypothalamus, Pituitary Gland, and Pineal Gland.

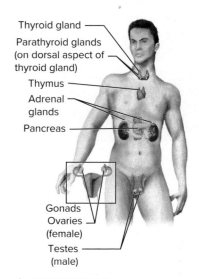

▲ **FIGURE 12.2**
Major Endocrine Glands.

Hypothalamus (LO 12.2 and 12.4)

The hypothalamus, which is the size of an almond, is located in the brain just above the pituitary gland. It connects the brain to the endocrine system through blood vessels between the hypothalamus and the pituitary gland, thus enabling hypothalamic hormones to control pituitary hormone secretion. Six of them are local hormones that regulate the production of hormones by the anterior pituitary gland (see page 334). Two of them, **oxytocin** and **antidiuretic hormone (ADH),** are transported to the posterior pituitary, where they are stored until they are needed elsewhere in the body.

Pineal Gland (LO 12.2 and 12.4)

The pineal gland is located near the top of the brain's third ventricle, posterior to the hypothalamus. It secretes the feel-good hormone **serotonin** by day, and at night, converts it to **melatonin**, which helps to regulate sleep and wake cycles. This gland reaches its maximum size in childhood and may regulate the timing of puberty.

WORD	PRONUNCIATION	ELEMENTS		DEFINITION
antidiuretic (Note: This term has two prefixes)	**AN**-tih-die-you-**RET**-ik	S/ P/ P/ R/	-ic *pertaining to* anti- *against* -di- *complete* -uret- *urination*	An agent that decreases urine production
antidiuretic hormone	**AN**-tih-die-you-**RET**-ik **HOR**-mohn		hormone *Greek to set in motion*	Posterior pituitary hormone that decreases urine output by acting on the kidney
endocrine	**EN**-doh-krin	P/ R/CF	endo- *within* -crine *secrete*	A gland that produces an internal or hormonal secretion
endocrinology (Note: The "e" in crine *changes to "o" for better flow.*)	**EN**-doh-krih-**NOL**-oh-jee	S/	-logy *study of*	Medical specialty concerned with the production and effects of hormones
endocrinologist	**EN**-doh-krih-**NOL**-oh-jist	S/	-logist *one who studies, specialist*	A medical specialist in endocrinology
erythropoietin	eh-**RITH**-roh-**POY**-ee-tin	S/ R/CF	-poietin *the maker* erythr/o- *red*	Protein secreted by the kidney that stimulates red blood cell production
hormone	**HOR**-mohn		Greek *to set in motion*	Chemical formed in one tissue or organ and carried by the bloodstream to stimulate or inhibit a function of another tissue or organ
hormonal (adj)	hor-**MOHN**-al	S/ R/	-al *pertaining to* hormon- *hormone*	Pertaining to hormones
hypothalamus	high-poh-**THAL**-ah-muss	S/ P/	-us *pertaining to* hypo- *below*	An endocrine gland in the floor and wall of the third ventricle of the brain
hypothalamic (adj)	high-poh-thal-**AM**-ik	S/ R/	-ic *pertaining to* -thalam- *thalamus*	Pertaining to the hypothalamus
leptin	**LEP**-tin	S/ R/	-in *chemical compound* lept- *thin, small*	Hormone secreted by adipose tissue
melatonin	mel-ah-**TONE**-in	S/ R/ R/	-in *substance* mela- *black* -ton- *tension, pressure*	Hormone formed by the pineal gland
oxytocin	**OCK**-see-**TOH**-sin	S/ R/ R/	-in *substance* oxy- *oxygen* -toc- *labor and childbirth*	Pituitary hormone that stimulates the uterus to contract
pineal	**PIN**-ee-al		Latin *like a pine cone*	Pertaining to the pineal gland
pituitary	pih-**TYU**-ih-**TAIR**-ee	S/ R/	-ary *pertaining to* pituit- *pituitary*	Pertaining to the pituitary gland
prostaglandin	**PROS**-tah-**GLAN**-din	S/ R/ R/	-in *chemical* prosta- *prostate* -gland- *gland*	Hormone present in many tissues, but first isolated from the prostate gland
serotonin	ser-oh-**TOH**-nin	S/ R/CF R/	-in *substance* ser/o- *serum* -ton- *tension, pressure*	Neurotransmitter in central and peripheral nervous systems

Pituitary Gland (LO 12.2, 12.3, and 12.4)

Each hormone plays its part in maintaining the body's homeostasis, but the pituitary gland and hypothalamus work together and often influence hormone production in the other endocrine glands. The pituitary gland is suspended from the hypothalamus, and has two components:

- A large anterior lobe; and
- A small posterior lobe.

ACTH	adrenocorticotropic hormone
CRH	cortico-releasing hormone
FSH	follicle-stimulating hormone
GH	growth hormone
GHRH	growth hormone-releasing hormone
GnRH	gonadotropin-releasing hormone
LH	luteinizing hormone
OT	oxytocin
PTH	parathyroid hormone
PRL	prolactin
T3	triiodothyronine
T4	tetraiodothyronine (thyroxine)
TRH	thyrotropin-releasing hormone
TSH	thyroid-stimulating hormone

There are six **anterior-lobe hormones,** which are listed here with their functions. Releasing and inhibiting hormones secreted by the hypothalamus *are shown in italics.*

1. **Follicle-stimulating hormone (FSH)** stimulates target cells in the ovaries to develop eggs, as well as sperm production in the testes.

2. **Luteinizing hormone (LH)** stimulates ovulation. It also encourages a corpus luteum (a yellow tissue mass) to form in the ovary *(see Chapter 15)* to secrete estrogen and progesterone. In the male, LH stimulates testosterone production *(see Chapter 14).* Both FSH and LH production are stimulated by *gonadotropin-releasing hormone (GnRH)* of the hypothalamus.

3. **Thyroid-stimulating hormone (TSH),** or **thyrotropin,** stimulates the growth of the thyroid gland and the production of the chief thyroid hormone, thyroxine. TSH production is stimulated by *thyrotropin-releasing hormone (TRH)* of the hypothalamus.

4. **Adrenocorticotropic hormone (ACTH),** or **corticotropin,** stimulates the adrenal glands to produce hormones called **corticosteroids,** including **hydrocortisone (cortisol)** and **cortisone.** ACTH production is stimulated by *cortico-releasing hormone (CRH)* of the hypothalamus.

5. **Prolactin (PRL)** encourages the mammary glands to produce milk after pregnancy. In the male, it sensitizes the testes to LH, which enhances testosterone production. Prolactin production is stimulated by *thyrotropin-releasing hormone (TRH)* of the hypothalamus.

6. **Growth hormone (GH),** or **somatotrophin,** stimulates cells to enlarge and divide. The body produces at least a thousand times more GH than any other pituitary hormone. This production of growth hormone is stimulated by *growth hormone-releasing hormone (GHRH)* of the hypothalamus.

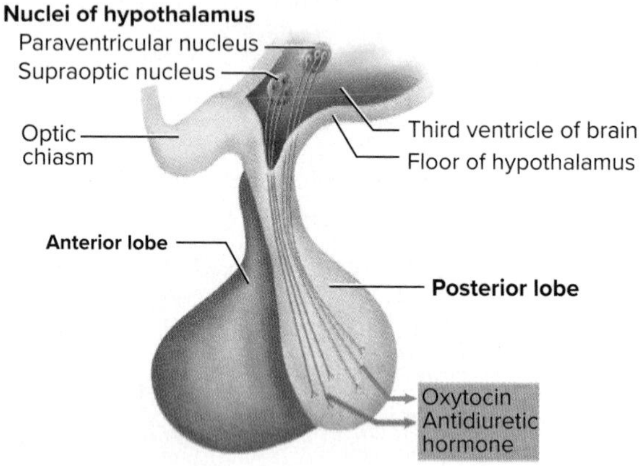

Tropic hormones are hormones that stimulate other endocrine glands to produce their hormones. FSH and LH are called **gonadotropins** because they stimulate **gonadal** (reproductive organ) functions.

In addition to the six anterior-lobe hormones, there are the **posterior-lobe hormones.** These hormones are produced in the hypothalamus and stored and released in the pituitary posterior lobe *(Figure 12.3).* The two types of posterior-lobe hormones and their functions are:

1. **Oxytocin (OT)** in childbirth stimulates uterine contractions, and in lactation, forces milk to flow down ducts to the nipple. In both sexes, its production increases during social interaction and sexual intercourse to create feelings of satisfaction and emotional bonding.

2. **Antidiuretic hormone (ADH),** also called **vasopressin,** reduces the volume of urine produced by the kidneys.

▲ **FIGURE 12.3**
Hormones of the Posterior Lobe of the Pituitary Gland.

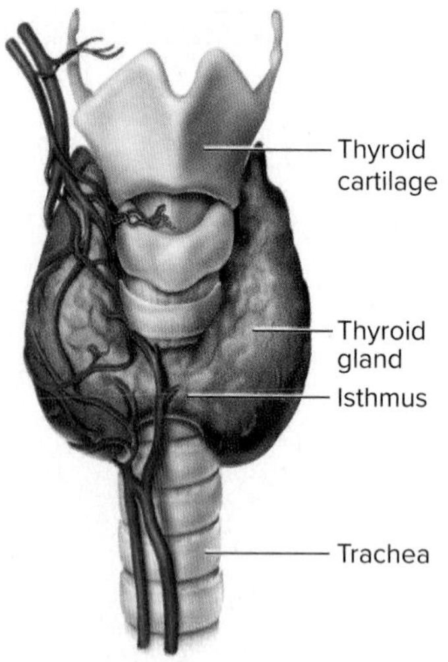

▲ **FIGURE 12.4**
Anatomy of the Thyroid Gland.

Thyroid Gland (LO 12.3 and 12.4)

Shaped like a bow tie and measuring about 2 inches wide, the **thyroid** gland lies just beneath the skin of the neck and below the thyroid cartilage ("Adam's apple"). Two lobes extend up on either side of the trachea (or windpipe) and are joined by an isthmus *(Figure 12.4).*

Cells in the thyroid gland secrete the two thyroid hormones **T3** and **T4.** The latter is known as **thyroxine.** The term **thyroid hormone** refers to T3 and T4 collectively, and it performs the following functions:

* **Stimulates** almost every tissue in the body to produce proteins;

* **Increases** the amount of oxygen that cells use; and

* **Controls** the speed of the body's chemical functions, known as the **metabolic rate.**

The thyroid gland also produces the hormone **calcitonin,** which promotes calcium deposition and bone formation.

Parathyroid Glands (LO 12.3 and 12.4)

Most people have four **parathyroid** glands, and these are partially embedded in the posterior surface of the thyroid gland. The parathyroid glands secrete **parathyroid hormone (PTH).** PTH stimulates bone resorption to bring calcium back into the blood, and calcitonin takes calcium from the blood to stimulate bone deposition *(see Chapter 4).*

WORD	PRONUNCIATION	ELEMENTS		DEFINITION
adrenocorticotropic	ah-**DREE**-noh-**KOR**-tih-koh-**TROH**-pik	S/ R/CF R/CF	**-tropic** *a turning, change* **adren/o-** *adrenal gland* **-cortic/o-** *from the cortex*	Hormone of the anterior pituitary that stimulates the cortex of the adrenal gland to produce its own hormones
corticosteroid	**KOR**-tih-koh-**STAIR**-oyd	S/ R/CF	**-steroid** *steroid* **cortic/o-** *from the cortex*	A hormone produced by the adrenal cortex
corticotropin	**KOR**-tih-koh-**TROH**-pin	S/ R/CF	**-tropin** *stimulation* **cortic/o-** *from the cortex, cortex*	Pituitary hormone that stimulates the cortex of the adrenal gland to secrete cortisone
cortisone	**KOR**-tih-sohn	S/ R/	**-one** *hormone* **cortis-** *from the cortex*	A corticosteroid produced in small amounts by the adrenal cortex
gonadotropin	**GO**-nad-oh-**TROH**-pin	S/ R/CF	**-tropin** *stimulation* **gonad/o-** *testis, ovary*	Any hormone that stimulates gonadal function
gonad	**GO**-nad		**gonad** Latin *seed*	An organ that produces sex cells; a testis or an ovary
hydrocortisone cortisol (syn)	high-droh-**KOR**-tih-sohn	S/ R/CF R/	**-one** *hormone* **hydr/o-** *water* **-cortis-** *from the cortex*	Potent glucocorticoid with anti-inflammatory properties
prolactin	pro-**LAK**-tin	S/ P/ R/	**-in** *substance* **pro-** *before* **-lact-** *milk*	Pituitary hormone that stimulates the production of milk
somatotrophin growth hormone, GH (syn)	**SO**-mah-toh-**TROH**-fin	S/ R/CF	**-trophin** *stimulation* **somat/o-** *the body*	Hormone of the anterior pituitary that stimulates the growth of body tissues
thyrotropin	thigh-roe-**TROH**-pin	S/ R/CF	**-tropin** *stimulation* **thyr/o-** *thyroid*	Hormone from the anterior pituitary gland that stimulates function of the thyroid gland
tropin (noun) trophin (alt) tropic (adj)	**TROH**-pin **TROH**-fin **TROH**-pik	 S/ R/	Greek *a turning* Greek *nourishment* **-ic** *pertaining to* **trop-** *turning*	Hormone Hormone Tropic hormones stimulate other endocrine glands to produce hormones

Thymus Gland (LO 12.3 and 12.4)

The **thymus** gland is located in the mediastinum *(Figure 12.5)*. This gland is large in children and over time, decreases in size until it becomes mostly fibrous tissue in the elderly. It secretes a group of hormones that stimulate the production of T lymphocytes (see *Chapter 7*).

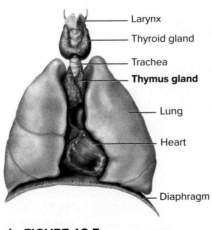

— Larynx
— Thyroid gland
— Trachea
— **Thymus gland**
— Lung
— Heart
— Diaphragm

▲ **FIGURE 12.5**
Position of the Thymus Gland.

WORD	PRONUNCIATION	ELEMENTS		DEFINITION
calcitonin	kal-sih-**TONE**-in	S/ R/CF R/	-in *substance* calc/i- *calcium* -ton- *tension, pressure*	Hormone produced by the thyroid gland that moves calcium from blood to bones
parathyroid	pair-ah-**THIGH**-royd	S/ P/ R/	-oid *resembling* para- *adjacent, beside* -thyr- *thyroid*	Endocrine glands embedded in the back of the thyroid gland
thymus	**THIGH**-mus		Greek *sweetbread*	Endocrine gland located in the mediastinum
thyroid	**THIGH**-royd		Greek *an oblong shield*	Endocrine gland in the neck; or a cartilage of the larynx
thyroxine	thigh-**ROCK**-sin	S/ R/ R/	-ine *pertaining to* thyr- *thyroid gland* -ox- *oxygen*	Thyroid hormone T4, tetraiodothyronine

Adrenal Glands (LO 12.4)

An **adrenal (suprarenal)** gland is anchored like a cap on the upper pole of each kidney *(Figure 12.6 inset).* The outer layer of the gland—the adrenal cortex *(Figure 12.6)*—synthesizes more than 25 **steroid** hormones known collectively as **adrenocortical** hormones, or corticosteroids. These hormones include:

1. **Glucocorticoids**, mainly **hydrocortisone (cortisol)**, which help regulate blood glucose levels, particularly in response to stress. They also have an anti-inflammatory effect, and are often found in dermatologic lotions and ointments;

2. **Mineralocorticoids**, mostly **aldosterone,** which promote sodium retention and potassium excretion by the kidneys; and

3. **Sex steroids,** which include a weak androgen that is converted to testosterone *(see Chapter 14)* and estrogen *(see Chapter 15).*

The inner layer of the adrenal gland, the adrenal medulla *(Figure 12.6),* also secretes hormones. These hormones are called **catecholamines**, and principally include **epinephrine (adrenaline)** and **norepinephrine (noradrenaline)**. These hormones prepare the body for physical activity and are responsible for the "flight or fight" response. The pancreas measures approximately 6 inches in length, rests across the back of the abdomen, and has many important functions, including the secretion of digestive juices and the production of hormones.

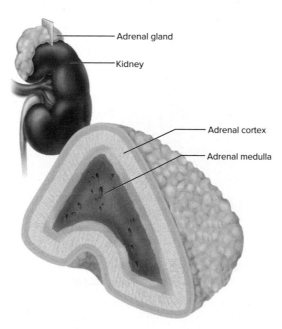

▲ **FIGURE 12.6**
Adrenal Gland.

WORD	PRONUNCIATION	ELEMENTS		DEFINITION
adrenal suprarenal (syn)	ah-**DREE**-nal	S/ P/ R/ P/	-al *pertaining to* ad- *to, toward* -ren- *kidney* supra- *above*	Endocrine gland on the upper pole of each kidney
adrenaline epinephrine (syn)	ah-**DREN**-ah-lin ep-ih-**NEF**-rin	S/ P/ R/	-ine *pertaining to* epi- *above* -nephr- *kidney*	Main catecholamine produced by the adrenal medulla
adrenocortical	ah-dree-noh-**KOR**-tih-kal	S/ R/CF R/	-al *pertaining to* adren/o- *adrenal* -cortic- *cortex*	Pertaining to the cortex of the adrenal gland
aldosterone	al-**DOS**-ter-own	S/ R/CF R/	-one *hormone* ald/o- *organic compound* -ster- *steroid*	Mineralocorticoid hormone of the adrenal cortex
catecholamine	kat-eh-**COAL**-ah-meen	S/ R/	-amine *nitrogen-containing substance* catechol- *tyrosine containing*	Major elements produced by the adrenal cortex in the stress response; including epinephrine and norepinephrine
epinephrine adrenaline (syn)	ep-ih-**NEF**-rin	S/ P/ R/	-ine *pertaining to* epi- *above* -nephr- *kidney*	Main catecholamine produced by the adrenal medulla
glucocorticoid	glu-co-**KOR**-tih-koyd	S/ R/ R/CF	-oid *resembling* -cortic- *cortisone* gluc/o- *glucose*	Hormone of the adrenal cortex that helps regulate glucose metabolism
hydrocortisone cortisol (syn)	high-droh-**KOR**-tih-sohn	S/ R/CF R/	-one *hormone* hydr/o- *water* -cortis- *cortisone*	Potent glucocorticoid with anti-inflammatory properties
mineralocorticoid	**MIN**-er-al-oh-**KOR**-tih-koyd	S/ R/CF R/	-oid *resemble* mineral/o- *inorganic material* -cortic- *cortex*	Hormone of the adrenal cortex that influences sodium and potassium metabolism
norepinephrine (Note: *Two prefixes* noradrenaline (syn)	**NOR**-ep-ih-**NEFF**-rin	S/ P/ P/ R/	-ine *pertaining to* nor- *normal* -epi- *above* -nephr- *kidney*	Catecholamine hormone of the adrenal gland that is a sympathetic neurotransmitter
steroid	**STAIR**-oyd	S/ R/	-oid *resembling* ster- *solid*	Large family of chemical substances found in many drugs, hormones, and body components

The Pancreas (LO 12.2 and 12.4)

The location and structure of the pancreas are further detailed in *Chapter 9*. Most of your pancreas is an **exocrine** gland (external secretion gland) that secretes digestive juices through a duct *(Figure 12.7a)*. Scattered throughout the pancreas are clusters of endocrine cells grouped around blood vessels. These clusters are called **pancreatic islets (islets of Langerhans)**. Within the islets are three distinct cell types *(Figure 12.7b)*:

1. **Alpha cells:** Secrete the hormone **glucagon** in response to low blood **glucose**. Glucagon's actions are:
   a. In the liver, to stimulate **gluconeogenesis**, **glycogenolysis**, and the release of glucose into the bloodstream; and
   b. In adipose tissue, to stimulate fat catabolism and the release of free fatty acids.
2. **Beta cells:** Secrete **insulin** in response to a high blood glucose level. Insulin has the opposite effects to those of glucagon, and its actions are:
   a. In muscle and fat cells, to enable them to absorb glucose, and to store glycogen and fat; and
   b. In the liver, to stimulate the conversion of glucose to glycogen.
3. **Delta cells:** Secrete **somatostatin**, which acts within the pancreas to prevent the secretion of glucagon and insulin.

Keynotes

- Glucagon is not the only hormone that raises blood glucose; epinephrine, hydrocortisone, and growth hormone do as well.
- Insulin is the only hormone that lowers blood glucose.

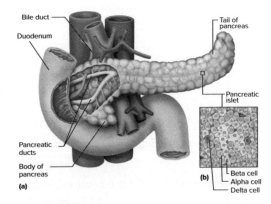

▲ **FIGURE 12.7**
Pancreas. (a) Anatomy of the pancreas.
(b) Alpha, beta, and delta cells.

WORD	PRONUNCIATION	ELEMENTS		DEFINITION
exocrine	EK-soh-krin	P/ R/CF	exo- *outward* -crine *secrete*	A gland that secretes outwardly through excretory ducts
glucagon	GLU-kah-gon	S/ R/	-agon *to fight* gluc- *sugar, glucose*	Pancreatic hormone that supports blood glucose levels
gluconeogenesis	GLU-koh-nee-oh-JEN-eh-sis	S/ P/ R/CF	-genesis *creation* -neo- *new* gluc/o- *sugar, glucose*	Formation of glucose from noncarbohydrate sources
glucose	GLU-kose	S/ R/	-ose *full of* gluc- *sugar, glucose*	The final product of carbohydrate digestion and the main sugar in the blood
glycogenolysis	GLYE-koh-jen-NOL-ih-sis	S/ R/CF R/CF	-lysis *separate, dissolve* glyc/o- *glycogen* -gen/o- *create*	Conversion of glycogen to glucose
insulin	IN-syu-lin	S/ R/	-in *a substance* insul- *an island*	Hormone produced by the islet cells of the pancreas
pancreatic islets islets of Langerhans (syn)	pan-kree-AT-ik EYE-lets EYE-lets of LAHNG-er-hahnz	S/ R/ S/ R/	-ic *pertaining to* pancreat- *pancreas* -et *little* isl- *island* Paul Langerhans, 1847–1888, German anatomist	Areas of pancreatic cells that produce insulin and glucagon
somatostatin	SOH-mah-toh-STAT-in	S/ R/CF	-statin *inhibit* somat/o- *body*	Hormone that inhibits release of growth hormone and insulin

EXERCISES

A. Identify *organs, hormones, and functions of the hormones of the endocrine system. Fill in the blanks.*   **LO 12.2 and 12.4**

1. The _____ is the connection between the brain and the endocrine system via blood vessels.

2. How many hormones does the hypothalamus secrete that control anterior pituitary gland hormone secretion? _____

3. The hormone secreted by fat cells that suppresses appetite: _____

4. The hormone that stimulates uterine contractions: _____

B. Elements *remain your best tool for understanding medical terms. The elements are listed in column 1. Identify the type of element in column 2, its meaning in column 3, and an example of a term related to the anatomy of the endocrine system containing that element in column 4. Fill in the chart.*   **LO 12.1 and 12.2**

Element	Type of Element (P, R, CF, or S)	Meaning of Element	Medical Term Containing This Element
anti	1.	2.	3.
di	4.	5.	6.
ton	7.	8.	9.
hypo	10.	11.	12.
logy	13.	14.	15.
mela	16.	17.	18.

C. Identify *the meaning of the word element. Select the correct answer.*   **LO 12.1 and 12.4**

1. The meaning of the suffix in the term cortisone:
   a. before   b. hormone   c. seed   d. cortex   e. inflammation

2. The meaning of the suffix in the term gonadotropin:
   a. thyroid   b. hormone   c. testis   d. substance   e. stimulation

3. The meaning of the combining form in the term somatotrophin:
   a. body   b. stimulation   c. water   d. growth   e. hormone

D. Abbreviations *will be your answers in this matching exercise. Match the correct abbreviation to its description.* **LO 12.3 and 12.4**

_____ **1.** stimulates ovulation   **A.** LH

_____ **2.** stimulates production of corticosteroids   **B.** ADH

_____ **3.** stimulates uterine contractions   **C.** ACTH

_____ **4.** stimulates ovaries to develop eggs   **D.** TSH

_____ **5.** reduces volume of urine   **E.** OT

_____ **6.** stimulates production of thyroxin   **F.** FSH

E. Describe the functions of the pancreas. *Select the correct answer for each of the following statements.* **LO 12.2 and 12.4**

1. The effect of glucagon is:

  a. decrease blood sugar levels   **b.** increase blood sugar levels

2. Glucagon is secreted by the _____ cells.

  a. alpha   **b.** beta   **c.** delta

3. Clusters of alpha, beta, and delta cells in the pancreas are called:

  a. pancreatic clusters   **b.** pancreatic islets   **c.** pancreatitis   **d.** gluconeogenesis

4. The process of gluconeogenesis will cause blood sugar levels to:

  a. increase   **b.** decrease   **c.** stay the same

5. Storage of glycogen is stimulated by the hormone:

  a. somatostatin   **b.** glucagon   **c.** insulin

F. Build the correct medical term *that matches the definition. Insert each missing element on the line, and label what type of element it is under the line. Then answer question 5.* **LO 12.1, 12.2, and 12.4**

1. Conversion of glycogen to glucose: _____ / _____ /lysis

2. Main sugar in the blood: _____ /ose

3. Hormone that inhibits release of GH and insulin: _____ /statin

4. The formation of glucose from noncarbohydrate sources: gluco/_____ /genesis

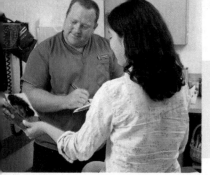

Section 12.2

Disorders of the Endocrine System

Disorders of Pituitary Hormones (LO 12.5)

Overproduction of Pituitary Hormones (LO 12.5)

Overproduction of growth hormone stimulates excessive growth of bones and muscles. It is almost always caused by a benign pituitary **adenoma.**

In children, excessive production starts before the growth plates of the long bones have closed. The long bones grow enormously, producing **gigantism** *(Figure 12.8).*

In adults, excessive growth hormone produces **acromegaly** *(Figure 12.9).* Signs include enlarged hands and feet, protruding jaw, coarse hair, and sweating.

A **prolactinoma** is a benign prolactin-secreting tumor of the pituitary gland in both men and women. It can lead to breast milk production in women who are not breast-feeding and produce scanty menstrual periods. In men it leads to breast milk production and impotence.

Underproduction of Pituitary Hormones (LO 12.3 and 12.5)

Hypopituitarism is uncommon. It can be caused by a pituitary tumor and cause a decline in the production of several hormones at the same time, a condition called **panhypopituitarism.**

Pituitary dwarfism can be caused by an underproduction of growth hormone that can be present at *(Figure 12.10).*

Diabetes insipidus (DI) results from a decreased production of ADH, which helps regulate the amount of water in the body. (Diabetes mellitus is an entirely different disorder; see Disorders of Pancreatic Hormones: Diabetes Mellitus.) Diabetes insipidus can result from insufficient production of ADH in the hypothalamus or failure of the pituitary gland to release it.

Abbreviation

DI   diabetes insipidus

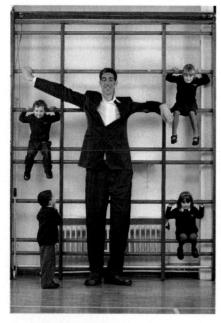

▲ **FIGURE 12.8**
Pituitary Gigantism.

Solent News/Shutterstock

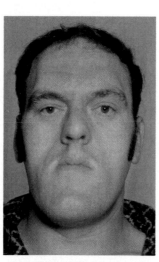

▲ **FIGURE 12.9**
Man with Acromegaly,
Age 52.

Clinical Photography, Central Manchester
University Hospitals NHS Foundation Trust,
UK/Science Source

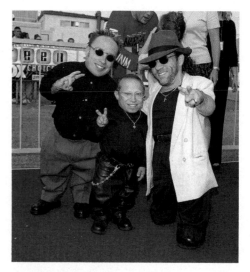

▲ **FIGURE 12.10**
Pituitary Dwarfism.

Frank Trapper/Getty Images

WORD	PRONUNCIATION	ELEMENTS		DEFINITION
acromegaly	ak-roh-**MEG**-ah-lee	P/ R/	**acro-** *highest point, extremity* **-megaly** *enlargement*	Enlargement of the head, face, hands, and feet due to excess growth hormone in an adult
adenoma	**AD**-eh-**NOH**-mah	S/ R/	**-oma** *tumor* **aden-** *gland*	A benign neoplasm of epithelial tissue
diabetes insipidus	die-ah-**BEE**-teez in-**SIP**-ih-dus	S/ P/ R/	**diabetes** Greek *siphon* **-us** *pertaining to* **in-** *not, without* **-sipid-** *flavor*	Excretion of large amounts of dilute urine as a result of inadequate ADH production
dwarfism	**DWORF**-izm	S/ R/	**-ism** *condition* **dwarf-** *miniature*	Short stature due to underproduction of growth hormone
gigantism	jie-**GAN**-tizm	S/ R/	**-ism** *condition* **gigant-** *giant*	Abnormal height and size of entire body
hypopituitarism	**HIGH**-poh-pih-**TYU**-ih-tah-rizm	S/ P/ R/	**-ism** *condition* **hypo-** *deficient* **-pituitar-** *pituitary*	Condition of one or more deficient pituitary hormones
panhypopituitarism	pan-**HIGH**-poh-pih-**TYU**-ih-tah-rizm	S/ P/ P/ R/	**-ism** *condition* **pan-** *all* **-hypo-** *deficient* **-pituitar-** *pituitary*	Deficiency of all the pituitary hormones
polyuria	pol-ee-**YOU**-ree-ah	S/ P/ R/	**-ia** *condition* **poly-** *excessive* **-ur-** *urine*	Excessive production of urine
prolactinoma	proh-lak-tih-**NOH**-mah	S/ S/ P/ R/	**-oma** *tumor* **-in-** *chemical compound* **pro-** *before, in front* **-lact-** *milk*	Prolactin-producing tumor

Disorders of the Thyroid and Parathyroid Glands (LO 12.5)

Hyperthyroidism (Thyrotoxicosis) (LO 12.5)

The symptoms of **hyperthyroidism** (excessive thyroid hormone production) are those of an increased body metabolism. These include tachycardia (rapid heart rate), hypertension, **hyperpyrexia**, sweating, shakiness, anxiety, weight loss despite increased appetite, and diarrhea. Weight loss may be severe, causing **emaciation.**

Graves disease is an autoimmune disorder *(see Chapter 7)* in which an antibody stimulates the thyroid to produce and secrete excessive amounts of thyroid hormone into the blood. It presents with **exophthalmos** (bulging of the eyes) *(Figure 12.11),* a **goiter** (an enlarged thyroid gland) *(Figure 12.12),* and a non-pitting, waxy edema of the lower leg.

Hypothyroidism (LO 12.2 and 12.5)

Hypothyroidism is the opposite of hyperthyroidism and results from an inadequate production of thyroid hormone. This decreases the body's metabolism. Primary hypothyroidism affects around 10% of older women. Symptoms develop gradually and include hair loss; dry, scaly skin; a puffy face and eyes; slow, hoarse speech; weight gain; constipation; and a high sensitivity to cold temperatures. No specific cause has been found.

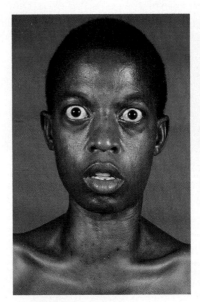

▲ **FIGURE 12.11**
Hyperthyroidism May Cause the Eyes to Protrude (Exophthalmos).

Dr. M.A. Ansary/Science Source

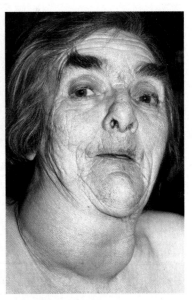

▲ **FIGURE 12.12**
Elderly Woman with Hypothyroidism and Goiter.

Dr P. Marazzi/Science Source

Severe hypothyroidism is called **myxedema**. In developing countries, a common cause of this is a lack of **iodine** in the diet. In the United States, iodine is added to table salt to prevent hypothyroidism. Iodine is also found in dairy products and seafood.

Thyroiditis is an inflammation of the thyroid gland. It presents most commonly as **Hashimoto disease,** an autoimmune disease with lymphocytic infiltration of the gland. Hypothyroidism results, necessitating lifelong thyroid hormone replacement therapy.

Cretinism *(Figure 12.13)* is a congenital form of thyroid deficiency that severely retards mental and physical growth. If diagnosed and treated early with thyroid hormones, the patient can achieve significant improvement.

Thyroid cancer usually presents as a symptomless nodule in the thyroid gland. It can metastasize (spread) to cervical and mediastinal lymph nodes, and to the liver, lungs, and bones.

Disorders of the Parathyroid Glands (LO 12.3 and 12.5)

Hypoparathyroidism is a deficiency of parathyroid hormone (PTH) that lowers levels of blood calcium (**hypocalcemia**). Most symptoms of this are neuromuscular (in nerve and muscle tissue), ranging from tingling in the fingers, to muscle cramps, to the painful muscle spasms of **tetany** (not **tetanus,** which is caused by a toxin acting on the central nervous system).

Hyperparathyroidism is an excess of PTH and is more common than hypoparathyroidism. It is usually caused by one of the four glands enlarging and working out of pituitary control. It leads to calcium depletion in bones (making bones brittle), high blood calcium levels (**hypercalcemia),** and kidney stones.

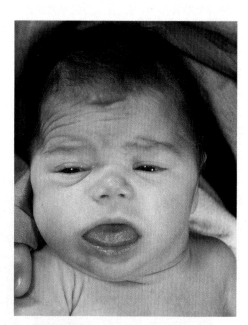

▲ **FIGURE 12.13**
Infant with Cretinism.

Mediscan/Alamy Stock Photo

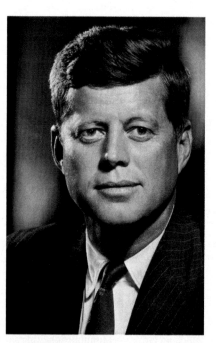

▲ **FIGURE 12.14**
John F. Kennedy.

Bettmann/Getty Images

WORD	PRONUNCIATION	ELEMENTS		DEFINITION
cretin cretinism	**KREH**-tin **KREH**-tin-izm	S/ R/	French *cretin* -ism *condition, process* cretin- *cretin*	Severe congenital hypothyroidism Condition of severe congenital hypothyroidism
emaciation	ee-may-see-**AY**-shun	S/ R/CF	-ation *process* emac/i- *make thin*	Abnormal thinness
emaciated (adj)	ee-may-see-**AY**-ted	S/	-ated *pertaining to a condition*	Pertaining to or suffering from emaciation
exophthalmos	ek-sof-**THAL**-mos	P/ R/	ex- *out* -ophthalmos *eye*	Protrusion of the eyeball
goiter	**GOY**-ter		Latin *throat*	Benign enlargement of the thyroid gland
Graves disease	**GRAVZ** diz-**EEZ**		Robert Graves, Irish physician, 1796–1853	Hyperthyroidism with toxic goiter
Hashimoto disease	hah-shee-**MOH**-toh diz-**EEZ**		Hakaru Hashimoto, Japanese surgeon, 1881–1934	Autoimmune disease of the thyroid gland
hypercalcemia	**HIGH**-per-kal-**SEE**-mee-ah	S/ P/ R/	-emia *condition of the blood* hyper- *above, excessive* -calc- *calcium*	High level of calcium in the blood
hypocalcemia	**HIGH**-poh-kal-**SEE**-mee-ah	P/	hypo- *deficient*	Low level of calcium in the blood
hyperparathyroidism (Note: *Two suffixes and two prefixes*)	**HIGH**-per-par-ah-**THIGH**-royd-izm	S/ S/ P/ P/ R/	-ism *condition* -oid- *resembling* hyper- *excessive* -para- *adjacent* -thyr- *thyroid*	Excessive levels of parathyroid hormone
hypoparathyroidism	**HIGH**-poh-par-ah-**THIGH**-royd-izm	P/	hypo- *deficient, below*	Deficient levels of parathyroid hormone
hyperpyrexia	**HIGH**-per-pie-**REK**-see-ah	S/ P/ R/	-ia *condition* hyper- *excessive* -pyrex- *fever*	Extremely high body temperature or fever
hyperthyroidism (Note: *Two suffixes*) thyrotoxicosis (syn)	high-per-**THIGH**-royd-izm	S/ S/ P/ R/	-ism *condition* -oid- *resembling* hyper- *excessive* -thyr- *thyroid*	Excessive production of thyroid hormones
hypothyroidism (Note: *Two suffixes*)	high-poh-**THIGH**-royd-izm	S/ S/ P/ R/	-ism *condition* -oid- *resembling* hypo- *deficient, below* -thyr- *thyroid*	Deficient production of thyroid hormones
iodine	**EYE**-oh-dine or **EYE**-oh-deen	S/ R/	-ine *pertaining to* iod- *violet*	Chemical element, the lack of which causes thyroid disease
myxedema	miks-eh-**DEE**-muh	P/ R/	myx- *mucus* -edema *swelling*	Nonpitting, waxy edema of the skin in hypothyroidism
tetany	**TET**-ah-nee		Greek *convulsive tension*	Severe muscle twitches, cramps, and spasms
thyroiditis	thigh-roy-**DIE**-tis	S/ S/ R/	-itis *inflammation* -oid- *resembling* thyr- *thyroid*	Inflammation of the thyroid gland
thyrotoxicosis hyperthyroidism (syn)	**THIGH**-roe-toks-ih-**KOH**-sis	S/ R/CF R/CF	-sis *condition* thyr/o- *thyroid* -toxic/o- *poison*	Disorder produced by excessive thyroid hormone production

Disorders of the Adrenal Glands (LO 12.3 and 12.5)

Adrenocortical hypofunction, most commonly seen as **Addison disease,** is caused by the wasting away of the adrenal cortex. Symptoms are weakness, fatigue, increased susceptibility to infection, and diminished resistance to stress. This disorder is treated with hormone replacement therapy, which John F. Kennedy received until he died *(Figure 12.14).*

Adrenocortical hyperfunction most commonly appears as **Cushing syndrome.** Excess production of the steroid hormones produces "moon" **facies** (facial features and expressions), muscle wasting and weakness, kidney stones, and reduced resistance to infection. Most cases are due to a pituitary tumor secreting too much ACTH, causing the adrenal glands to produce an excess of steroids. Sometimes, Cushing syndrome can be produced by the administration of excess steroid medications.

Hypersecretion of androgens is called **adrenal virilism** or **adrenogenital syndrome.** In adult women, manifestations include **hirsutism,** baldness, acne, deepened voice, decreased breast size, and other signs of masculinization.

WORD	PRONUNCIATION		ELEMENTS	DEFINITION
Addison disease	ADD-ih-son diz-EEZ	P/ R/	Thomas Addison, 1793–1860, English physician dis- apart -ease normal function	An autoimmune disease leading to decreased production of adrenocortical steroids
adrenalectomy	ah-DREE-nal-EK-toh-mee	S/ S/ P/ R/	-ectomy surgical excision -al- pertaining to ad- near, toward -ren- kidney gland Latin glans, acorn	Removal of part or all of an adrenal gland
adrenogenital syndrome	ah-DREE-noh-JEN-it-al SIN-drome	S/ R/CF R/ P/ R/	-al pertaining to adren/o- adrenal gland -genit- primary male or female sex organs syn- together -drome course	Hypersecretion of androgens from the adrenal gland
Cushing syndrome	KUSH-ing SIN-drome	P/ R/	Harvey Cushing, 1869–1939, American neurosurgeon syn- together -drome course	Hypersecretion of cortisol (hydrocortisone) by the adrenal cortex
facies	FASH-eez		Latin appearance	Facial expression and features characteristic of a specific disease
hirsutism	HER-sue-tizm		Latin shaggy	Excessive body and facial hair
virilism	VIR-ih-lizm	S/ R/	-ism condition, process viril- masculine	Development of masculine characteristics by a woman or girl

Keynote

• Type 2 diabetes used to only be common in those over the age of 30, but is now often seen also in obese adolescents and younger adults.

Abbreviations

DM	diabetes mellitus
IDDM	insulin-dependent diabetes mellitus
LADA	latent autoimmune diabetes in adults
MODY	mature-onset diabetes of the young
NIDDM	non-insulin-dependent diabetes mellitus

Disorders of Pancreatic Hormones:
Diabetes Mellitus (DM) (LO 12.3 and 12.5)

Diabetes mellitus is a condition characterized by hyperglycemia, resulting from an impairment of insulin secretion and/or insulin action. Diabetes affects the body's ability to make use of the energy found in food, disrupting the normal process of carbohydrate, fat, and protein metabolism. It is the world's most prevalent metabolic disease and the leading cause of blindness, renal failure, and gangrene of the lower extremities. There is a spectrum of diabetes types, including

1. **Type 1 diabetes,** also called **insulin-dependent diabetes mellitus (IDDM),** accounts for 10% to 15% of all cases of DM. It is the predominant type of DM found in patients under the age of 30. When symptoms become apparent, 90% of the pancreatic insulin-producing cells have already been destroyed by **autoantibodies** (antibodies that attack the patient's own system).

2. **Type 2 diabetes,** also called **non-insulin-dependent diabetes mellitus (NIDDM),** accounts for up to 95% of all DM cases. Over 37 million people in the United States, about 1 in 10 have been diagnosed with type 2 DM. Not only is there an impairment of insulin response, but there is also a decreased glucose uptake by tissues due to insulin resistance. In addition to contributing to type 2 DM, insulin resistance leads to other common disorders like hypertension, hyperlipidemia, and coronary artery disease.

3. **Latent autoimmune diabetes in adults (LADA or Type 1.5)** accounts for roughly 10% of people with diabetes. It occurs in adults who have the same autoantibodies as Type 1 diabetics, but there is no need for insulin treatment in the first 6 months after diagnosis. It is a more slowly progressing variation of Type 1 diabetes.

4. **Gestational diabetes** occurs in about 5% of pregnancies. While most cases of gestational diabetes resolve after the pregnancy, a woman who has this complication of pregnancy has a 30% chance of developing type 2 DM within 10 years.

5. **Mature-onset diabetes of the young (MODY)** is a selection of genetically linked forms of diabetes usually found in thin people under 55 years of age. Many forms of MODY will respond to small doses of insulin or to sulfonylurea drugs.

Source: https://www.cdc.gov/diabetes/library/spotlights/diabetes-facts-stats.html

WORD	PRONUNCIATION	ELEMENTS		DEFINITION
acetone	**ASS**-eh-tone		Latin *vinegar*	Ketone that is found in blood, urine, and breath when diabetes mellitus is out of control
dehydration	dee-high-**DRAY**-shun	S/ P/ R/	-ation *a process* de- *without* -hydr- *water*	Process of losing body water
ketoacidosis	**KEY**-toh-ass-ih-**DOE**-sis	S/ R/CF R/	-osis *condition* ket/o- *ketone* -acid- *acid*	Excessive ketones in the blood, making it acidic
ketone ketosis	**KEY**-tone key-**TOH**-sis	S/ R/	Greek *acetone* -osis *condition* ket- *ketone*	Chemical formed in uncontrolled diabetes or in starvation Excessive production of ketones
lethargy lethargic (adj)	**LETH**-ar-jee le-**THAR**-jik		Greek *drowsiness*	Abnormal drowsiness in depth or length of time
metabolic acidosis	met-ah-**BOL**-ik ass-ih-**DOE**-sis	S/ R/ S/ R/	-ic *pertaining to* metabol- *change* -osis *condition* acid- *acid*	Decreased pH in blood and body tissues as a result of an upset in metabolism

Hypoglycemia (LO 12.3 and 12.5)

Hypoglycemia is present when blood glucose is below 70 mg/dL. Because brain metabolism depends primarily on glucose, the brain is the first organ affected by hypoglycemia. This disorder presents clinically as an impaired mental efficiency, followed by shakiness, anxiety, confusion, tremor, seizures, and, if untreated, loss of consciousness. Symptomatic hypoglycemia is sometimes called **insulin shock.** Low blood glucose can be raised to normal in minutes by taking 10 to 20 g carbohydrate (3 to 4 ounces), such as orange, apple, or grape juice, or a sugar-containing soft drink.

Hyperglycemia (LO 12.3 and 12.5)

In **hyperglycemia**, the classic symptoms are **polyuria** (excessive urination), **polydipsia** (excessive thirst), and **polyphagia** (excessive hunger), with unexplained weight loss.

Symptomatic hyperglycemia is how type 1 DM usually presents. Type 2 DM can be symptomatic or asymptomatic, and is often found during a routine health exam.

Because of high glucose levels, hyperglycemia damages capillary endothelial cells in the retina, renal glomerulus *(see Chapter 13),* and neurons in peripheral nerves *(see Chapter 10).* Of all diabetics, 85% develop some degree of **diabetic retinopathy**; 30% develop diabetic **nephropathy**, which can progress to end-stage renal disease *(see Chapter 13).* Diabetic **neuropathy** causes sensory defects with numbness, tingling, and **paresthesias** (abnormal skin sensations) in the feet and/or hands.

In larger blood vessels, hyperglycemia contributes to endothelial cell-lining damage and atherosclerosis. Coronary artery disease and peripheral vascular disease with claudication *(see Chapter 6)* are complications. Hyperglycemia is the most common cause of foot ulcers and gangrene of the lower extremity, sometimes requiring **amputation**. The risk of infection is increased by the cellular hyperglycemia and the circulatory deficits.

The complications of hyperglycemia can be kept at bay by stringent control of blood glucose levels.

Diabetes Ketoacidosis (LO 12.3 and 12.5)

Diabetic ketoacidosis (DKA) is a state of marked hyperglycemia with dehydration, **metabolic acidosis** (abnormal increase in blood acidity), and **ketone** formation. This is seen mostly in type 1 DM and usually results from a lapse in insulin treatment, an acute infection, or a trauma that makes the usual insulin treatment inadequate.

DKA presents with polyuria, vomiting, and **lethargy** and can progress to coma. The ketone **acetone** can be smelled on the breath. DKA is a medical emergency, and there is a 2% to 5% mortality rate from circulatory collapse if the DKA is not promptly controlled.

Diabetic coma is a severe medical emergency, caused by hyperglycemia.

Insulin shock is another severe medical emergency, caused by hypoglycemia.

A blood glucose test will differentiate hypoglycemia from hyperglycemia.

Keynotes

- The brain is the first organ affected by hypoglycemia.
- Hyperglycemia causes damage to vascular endothelial cells at the microvascular and macrovascular levels.
- Untreated hyperglycemia can progress to diabetic coma.
- Diabetic ketoacidosis (DKA) is a medical emergency.
- Maintaining normal plasma glucose levels is the basis for good management of DM.
- Many insulin-dependent diabetics need multiple subcutaneous insulin injections each day.

Abbreviation

DKA   diabetic ketoacidosis

WORD	PRONUNCIATION		ELEMENTS	DEFINITION
amputation	am-pyu-**TAY**-shun	S/ R/	**-ation** *a process* **amput-** *to prune, lop off*	Process of removing a limb, part of a limb, a breast, or other projecting part
autoantibody (Note: *Two prefixes*)	awe-toh-**AN**-tee-bod-ee	P/ P/ R/	**auto-** *self, same* **-anti-** *against* **-body** *body*	Antibody produced in response to an antigen from the host's own tissue
coma comatose (adj)	**KOH**-mah **KOH**-mah-tohs	S/ R/	Greek *deep sleep* **-ose** *full of* **comat-** *coma*	State of deep unconsciousness In a state of coma
diabetes mellitus diabetic (adj)	dye-ah-**BEE**-teez **MEL**-ih-tus dye-ah-**BET**-ik	S/ R/	**diabetes,** Greek *a siphon* **mellitus,** Latin *sweetened with honey* **-ic** *pertaining to* **diabet-** *diabetes*	Metabolic syndrome caused by absolute or relative insulin deficiency and/or ineffectiveness Pertaining to or suffering from diabetes
hyperglycemia hyperglycemic (adj)	**HIGH**-per-gly-**SEE**-me-ah **HIGH**-per-gly-**SEE**-mik	S/ P/ R/ S/	**-emia** *a blood condition* **hyper-** *above* **-glyc-** *glucose* **-emic** *pertaining to a blood condition*	High level of glucose (sugar) in the blood Pertaining to or having hyperglycemia
hypoglycemia hypoglycemic (adj)	**HIGH**-poh-gly-**SEE**-me-ah **HIGH**-poh-gly-**SEE**-mik	S/ P/ R/ S/	**-emia** *a blood condition* **hypo-** *below, deficient* **-glyc-** *glucose* **-emic** *pertaining to a blood condition*	Low level of glucose (sugar) in the blood Pertaining to or suffering from low blood sugar
nephropathy	neh-**FROP**-ah-thee	S/ R/CF	**-pathy** *disease* **nephr/o-** *kidney*	Any disease of the kidney
neuropathy	nyu-**ROP**-ah-thee	S/ R/	**-pathy** *disease* **neur/o-** *nerve*	Any disease of the nervous system
paresthesia paresthesias (pl)	pair-es-**THEE**-ze-ah	S/ P/ R/	**-ia** *condition* **par-** *abnormal* **-esthes-** *sensation*	An abnormal sensation; e.g., tingling, burning, pricking
polydipsia	pol-ee-**DIP**-see-ah	S/ P/ R/	**-ia** *condition* **poly-** *many, excessive* **-dips-** *thirst*	Excessive thirst
polyphagia	pol-ee-**FAY**-jee-ah	S/ P/ R/	**-ia** *condition* **poly-** *many, excessive* **-phag-** *eat*	Excessive eating
polyuria	pol-ee-**YOU**-ree-ah	S/ P/ R/	**-ia** *condition* **poly-** *many, excessive* **-ur-** *urine*	Excessive production of urine
retinopathy	ret-ih-**NOP**-ah-thee	S/ R/CF	**-pathy** *disease* **retin/o-** *retina of the eye*	Degenerative disease of the retina

EXERCISES

 ## Case Report 12.1

You are . . .

. . . a registered nurse working with **endocrinologist** Sabina Khalid, MD, in the Endocrinology Clinic at Fulwood Medical Center.

You are communicating with . . .

. . . Mrs. Gina Tacher, a 33-year-old schoolteacher. She complains of coarsening of her facial features and enlargement of the bones of her hands. Over the past 10 years, Mrs. Tacher's nose and jaw have increased in size and her voice has become husky. She has brought photos of herself at ages 9 and 16. She reports no other health problems.

Dr. Khalid's examination of Mrs. Tacher shows a protruding mandible (jaw) and an enlarged, deeply grooved tongue. Her feet and hands are enlarged, her ribs are thickened, and her heart is enlarged. X-rays show a thickened skull and enlarged nasal sinuses. Blood tests display high growth hormone levels. CT and MRI scans show a tumor in the **pituitary** gland, and as a result, Mrs. Tacher is scheduled for surgery to remove the tumor.

A. Given *the description, insert the abbreviation for the hormone. Fill in the blanks.*   **LO 12.2, 12.5, and 12.8**

1. Lack of this hormone would increase urine production. _____

2. This hormone will be increased with thyrotropin-secreting adenomas. _____

3. Helps distinguish corticotropin pituitary tumors from adrenal gland tumors. _____

Case Report 12.2

You are...

... an EMT working in the Emergency Department at Fulwood Medical Center at 0200 hours in the morning.

You are communicating with...

... the parents of Ms. Norma Leary, a 22-year-old college student who is living with her parents for the summer. Ms. Leary is **emaciated**, extremely agitated, and at times disoriented and confused. Her parents tell you that in the past 3 or 4 days she has been coughing and not feeling well. In the past 12 hours, she has become feverish and been complaining of a left-sided chest pain. Upon questioning, the parents reveal that prior to this acute illness, Ms. Leary had lost about 20 pounds in weight, although she was eating voraciously. Her **VS** are T 105.2, P 160 and irregular, R 24, BP 160/85.

You call for Dr. Hilinski, an emergency physician, STAT. On his initial examination, he believes that the patient is in thyroid storm, which is a medical emergency. There are no immediate laboratory tests that can confirm this diagnosis.

Thyroid storm is the condition Ms. Norma Leary presented with in the Emergency Department. It is the most extreme state of **hyperthyroidism**, with severely exaggerated effects of the thyroid hormones causing **hyperpyrexia**, **tachycardia**, agitation, and delirium. The weight loss prior to her illness becoming acute was part of her undiagnosed hyperthyroidism.

B. Review *Case Report 12.2, then select the correct answer that answers each question or completes the statement.*   **LO 12.5 and 12.9**

1. What does the term **emaciated** mean?

   a. exhausted

   b. anxious

   c. irritated

   d. thin

2. After reviewing her vital signs, what term describes Ms. Leary's heart rate?

   a. hypotensive

   b. febrile

   c. tachycardic

   d. bradypneic

3. Ms. Leary's signs and symptoms are due to:

   a. decreased thyroid hormones

   b. increased thyroid hormones

   c. dehydration

   d. overhydration

4. The thyroid storm:

   a. came about suddenly

   b. has been occurring for a long period of time

   c. is diagnosed with a measure of serum electrolytes

   d. requires an MRI to confirm Dr. Hilinski's diagnosis

C. Construct *terms related to anatomy and function of the thyroid gland, parathyroid glands, and the thymus gland. Fill in the blanks.*   **LO 12.1, 12.3, 12.5, and 12.9**

1. Thyroid hormone T4: _____/_____/ine

2. Abnormal thinness: _____/_____

3. Endocrine glands embedded in the back of the thyroid: _____/_____/oid

4. Hormone that moves calcium from the blood into the bone: _____/_____/_____

D. Elements: One word or phrase in each of the descriptions in the following questions is in bold. *This is your clue to finding the correct medical term in the word bank. Fill in the blanks with the language of endocrinology. Not all terms will be used.*   **LO 12.2 and 12.5**

thyroiditis   tetany   hyperparathyroidism   hypoparathyroidism   thyrotoxicosis   hyperthyroidism   myxedema   thyroidectomy

1. **Excessive production** of thyroid hormones: _____

2. **Swelling** with a waxy substance: _____

3. **Deficient** of production of parathyroid hormone: _____

4. **Inflammation** of the thyroid gland: _____

5. **Removal** of the thyroid gland: _____

E. Diabetes *is the world's most prevalent metabolic disease. Many patients have diabetes as a concurrent condition with other health problems, which always makes it a consideration in treatment and the prescribing of medications. Test your knowledge of this disease by answering the following questions. Select the correct answer that completes each statement.*   **LO 12.5**

1. Diabetes is the leading cause of:

   a. blindness   **b.** renal failure   **c.** gangrene   **d.** all of these

2. The first organ affected by hypoglycemia is the:

   a. kidney   **b.** heart   **c.** pancreas   **d.** brain   **e.** liver

3. Impairment of insulin response and decreased insulin effectiveness is termed insulin:

   a. production   **b.** resistance   **c.** autoantibodies   **d.** control   **e.** conversion

4. Most cases of gestational diabetes resolve after:

   a. medication   **b.** treatment   **c.** testing   **d.** pregnancy   **e.** surgery

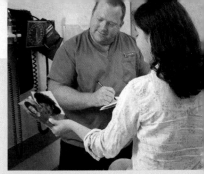

Section 12.3

Diagnostic and Therapeutic Procedures and Pharmacology for Disorders of the Endocrine System

Rick Brady/McGraw Hill

Endocrinologists are physicians that specialize in **endocrinology,** the study of the organs and tissues that release hormones into the blood to affect other tissues and organs in the body. They, along with **internists, endocrine physician assistants,** and **endocrine nurse practitioners,** diagnose and treat people with hormone imbalances.

Pituitary Diagnostic Procedures (LO 12.3, 12.6, and 12.9)

Visual field tests can assist in the identification of potential pituitary tumor as the tumor presses on the **optic chiasma** causing loss of vision in the peripheral visual fields.

Levels of pituitary hormones in the blood and/or urine can be measured directly to help confirm the presence of a hormone-producing pituitary adenoma.

Examples are the levels of **growth hormone** and **insulinlike growth factor-1 (IGF-1).** When growth hormone levels are high, they cause the liver to produce more IGF-1. When both levels are very high, a pituitary tumor is the diagnosis. If the levels are only slightly increased, a **glucose suppression test** is performed. Ingestion of a large amount of sugar normally leads to a drop in growth hormone levels. If growth hormones remain high, a pituitary adenoma is the cause. High levels of growth hormone are found in gigantism, beginning in children, and acromegaly, beginning in adults.

Blood prolactin levels can be measured to check for a prolactinoma; **ACTH (corticotropin)** levels help distinguish ACTH-secreting pituitary tumors from adrenal gland tumors: **TSH (thyrotropin)** levels usually identify thyrotropin-secreting adenomas.

Diabetes insipidus, caused by failure in production of **ADH (antidiuretic hormone)** by the hypothalamus or by failure of the posterior pituitary to release it due to an adenoma, is diagnosed primarily by measurement of the amount of urine and its **osmolality.**

Magnetic resonance imaging (MRI) can show pituitary tumors greater than 3 mm across.

Biopsy of the tumor is sometimes needed to make a firm diagnosis. When pituitary tumors are removed surgically, they are examined under a microscope to confirm the exact diagnosis.

Pituitary Therapeutic Procedures (LO 12.6)

Surgical removal of a pituitary tumor is necessary if the tumor is pressing on the optic nerves or overproducing hormones. In 99% of cases, this is performed by an **endoscopic transnasal transsphenoidal approach** in which the surgery is performed through the nose and sphenoid sinus using an **endoscope. Craniotomy,** in which a very large tumor is removed through the upper part of the skull, is occasionally necessary. The surgery can be made more efficient by using **image-guided stereotactic surgery** in which advanced computers create a three-dimensional image of the tumor to guide the surgeon.

Radiation therapy can be used alone, after surgery, or if the tumor persists or returns after surgery. Methods of radiation therapy include:

- **Gamma knife stereotactic radiosurgery,** which delivers a single high-dose radiation beam the size and shape of the tumor using special brain-imaging techniques.

- **Proton beam therapy,** which delivers positively charged ions (protons) rather than X-rays in beams that are finely controlled with minimal risk to surrounding healthy tissues.

- **External beam radiation,** which delivers X-rays in small increments, usually five times a week over a 4-to-6-week period. It may damage surrounding healthy pituitary and brain tissues.

Abbreviations

ACTH	adrenocorticotropic hormone, corticotropin
ADH	antidiuretic hormone
IGF-1	insulinlike growth factor-1
MRI	magnetic resonance imaging

Keynote

- Pituitary tumors present with symptoms that lead to a complete medical history and physical examination, blood and urine tests, and X-rays.

WORD	PRONUNCIATION		ELEMENTS	DEFINITION
analog	AN-ah-log		Greek *proportionate*	A compound that resembles another in structure but not in function; analog is a means of the transmission of continuous information to our senses, in contrast with the digital transmission of only zeros and ones.
biopsy (*Note:* the extra "o" *in the root bio is dropped from the spelling.*)	BIE-op-see	S/ R/	-opsy *to view* bio- *life*	Process of removing tissue from living patients for microscopic examination
craniotomy	kray-nee-**OT**-oh-mee	S/ R/	-tomy *incision* crani/o- *cranium*	Incision of the skull
chiasm chiasma (alt)	KIE-asm kie-**AZ**-mah		Greek *cross*	X-shaped crossing of the two optic nerves at the base of the brain
endoscope endoscopic (adj)	EN-doh-skope EN-doh-**SKOP**-ik	P/ R/ S/	endo- *inside* -scope *instrument for viewing* -ic *pertaining to*	Instrument for viewing the inside of a tubular or hollow organ Pertaining to an endoscope.
gamma knife	GAM-ah NIFE		gamma *third letter in Greek alphabet* knife *Old English knife*	A minimally invasive radiosurgical system
optic	OP-tik	S/ R/	-ic *pertaining to* opt- *vision*	Pertaining to the eye
osmolality	OZ-moh-**LAL**-ih-tee	S/ S/ R/	-ity *state* -al- *pertaining to* osmol- *concentration*	The concentration of a solution
proton	PROH-ton		Greek *first*	The positively charged unit of the nuclear mass
stereotactic	STAIR-ee-oh-**TAK**-tik	S/ R/CF R/	-ic *pertaining to* stere/o- *three- dimensional* -tact- *orderly arrangement*	Pertaining to a precise three-dimensional method to locate a lesion or a tumor
transnasal	trans-**NAY**-zal	S/ P/ R/	-al *pertaining to* trans- *across, through* -nas- *nose*	Through the nose
transsphenoid	trans-**SFEE**-noyd	S/ P/ R/CF	-oid *resembling* trans- *through* -sphen/o- *wedge*	Through the sphenoid sinus

Pituitary Medications and Hormone Replacement Therapy (LO 12.3 and 12.6)

Chemotherapy medications, as with other forms of cancer, can also be administered to certain patients diagnosed with a pituitary tumor.

Medications can help to block excessive hormone secretion and sometimes reduce pituitary tumor size:

- **Growth hormone-secreting tumors** have two types of drugs used if surgery has been unsuccessful in normalizing growth hormone production. **Somatostatin analogs** *(Sandostatin, Somatuline Depot)* cause a decrease in growth hormone production and are given by injection every four weeks. The second type, **pegvisomant** *(Somavert),* blocks the effect of excess growth hormone, is given by daily injection, and may cause liver damage.

- **Prolactin-secreting tumors (prolactinomas)** are treated with two drugs, **cabergoline** *(Dostinex)* and **bromocriptine** *(Parlodel),* that decrease prolactin secretion, but they can have serious side effects, including developing compulsive behaviors.

Pituitary hormone replacement therapy is needed after surgery or radiation therapy to maintain normal hormone levels. The medication taken depends on the hormones that need to be replaced, which include adrenocorticotropic hormone (ACTH), thyroxine, estrogen and progesterone, testosterone, antidiuretic hormone (ADH), and synthetic growth hormones. Treatment of diabetes insipidus is with vasopressin or desmopressin, synthetic modified forms of ADH. They are taken as a nasal spray several times daily, the dose being adjusted to maintain a normal urine output.

Diagnostic Procedures for Disorders of the Thyroid Gland (LO 12.3, 12.5, and 12.6)

Blood tests

Thyroid-stimulating hormone (TSH) levels in the blood are low if the gland is overactive.

Thyroid hormone levels in the blood detail the activity of the gland; the levels are high if the gland is overactive.

Antithyroid antibodies are associated with autoimmune inflammatory diseases of the thyroid.

Serum calcitonin level is elevated in medullary carcinoma.

Isotopic thyroid scans detail the nature of the thyroid enlargement and the function of the gland.

Fine needle aspiration biopsy distinguishes benign from malignant nodules.

Ultrasonography reveals the size of the gland and the presence of nodules.

Therapeutic Procedures for Disorders of the Thyroid Gland (LO 12.3, 12.5, and 12.6)

Radioactive iodine (I-131) therapy uses the **isotope** of iodine that emits radiation to treat hyperthyroidism and thyroid cancer. When a small dose of the isotope is swallowed, it is absorbed into the bloodstream, taken up from the blood, and concentrated by the cells of the thyroid gland, where it begins destroying the gland's cells.

Levothyroxine (T4) tablet once daily should adequately treat hypothyroidism. For hypothyroidism due to destruction of thyroid cells, TSH levels are monitored. For central (pituitary or hypothalamic) hypothyroidism, **T4** levels are used for monitoring.

Thyroid surgery is indicated for a variety of conditions including cancerous and benign nodules, goiters, and overactive thyroid glands. The types of surgery that can be performed include:

- **Lobectomy**: removal of half of the thyroid gland **(hemi-lobectomy).**

- **Total thyroidectomy:** removal of all thyroid tissue.

- **Near-total thyroidectomy:** removal of all but a very small part of the gland.

- **Endoscopic thyroidectomy:** performed through a single small incision using a flexible lighted tube and video monitor to guide the surgical procedure.

- **Laser ablation:** a minimally invasive procedure used to remove benign thyroid nodules using ultrasound guidance without affecting the surrounding organ.

Word Analysis and Definition

S = Suffix   P = Prefix   R = Root   R/CF = Combining Form

WORD	PRONUNCIATION		ELEMENTS	DEFINITION
ablation	ab-**LAY**-shun	S/ R/	-ion *process* ablat- *take away*	Removal of tissue to destroy its function
aspiration	**AS**-pih-**RAY**-shun	S/ R/	-ion *process* aspirat- *breathe in*	Removal by suction of fluid or gas from a body cavity
isotope isotopic (adj)	**EYE**-so-tope **EYE**-so-**TOH**-pik	P/ R/ S/ R/	iso- *equal* -tope *part* -ic *pertaining to* -top- *part*	Radioactive element; some of these elements are used in diagnostic procedures Of identical chemical composition
lobectomy hemi-lobectomy (syn)	loh-**BEK**-toh-mee **HEM**-ee-loh-**BEK**-toh-mee	S/ R/ P/	-ectomy *surgical excision* -lob- *lobe* hemi- *half*	Surgical removal of a lobe of the lungs or the thyroid gland
radioactive iodine	**RAY**-dee-oh-**AK**-tiv **EYE**-oh-dine	S/ R/CF R/	-ive *pertaining to* radi/o- *radiation* -act- *performance* iodine *nonmetallic element*	Any of the various tracers that emit alpha, beta, or gamma rays
thyroidectomy	thigh-roy-**DEK**-toh-me	S/ S/ R/CF	-ectomy *surgical excision* -oid- *resembling* thyr/o- *thyroid*	Surgical removal of the thyroid gland
ultrasonography	**UL**-trah-soh-**NOG**-rah-fee	S/ P/ R/CF	-graphy *recording* ultra- *beyond* -son/o- *sound*	Delineation of deep structures using sound waves

Thyroid Pharmacology (LO 12.3, 12.5, and 12.6)

Antithyroid medications prevent formation of thyroid hormones in the gland's cells.

Propylthiouracil and **methimazole** both decrease the amount of thyroid hormone produced by the gland's cells and can be used to treat hyperthyroidism. Unfortunately, they both have the major and frequent side effects of agranulocytosis and aplastic anemia.

Teprotumumab is a newer medication in the monoclonal antibody category, used to treat thyroid eye conditions and Graves disease.

Thyroid replacements are:

- L-thyroxine. This synthetic T4 is a preferred replacement.

- Liothyronine sodium. This synthetic T3 has a rapid turnover and has to be monitored frequently.

Diagnostic Procedures for Disorders of the Adrenal Glands (LO 12.3 and 12.5)

Amniocentesis and **chorionic villus sampling** can diagnose **congenital adrenal hyperplasia** in the fetus and in the newborn through a heel stick to obtain a blood sample. The test detects elevated levels of 17-hydroxy-progesterone (17-HP) and, as with all screening tests, a confirmatory test(s) has to be performed. Treatment can then be started in the womb or immediately after birth.

Cushing syndrome can be confirmed if elevated cortisol is found in any of the following:

- Blood;

- 24-hour urine collection; and

- Evening collection of saliva.

Suppression of cortisol production by the synthetic steroid dexamethasone supports the diagnosis of Cushing syndrome.

Addison disease can be diagnosed based on routine blood tests showing hypercalcemia, hypoglycemia, **hyponatremia**, and **hyperkalemia**; the diagnosis is confirmed by the ACTH stimulation test, in which the synthetic pituitary ACTH hormone **tetracosactide** fails to stimulate the production of cortisol.

Therapeutic Procedures for Disorders of the Adrenal Glands (LO 12.5 and 12.6)

Congenital adrenal hyperplasia, when diagnosed in a female fetus, can require the pregnant mother to take a **corticosteroid** drug such as **dexamethasone** during pregnancy. This drug crosses the placenta to reduce the secretion of the fetal male hormones and allow the female genitals to develop normally. When diagnosed in childhood, dexamethasone or hydrocortisone are needed daily, and in some infant girls who have **ambiguous external genitalia,** reconstructive surgery to correct the appearance and function of the **genitals** is performed.

Addison disease requires lifelong replacement of the absent hormones by taking oral corticosteroids such as hydrocortisone and fludrocortisone.

Adreno cortical carcinomas or benign adenomas are usually treated with surgery.

Adrenal Pharmacology (LO 12.6 and 12.8)

The **adrenal medulla** secretes **epinephrine (adrenaline).** The **adrenal cortex** synthesizes **steroids** from cholesterol. The outer zona glomerulosa secretes **mineralocorticoids**, which regulate salt and water metabolism (aldosterone) by affecting excretory organs such as the kidney, colon, salivary glands, sweat glands, and brain. The middle zona fasciculata synthesizes **glucocorticoids**, which regulate normal metabolism and resistance to stress (cortisol) by affecting every organ in the body including the brain. The inner zona reticularis secretes adrenal **androgens** that control the development and activity of the male sex organs and male secondary sex characteristics. Androgens are the precursor of all **estrogens**. The primary androgen is testosterone, present in males and females.

WORD	PRONUNCIATION		ELEMENTS	DEFINITION
ambiguous	am-**BIG**-you-us		Latin *to wander*	Uncertain
androgen	**AN**-droh-jen	S/ R/CF	-gen *to produce* andr/o- *male*	Hormone that produces masculine characteristics
cortex	**KOR**-teks		Latin *outer covering*	Outer portion of an organ
genital	**JEN**-ih-tal	S/ R/	-al *pertaining to* genit- *primary male or female sex organs*	Relating to the primary male or female sex organs
hyperkalemia	**HIGH**-per-kah-**LEE**-me-ah	S/ P/ R/	-emia *blood condition* hyper- *excess* -kal- *potassium*	An excessive amount of potassium in the blood
hyponatremia	**HIGH**-poh-nah-**TREE**-me-ah	S/ P/ R/	-emia *condition of the blood* hypo- *below, deficient* -natr- *sodium*	Low level of sodium in the blood
hyperplasia	high-per-**PLAY**-zee-ah	S/ P/ R/	-ia *condition* hyper- *excessive* -plas- *formation*	Increase in the number of cells in a tissue or organ
medulla	meh-**DULL**-ah		Latin *marrow*	Central part of a structure surrounded by cortex
steroid	**STER**-oyd	S/ R/	-oid *resemble* ster- *solid*	Large family of chemical substances found in hormones, body components, and drugs

Diagnosis and Treatment of Diabetes Mellitus (LO 12.3 and 12.6)

Criteria for the Diagnosis of Diabetes Mellitus (LO 12.3 and 12.6)

The accepted **criteria** for the diagnosis of diabetes mellitus (**DM**) include either a fasting (8 hours) plasma glucose of 126 mg/dL or greater; or symptoms (polyuria, polydipsia, polyphagia, unexplained weight loss) and a random plasma glucose of 200 mg/dL or higher.

Treatment of Diabetic Ketoacidosis (LO 12.3 and 12.6)

Insulin to decrease blood glucose levels, and **intravenous (IV) saline** and **electrolytes** to replace fluid and electrolytes lost via polyuria.

Treatment of Diabetes Mellitus (LO 12.3, 12.5, 12.6, and 12.9)

The basic principle of diabetes treatment is to avoid hyperglycemia and hypoglycemia. **Certified Diabetic Educators** work alongside people with diabetes to formulate individualized plans to best manage their diabetes. The areas of treatment are as follows:

Abbreviations

BUN	blood urea nitrogen
HbA1c	glycosylated hemoglobin, hemoglobin A1c

- **Diet and exercise** to achieve weight reduction of 2 pounds per week in overweight type 2 DM patients is essential.
- **Patient education** is necessary so that the patient understands the disease process, can recognize the indications for seeking immediate medical care, and will follow a foot care regimen.
- **Plasma glucose monitoring** is an essential skill that all diabetics must learn. Patients on insulin must learn to adjust their insulin doses. Home glucose analyzers use a drop of blood obtained from the fingertip or forearm by a spring-powered lancet. The frequency of testing varies individually.
- **Assessment of the patient** should be performed on routine physician visits for symptoms or signs of complications.
- **Periodic laboratory evaluation** includes **BUN** and serum creatinine (kidney function), lipid profile, ECG, and an annual complete ophthalmologic evaluation.

Glycosylated hemoglobin (HbA1c) is used to monitor plasma glucose control during the preceding 2 to 3 months.

Oral antidiabetic drugs are used for type 2 DM but not type 1 DM. There are numerous drugs available, and they produce their effect in four main ways:

- Decrease glucose production by the liver. **Biguanides**—metformin (Glucophage)—act in this way.

- Stimulate the beta cells of the pancreas to produce more insulin. Second-generation sulfonylureas, including glipizide (Glucotrol) and glyburide (Micronase), are the current first line treatment of type 2 diabetes for patients who do not tolerate **Metformin. Meglitinides**—repaglinide (Prandin)—act in the same way.

- Block the breakdown of starches in the intestine. **Alpha-glucosidase inhibitors**—acarbose (Precose)—act in this way.

- Increase insulin production and decrease glucose production. **DPP-4 inhibitors**—sitagliptin (Januvia)—are an example of this type.

- Acts on the kidney to excrete glucose in the urine, thereby reducing blood glucose levels—empagliflozin *(Jardiance)* tablets are taken once in the morning.

- Once-weekly injection that reduces blood sugar by increasing the amount of insulin released, slowing how fast food moves through the stomach, and blocking the release of glucagon. Dulaglutide *(Trulicity)* and semaglutide *(Ozempic)* are examples.

- Another form of semaglutide is *Rybelsus.* It is a pill taken once per day.

Combinations of these different-acting drugs are often used.

Injectable insulin preparations are used in type 1 DM and sometimes in type 2 DM. They are classified by their speed of action.

The injectable insulins are supplied in vials, cartridges, and prefilled pens.

For some patients requiring frequent doses of insulin, continuous subcutaneous insulin infusion is given by an implanted battery-powered, programmable pump *(Figure 12.15)*. This pump provides continuous insulin through a small needle in the abdominal wall.

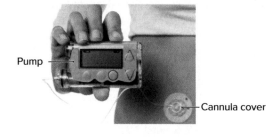

Pump

Cannula cover

◀ **FIGURE 12.15**
Photograph of Insulin Pump—with Cannula Inserted in the Subcutaneous Tissue of the Abdominal Wall.

Oscar Gimeno Baldo/Alamy Stock Photo

WORD	PRONUNCIATION	ELEMENTS		DEFINITION
blood urea nitrogen (BUN)	BLUD you-**REE**-ah **NIE**-troh-jen	S/ R/CF	Old English *fluid which circulates in the arteries and veins* Greek *urine* **-gen** *create, produce, form* nitr/o- *nitrogen*	Laboratory measurement of the amount of urea in the blood; provides rough estimation of kidney function
criterion criteria (pl)	kri-**TEER**-ee-on kri-**TEER**-ee-ah		Greek *a standard*	Standard or rule for judging
electrolyte	ee-**LEK**-troh-lite	S/ R/CF	-lyte *soluble* electr/o- *electricity*	Substance that, when dissolved in a suitable medium, forms electrically charged particles
glycosylated hemoglobin (Hb A1c)	**GLIE**-koh-sih-lay-ted **HEE**-moh-**GLOH**-bin	S/ R/CF R/CF R/	-sylated *linked* glyc/o- *glucose* hem/o- *blood* -globin *protein*	Hemoglobin A fraction linked to glucose; used as index of glucose control
intravenous	IN-trah-**VEE**-nus	S/ P/ R/	-ous *pertaining to* intra- *within, inside* -ven- *vein*	Inside a vein
saline	**SAY**-leen		Latin *salt*	Salt solution, usually sodium chloride

EXERCISES

Case Report 12.3

John Fitzgerald Kennedy (JFK) (1917–1963) was elected president of the United States of America in 1960 at the age of 43. He had health problems from the age of 13, when he was first diagnosed as having **colitis**. At age 27, he had lower back pain that necessitated lower back surgery. He was then diagnosed as having adrenal gland insufficiency (**Addison disease**) with osteoporosis of his lumbar spine. This required lower back surgery on three more occasions. JFK received adrenal hormone replacement therapy for the rest of his life, together with pain medication for his lower back pain, until his assassination in Dallas, Texas, in 1963. In medical retrospect, instead of colitis, JFK probably had **celiac** disease *(see Chapter 9),* which has strong associations with Addison disease.

A. Review *Case Report 12.3 before answering the questions. Correctly answer each question. Fill in the blanks.*   **LO 12.2, 12.5, 12.6, 12.8, and 12.9**

1. Did Kennedy's adrenal glands produce too much or too little hormone? _____

2. *Adrenal gland insufficiency* is also known as _____ .

3. What lumbar spine problem did Kennedy also have? _____

4. What was used to treat Kennedy's adrenal gland insufficiency? _____

5. What other disease has a *strong association* with Addison disease? _____

Case Report 12.4

You are ...

... a certified medical assistant working with Susan Lee, MD, in her Primary Care Clinic at Fulwood Medical Center.

You are communicating with . . .

. . . Mrs. Martha Jones, who is here for her monthly checkup. She is a 53-year-old type 2 diabetic on insulin. Mrs. Jones has **diabetic retinopathy** and **diabetic neuropathy** of her feet. Bariatric surgery enabled her to reduce her weight from 275 to 156 pounds. The time is 0930 hrs. She is complaining of having a cold and cough for the past few days. Now, she is feeling drowsy and nauseous and has a dry mouth. As you talk with her, you notice that her speech is slurred. She cannot remember if she gave herself her morning insulin. Examination of her lungs reveals **rales** (wet, crackly lung noises) at her right base.

Her VS: T 97.8, P 127, R 20, BP 102/53. You perform her blood **glucose** measurement. The reading is 604 milligrams per deciliter (mg/dL). A recommended value 2 hours after breakfast is < 145 mg/dL.

Mrs. Martha Jones is in the early stages of a diabetic **ketoacidosis** coma, probably initiated by a right lower-lobe pneumonia. A urine specimen was obtained. Dr. Lee was notified. Blood was taken for a full chemistry panel, and arterial blood gases were drawn. Dr. Lee treated Mrs. Jones immediately with an IV infusion of **saline** solution and IV **insulin**. She was admitted to the hospital.

B. Define the word elements to quickly decipher the meaning of the medical term. *Knowing the meaning of the word elements makes short work of defining medical terms. Identify the meaning of the element in the first column with its correct meaning in the second column. Fill in the blanks.* **LO 12.1, and 12.8**

_____	**1.** *osmol-*	**a.**	tumor
_____	**2.** *-oma*	**b.**	gland
_____	**3.** *bio-*	**c.**	to view
_____	**4.** *-opsy*	**d.**	concentration
_____	**5.** *aden-*	**e.**	life

C. Medications: Diabetics will deal with medications for the rest of their lives. *Select the one drug that is the correct answer for each statement.* **LO 12.4 and 12.6**

1. Act(s) by stimulating the beta cells to secrete insulin:

    a. metformin   **b.** sulfonylureas   **c.** alpha-glucosidase inhibitors

2. Suppress(es) hepatic glucose production:

    a. metformin   **b.** meglitinides   **c.** glipizide

3. Blocks the breakdown of starches in the intestine:

    a. acarbose   **b.** repaglinide   **c.** sitagliptin

D. Test your knowledge of the treatment of patients with diabetes mellitus by identifying statements as T for true and F for false. **LO 12.5 and 12.6**

1. All patients with diabetes mellitus should follow the same plasma glucose monitoring schedule.   **T**   **F**

2. An important part of self-monitoring is foot care.   **T**   **F**

3. Ketosis can be treated at home.   **T**   **F**

4. The HbA1c is a record of blood sugar control over the preceding 6 to 8 months.   **T**   **F**

5. Glucophage works by consuming glucose in the blood.   **T**   **F**

E. Explain *the therapeutic procedures for disorders of the pituitary gland. Select the correct answer to complete the sentence or answer the question.* **LO 12.6**

1. Treatment of pituitary tumors is aimed at:

    a. shrinking or removing the tumor

    b. increasing pituitary hormone levels

    c. hormone replacement therapy

    d. suppressing adrenal gland secretion

2. Large pituitary tumors may require a:

    a. Oral corticosteroids   **b.** craniotomy   **c.** lithotripsy   **d.** lobectomy

3. After treatment of pituitary tumors, what type of therapy is often begun to maintain normal hormone levels?

   a. physical   **b.** occupational   **c.** radiation   **d.** hormone-replacement

F. Identify *the word elements of medical terms will help you understand the purpose of the procedure. Choose the correct answer.*   **LO 12.1 and 12.6**

1. The suffix of the term **endoscopic** means

   a. process of viewing   **b.** use of a microscope   **c.** across   **d.** pertaining to

2. The suffix in the term **transsphenoid** means:

   a. pertaining to   **b.** bony projection   **c.** resembling   **d.** across   **e.** butterfly

3. The suffix in the term **craniotomy** means:

   a. incision into   **b.** removal of   **c.** skull   **d.** treatment of   **e.** covering

G. Certain kinds of tests are performed for the purpose of arriving at the correct diagnosis for treatment. *Select the correct diagnostic test for each described condition.*   **LO 12.5 and 12.6**

1. Is associated with autoimmune inflammatory disease of the thyroid:

   a. serum calcitonin levels   **c.** antithyroid antibodies hormone levels

   b. thyroid-stimulating hormone levels   **d.** fine needle aspiration biopsy

2. Blood test to measure activity of the thyroid gland:

   a. serum calcitonin levels   **c.** antithyroid hormone levels

   b. thyroid hormone levels   **d.** fine needle aspiration biopsy

3. Level becomes elevated in medullary carcinoma:

   a. serum calcitonin levels   **c.** antithyroid hormone levels

   b. thyroid-stimulating hormone levels   **d.** fine needle aspiration biopsy

4. Reveals the size of the gland and the presence of nodules:

   a. radioactive iodine therapy   **c.** ultrasonography

   b. fine needle aspiration biopsy   **d.** serum calcitonin levels

5. Distinguishes benign from malignant nodules:

   a. radioactive iodine therapy   **c.** ultrasonography

   b. fine needle aspiration biopsy   **d.** isotopic thyroid scans

6. Details the nature of the thyroid enlargement and the function of the gland:

   a. isotopic thyroid scans   **c.** ultrasonography

   b. fine needle aspiration biopsy   **d.** serum calcitonin levels

H. Explain the therapeutic procedures for disorders of the adrenal glands. *Select the correct answer for each statement.*   **LO 12.6**

1. Treatment for this condition requires lifelong hormone replacement with hydrocortisone:

   a. pheochromocytoma

   b. Addison disease

   c. Cushing syndrome

   d. adrenal cortex carcinoma

2. In this condition, it is the mother who takes medication to treat the fetal condition:

   a. congenital adrenal hyperplasia

   b. pheochromocytoma

   c. Addison disease

   d. Cushing syndrome

3. A condition that is often treated with laparoscopic surgery and removal of the adrenal tumor:

   a. Cushing syndrome

   b. Addison disease

   c. pheochromocytoma

   d. congenital adrenal hyperplasia

I. **Pronunciation is important whether you are saying the word or listening to a word from a coworker.** Identify the proper pronunciation of the following medical terms. Correctly spell the term. **LO 12.1, 12.2, 12.3, and 12.9**

1. The correct pronunciation for the formation of glucose from noncarbohydrate sources

   a. **GLU**-koh-nee-oh-**JEN**-eh-sis

   b. glue-**KOH**-nee-**OH**-jen-ee-sis

   c. ak-roh-**MEG**-ah-lee

   d. ak-roh-mega-**AH-LEE**

   Correctly spell the term: _____

2. The correct pronunciation for thyroid hormone T4, tetraiodothyronine

   a. thigh-**ROCK**-seen

   b. **THIGH**-rok-sin

   c. kal-sih-**TONE**-in

   d. kal-**SIH**-toh-nine

   Correctly spell the term: _____

3. The correct pronunciation for one of the catecholamines

   a. kor-**tik**-oyd

   b. **KOR**-tih-koyd

   c. ep-**EE**-nefr-in

   d. ep-ih-**NEF**-rin

   Correctly spell the term: _____

4. The correct pronunciation for inflammation of the thyroid gland

   a. thigh-roy-**DIE**-tis

   b. thigh-ro-id-**EYE**-tis

   c. ant-**EE**-thigh-royd

   d. an-tee-**THIGH**-royd

   Correctly spell the term: _____

5. The correct pronunciation for excessive body and facial hair

   a. hair-**SUIT**-izm

   b. **HER**-sue-tizm

   c. **VIR**-ih-lizm

   d. vire-**LYE**-izm

   Correctly spell the term: _____

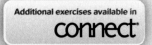
Additional exercises available in
Chapter Review exercises, along with additional practice items, are available in Connect!

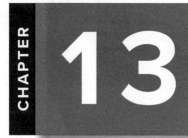

CHAPTER 13

The Urinary System
The Essentials of the Language of Urology

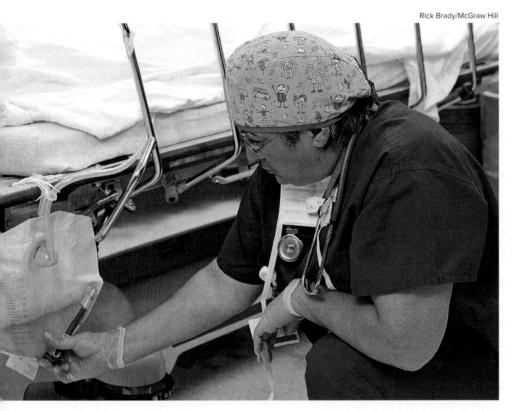

Rick Brady/McGraw Hill

Learning Outcomes

To understand and assess patients with urinary system conditions, define and recognize areas of concern, communicate with the other health care professionals involved in the care of these patients, and document a patient's progress, you need to be able to:

LO 13.1 Use **roots, combining forms, suffixes,** and **prefixes** to construct and analyze (deconstruct) medical terms related to the urinary system.

LO 13.2 Spell and pronounce correctly medical terms related to the urinary system to communicate them with accuracy and precision in any health care setting.

LO 13.3 Define accepted abbreviations related to the urinary system.

LO 13.4 Identify and describe the anatomy and physiology of the urinary system.

LO 13.5 Identify and describe disorders and pathological conditions related to the urinary system.

LO 13.6 Describe the diagnostic and therapeutic procedures and the pharmacologic agents used for disorders of the urinary system.

LO 13.7 Apply your knowledge of medical terms relating to the urinary system to documentation, medical records, and medical reports.

LO 13.8 Translate the medical terms relating to the urinary system into everyday language to communicate clearly with patients and their families.

In your future career, being able to communicate comfortably, accurately, and effectively with the health professionals involved in the diagnosis and treatment of problems with the urologic system is key. You may work directly and/or indirectly with one or more of the following:

- **Urologists** are specialists in the diagnosis and treatment of diseases of the urinary system.
- **Nephrologists** are specialists in the diagnosis and treatment of diseases of the kidney.
- **Urologic nurses** and **nurse practitioners** are registered nurses with advanced academic and/or clinical experience in urology.

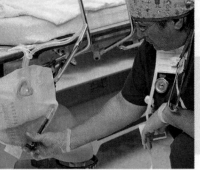

Rick Brady/McGraw Hill

- The kidney removes waste products from the blood by a process of filtration.

- Each renal cortex contains about 1 million nephrons, the functional filtration unit of the kidney.

- The filtrate from the kidney's filtration process is urine. It consists of excess water, electrolytes, and urea.

Your body's metabolism continually produces metabolic waste products. If these wastes are not eliminated, they will poison your body. Your **urinary** system, also called the **urinary tract**, carries the major burden of excreting these wastes, and within this system, the kidney is the organ that does the actual eliminating.

Urinary System (LO 13.4)

Your **urinary system** *(Figure 13.1)* consists of **six organs:**

- Two **kidneys**
- Two **ureters**
- A single **urinary bladder**
- A single **urethra**

The process of removing metabolic wastes is called excretion, and it is essential in maintaining your body's homeostasis *(see Chapter 2)*. Metabolic wastes include carbon dioxide, excess water and electrolytes, **nitrogenous** compounds including **ammonia** (from the breakdown of proteins), and **urea**. If these wastes are not eliminated, they will poison the entire body.

The Kidneys (LO 13.4)

Each of your kidneys is a bean-shaped organ about the size of your clenched fist. One kidney is located on each side of the vertebral column and lies against the deep muscles of your back *(Figure 13.1)*.

Waste-laden blood enters your kidney at its **hilum** (an area for incoming nerves and vessels) *(Figure 13.2)* through the **renal** artery. Excess water, urea, and other waste products are **filtered** from the blood by the more than 1 million **nephrons** in each kidney's cortex. The renal artery *(Figure 13.2)* divides into smaller and smaller arterioles, each of which then enters a nephron and divides into a network of capillaries known as a **glomerulus** *(Figure 13.3)*, which is encased in the **glomerular capsule** (Bowman's capsule). Because the blood is under pressure and the capillaries are permeable, much

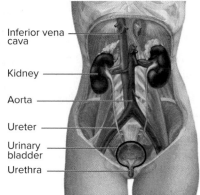

Inferior vena cava

Kidney

Aorta

Ureter

Urinary bladder

Urethra

▲ **FIGURE 13.1**
Urinary System.

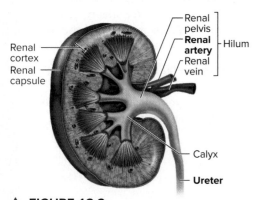

Renal cortex
Renal capsule

Renal pelvis
Renal artery
Renal vein
— Hilum

Calyx

Ureter

▲ **FIGURE 13.2**
Section of Kidney.

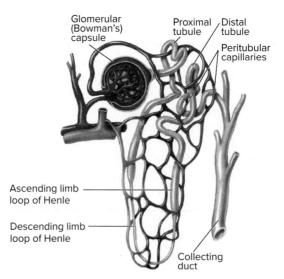

Glomerular (Bowman's) capsule

Proximal tubule

Distal tubule

Peritubular capillaries

Ascending limb loop of Henle

Descending limb loop of Henle

Collecting duct

▲ **FIGURE 13.3**
Nephron.

of the fluid from the blood filters through the capillary walls into the surrounding renal tubules, including the nephron loop (loop of Henle). The tubules join to form the collecting duct, and collecting ducts join to form **calyces,** which join to form the **ureter** *(Figure 13.2).* The ureters carry the **filtrate**, now called **urine**, from the kidneys to the urinary **bladder.**

The **excretion functions** of the **kidneys** are to:

- **Filter** blood to eliminate wastes;
- **Regulate** blood volume and pressure by eliminating or conserving water; and
- **Maintain** homeostasis by controlling the amounts of water and electrolytes that are eliminated.

Word Analysis and Definition

S = Suffix   P = Prefix   R = Root   R/CF = Combining Form

WORD	PRONUNCIATION	ELEMENTS		DEFINITION
ammonia	ah-**MOAN**-ih-ah	S/ R/	-ia *condition* ammon- *ammonia*	Toxic breakdown product of amino acids (proteins)
bladder	**BLAD**-er		Old English *bladder*	Hollow sac that holds fluid; e.g., urine or bile
calyx calyces (pl) calices (syn)	**KAY**-licks **KAL**-lih-seez		Greek *cup of a flower*	Funnel-shaped structure
filter (noun or verb)	**FIL**-ter		Latin *strain through material*	Porous substance used to separate liquids and gases from particulate matter; or to subject a substance to the action of a filter
filtrate	**FIL**-trate	S/ R/	-ate *composed of, pertaining to* filtr- *strain through*	Liquid that has passed through a filter
filtration	fil-**TRAY**-shun	S/	-ation *process*	Process of passing liquid through a filter
glomerulus glomeruli (pl) glomerular (adj)	glo-**MAIR**-you-lus glo-**MAIR**-you-lie glo-**MAIR**-you-lar	R/ S/	Latin *small ball of yarn* glomerul- *glomerulus* -ar *pertaining to*	Plexus of capillaries; part of a nephron Pertaining to or affecting a glomerulus or glomeruli
hilum hila (pl)	**HIGH**-lum **HIGH**-lah		Latin *small bit*	The opening where the nerves and blood vessels enter and leave an organ
kidney	**KID**-nee		Old English *kidney*	Organ of excretion
nephron	**NEF**-ron		Greek *kidney*	Filtration unit of the kidney; composed of glomerulus and renal tubule
nephrology	neh-**FROL**-oh-jee	S/ R/CF	-logy *study of* nephr/o- *kidney*	Medical specialty that studies the kidney
nephrologist	neh-**FROL**-oh-jist	S/	-logist *one who studies, specialist*	Medical specialist in disorders and diseases of the kidney
nitrogenous (adj)	ni-**TRO**-jen-us	S/ R/CF R/	-ous *pertaining to* nitr/o- *nitrogen* -gen- *create*	Containing or generating nitrogen
peristalsis	pair-ih-**STAL**-sis	P/ R/	peri- *around* -stalsis *constrict*	Waves of alternate contraction and relaxation of the muscle wall of a tube
renal (adj)	**REE**-nal	S/ R/	-al *pertaining to* ren- *kidney*	Pertaining to the kidney
tract	**TRACKT**		Latin *tractus*	An elongated pathway
urea	you-**REE**-ah		Greek *urine*	End product of nitrogen metabolism
ureter	you-**REE**-ter		Greek *urinary canal*	Tube that connects each kidney to the urinary bladder
ureteral (adj)	you-**REE**-ter-al	S/ R/	-al *pertaining to* ureter- *ureter*	Pertaining to a ureter
urethra (**Note:** *One "e" = one tube.*)	you-**REE**-thra	R/	Greek *passage for urine* urethr- *urethra*	Tube that carries urine from bladder to outside
urethral (adj)	you-**REE**-thral	S/	-al *pertaining to*	Pertaining to the urethra
urine urinary (adj)	**YUR**-in **YUR**-in-air-ee	S/ R/	Latin *urine* -ary *pertaining to* urin- *urine*	Fluid and dissolved substances excreted by the kidney Pertaining to urine
urinate (verb) urination	**YUR**-in-ate yur-ih-**NAY**-shun	S/ S/	-ate *composed of, pertaining to* -ation *process*	To pass urine Process of passing urine
urology	yur-**ROL**-oh-jee	S/ R/CF	-logy *study of* ur/o- *urinary system*	Medical specialty that studies the urinary system
urologist	yur-**ROL**-oh-jist	S/	-logist *one who studies, specialist*	Specialist in urology
urological (adj)	yur-roh-**LOJ**-ik-al	S/	-ical *pertaining to*	Pertaining to urology

The Ureters (LO 13.4)

Each ureter is a muscular tube, about 10 inches long and ¼ inch wide. The ureters carry urine from the renal pelvis to the urinary bladder. Each ureter lies on the posterior abdominal wall.

The ureters pass obliquely through the bladder's muscle wall. As pressure builds in the filling bladder, the muscle wall compresses the ureters and prevents urine from being forced back up the ureters to the kidneys **(reflux).**

In addition to gravity, intermittent muscular **peristaltic** waves, originating in the renal pelvis, squeeze urine down the ureters and squirt it into the bladder.

The Urinary Bladder and Urethra (LO 13.5)

The urinary bladder is a temporary storage place for urine before it is *voided* through the *urethra*. A moderately full bladder contains about 500 mL (1 pint) of urine. The maximum capacity of the bladder is around 750 to 800 mL (1½ pints). *Urination*, or emptying of the bladder, is also called *micturition*.

Urinary Bladder (LO 13.4)

The urinary bladder is a hollow, muscular organ on the floor of the pelvic cavity, posterior to the pubic symphysis *(Figure 13.4).*

Urethra (LO 13.4)

The urethra, a thin-walled tube, transports urine from the floor of the bladder to the outside. The base of the bladder's muscular wall is thickened to form the **internal urethral sphincter.** As the urethra passes through the skeletal muscles of the pelvic floor, the **external urethral sphincter** provides voluntary control of urination.

In the male *(Figure 13.4a),* the urethra is 7 to 8 inches long and passes through the penis. In the female *(Figure 13.4b),* the urethra is only about 1½ inches long, and it opens to the outside just above the vagina.

In both the male and female, the opening of the urethra to the outside is called the **external urinary meatus.**

Micturition (LO 13.4)

When the bladder contains about 200 mL or 7 fluid ounces (just less than a cup) of urine, stretch receptors in its wall trigger the **micturition reflex**. Parasympathetic nerves stimulate the bladder's muscle wall to contract and the internal sphincter to relax, and the need to urinate feels urgent. However, **voluntary** control of the external sphincter can keep that sphincter contracted and can hold urine in the bladder until urination is initiated voluntarily.

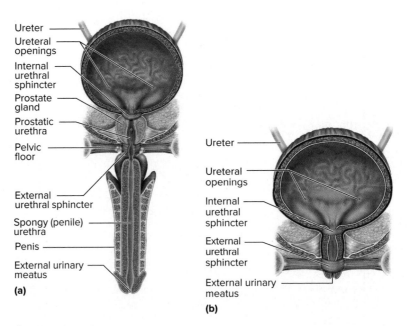

▲ **FIGURE 13.4** Urinary Bladder.
(a) Male anatomy. (b) Female anatomy.

S = Suffix   P = Prefix   R = Root   R/CF = Combining Form

WORD	PRONUNCIATION		ELEMENTS	DEFINITION
meatus	me-**AY**-tus		Latin *a passage*	The external opening of a passage
micturition (noun)	mik-choo-**RISH**-un	S/ R/	-ition *process* mictur- *pass urine*	Act of passing urine
micturate (verb)	**MIK**-choo-rate	S/	-ate *pertaining to*	Pass urine
reflex	**REE**-fleks		Latin *to bend back*	An involuntary response to a stimulus
sphincter	**SFINK**-ter		Greek *a band*	A band of muscle that encircles an opening; when it contracts, the opening squeezes closed
void (verb)	**VOYD**		Latin *to empty*	To evacuate urine or feces
voluntary involuntary	**VOL**-un-tare-ee in-**VOL**-un-tare-ee	P/	Latin *voluntary* in- *not*	Acting in obedience to the will Independent of or contrary to the will

EXERCISES

A. Construct *the following terms related to the urinary system by inserting the correct elements. Fill in the blanks.*   **LO 13.1 and 13.4**

1. specialist in the urinary system: _____ / _____

2. containing or generating nitrogen: _____ / _____ / _____

3. pertaining to the ureter: _____ / _____

4. study of diseases of the kidney: _____ / _____

5. pertaining to the kidney: _____ / _____

6. liquid that has passed through a filter: _____ / _____

B. Employ the *language of urology* **to correctly match the medical term to the brief description**   **LO 13.4**

_____	1. hollow sac that holds fluids	**a.** kidney
_____	2. organ of excretion	**b.** ureter
_____	3. connects kidney to bladder	**c.** urethra
_____	4. canal leading from bladder to outside the body	**d.** bladder

C. Describe the structures of the bladder and urethra. *Indicate if the following statements are accurate. If the statement is true, choose T. If the statement is false, choose F.*   **LO 13.4**

1. The length of the urethra is the same for males and females.   T   F

2. Micturition, voiding, and urination are synonyms.   T   F

3. Humans have control over the micturition reflex.   T   F

4. In both males and females, urine exits the urinary meatus.   T   F

5. There are two urethral sphincters.   T   F

6. The presence of 100 mL of urine in the bladder triggers the urge to void.   T   F

D. Correct pronunciation of medical terms is necessary when communicating to health care professional and to the patient and their friends and family members. *Choose the correct answer to the following questions.*   **LO 13.2**

1. In the term urethra, the letter "e" is pronounced like the letter "e" in:
   a. bet   **b.** new   **c.** break   **d.** me

2. The bolded letter "o" in the following term nephr**o**logy is pronounced like the "o" in:
   a. throat   **b.** rot   **c.** goose   **d.** boy

3. **Identify the only correct pronunciation of the medical term.**
   a. meatus–**MEET**-us   **b.** ureteral–your-ih-**TER**-al   **c.** sphincter - **SKINK**-ter   **d.** micturate – **MIK**-choo-rate

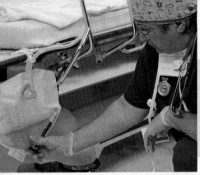

Section 13.2

Disorders of the Urinary System

Keynotes

- 25% to 30% of all renal cancers relate directly to smoking.
- As little as 1 milliliter of blood will turn the urine red.
- The acute form of glomerulonephritis has a 100% recovery rate.

Abbreviations

ARF	acute renal failure
CKD	chronic kidney disease
CRF	chronic renal failure
ESRD	end-stage renal disease
NSAID	nonsteroidal anti-inflammatory drug
PKD	polycystic kidney disease
UTI	urinary tract infection

Keynotes

- Diabetes and hypertension (high blood pressure) are the primary causes of renal failure.
- Acute renal failure is potentially reversible.
- Chronic renal failure has no cure and in latter stages may require blood filtration via dialysis.

Disorders of the Kidneys (LO 13.5)

Renal cell carcinoma, the most common form of kidney cancer, occurs about twice as often in men as in women. The cancer develops in the lining cells of the renal tubules, which can cause hematuria.

Wilms tumor, or **nephroblastoma**, is a malignant childhood kidney tumor, usually occurring between the ages of 3 and 4. It is treated effectively with a combination of surgery and chemotherapy.

Renal adenomas (benign kidney tumors) are usually asymptomatic (produce no symptoms), are discovered by chance, and are not life threatening.

Hematuria (blood in the urine) can be caused by lesions or stones anywhere in the urinary system. These lesions may result from trauma, infections, and congenital diseases like sickle cell anemia.

Acute glomerulonephritis is an inflammation of the kidney's filtration unit (the nephron). It damages the glomerular capillaries and allows protein and red blood cells to leak into the urine. It can develop rapidly after a strep throat infection, especially in children.

Chronic glomerulonephritis can occur with no history of kidney disease and present as kidney failure. It also occurs in **diabetic nephropathy** and can be associated with autoimmune diseases like systemic lupus erythematosus (an inflammatory, autoimmune disease).

Nephrotic syndrome is caused by different disorders that damage the kidneys, causing large amounts of protein to leak into the urine, so the level of protein in the blood drops. The most obvious symptom of nephrotic syndrome is fluid retention, with edema of the ankles and legs. Minimal change disease *(Table 13.1)* is the most common cause in children. Focal segmental glomerulosclerois (FSGS) *(Table 13.1)* is the most common cause in adults.

Interstitial nephritis is an inflammation (often acute and temporary) of the kidney tissue between the renal tubules. It can be an allergic reaction to or a side effect of drugs like penicillin or ampicillin, **NSAIDs,** and diuretics.

Pyelonephritis is an infection of the renal parenchyma, calyces, and pelvis. This usually occurs as part of a total urinary tract infection **(UTI,)** beginning in the urinary bladder *(see the next lesson in this chapter).* It has a high mortality rate in the elderly and in people with a compromised immune system.

Polycystic kidney disease (PKD) is an inherited disease. Large fluid-filled cysts grow within the kidneys and press against the kidney tissue. Eventually, the kidneys cannot function effectively.

Acute renal failure (ARF) describes the sudden inability of the kidneys to filter waste products from the blood. Initially, **oliguria** presents with eventual **anuria**, resulting in confusion, seizures, and coma.

The causes of acute renal failure include: severe burns; trauma; septicemia; toxins like mercury and excess alcohol; excessive amounts of drugs like aspirin and ibuprofen; and antibiotics like streptomycin and gentamycin.

When caring for a patient who has ARF, the goal is to treat the underlying disease. **Dialysis** may be necessary while the kidneys are healing.

Chronic renal failure (CRF), or **chronic kidney disease (CKD),** is a result of the gradual loss of renal function. Symptoms and signs may not appear until the kidney's level of functioning is less than 25% of normal. The main causes of chronic renal failure are diabetes, hypertension, kidney disease (including chronic glomerulonephritis, nephrotic syndrome), and heart failure.

Uremia is the result of an accumulation of excess nitrogenous waste products in the blood, as seen in renal failure.

End-stage renal disease (ESRD) means the kidneys are functioning at less than 10% of their normal capacity. At this point, life cannot be maintained, and either dialysis or a kidney transplant is needed.

Table 13.1 Types of Nephrotic Syndrome (LO 13.4)

Disease (as Seen on Biopsy)	Description
Minimal change disease	Most common in children; responds to steroids
Focal segmental glomerulosclerosis (FSGS)	Cause unknown; little response to treatment
Membranous nephropathy	Cause unknown; may respond to immunosuppressive treatment
Diabetes	Occurs if blood sugar has been poorly controlled

WORD	PRONUNCIATION	ELEMENTS		DEFINITION
adenoma	AD-eh-NOH-mah	S/ R/	-oma *tumor* aden- *gland*	A benign neoplasm of epithelial tissue
anuria	an-YOU-ree-ah	S/ P/ R/	-ia *condition* an- *a lack of, no* -ur- *urine*	Absence of urine production
carcinoma	kar-sih-NOH-mah	S/ R/	-oma *tumor, mass* carcin- *cancer*	A malignant and invasive epithelial tumor
glomerulonephritis	glo-MER-you-low-nef-RYE-tis	S/ R/CF R/	-itis *inflammation* glomerul/o- *glomerulus* -nephr- *kidney*	Infection of the glomeruli of the kidney
hematuria	he-mah-TYU-ree-ah	S/ R/	-uria *urine* hemat- *blood*	Blood in the urine
interstitial	in-ter-STISH-al	S/ R/	-al *pertaining to* interstiti- *space between cells*	Pertaining to spaces between cells in an organ or tissue
nephroblastoma Wilms tumor	NEF-roh-blas-TOE-mah VILMZ TOO-mor	S/ R/CF R/	-oma *tumor, mass* nephr/o- *kidney* -blast- *immature cell* Max Wilms, German surgeon, 1867–1918	Cancerous kidney tumor of childhood
nephropathy	neh-FROP-ah-thee	S/ R/CF	-pathy *disease* nephr/o- *kidney*	Any disease of the kidney
nephrotic syndrome nephrosis (*same as* nephrotic syndrome)	neh-FROT-ik SIN-drohm neh-FROH-sis	S/ R/CF S/ R/	-tic *pertaining to* nephr/o- *kidney* -osis *condition* nephr- *kidney*	Glomerular disease with marked loss of protein
nephritis	neh-FRY-tis	S/ R/	-itis *inflammation* nephr- *kidney*	Inflammation of the kidney
oliguria	ol-ih-GYUR-ee-ah	S/ P/ R/	-ia *condition* olig- *scanty* -ur- *urine*	Overall low production of urine
polycystic	pol-ee-SIS-tik	S/ P/ R/	-ic *pertaining to* poly- *many* -cyst- *sac, bladder, cyst*	Composed of many cysts
pyelonephritis	PIE-eh-loh-neh-FRY-tis	S/ R/CF R/	-itis *inflammation* pyel/o- *renal pelvis* -nephr- *kidney*	Inflammation of the kidney and renal pelvis
uremia	you-REE-me-ah	S/ R/	-emia *a blood condition* ur- *urine*	An accumulation of nitrogenous waste products within blood

Disorders of the Ureters (LO 13.5)

Kidney and Ureteral Stones (Nephrolithiasis) (LO 13.5)

Stones (**calculi**) begin in the pelvis of the kidney as a tiny grain of undissolved material, usually the minerals uric acid or calcium oxalate *(Figure 13.5)*. When the urine flows out of the kidney, this grain of material is left behind. Over time, more material is deposited and a stone is formed. Most stones enter one of the ureters while they are still small enough to pass down the ureter into the bladder and out of the body in urine. **Calculi** in the kidney are asymptomatic. Symptoms of calculi in the ureter typically starts as acute **flank** pain and then progresses to **spasmodic** pain that radiates to the **groin**.

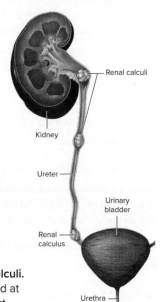

▶ **FIGURE 13.5** Renal Calculi. Calculi can become lodged at sites along the urinary tract.

S = Suffix P = Prefix R = Root R/CF = Combining Form

WORD	PRONUNCIATION		ELEMENTS	DEFINITION
calculus calculi (pl)	KAL-kyu-lus KAL-kyu-lie		Latin *pebble*	Small stone
flank	FLANK		Latin *broad*	Side of the body between the pelvis and the ribs
groin	GROYN		Old English *groin*	Crease where the thigh joins the abdomen
hydronephrosis	HIGH-droh-neh-FRO-sis	S/ R/CF R/CF	-osis *condition* hydr/o- *water* -nephr/o- *kidney*	Dilation of the pelvis and calyces of a kidney
hydronephrotic (adj)	HIGH-droh-neh-FROT-ik	S/	-tic *pertaining to*	Pertaining to or suffering from the dilation of the pelvis and calyces of the kidney
nephrolithiasis	NEF-roe-lih-THIGH-ah-sis	S/ R/CF R/	-iasis *condition, state of* nephr/o- *kidney* -lith- *stone*	Presence of a kidney stone

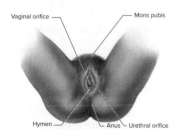

▲ **FIGURE 13.6**
Female External Genitalia.

(labels: Vaginal orifice, Mons pubis, Hymen, Anus, Urethral orifice)

Keynotes

- 7–10 million doctor visits each year are for UTIs.
- Incontinence is not considered normal past infancy and can be treated.
- Cigarette smoking contributes to more than 50% of bladder cancers.

Disorders of the Urinary Bladder and Urethra (LO 13.5)

Urinary Tract Infection (UTI) (LO 13.5)

A urinary tract infection occurs when bacteria invade and multiply in the urinary tract. The bacteria's point of entry is through the urethra. Women are more prone to UTIs than men. Once UTIs have occurred, they often recur. The female urethra is shorter than that of the male and opens to the surface near the anus *(Figure 13.6)*. This is why bacteria from the GI tract, like *E. coli,* can more easily invade the female urethra.

An infection of the urethra is called **urethritis**; **cystitis** is an infection of the urinary bladder. If cystitis is untreated, infection can spread up the ureters to the renal pelvis, causing **pyelitis**. The infection can then travel to the renal cortex and nephrons, causing pyelonephritis.

Pyelonephritis, an inflammation of the renal parenchyma, calyces, and pelvis, is commonly caused by bacterial infection that has spread up the urinary tract, often in association with structural abnormalities in the urinary tract, kidney stones, prostate disease, or **vesicoureteral reflux.** 70% to 80% of the infections are caused by *E. coli* and require aggressive, appropriate antibiotic therapy.

Symptoms of a UTI include **dysuria, suprapubic** pain, and hematuria. The diagnosis of a UTI can be made through a urinalysis. A culture of the infection-causing organism and testing of its sensitivity to different antibiotics allows the prescription of appropriate antibiotic therapy. Cranberry juice can make the urine more acidic and resistant to infection but is not a current recommendation as a single preventative or curative treatment.

Urinary Incontinence (LO 13.5)

Urinary incontinence is a result of a loss of bladder control. Millions of adults in America have this condition. Urinary incontinence is most common in women over the age of 50, and it's also seen frequently in elderly men. However, aging alone is not a cause of urinary incontinence.

- **Stress** incontinence is the loss of urine when pressure is exerted on the bladder by coughing, laughing, exercising, or lifting.
- **Urge** incontinence is a sudden, intense urge to urinate followed by an involuntary loss of urine.
- **Overflow** incontinence is the frequent or constant dribbling of urine. It can occur with a damaged bladder; blocked urethra; nerve damage from diabetes, multiple sclerosis, or spinal cord injury; and in men with prostate gland hypertrophy.
- **Functional incontinence** occurs in older adults when a physical or mental impairment prevents them from getting to the toilet in time.
- **Mixed incontinence** is when there are more than one type of incontinence producing symptoms.
- **Total incontinence** is the continuous leakage of urine day and night.

Urinary Retention (LO 13.5)

Urinary retention is the abnormal, involuntary holding of urine in the bladder. **Acute retention** can be caused by an obstruction in the urinary system, like an enlarged prostate in the male or neurologic problems, like multiple sclerosis. **Chronic retention** can be caused by any untreated obstruction in the urinary tract, such as an enlarged prostate gland in males and urethritis in any person.

Bladder Cancer (LO 13.5)

Bladder cancer is most common in smokers, males, and persons over 55 years of age.

Enuresis (LO 13.5)

Enuresis is involuntary micturition during sleep twice a week or more in older children five years or older. It usually resolves on its own and does not require treatment.

Word Analysis and Definition

S = Suffix   P = Prefix   R = Root   R/CF = Combining Form

WORD	PRONUNCIATION	ELEMENTS		DEFINITION
cystitis	sis-**TIE**-tis	S/ R/	-itis *inflammation* cyst- *bladder*	Inflammation of the urinary bladder
dysuria	dis-**YOU**-ree-ah	S/ P/ R/	-ia *condition* dys- *bad, difficult* -ur- *urine*	Difficulty or pain with urination
enuresis	en-you-**REE**-sis	S/ R/	-esis *condition* enur- *urinate*	Involuntary bedwetting
incontinence	in-**KON**-tin-ence	S/ P/ R/	-ence *state of* in- *not* -contin- *hold together*	Inability to prevent discharge of urine or feces
incontinent (adj)	in-**KON**-tin-ent	S/	-ent *pertaining to*	Denoting incontinence
pyelitis	pie-eh-**LYE**-tis	S/ R/	-itis *inflammation* pyel- *renal pelvis*	Inflammation of the renal pelvis
pyelonephritis	**PIE**-eh-loe-neh-**FRIE**-tis	S/ R/ R/CF	-itis *inflammation* -nephr- *kidney* pyel/o- *pelvis*	inflammation of the kidney and renal pelvis
retention	ree-**TEN**-shun		Latin *hold back*	Holding back in the body what should normally be discharged (e.g., urine)
suprapubic	**SOO**-prah-**PYU**-bik	S/ P/ R/	-ic *pertaining to* supra- *above* -pub- *pubis*	Above the symphysis pubis
urethritis	you-ree-**THRI**-tis	S/ R/	-itis *inflammation* urethr- *urethra*	Inflammation of the urethra
vesicoureteral reflux	**VES**-ih-koh-you-**REE**-ter-al **REE**-flucks	S/ R/CF R/ P/ R/	-al *pertaining to* vesic/o- *bladder* -ureter- *ureter* re- *back* -flux *flow*	Backward flow of urine from the bladder into the ureter.

EXERCISES

 Case Report 13.1

You are . . .

. . . a surgical physician assistant working with **urologist** Phillip Johnson, MD, at Fulwood Medical Center.

You are communicating with . . .

. . . Mr. Ichiro Cho, a 58-year-old school principal. You are making your afternoon hospital visits to Dr. Johnson's patients. Earlier today, you assisted at Mr. Cho's surgery. A **laparoscopic** radical **nephrectomy** (kidney removal) for a **TNM** Stage I **renal** cell carcinoma (cancer) with no evidence of local invasion or lymph node involvement was performed. Your job is to assess Mr. Cho's postoperative state and determine whether postoperative complications exist.

Mr. Ichiro Cho had been well until a few months before his surgery, when he noticed a vague, aching pain in the left side of his abdomen. One week prior to his surgery, he suddenly passed bright red urine. A urinalysis showed red blood cells (**hematuria**) and a physical examination revealed an enlarged left kidney. **Intravenous pyelogram (IVP)** (Figure 13.8) and other imaging tests showed a tumor 3 inches in diameter in the center of his left kidney. His bone scan was normal, indicating no metastases to the bones.

A. After reading Case Report 13.1 *answer the following questions. Select the correct answer.* **LO 13.6 and 13.8**

1. "Bright red urine" would indicate the presence of _____ in the urine.

   a. pus   **b.** blood   **c.** cancer cells   **d.** crystals   **e.** sugar

2. The diagnostic test that analyzed the contents of the urine:

   a. bone scan   **b.** pyelogram   **c.** nephrectomy   **d.** palpation   **e.** urinalysis

3. Which diagnostic test determined that Mr. Cho did not have bone metastases?

   a. intravenous pyelogram   **b.** radical nephrectomy   **c.** bone scan   **d.** PET scan   **e.** urinalysis

4. Has the cancer spread to other parts of the body?

   a. Yes   **b.** No

B. Differentiate *the types of kidney disorders. Match the kidney disorder in the first column with its correct description in the second column. Fill in the blanks.* **LO 13.5**

_____	**1.** renal adenoma	**a.** condition diagnosed only in children
_____	**2.** nephroblastoma	**b.** malignant condition of the kidney; develops in the cells of the renal tubules
_____	**3.** nephrotic syndrome	**c.** can develop as a result of strep throat infection
_____	**4.** renal cell carcinoma	**d.** benign and usually asymptomatic
_____	**5.** acute glomerulonephritis	**e.** condition that causes leakage of proteins into the urine; edema of the ankles and legs is a common sign

---

Case Report 13.2

You are . . .

. . . a medical assistant working in the office of Dr. Susan Lee, a primary care physician, at Fulwood Medical Center.

You are communicating with . . .

. . . Mrs. Caroline Dobson, a 32-year-old homemaker. You have asked her the reason for her visit to the office today.

Mrs. Dobson: "Since yesterday afternoon, I've had a lot of pain low down in my belly and in my lower back. I keep having to go to the bathroom every hour or so to pee. It's often difficult to start, and it burns as it comes out. I've had this problem twice before when I was pregnant with my two kids, so I've started drinking cranberry juice. I've been shivering since I woke up this morning, and the last urine I passed was pink. Was that due to the cranberry juice?"

Mrs. Dobson described many of the symptoms of cystitis. She had **suprapubic** and lower back pain. She had increased frequency of micturition with **dysuria** (difficulty with and pain or burning on urination). Her pink urine is probably **hematuria**.

C. Read *Case Report 13.2 and review all the terms and elements related to the urinary bladder and urethra. Fill in the blanks.* **LO 13.2, 13.5, and 13.7**

1. Is Mrs. Dobson suffering from enuresis? _____

2. Has Mrs. Dobson ever had this condition before? _____

3. If Dr. Lee feels that Mrs. Dobson might need a referral to a specialist, what kind of specialist would she recommend? _____

4. Which two medical terms are used to correctly document Mrs. Dobson's use of the words "to pee"? _____

5. What substance may be in Mrs. Dobson's urine, as indicated by the urine's pink color? _____

D. Apply your knowledge *of the language of urology to answer the following questions relating to chapter and lesson objectives. Fill in the blanks.* **LO 13.2 and 13.4**

1. Describe the location, structure, and function of the urinary bladder:

   Location: _____

   Structure: _____

   Function: _____

2. What is the function of a sphincter? _____

3. Which of the two urethral sphincters is voluntary? _____

   _____

4. What is the medical term that is used to describe the external opening of the urethra? _____

   _____

E. Define *the different types of disorders related to the urinary bladder and urethra. Choose the correct answer that completes each statement.* **LO 13.5**

1. The portal of entry for bacteria to infect the urinary bladder is the:

   a. urethra   **b.** ureter   **c.** blood   **d.** kidney

2. The medical term that defines infection of the bladder is:

   a. pyelitis   **b.** cystitis   **c.** incontinence   **d.** retention

3. Diagnosis of a specific bladder infection is confirmed via:

   a. blood test   **b.** X-ray of the bladder   **c.** ultrasound   **d.** urinalysis

4. The medical term incontinence is defined as a(n)

   a. inability to empty the bladder   **c.** loss of bladder control

   b. loss of the micturition reflex   **d.** infection of the bladder and urethra

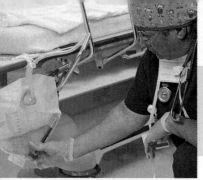

Rick Brady/McGraw Hill

Section 13.3

Diagnostic and Therapeutic Procedures of the Urinary System

Diagnostic Procedures (LO 13.6)

Urinalysis (LO 13.3 and 13.6)

A **dipstick** (a plastic strip bearing paper squares of reagent) is the most cost-effective method of screening urine *(Figure 13.7)*. After the stick is dipped into the urine specimen, the color change in each segment of the dipstick is compared to a color chart on the container. Dipsticks can screen for pH, specific gravity, protein, blood, glucose, ketones, bilirubin, **nitrite**, and leukocyte esterase *(see below)*.

A **routine urinalysis (UA)** in the lab can include the following tests:

- **Visual observation** examines color and clarity. Normal, healthy urine is pale yellow or amber in color and clear. Cloudiness indicates excess cells or cellular material. Red and cloudy indicates red blood cells.
- **Odor** of normal urine has a slight "nutty" scent. Infected urine has a foul odor. **Ketosis** gives urine a fruity odor.
- **pH** measures how acidic or alkaline urine is.
- **Specific gravity (SG)** measures how dilute or concentrated the urine is.
- **Protein** is not normally detected in urine; its presence (**proteinuria**) indicates infection or urinary tract disease.
- **Glucose** in the urine (**glycosuria**) is a spillover of sugar into the urine when the nephrons are damaged or diseased, or blood sugar is high in uncontrolled diabetes.
- **Ketones** are present in the urine in diabetic **ketoacidosis** *(see Chapter 12)* or in starvation when fat is used for energy in place of carbohydrates.
- **Leukocyte esterase** indicates the presence of white blood cells in the urine, which can point to a UTI.
- **Urine culture** from a clean-catch specimen *(see box)* is the definitive test for a UTI.

A **microscopic urinalysis** is performed on the solids deposited by centrifuging a specimen of urine. It can reveal:

- **Red blood cells (RBCs), white blood cells (WBCs),** and renal tubular epithelial cells stick together to form **casts;** WBCs stick together to form casts and bacteria.

Other Diagnostic Procedures (LO 13.3 and 13.6)

Other diagnostic procedures used to test for urinary bladder and urethra infections include:

- **KUB.** An X-ray of the abdomen shows the kidneys, ureters, and bladder.
- **Intravenous pyelogram (IVP).** A contrast material containing iodine is injected intravenously, and its progress through the urinary tract is recorded on a series of X-ray images *(Figure 13.8).*

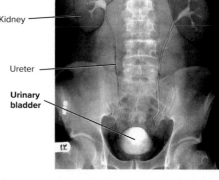

Kidney

Ureter

Urinary bladder

▲ **FIGURE 13.8**
Colored Intravenous Pyelogram (IVP).

Science History Images/Alamy Stock Photo

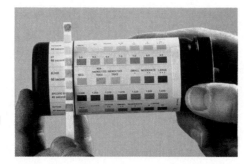

▶ **FIGURE 13.7**
Urinalysis Dipstick Being Compared against Color Chart on Container.

Saturn Stills/Science Source

- **Retrograde pyelogram.** Contrast material is injected through a urinary catheter into the ureters and kidneys to locate stones and other obstructions.

- **Voiding cystourethrogram (VCUG).** Contrast material is inserted into the bladder through a catheter and X-rays are taken as the patient voids.

- **CT scan.** X-ray images show cross-sectional views of the kidneys and bladder.

- **MRI.** Magnetic fields are used to generate cross-sectional images of the urinary tract.

- **Ultrasound imaging.** High-frequency sound waves and a computer generate noninvasive images of the kidneys.

- **Renal angiogram.** X-rays with contrast material are used to assess blood flow to the kidneys.

- **Cystoscopy.** A pencil-thin, flexible, tube-like optical instrument is inserted through the urethra into the bladder to examine the bladder's lining and to take a biopsy if needed *(Figure 13.9)*.

Abbreviation

VCUG voiding cystourethrogram

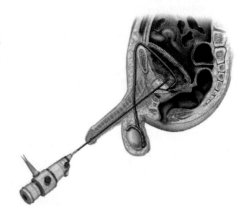

▲ **FIGURE 13.9**
Cystoscopy.

Word Analysis and Definition

S = Suffix   P = Prefix   R = Root   R/CF = Combining Form

WORD	PRONUNCIATION	ELEMENTS		DEFINITION
cast	KAST		Latin *pure*	A cylindrical mold formed by materials in tubules
cystoscope	SIS-toh-skope	S/ R/CF	-scope *instrument for viewing* cyst/o- *bladder*	An endoscope inserted to view the inside of the bladder
cystoscopy	sis-TOS-koh-pee	S/	-scopy *to examine*	The process of using a cystoscope
cystourethrogram	sis-toh-you-REETH-roe-gram	S/ R/CF R/CF	-gram *a record* cyst/o- *bladder* -urethr/o- *urethra*	X-ray image during voiding to show structure and function of bladder and urethra
dipstick	DIP-stik			A strip of plastic or paper bearing squares of reagent that change color to indicate presence of chemicals
glycosuria (**Note:** *The "s" is added to make the word flow.*)	GLYE-koh-SYU-ree-ah	S/ R/CF R/	-ia *condition* glyc/o- *glucose* -ur- *urinary system*	Presence of glucose in urine
ketone	KEY-tone		Greek *acetone*	Chemical formed in uncontrolled diabetes or in starvation
ketosis	key-TOE-sis	S/ R/CF	-sis *abnormal condition* ket/o- *ketones*	Excess production of ketones
ketoacidosis	KEY-toe-as-ih-DOE-sis	R/CF	-acid/o- *acid, low pH*	Excessive production of ketones, making the blood acidic
nitrite	NI-trite		Greek *niter, saltpeter*	Chemical formed in urine by *E. coli* and other microorganisms, indicative of UTI
proteinuria	pro-tee-NYU-ree-ah	S/ R/ R/	-ia *condition* protein- *protein* -uri- *urine*	Presence of protein in urine
pyelogram	PIE-el-oh-gram	S/ R/CF	-gram *record, recording* pyel/o- *renal pelvis*	X-ray image of renal pelvis and ureters using contrast media
retrograde	RET-roh-grade	P/ R/	retro- *backward* -grade *going*	Reversal of a normal flow; for example, back from the bladder into the ureters
urinalysis	you-rih-NAL-ih-sis	S/ R/CF	-lysis *to separate* urin/a- *urine*	Examination of urine to separate it into its elements and define their kind and/or quantity

Abbreviations

CAPD	continuous ambulatory peritoneal dialysis
CCPD	continuous cycling peritoneal dialysis
ESWL	extracorporeal shock wave lithotripsy

Therapeutic Procedures (LO 13.6)

Renal Stones (LO 13.5)

Renal stones are of four types: calcium oxalate stones are the most common; uric acid stones are more common in men; struvite stones occur mostly in women with UTIs; cystine stones are very rare. For renal stones that do not pass down the ureter into the bladder and out of the body in urine, there are several treatment options:

- **Watchful waiting.** With pain medication to relieve symptoms, the hope is that the stone can be passed.
- **Extracorporeal shock** wave **lithotripsy (ESWL).** With ESWL, a machine called a **lithotripter** from outside the body generates sound waves that crumble the stone into small pieces that can pass down the ureter into the bladder and be voided.
- **Ureteroscopy.** A small, flexible **ureteroscope** is passed through the urethra and bladder into the ureter. Devices can be passed through the endoscope to remove or fragment the stone.
- **Ureteral stent.** Silicone or plastic tube inserted into ureter to hold ureter open so that urine can flow around a kidney stone or stone fragments.
- **Percutaneous nephrolithotomy.** A **nephroscope** is inserted through the skin and into the kidney to locate and remove the stone.
- **Open surgery.** A surgical incision is made to expose the ureter and remove the stone; this is rarely done.

Kidney Failure (LO 13.5)

Dialysis is an artificial method of removing waste materials and excess fluid from the blood in end-stage renal disease. It is not a cure, but can prolong life. There are several types of kidney dialysis: In treatment of acute renal failure (ARF), the goal is to treat the underlying disease. Dialysis may be necessary while the kidneys are healing.

- **Hemodialysis** *(Figure 13.10)* filters the blood through an artificial kidney machine (**dialyzer**). Most patients require 12 hours of dialysis weekly, usually in three sessions.
- **Peritoneal dialysis** uses a solution that is infused into and drained out of the patient's abdominal cavity through a small flexible catheter implanted into the patient's abdominal cavity. The dialysis solution extracts wastes and excess fluid from the blood through the network of capillaries in the peritoneal lining of the abdominal cavity.
- **Continuous ambulatory peritoneal dialysis (CAPD)** *(Figure 13.11)* is performed by the patient at home usually four times each day, seven days a week.
- **Continuous cycling peritoneal dialysis (CCPD)** uses a machine to automatically infuse dialysis solution into and out of the abdominal cavity during sleep.

A **kidney transplant** provides a better quality of life than dialysis, provided a suitable donor can be found. A **sibling** or blood relative can often qualify as a donor. If not, tissue banks across the country can search for a kidney from a fatal accident victim or a donor who has died from a non-kidney-related condition.

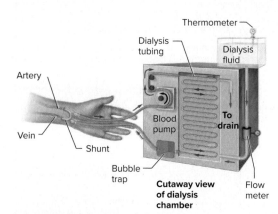

▲ **FIGURE 13.10**
Hemodialysis.

Nephrectomy (LO 13.5)

A **nephrectomy** is the removal of a kidney, entirely or partially. Nephrectomies are typically performed to treat renal carcinomas. Surgical methods to perform nephrectomies are open, laparoscopic, or via a robotic system.

- **Radical nephrectomy** is the removal of the entire kidney and surrounding tissues to treat renal carcinoma.
- A **donor nephrectomy** is the removal of a healthy kidney from a person so that it can be given to a person needing a healthy kidney.
- **Partial nephrectomy** is the removal of the diseased tissue of the kidney while leaving the healthy kidney tissue.

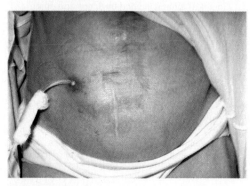

▲ **FIGURE 13.11**
Continuous Ambulatory Peritoneal Dialysis.

Mediscan/Alamy Stock Photo

Urinary Bladder (LO 13.5)

Cystoscopy can be used therapeutically to remove stones and to perform a transurethral resection of the prostate (**TURP**) to remove tissue from the inner portion of the prostate gland in men with benign prostatic hyperplasia (**BPH**).

For acute or chronic lower urinary tract obstruction in which the urethra is blocked, a flexible urethral catheter (**Foley catheter**) is passed into the bladder. The catheter can be left indwelling, or the patient can perform clean intermittent catheterization. If a Foley catheter cannot be passed, a suprapubic tube can be placed through the lower anterior abdominal wall into the bladder.

Treatment for urinary incontinence depends on the cause. If a medical or surgical problem is present, the incontinence can be resolved with proper treatment. **Bladder training** and **biofeedback** lengthen the time between the urges to urinate. **Kegel exercises** strengthen the muscles of the pelvic floor. Medications, for example, oxybutynin, are used for urge incontinence. Surgery can pull up the bladder and secure it if pelvic floor muscles are weak (**cystopexy**). Absorbent underclothing is also available for those with untreatable or continuing incontinence.

Word Analysis and Definition

S = Suffix   P = Prefix   R = Root   R/CF = Combining Form

WORD	PRONUNCIATION		ELEMENTS	DEFINITION
ambulatory	**AM**-byu-lah-tor-ee	S/ R/	-ory *relating to* ambulat- *walk*	Relating to walking
catheter	**KATH**-eh-ter		Greek *to send down*	Hollow tube that allows passage of fluid into or out of a body cavity, organ, or vessel
cystopexy	**SIS**-toh-pek-see	S/ R/CF	-pexy *surgical fixation* cyst/o- *bladder*	Surgical procedure to support the urinary bladder
dialysis	die-**AL**-ih-sis	P/ R/	dia- *complete* -lysis *to separate*	An artificial method of filtration to remove excess waste materials and water from the body.
dialyzer	**DIE**-ah-**LIE**-zer	S/	-lyzer *separator*	Machine that performs dialysis.
hemodialysis	**HEE**-moh-die-**AL**-ih-sis	R/CF	hem/o- *blood*	An artificial machine-based method to remove wastes from the blood
extracorporeal	**EKS**-trah-kor-**POH**-ree-al	S/ P/ R/	-eal *pertaining to* extra- *outside* -corpor- *body*	Outside the body
Kegel exercises	**KEE**-gal **EKS**-er-size-ez		Arnold Kegel, 1894–1981, American gynecologist	Contraction and relaxation of the pelvic floor muscles to improve urethral and rectal sphincter function
lithotripsy	**LITH**-oh-trip-see	S/ R/CF	-tripsy *to crush* lith/o- *stone*	Crushing stones by sound waves
lithotripter	**LITH**-oh–trip-ter	S/	-tripter *crusher*	Instrument that generates sound waves for lithotripsy
nephrolithotomy	**NEF**-roh-lih-**THOT**-oh-mee	S/ R/CF R/CF	-tomy *surgical incision* nephr/o- *kidney* -lith/o- *stone*	Incision to remove a renal stone
nephrectomy	neh-**FREK**-toe-me	S/ R/	-ectomy *surgical excision* nephr- *kidney*	Surgical removal of a kidney
nephroscope	**NEF**-roh-skope	S/ R/CF	-scope *instrument for viewing* nephr/o- *kidney*	Endoscope to view the inside of the kidney
nephroscopy	neh-**FROS**-koh-pee	S/	-scopy *to examine*	Visual examination of the kidney
percutaneous	**PER**-kyu-**TAY**-nee-us	S/ P/ R/CF	-us *pertaining to* per- *through* -cutane/o- *skin*	Pertaining to through the skin
sibling	**SIB**-ling	S/ R/	-ling *small* sib- *relative*	Brother or sister
transplant	**TRANZ**-plant	P/ R/	trans- *across* -plant *insert, plant*	The act of transferring tissue from one person to another
ureteroscope	you-**REE**-ter-oh-skope	S/ R/CF	-scope *instrument for viewing* ureter/o *ureter*	Endoscope to view the inside of the ureter
ureteroscopy	you-**REE**-ter-**OS**-koh-pee	S/	-scopy *to examine*	Endoscopic examination of the inside of the ureter

Urinary Tract Pharmacology (LO 13.2 and 13.6)

The kidneys represent approximately 0.5% of total body weight but receive about 25% of the total arterial blood pumped by the heart. When necessary, **diuretics** are prescribed to increase the output of urine in order to maintain homeostasis. There are several types of diuretics:

1. **Thiazides** are medium-potency diuretics used in heart failure and certain cases of hypertension. Examples are indapamide (*Natrilix*) and hydrochlorothiazide (*Microzide*). A major side effect is **hypokalemia** (low levels) of potassium.

2. **Loop diuretics** have a strong but brief diuresis period and are the most potent diuretics available. The most commonly used is furosemide (*Lasix*), and it also has a major side effect of potassium loss.

3. **Potassium-sparing diuretics** such as spironolactone (*Aldactone*), which has been used since 1959 and is gradually being replaced by newer agents such as eplerenone (*Inspra*), are used for reducing cardiovascular risk following myocardial infarction. **Hyperkalemia** can be a side effect. Not all of these are potent diuretics.

4. An **osmotic diuretic,** such as mannitol (*Osmitrol*), is given intravenously and used occasionally to prevent renal failure or decrease intracranial pressure in patients with head injury.

Alcohol also acts as a diuretic.

Uric acid, in the form of sodium urate crystals, contributes to the formation of kidney stones and produces the pain of gout when deposited in joints. **Uricosuric agents,** such as probenecid (*Benemid*), increase the excretion of uric acid by the kidneys and are used to prevent recurrences of kidney stones and to treat gout. Allopurinol (*Aloprim*) is another common medication used to prevent uric acid accumulation and avoid formation of kidney stones.

Medications used to treat incontinence include:

- **Anticholinergics** calm an overactive bladder and include oxybutynin (*Ditropan*), tolterodine (*Detrol*), and darifenacin (*Enablex*).

- **Antidepressants** imipramine (*Tofranil*) and duloxetine (*Cymbalta*) may be used to treat stress incontinence.

Word Analysis and Definition

S = Suffix   P = Prefix   R = Root   R/CF = Combining Form

WORD	PRONUNCIATION		ELEMENTS	DEFINITION
anticholinergic	AN-tee-koh-lih-NER-jik	S/ P/ R/ R/	-ic *pertaining to* anti- *against* -cholin- *choline* -erg- *work*	Antagonistic to parasympathetic nerve fibers
antidepressant	AN-tee-dee-PRESS-ant	S/ P/ P/ R/	-ant *pertaining to* anti- *against* -de- *without* -press- *press close, press down*	An agent used to counteract depression
diuretic (adj) (**Note:** *The "a" is dropped from dia to enable the word to flow.*) diuresis (noun)	die-you-RET-ik die-you-REE-sis	S/ P/ R/ S/	-etic *pertaining to* di(a)- *complete* -ur- *urine* -esis *condition*	Agent that increases urine output Excretion of large volume of urine
hyperkalemia	HIGH-per-kah-LEE-me-ah	S/ P/ R/	-emia *blood condition* hyper- *excess* -kal- *potassium*	An excessive amount of potassium in the blood
osmosis osmotic (adj)	os-MOH-sis os-MOT-ik	S/ R/ S/	-sis *process* osmo- *push* -tic *pertaining to*	The passage of a solvent across a cell membrane Relating to the process by which a liquid (usually water) moves across a membrane
potent	POH-tent		Latin *power*	Possessing strength, power
thiazide	THIGH-ah-zide	S/ R/	-ide *having a special quality* thiaz- *blue dye*	Abbreviated form of benzothiadiazide, a class of diuretic
uric acid uricosuric	YUR-ik ASS-id YUR-ih-koh-SU-rik	 S/ R/CF	Latin *relating to urine* -suric *excess* uric/o- *urine*	A chemical of white crystals poorly soluble in urine Pertaining to excessive amounts of uric acid in urine

EXERCISES

Case Report 13.3

Clinical Note Emergency Department, Fulwood Medical Center 9/12/19

Mr. Cho a 37-year-old construction worker, presented at 1520 hrs. He complained of a sudden onset of excruciating pain in his right abdomen and back an hour previously, while at work. The pain is **spasmodic** and radiates down into his **groin**.

He has vomited once, and keeps having the urge to urinate. He has no previous medical history of significance.

VS: T 99.4°F, P 114, R 28, BP 130/86.

Patient's abdomen is slightly distended, with tenderness in the right upper and lower quadrants and **flank**. A **dipstick** test showed blood in his urine.

Provisional diagnosis by Kiara Eagle, MD: stone in the right ureter.

An IV line was started, and 2 mg of morphine sulfate was given by IV push at 1540 hrs. He is going to X-ray STAT for KUB and IVP.

Mr. Cho's KUB (X-ray of **k**idney, **u**reter, and **b**ladder) showed a suspicious lesion halfway down his right ureter. IVP (**i**ntra**v**enous **p**yelogram) confirmed that this was a stone (renal **calculus**) blocking the ureter and showed the pelvis of the right kidney to be slightly dilated.

Mr. Cho's stone was large enough to be lodged in the ureter, blocking the flow of urine, with the backflow pressure leading to **hydronephrosis** of the kidney.

Mr. Cho was kept in the hospital overnight with IV pain medication but did not pass the stone. **Extracorporeal shock wave lithotripsy (ESWL)** was successful in crushing the stone. He urinated through a strainer so that the stone fragments could be recovered and chemically analyzed.
—Andrea Facundo, EMT-P, 1555 hrs.

A. After reading Case Report 13.3 *answer the following questions. Select the correct answer to complete each statement or answer each question.* **LO 13.3, 13.4, 13.5, 13.6, 13.7, and 13.8**

1. If Mr. Cho's pain had a "sudden onset," it is termed:

    a. acute   **b.** chronic

2. Where is the renal calculus located?

    a. the organ that filters blood to make urine   **c.** tube that leads from the bladder to the outside of the body

    b. the organ that breaks down toxins   **d.** tube that leads from the kidney to the bladder

3. Which of the following is the treatment that assisted in removing the renal calculus?

    a. IVP   **b.** ESWL   **c.** KUB   **d.** EMT-P

B. Match *the element in the first column with the correct meaning in the second column.* **LO 13.1**

_____ 1. extra-   **a.** body

_____ 2. lith/o   **b.** crushing

_____ 3. corpor   **c.** water

_____ 4. -tripsy   **d.** stone

_____ 5. hydr/o   **e.** outside

C. Abbreviations *are commonly used in written and verbal communication. Demonstrate your understanding of kidney disorders by selecting the correct kidney disorder abbreviation that completes each sentence. Not all terms will be used.* **LO 13.3 and 13.5**

    CRF   **ARF**   **PKD**   **ESRD**

1. An athlete has sprained her knee. She self-treats it with very large doses of ibuprofen, which can lead to _____ .

2. Diabetes that is not well managed over prolonged periods will likely lead to _____ .

3. An inherited disease in which fluid-filled sacs are present within the kidney is known as _____ .

D. Identify *the meanings of the word elements in each term. Select the correct answer that completes each statement.* **LO 13.1 and 13.5**

1. The meaning of the prefix in the term *transplant* is:

    a. across   **b.** condition   **c.** insert   **d.** remove

2. The meaning of the prefix in the term *oliguria* is:

    a. urine   **b.** scanty   **c.** condition   **d.** blood

3. The meaning of the root in the term *dialysis* is:

    a. urine   **b.** condition   **c.** destruction   **d.** inflammation

4. The prefix *an-* means:

    a. in addition to   **b.** move across   **c.** surgically remove   **d.** lack of

5. The prefix *poly-* means:

    a. sac   **b.** fluid   **c.** scanty   **d.** many

E. Apply your knowledge *of medical language to this exercise. Select the best answer.* **LO 13.6**

1. An X-ray image taken during voiding:

    a. retrograde pyelogram   **b.** angiogram   **c.** cystourethrogram

2. Presence of glucose in urine:

    a. hematuria   **b.** polyuria   **c.** glycosuria

3. Urine collection method to test for proteinuria:

    a. catheterization   **b.** 24 hour   **c.** clean catch

4. Reversal of normal flow:

    a. reflex   **b.** retrograde   **c.** regenerate

5. Excessive ketones in the blood, making it acidic:

    a. ketosis   **b.** ketoacidosis   **c.** ketone

6. Examination of urine to determine its quality and elements:

    a. urinalysis   **b.** cystourethrogram   **c.** retrograde pyelogram

F. Demonstrate your knowledge *of abbreviations and the medical terms they represent. Insert the medical terms that each abbreviation represents. Fill in the blanks.* **LO 13.2, 13.3, and 13.6**

1. KUB _____

2. UA _____

3. IVP _____

4. VCUG _____

G. Employ *the language of urology and match the correct diagnostic procedure in the first column with the correct statement in the second column.* **LO 13.3 and 13.6**

_____	1. KUB	a. uses contrast material
_____	2. cystoscopy	b. X-ray
_____	3. renal angiogram	c. invasive procedure to view the inside of the urinary bladder
_____	4. CT scan	d. cross-sectional views
_____	5. ultrasound imaging	e. noninvasive procedure that uses sound waves to view internal structures

H. Abbreviations are used in written and verbal communication. *Complete each sentence with the correct abbreviations. Use the provided abbreviations to fill in the blanks.* **LO 13.3 and 13.6**

> **BPH**   **CAPD**   **CCPD**   **ESWL**   **TURP**

1. The nephrologist recommended that the patient have _____ to assist in the passing of his kidney stones.

2. Because of his _____, Mr. Plaza suffered from overflow incontinence.

3. Mrs. Doskos prefers to receive her dialysis while she sleeps, and therefore the nephrologist recommended _____ to dialyze her blood.

4. _____ is used to remove sections of an enlarged prostate.

5. _____ allows the patient to walk around while receiving dialysis.

I. Construct terms using word elements. *Given the definition, complete each medical term with the correct missing element. Fill in the blanks. The first one has been done for you.* **LO 13.1 and 13.6**

1. Relating to walking   ambulat/ory

2. Surgical procedure to support the urinary bladder.   cysto/ _____

3. Visual examination of the kidney.   _____ /scopy

4. Pertaining to through the skin.   _____ /cutaneo/us

5. Incision to remove a stone.   nephro/litho/ _____

6. Artificial method to remove wastes from the blood.   _____ /dia/lysis

J. Deconstruct *the following medical terms into their elements.* **LO 13.1**

1. osmotic _____ / _____
   R, R/CF   S

2. uricosuric _____ / _____
   R, R/CF   S

3. antidepressant _____ / _____ / _____ / _____
   P   P   R, R/CF   S

4. hyperkalemia _____ / _____ / _____
   P   R, R/CF   S

5. thiazide _____ / _____
   R, R/CF   S

Additional exercises available in **connect**

Chapter Review exercises, along with additional practice items, are available in Connect!

14 CHAPTER

The Male Reproductive System

The Essentials of the Language of the

Male Reproductive System

Learning Outcomes

You must be able to understand the medical language related to the male reproductive system to care for patients with male reproductive disorders and conditions. You will also need to document the patient's care. To participate effectively in this process, you must be able to:

LO 14.1 Use roots, combining forms, suffixes, and prefixes to construct and analyze (deconstruct) medical terms related to the male reproductive system.

LO 14.2 Spell and pronounce correctly medical terms related to the male reproductive system in order to communicate them with accuracy and precision in any health care setting.

LO 14.3 Define accepted abbreviations related to the male reproductive system.

LO 14.4 Relate the anatomy of the penis, perineum, scrotum, testes, and spermatic cords and their functions.

LO 14.5 Relate the anatomy and anatomical positions of the five accessory glands of the male reproductive system to their functions.

LO 14.6 Identify and describe disorders and pathological conditions related to the male reproductive system.

LO 14.7 Explain the causes of male infertility and their treatments.

LO 14.8 Identify sexually transmitted diseases, their prevention, and treatments.

LO 14.9 Describe diagnostic and therapeutic procedures and pharmacology used to treat disorders of the male reproductive system.

LO 14.10 Identify health professionals involved in the care of patients with male reproductive system diseases and disorders.

LO 14.11 Apply your knowledge of medical terms relating to the male reproductive system to documentation, medical records, and medical reports.

LO 14.12 Translate the medical terms relating to the male reproductive system into everyday language in order to communicate clearly with patients and their families.

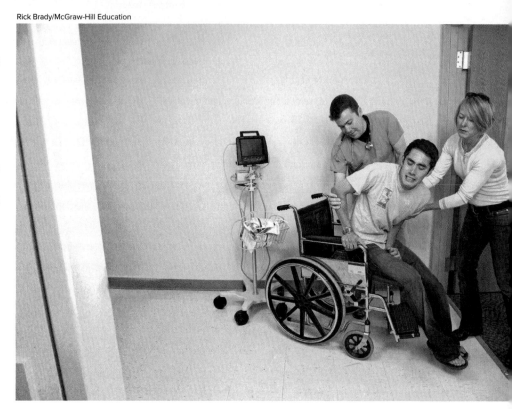

The health professionals involved in the diagnosis and treatment of patients with problems of the urinary system include:

• **Urologists,** who are specialists in the diagnosis and treatment of patients with diseases of the urinary system.

• **Nephrologists,** who are specialists in the diagnosis and treatment of diseases of the kidney.

• **Urologic nurses and nurse practitioners,** who are registered nurses with advanced academic and clinical experience in urology.

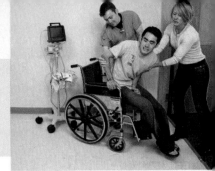

Section 14.1

The Male Reproductive System

Rick Brady/McGraw-Hill Education

Unlike every other organ system, the reproductive system is not essential for an individual human to survive. However, without the reproductive system, the human species could not survive.

Male Reproductive System (LO 14.4 and 14.5)

The **male reproductive organ system** *(Figure 14.1)* consists of the primary and secondary sex organs, and the accessory glands. These are categorized as follows:

1. The **primary sex organs,** or **gonads,** are the two **testes.**
2. The **secondary sex organs** include:
   a. The **penis**;
   b. The **scrotum**; and
   c. A system of ducts, including the **epididymis, ductus (vas) deferens,** and **urethra**.
3. The accessory glands include:
   a. The **prostate**;
   b. The **seminal vesicles**; and
   c. The **bulbourethral glands.**

Perineum (LO 14.4)

The external **genitalia** (penis, scrotum, and testes) occupy the **perineum,** a diamond-shaped region between the thighs. The perineum borders the pubic symphysis anteriorly and the coccyx posteriorly *(Figure 14.2)*. The anus is also in the perineum.

Scrotum (LO 14.4)

The scrotum is a skin-covered sac situated just behind the penis at the front of the upper thighs. It is divided into two compartments. Each compartment contains a testis. The scrotum's function is to provide a cooler environment for the testes than that inside the body. Sperm are best produced and stored at a few degrees cooler than that of the male's internal body temperature.

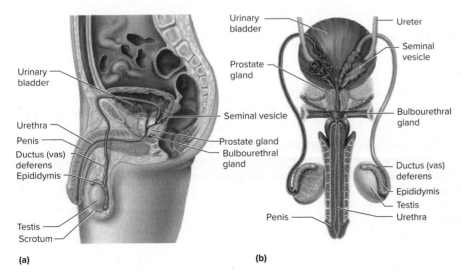

(a)   (b)

▲ **FIGURE 14.1** Male Reproductive System.
(a) Male pelvic cavity, midsagittal section. (b) Male reproductive organs.

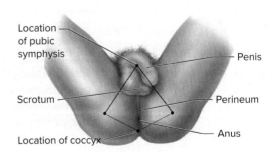

▲ **FIGURE 14.2** Male Perineum.

WORD	PRONUNCIATION	ELEMENTS		DEFINITION
bulbourethral	BUL-boh-you-REE-thral	S/ R/CF R/	-al *pertaining to* bulb/o- *bulb* -urethr- *urethra*	Pertaining to the bulbous penis and urethra
ductus deferens (*same as* vas deferens)	DUK-tus DEH-fuh-renz VAS		ductus, Latin *to lead* deferens, Latin *carry away* vas, Latin *vessel, canal*	Tube that receives sperm from the epididymis
epididymis	EP-ih-DID-ih-miss	P/ R/	epi- *above* -didymis *testis*	Coiled tube attached to testis
genitalia (Note: *Two suffixes*) genital (adj)	JEN-ih-TAY-lee-ah JEN-ih-tal	S/ S/ R/	-ia *condition* -al- *pertaining to* genit- *primary male or female sex organs*	External and internal organs of reproduction Pertaining to reproduction or to the male or female sex organs
gonad gonads (pl) gonadal (adj)	GO-nad GO-nadz go-NAD-al	R/ S/	Greek *seed* gonad- -al *pertaining to*	Testis or ovary Pertaining to the testis or ovary
penis penile (adj)	PEE-nis PEE-nile	S/ R/	Latin *tail* -ile *pertaining to* pen- *penis*	Conveys urine and semen to the outside Pertaining to the penis
perineum perineal (adj)	PER-ih-NEE-um PER-ih-NEE-al	S/ R/	Greek *perineum* -al *pertaining to* perine- *perineum*	Area between the thighs, extending from the coccyx to the pubis Pertaining to the perineum
scrotum scrotal (adj)	SKRO-tum SKRO-tal	S/ R/	Latin *scrotum* -al *pertaining to* scrot- *scrotum*	Sac containing the testes Pertaining to the scrotum
seminal vesicle	SEM-in-al VES-ih-kull	S/ R/ S/ R/	-al *pertaining to* semin- *semen* -le *small* vesic- *sac containing fluid*	Sac of the ductus deferens that produces seminal fluid
testicle testicular (adj) testis testes (pl)	TES-tih-kul tes-TICK-you-lar TES-tis TES-teez	S/ R/	Latin *small testis* -ar *pertaining to* testicul- *testicle* Latin *testis*	One of the male reproductive glands Pertaining to the testicle Same as testicle
urethra (Note: *one "e" = one tube.*) urethral	you-REE-thra you-REE-thral	R/ S/	Greek *passage for urine* urethr- *urethra* -al *pertaining to*	Tube that carries urine from bladder to outside Pertaining to the urethra

Testes and Spermatic Cord (LO 14.4)

Testes (LO 14.4)

In the adult male, each testis is an asymmetrical oval organ that measures about 2 inches long and ¾ of an inch wide *(Figure 14.3)*. Each testis is covered by a serous membrane—the **tunica vaginalis**—which has outer and inner layers that are separated by serous fluid.

Inside the testis are some 250 lobules (small lobes); each contains three or four **seminiferous tubules**, which produce **semen**. Within these tubules are several layers of germ cells that are in the process of developing into sperm. Between the seminiferous tubules are the interstitial (occurring between tissues) cells. These cells produce hormones called **androgens**.

Testosterone is the major androgen produced by the interstitial cells of the testes. Its effects include the stimulation of the following activities:

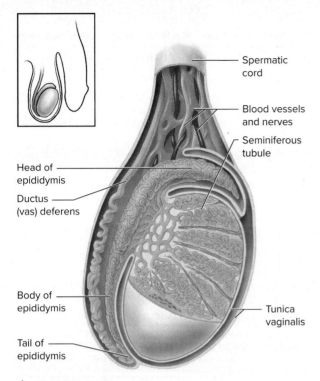

▲ **FIGURE 14.3**
The Testis and Associated Structures.

Labels on Figure 14.3:
Spermatic cord
Blood vessels and nerves
Seminiferous tubule
Head of epididymis
Ductus (vas) deferens
Body of epididymis
Tail of epididymis
Tunica vaginalis

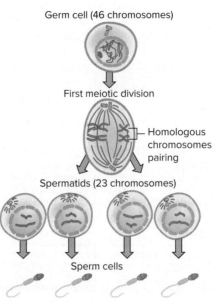

▲ **FIGURE 14.4** Spermatogenesis.

Labels on Figure 14.4:
Germ cell (46 chromosomes)
First meiotic division
Homologous chromosomes pairing
Spermatids (23 chromosomes)
Sperm cells

1. **Spermatogenesis** *(Figure 14.4)*, which is the process of production of **spermatozoa** (**sperm**).
2. The development of the male secondary sex characteristics at puberty, which include:
   a. Enlargement of the testes, scrotum, and penis.
   b. Development of the pubic, axillary, body, and facial hair.
   c. Secretion of sebum in skin, which can result in acne *(Chapter 3)*.
3. A burst of growth at puberty, including an increased muscle mass, a higher basal metabolic rate **(BMR),** and a larger larynx (which deepens the voice).
4. Stimulating the brain to generate the male's **libido** (sex drive).

Spermatic Cord (LO 14.4)

The blood vessels and nerves to the testes—which arise in the abdominal cavity—pass through the **inguinal canal,** or groin, where they join with connective tissue. This forms the **spermatic cord** that suspends each testis in the scrotum *(Figure 14.3)*. The left testis is suspended lower than the right. Within the cord exist:

• an artery;
• a **plexus** of veins;
• nerves;
• a thin muscle; and
• the ductus (vas) deferens into which sperm are deposited when they leave the testis.

Sperm (LO 14.4)

A mature sperm has a pear-shaped head and a long tail. The sperm's head contains three segments *(Figure 14.5):*

• The **nucleus**, which contains 23 chromosomes;
• The **cap,** which contains enzymes used to penetrate the egg; and
• The **basal body** of the tail.

The tail is further divided into three segments and is responsible for movement as the sperm swims up the female reproductive tract.

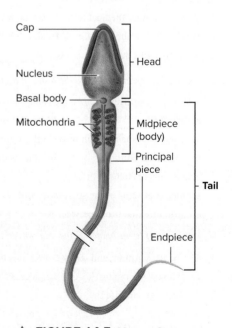

Labels on Figure 14.5:
Cap
Head
Nucleus
Basal body
Mitochondria
Midpiece (body)
Principal piece
Tail
Endpiece

▲ **FIGURE 14.5** Mature Sperm.

Word Analysis and Definition

S = Suffix   P = Prefix   R = Root   R/CF = Combining Form

WORD	PRONUNCIATION		ELEMENTS	DEFINITION
androgen	AN-droh-jen	S/ R/CF	-gen *create, produce* andr/o- *masculine*	Hormone that promotes masculine characteristics
inguinal	IN-gwin-al	S/ R/	-al *pertaining to* inguin- *groin*	Pertaining to the groin
libido	lih-BEE-doh		Latin *lust*	Sexual desire
plexus plexuses (pl)	PLEK-sus PLEK-sus-ez		Latin *braid*	A weblike network of joined nerves
semen seminiferous (adj)	SEE-men sem-ih-NIF-er-us	S/ R/ R/	Latin *seed* -ous *pertaining to* semin/i- *semen* -fer- *to bear, carry*	Penile ejaculate containing sperm and seminal fluid Pertaining to carrying semen
sperm spermatozoa (pl) spermatic (adj) spermatogenesis	SPERM SPER-mat-oh-ZOH-ah SPER-mat-ik SPER-mat-oh-JEN-eh-sis	S/ R/CF S/ S/	Greek *seed* -zoa *animal* spermat/o- *sperm* -ic *pertaining to* -genesis *creation,* *formation*	Mature male sex cell Sperm (plural) Pertaining to sperm The process by which male germ cells differentiate into sperm
testosterone	tes-TOSS-ter-own	S/ R/CF	-sterone *steroid* test/o- *testis*	Powerful androgen produced by testes
tunica vaginalis	TYU-nih-kah vaj-ih-NAHL-iss	S/ R/	tunica, Latin *coat* -alis *pertaining to* vagin- *sheath, vagina*	Covering, particularly of a tubular structure The tunica vaginalis is the sheath of the testis and epididymis

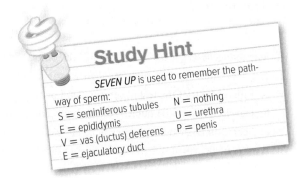

Study Hint

SEVEN UP is used to remember the pathway of sperm:

S = seminiferous tubules   N = nothing
E = epididymis   U = urethra
V = vas (ductus) deferens   P = penis
E = ejaculatory duct

EXERCISES

A. Write *the correct medical term to answer the question.* **LO 14.2, 14.3, and 14.4**

1. What is the name of the serous membrane that covers the testis? _____

2. The term *seminiferous* pertains to: _____

3. What is another medical term for sex drive? _____

4. What does the abbreviation BMR stand for? _____

5. What structure supports the testes? _____

B. Use *medical terms related to the testes and spermatic cord. Select the correct answer to complete each statement.* **LO 14.4 and 14.5**

1. The major androgen of the male reproductive system:

   a. estrogen   **b.** testosterone   **c.** semen   **d.** cortisone   **e.** spermatid

2. That which suspends each testis in the scrotum is the:

   a. spermatic cord   **b.** ductus deferens   **c.** dartos muscle   **d.** interstitial cells   **e.** tunica

3. The ductus deferens is the:

   a. plexus of veins in the spermatic cord   **c.** the tube carries sperm through the spermatic cord

   b. structure that produces sperm   **d.** covering of each testis

C. Use *medical terms related to the anatomy of the male reproductive system. Select the correct answer to complete each statement.* **LO 14.4 and 14.5**

1. The penis, scrotum, and testes collectively are known as:

   a. primary sex organs   **b.** accessory glands   **c.** secondary sex organs   **d.** external genitalia   **e.** the perineum

2. The male gonads are the:

   a. scrotum   **b.** penis   **c.** prostate   **d.** ductus deferens   **e.** testes

3. The medical term that refers to the area between the thighs is the:

   a. perineum   **b.** raphae   **c.** spermatic cord   **d.** genitalia   **e.** varicocele

Section 14.2

Spermatic Ducts, Accessory Glands, and Penis

Rick Brady/McGraw-Hill Education

The male prostate and urethra have both **urological** and **reproductive** functions, as the flow of urine and semen goes through both organs. Disorders of the prostate and urethra produce symptoms and signs that arise in both areas.

Spermatic Ducts (LO 14.4)

As the sperm cells mature in the testes over a 60-day period, they move down the seminiferous tubules into the epididymis for storage. The epididymis adheres to the posterior side of the testis. It is a single-coiled duct or tube in which the sperm are stored for 12 to 20 days until they mature and become **motile** (capable of movement).

To be ejaculated, the sperm move into the ductus (vas) deferens, the **ejaculatory** duct, and finally the urethra to reach the outside of the body.

The ductus (vas) deferens is a muscular duct that travels up from the epididymis in the scrotum, passes behind the urinary bladder, and joins with the duct of the seminal vesicle to form the ejaculatory duct, which empties sperm and semen into the urethra.

Accessory Glands (LO 14.5)

The five accessory glands *(Figure 14.6)* are:

1. The two **seminal vesicles**, located on the posterior surface of the urinary bladder, hold fluid that mixes with the sperm in the vas deferens. The fluid contains glucose to provide nourishment for the sperm and has clotting properties that make the semen sticky.

2. The single **prostate gland** is close in size and shape to the average walnut. The prostate gland is located immediately below the bladder and anterior to the rectum. It surrounds the urethra and the ejaculatory duct. It is composed of 30 to 50 glands that open directly into the urethra; these glands secrete fluid that nourishes and protects sperm. During ejaculation, the prostate squeezes this fluid into the urethra to form part of semen.

3. The two **bulbourethral glands** are located one on either side of the membranous urethra. Each gland has a short duct leading into the spongy (penile) urethra. When sexually aroused, the glands produce a fluid that neutralizes any acidity in the urethra to make a more hospitable environment in which the sperm can travel.

Keynotes

- Semen is derived from the secretions of several glands:
  - 5% comes from the testicles and epididymis (sperm).
  - 50% to 80%, from the seminal vesicles.
  - 15% to 33%, from the prostate gland.
  - 2% to 5%, from the bulbourethral glands.
- A normal sperm count is in the range of 75 to 150 million sperm per milliliter (mL) of semen. A normal ejaculation consists of 2 to 5 mL of semen.

Abbreviations

| CST | Certified Surgical Technologist |
| mL | milliliter |

▼ **FIGURE 14.6**
The Five Accessory Glands of the Male Reproductive System.

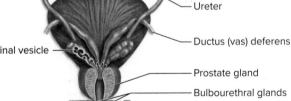

- Ureter
- Seminal vesicle
- Ductus (vas) deferens
- Prostate gland
- Bulbourethral glands

Word Analysis and Definition

S = Suffix   P = Prefix   R = Root   R/CF = Combining Form

WORD	PRONUNCIATION	ELEMENTS		DEFINITION
ejaculate (can be a verb or a noun)	ee-**JACK**-you-late	S/ R/	-ate *composed of, pertaining to* ejacul- *shoot out*	To expel suddenly; *or* the semen expelled in ejaculation
ejaculation (noun)	ee-**JACK**-you-**LAY**-shun	S/	-ation *process*	Process of expelling semen suddenly
ejaculatory (adj)	ee-**JACK**-you-lah-**TOR**-ee	S/	-atory *pertaining to*	Pertaining to ejaculation
motile (adj)	**MOH**-til	S/ R/	-ile *pertaining to* mot- *to move*	Capable of spontaneous movement
motility	moh-**TILL**-ih-tee	S/ R/	-ity *condition, state* motil- *to move*	The ability for spontaneous movement
prostate (**Note:** *not* **PROS**-trate, *which means exhausted*)	**PROS**-tate		Greek *one standing before*	Gland surrounding the beginning of the urethra
prostatic (adj)	pros-**TAT**-ik	S/ R/	-ic *pertaining to* prostat- *prostate*	Pertaining to the prostate

Penis (LO 14.4)

The **penis** *(Figure 14.7a)* is an important male external body structure, which is specifically designed to meet its two main functions:

- To enable urine to flow to the outside.
- To deposit semen in the female vagina around the cervix.

The external, visible part of the penis is composed of the **shaft** and the more sensitive **glans**. The external urethral meatus is located at the tip of the glans. The skin of the penis continues over the glans as the **prepuce**, otherwise known as the foreskin. A ventral fold of tissue called the **frenulum** attaches the foreskin to the glans. In the large portion of men who have been circumcised, the foreskin has been removed.

The shaft of the penis contains these three **erectile** vascular bodies *(Figure 14.7b)*:

- The paired **corpora cavernosa** (columns of erectile tissue found in the penis) are located dorsolaterally.
- The single **corpus spongiosum** is located inferiorly. It contains the urethra and goes on to form the glans.

Erection occurs when the corpora cavernosa fill with blood, causing the erectile bodies to distend and become rigid. It is a parasympathetic nervous system response to stimulation.

Ejaculation occurs when the sympathetic nervous system stimulates the smooth muscle of the ductus deferens, ejaculatory ducts, and the glands in the prostate to contract.

The Prepuce (Foreskin) and Urethra (LO 14.4)

The functions of the **prepuce** (foreskin) are to cover and protect the glans *(Figure 14.8a)*, and to produce smegma. **Smegma** is a lubricant containing lipids, cell debris, and some natural antibiotics.

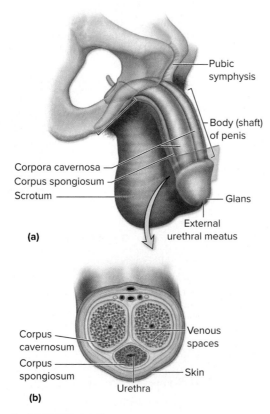

(a)

(b)

▲ **FIGURE 14.7** Anatomy of the Penis.
(a) External anatomy. (b) Cross-sectional view.

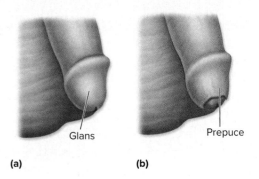

(a)   (b)

▲ **FIGURE 14.8** Prepuce.
(a) Uncircumcised penis.
(b) Circumcised penis.

WORD	PRONUNCIATION	ELEMENTS		DEFINITION
cavernosa	kav-er-**NOH**-sah	S/ R/	**-osa** *like* **cavern-** *cave*	Resembling a cave
corpus corpora (pl)	**KOR**-pus **KOR**-por-ah		Latin *body*	Major part of a structure
erectile	ee-**REK**-tile	S/ R/	**-ile** *pertaining to* **erect-** *to set up, straight*	Capable of erection or being distended with blood
erection	ee-**REK**-shun	S/	**-ion** *action, condition*	Distended and rigid state of an organ
frenulum	**FREN**-you-lum		Latin *small bridle*	Fold of mucous membrane between the glans and the prepuce
glans	GLANZ		Latin *acorn*	Head of the penis or clitoris
prepuce *(same as* **foreskin***)*	**PREE**-puce		Latin *foreskin*	Fold of skin that covers the glans penis
smegma	**SMEG**-mah		Greek *ointment*	Oily material produced by the glans and prepuce
spermicide	**SPER**-mih-side	S/ R/CF	**-cide** *destroy* **sperm/i-** *sperm*	Agent that destroys sperm
spermicidal (adj)	sper-mih-**SIGH**-dal	S/	**-al** *pertaining to*	Pertaining to the killing of sperm; *or* destructive to sperm
spongiosum	spun-jee-**OH**-sum	S/ R/	**-um** *tissue* **spongios-** *sponge*	Spongelike tissue

EXERCISES

A. Recall and review. *Become familiar with the terms pertaining to the spermatic ducts and accessory gland and how they depict clinical conditions related to the male reproductive system. Fill in the blanks.* **LO 14.1 and 14.5**

1. After leaving the testis, sperm are stored in the _____.

2. The _____ glands secrete a fluid that neutralizes the pH in the male urethra.

3. The walnut-sized gland of the male reproductive system is the _____ gland.

4. The structure that empties semen into the urethra is the _____ duct.

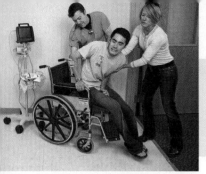

Rick Brady/McGraw-Hill Education

Disorders of the Testes (LO 14.4 and 14.6)

Testicular torsion is the twisting of a testis on its spermatic cord. The testicular artery in the twisted cord becomes blocked, and the blood supply to the testis is cut off. The condition occurs in men between puberty and age 25. In half the cases, it starts in bed at night.

Varicocele is a condition in which the veins in the spermatic cord become dilated and painful as with varicose veins often seen in the legs. If uncomfortable, it can be treated by surgically tying off the affected veins.

Hydrocele is a collection of excess fluid in the space between the visceral and parietal layers of the tunica vaginalis of the testis *(Figure 14.9)*. It is most common after age 40. The diagnosis can be confirmed by transillumination *(Figure 14.9)*, shining a bright light on the scrotal swelling to see the shape of the testis through the surrounding translucent excess fluid. If this condition does not resolve on its own a needle can be used to aspirate and remove the extra fluid.

Spermatocele is a collection of sperm in a sac formed in the epididymis, which is the sperm-containing tube attached to a testicle. It occurs in about 30% of men, is benign, and rarely causes symptoms. It does not require treatment unless it becomes uncomfortable.

Cryptorchism (cryptorchidism) occurs when a testis fails to descend from the abdomen into the scrotum before a boy is 12 months old.

Epididymitis is an inflammation of the epididymis; **epididymoorchitis** is an inflammation of the epididymis and testis. **Orchitis,** an inflammation of either testis (or both), is usually a consequence of epididymitis. In each of these cases, the inflammation is most commonly caused by a bacterial infection spreading from an infection in the urinary tract or prostate. These infections can also be caused by sexually transmitted diseases **(STDs),** also called sexually transmitted infections **(STIs)** like gonorrhea or chlamydia.

Mumps is a viral cause of orchitis. In males past puberty who develop mumps, 30% will develop orchitis, and 30% of those will develop resulting testicular atrophy. A bilateral infection can result in infertility. Mumps is avoidable by immunization in childhood.

Testicular cancer is the most common cancer in males aged 20 to 39 years. One of the first signs is often a lump in the testis, which may be found through testicular self-examination **(TSE).** Metastasis is uncommon, but it can be seen in the lungs, in the abdominal and cervical lymph nodes, and occasionally in the brain.

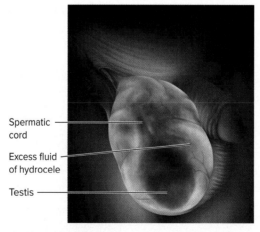

Spermatic cord

Excess fluid of hydrocele

Testis

▲ **FIGURE 14.9**
Transillumination of Hydrocele Showing Testis and Spermatic Cord.

Brian Evans/Science Source

WORD	PRONUNCIATION	ELEMENTS		DEFINITION
cryptorchism cryptorchidism (syn)	krip-**TOR**-kizm	S/ P/ R/	-ism *condition* crypt- *hidden* -orch- *testicle*	Failure of one or both testes to descend into the scrotum
epididymitis	**EP**-ih-did-ih-**MY**-tis	S/ R/	-itis *inflammation* epididym- *epididymis*	Inflammation of the epididymis
epididymoorchitis *(same as orchitis)* (**Note:** *One of the two consecutive "i"s is not used.*)	ep-ih-**DID**-ih-moh-or-**KIE**-tis	S/ R/CF R/	-itis *inflammation* epididym/o- *epididymis* -orchi- *testicle*	Inflammation of the epididymis and testicle
hydrocele	**HIGH**-droh-seal	S/ R/CF	-cele *swelling* hydr/o- *water*	Collection of fluid in the space of the tunica vaginalis
orchitis (**Note:** *One of the two consecutive "i"s is not used.*)	or-**KIE**-tis	S/ R/	-itis *inflammation* orchi- *testicle*	Inflammation of the testis
spermatocele	**SPER**-mat-oh-seal	S/ R/CF	-cele *swelling* spermat/o- *sperm*	Cyst of the epididymis that contains sperm
torsion	**TOR**-shun		Latin *to twist*	The act or result of twisting
varicocele	**VAIR**-ih-koh-seal	S/ R/CF	-cele *swelling* varic/o- *varicosity*	Varicose veins of the spermatic cord

Disorders of the Prostate Gland (LO 14.6)

Benign prostatic hyperplasia (BPH), also known as benign prostatic hypertrophy or **benign enlargement of the prostate (BEP)**—a noncancerous enlargement of the prostate—can cause symptoms starting around age 45; by age 80, up to 90% of men may have symptoms. This enlargement is one of **hyperplasia** (number of cells) rather than **hypertrophy** (size of cells), and it compresses the prostatic urethra to produce symptoms including:

- Difficulty starting and stopping the urine stream.
- **Nocturia** (excessive nighttime urination), **polyuria** (excessive urine production), and dysuria (difficulty or pain in urination).

    Prostatic cancer affects 10% of men over the age of 50, and its incidence is increasing. It forms hard nodules in the periphery of the gland and is often asymptomatic (produces no symptoms) in its early stages, as it does not compress the urethra.

    Prostatitis is an inflammation of the prostate gland that causes groin pain and difficulty and discomfort when urinating.

Male Infertility (LO 14.6 and 14.7)

Infertility is the inability of a couple to conceive after one year of unprotected intercourse. **Male infertility** is the man's inability to produce or deliver fully functioning sperm. The main causes of male infertility are:

- Impaired sperm production, due to cryptorchidism, anorchism (absence of one or both testes), testicular trauma, testicular cancer, or orchitis after puberty.
- Impaired sperm delivery, due to infections and blockage of spermatic ducts.
- **Sperm disorders,** in which sperm are underdeveloped, abnormally shaped, unable to move properly, produced in abnormally low numbers (**oligospermia**), or not produced at all (**azoospermia**).
- **Varicoceles**, in which the dilated scrotal veins impair sperm production by preventing proper drainage of blood within the testes.
- Testosterone deficiency (**hypogonadism**). Phthalates in plastics and dioxins in paper are examples of environmental endocrine disrupters that can contribute to testosterone deficiency.

Keynotes

- Erectile dysfunction occurs in some 30 million American men.
- Erectile dysfunction can be associated with diabetes, stroke, multiple sclerosis, hypertension, cigarette smoking, radiation therapy, drugs such as antidepressants and cholesterol-lowering medications, and loss of interest in one's sexual partner.
- Survival from prostate cancer is over 99% if it is detected before it spreads outside the gland.
- Male infertility is involved in up to 50% of couples attempting to conceive.
- Vasectomy is almost 100% successful in producing male sterility.

Abbreviations

BEP	benign enlargement of the prostate
BPH	benign prostatic hyperplasia
ED	erectile dysfunction
PSA	prostate-specific antigen

WORD	PRONUNCIATION		ELEMENTS	DEFINITION
azoospermia	a-zoh-oh-**SPER**-me-ah	S/ P/ R/ R/	-ia *condition* a- *without* -zoo- *animal* -sperm- *seed*	Absence of living sperm in the semen
oligospermia	**OL**-ih-go-**SPER**-me-ah	P/	oligo- *too few*	Deficient numbers of sperm in the semen
hyperplasia	**HIGH**-per-**PLAY**-zee-ah	S/ P/ R/	-ia *condition* hyper- *excessive* -plas- *molding, formation*	Increase in the *number* of cells in a tissue or organ
hypertrophy	high-**PER**-troh-fee	P/ R/	hyper- *excessive* -trophy *development*	Increase in the *size* of the cells in a tissue or organ
hypogonadism	**HIGH**-poh-**GOH**-nad-izm	S/ P/ R/	-ism *condition* hypo- *deficient* -gonad- *testis or ovary*	Deficient gonad production of sperm, eggs, or hormones
infertility	in-fer-**TIL**-ih-tee	S/ P/ R/	-ity *condition* in- *not* -fertil- *able to conceive*	Failure to conceive
nocturia	nok-**TYU**-ree-ah	S/ P/ R/	-ia *condition* noct- *night* -ur- *urine*	Excessive urination at night
polyuria	pol-ee-**YOU**-ree-ah	S/ P/ R/	-ia *condition* poly- *excessive* -ur- *urine*	Excessive production of urine
prostatitis	pros-tah-**TIE**-tis	S/ R/	-itis *inflammation* prostat- *prostate*	Inflammation of the prostate
transurethral	**TRANS**-you-**REE**-thral	S/ P/ R/	-al *pertaining to* trans- *across, through* -urethr- *urethra*	Procedure performed through the urethra

- Three million cases of chlamydia and trichomoniasis infections and and 1.6 million new gonorrhea infections are recognized annually in the United States and can be prevented by abstinence or by using a **condom**.

Disorders of the Penis (LO 14.6)

Disorders involving the penis range from minor injuries to STDs to cancer. These conditions are outlined below.

Trauma to the penis can vary from being caught in a pants' zipper to being fractured while erect during vigorous sexual activity.

Priapism is a persistent, painful erection that occurs when blood cannot escape from the erectile tissue. It can be caused by drugs like epinephrine, by blood clots, or by spinal cord injury.

Cancer of the penis occurs most commonly on the glans and is rare in circumcised men.

Erectile dysfunction (ED), or **impotence,** is the inability to achieve or maintain a satisfactory erection. Treatment is aimed at addressing any underlying disease.

Premature ejaculation is more common than erectile dysfunction. It occurs when a man ejaculates so quickly during intercourse that it causes distress or embarrassment to one or both partners.

Disorders of the Prepuce (LO 14.6)

- **Balanitis** is an infection of the glans and foreskin with bacteria or yeast.

- **Phimosis** is a condition in which the foreskin is tight because of a small opening and cannot be retracted over the glans for cleaning. This can lead to balanitis.

- **Paraphimosis** is a condition in which the retracted foreskin cannot be pulled forward to cover the glans.

Disorders of the Penile Urethra (LO 14.6)

Urethritis is an inflammation of the urethra. It can be caused by bacteria, STDs, viruses, and chemical irritants from **spermicides** and contraceptive gels.

Urethral stricture is scarring that narrows the urethra. It results from infection or injury.

Hypospadias is a congenital defect in which the opening of the urethra is on the undersurface of the penis instead of at the head of the glans. It can be corrected surgically.

Epispadias is a congenital defect in which the opening of the urethra is on the dorsum of the penis.

WORD	PRONUNCIATION	ELEMENTS		DEFINITION
balanitis	bal-ah-**NIE**-tis	S/ R/	-itis *inflammation* balan- *glans penis*	Inflammation of the glans and prepuce of the penis
epispadias	ep-ih-**SPAY**-dee-as	S/ P/ R/	-ias *condition* epi- *above* -spad- *tear or cut*	Condition in which the urethral opening is on the dorsum of the penis
hypospadias		P/	hypo- *below*	Urethral meatus on the underside of the penis
impotence	**IM**-poh-tence		Latin *inability*	Inability to achieve an erection
phimosis	fih-**MOH**-sis	S/ R/	-osis *condition* phim- *muzzle*	A condition where the prepuce cannot be retracted
paraphimosis	**PAR**-ah-fih-**MOH**-sis	P/	para- *abnormal*	Condition in which a retracted prepuce cannot be pulled forward to cover the glans
priapism	**PRY**-ah-pizm		Priapus, mythical Roman god of procreation	Persistent erection of the penis

Sexually Transmitted Diseases (STDs) (LO 14.3, 14.6, and 14.8)

According to the Centers for Disease Control and Prevention **(CDC)**, 15 million new cases of sexually transmitted diseases (STDs) are reported annually in the United States. Adolescents and young adults have the greatest risk of contracting STDs.

Chlamydia is known as the "silent" disease because up to 75% of infected women and men have no symptoms. When there are signs, a vaginal or penile discharge and irritation with dysuria (difficult or painful urination) are common.

Trichomoniasis ("trich") is caused by the parasite **Trichomonas** *vaginalis*. In women, it can produce a frothy yellow-green vaginal discharge with irritation and itching of the vulva. Because it is a "ping-pong" infection that goes back and forth between partners, both individuals should be treated.

Gonorrhea is spread by unprotected sex and can be passed on to a baby in childbirth, causing a serious eye infection. As with chlamydia, newborns receive antibiotic eyedrops to prevent eye infections from gonorrhea. Symptoms include a vaginal discharge, bleeding, and dysuria.

Syphilis is transmitted sexually and can spread through the bloodstream to every organ in the body. **Primary syphilis** begins 10 to 90 days after infection as an ulcer or **chancre** at the infection site. Four to ten weeks later, if the primary syphilis is not treated, **secondary syphilis** appears as a rash on the palms of the hands and the soles of the feet. Swollen glands and muscle and joint pain accompany the rash. **Tertiary syphilis** can occur years after the primary infection and cause permanent damage to the brain, with dementia.

Genital herpes simplex is a disease caused by the virus herpes simplex 2 **(HSV2)**. It manifests with painful genital sores *(Figure 14.10),* which can recur throughout life *(Figures 14.10 and 14.11).* **Herpes of the newborn** *(Figure 14.11)* occurs when a pregnant woman with genital herpes sores delivers her baby vaginally and transmits the virus to the baby.

Human papilloma virus (HPV) causes genital warts in both men and women. HPV can also cause changes to the cells in the cervix. Some strains of the virus can increase a woman's risk for cervical cancer.

Molluscum contagiosum is a virus that can be sexually transmitted and produces small, shiny bumps that contain a milky-white fluid. They can disappear and reappear anywhere on the body.

Human immunodeficiency virus (HIV) is a virus that attacks the immune system and usually leads to **acquired immune deficiency syndrome (AIDS)**. HIV is carried in body fluids and transmitted during unprotected sex. Sharing needles can spread the virus. The virus can also pass from an infected pregnant woman to her unborn child, so she must take medications to protect the baby. HIV damages the immune system, allowing infections to develop that the body would normally cope with easily. These are **opportunistic infections** and include herpes simplex, candidiasis, and syphilis.

Abbreviations

AIDS	acquired immunodeficiency syndrome
CDC	Centers for Disease Control and Prevention
HIV	human immunodeficiency virus
HPV	human papillomavirus
HSV2	herpes simplex virus 2

Vesicles

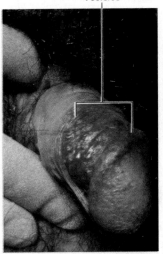

▲ **FIGURE 14.10**
Genital Herpes Simplex in Male.

Clinical Photography, Central Manchester University Hospitals NHS Foundation Trust, UK/Science Source

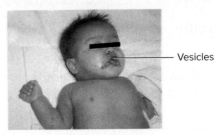

Vesicles

◀ **FIGURE 14.11**
Newborn Infant with Herpes Simplex.

Source: JD Millar/Centers for Disease Control and Prevention

WORD	PRONUNCIATION		ELEMENTS	DEFINITION
acquired immunodeficiency syndrome (AIDS)	ah-**KWIRED** **IM**-you-noh-dee-**FISH**-en-see	S/ R/CF R/	**acquired,** Latin *obtain* **-ency** *condition* **immun/o-** *immune response* **-defici-** *lacking, inadequate*	Infection with the HIV
	SIN-drohm	P/ R/	**syn-** *together* **-drome** *running*	Combination of signs and symptoms associated with a particular disease process
chancre	**SHAN**-ker		Latin *cancer*	Primary lesion of syphilis
chlamydia	klah-**MID**-ee-ah		Latin *cloak*	An STD caused by infection with *Chlamydia,* a species of bacteria
condom	**KON**-dom		Old English *sheath or cover*	A sheath or cover for the penis or vagina to prevent conception and infection
gonorrhea	gon-oh-**REE**-ah	S/ R/CF	**-rrhea** *flow, discharge* **gon/o-** *seed*	Specific contagious sexually transmitted infection
herpes simplex virus (HSV)	**HER**-peez **SIM**-pleks **VIE**-rus	R/	**herpes** Greek *spreading skin eruption* **virus** *poison*	An infection that manifests with painful, watery blisters on the skin and mucous membranes
human immunodeficiency virus (HIV)	**HYU**-man **IM**-you-noh-dee-**FISH**-en-see **VIE**-rus	R/ S/ R/CF R/	**human** *human being* **-ency** *condition* **immun/o-** *immune response* **-defici-** *lacking, inadequate* **virus,** Latin *poison*	Etiologic agent of acquired immunodeficiency syndrome (AIDS)
human papilloma virus (HPV)	**HYU**-man pap-ih-**LOW**-mah **VIE**-rus	R/ S/ R/	**human** *human being* **-oma** *tumor* **papill-** *pimple* **virus,** Latin *poison*	Causes warts on the skin and genitalia and can increase the risk for cervical cancer
molluscum contagiosum (**Note:** "S" in "sum" added to enable word to flow.) (*modern word contagious*)	moh-**LUS**-kum kon-**TAY**-jee-oh-sum	S/ R/ R/CF	**-um** *structure* **mollusc-** *soft* **contagi/o-** *transmissible by contact*	STD caused by a virus
opportunistic infection (**Note:** TWO suffixes)	**OP**-or-tyu-**NIS**-tik in-**FEK**-shun	S/ S/ R/	**-ic** *pertaining to* **-ist-** *agent, specialist* **opportun-** *take advantage of*	An infection that causes disease when the immune system is compromised for other reasons
syphilis	**SIF**-ih-lis		Principal character in a Latin poem	Sexually transmitted disease caused by a spirochete
Trichomonas	trik-oh-**MOH**-nas	R/CF R/	**trich/o-** *hair* **-monas** *single unit*	A parasite causing an STD
trichomoniasis	**TRIK**-oh-moh-**NIE**-ah-sis	S/ R/	**-iasis** *condition* **-mon-** *single*	Infection with *Trichomonas vaginalis*

EXERCISES

 ## Case Report 14.1

You are . . .

. . . an EMT-P working in the Emergency Department at Fulwood Medical Center.

You are communicating with . . .

. . . Joseph Davis, a 17-year-old high school senior, who has been brought in by his mother at 0400 hrs.

Joseph is complaining of **(c/o)** a sudden onset of pain in his left **testicle**, which began 3 hours earlier and woke him up. The pain is intense and caused him to vomit. VS: T 99.2°F, P 98, R 26, BP 137/75. An examination reveals his left testicle to be enlarged, warm, and tender. His abdomen is normal to palpation.

At your request, Dr. Helinski, the emergency physician on duty, examines Joseph immediately. He diagnoses a **torsion** (twisting) of the patient's left testicle.

Joseph Davis presented with typical symptoms and signs of testicular torsion. The affected testis rapidly became painful, tender, swollen, and inflamed. Emergency surgery was performed, and the testis and cord were manually untwisted through an incision in the scrotum. The testis was stitched to surrounding tissues to prevent a recurrence of the torsion.

A. Using *the information presented in Case Report 14.1, document the case in the patient's record. Use the following terms to fill in the blanks. One term will be used twice.* **LO 14.2 and 14.6**

testicular	testes	testicle

This patient presented to the ED because of pain in his left (1.) _____. Both (2.) _____ were examined, but the left (3.) _____ was enlarged, warm, and tender. The emergency physician on duty diagnosed (4.) _____ torsion. Patient will be scheduled for surgery immediately.

Case Report 14.2

You are . . .

. . . a certified surgical technologist (CST) working for urologist Phillip Johnson, MD, in the Urology Clinic at Fulwood Medical Center.

You are communicating with . . .

. . . Mr. Ronald Detrick, a 60-year-old man, who has been referred to the Urology Clinic.

Patient Interview

Mr. Detrick complains of having to get out of bed to urinate four or five times at night. He has difficulty starting urination, has a weak stream, and feels he is not emptying his bladder completely. He has lost interest in sex. His physical examination is unremarkable except that a digital rectal examination (DRE) reveals a diffusely enlarged **prostate** with no nodules.

B. Read *Case Report 14.2 and then answer the following questions. Fill in the blanks.* **LO 14.2, 14.3, 14.5, 14.6, 14.10, 14.11, and 14.12**

1. Does Mr. Detrick have a strong libido? _____

2. What does the abbreviation *DRE* mean? _____

3. Which gland had an abnormality? _____

4. Did Dr. Johnson find any other abnormalities? (yes or no) _____

5. What is responsible for Mr. Detrick's symptoms? _____

C. Construct *medical terms related to disorders of the testes. Fill in the blanks.* **LO 14.1, 14.2, 14.4, and 14.6**

1. Inflammation of the epididymis:_____/itis

2. Failure of a testicle to descend into the scrotum: _____/_____/ism

3. Swelling containing fluid: _____/cele

4. Inflammation of the testis: orch/_____

5. Varicose veins of the spermatic cord: varico/_____

D. Build your knowledge *of the language of the male reproductive system by correctly answering the questions regarding the elements in the following terms. Select the best answer.* **LO 14.1 and 14.6**

1. In the term *hydrocele,* the R/CF means:

   a. testis   **b.** water   **c.** sperm

2. In the term *cryptorchism,* the element *crypt-* means:

    a. outside of   **b.** behind   **c.** hidden

3. In the term *spermatocele,* the suffix means:

    a. water   **b.** swelling   **c.** sperm

4. In the term *epididymitis,* which element means inflammation?

    a. epi   **b.** epididym   **c.** itis

5. In the term *epididymoorchitis,* the element *orchi* means:

    a. threadlike   **b.** testicle   **c.** hidden

E. Translate *medical terms into everyday language. Use the terms below to correctly fill in the blanks. Not all terms will be used.* **LO 14.1, 14.2, 14.6, and 14.12**

ur-   -ia   -itis   -uria   -urism   -uritis

hyperplasia   hypertrophy   hypogonadism   nocturia   oligospermia   polyuria

The root (1) _____ means urine. The suffix (2) _____ means condition. Therefore when you read or hear the combination of (3) _____, it means a condition of urine.

The suffix (4) _____ means inflammation.

A person that produces a more than normal amount of urine has (5) _____. To be more specific with a urinary condition, when a person complains of having to urinate a lot at night, he/she has (6) _____. In men, these conditions may be due to (7) _____ of the prostate gland.

F. Remember *the definitions related to male infertility. Select the correct answer(s) to complete each statement.* **LO 14.6 and 14.7**

1. Male infertility is defined as the inability to: (choose two answers)

    a. produce sperm   **c.** secrete adequate amounts of prostatic fluid

    b. have unprotected sex   **d.** deliver fully functioning sperm

2. The term **hypogonadism** is defined as:

    a. undescended testicle(s)   **b.** lack of seminal fluid   **c.** testosterone deficiency   **d.** reduced production of sperm

3. A lack of sperm production can be caused by: (choose all that apply)

    a. dioxins in paper   **b.** decreased libido   **c.** dilated scrotal veins   **d.** absence of one or both testicles

G. Construct *the correct medical term to match the definition that is given. Insert the appropriate element on the line.* **LO 14.1, 14.2, 14.6, and 14.8**

1. Infection with *Trichomonas:* _____/ _____ / _____

2. Inflammation of glans and prepuce: _____ / _____

3. General term that means that an infection occurred due to a compromised immune system:

    _____ / _____ / _____

4. Contagious STD infection that can often be treated with one shot of antibiotics:

    _____ / _____

5. Term that means *soft structure:*

    _____ / _____

Section 14.4

Diagnostic and Therapeutic Procedures and Pharmacology

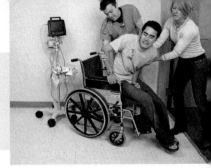

Rick Brady/McGraw-Hill Education

Diagnostic Procedures (LO 14.3 and 14.9)

A **digital rectal examination (DRE),** in which a lubricated, gloved finger is inserted into the rectum, is part of a routine physical examination in men and women. In men, it is used to check for enlargement or other abnormalities of the prostate gland.

Prostate-specific antigen (PSA) is a protein produced by cells of the prostate gland, and the PSA test measures the level of PSA in a man's blood. The level is increased in cancer of the prostate, benign prostatic hyperplasia (BPH), and acute prostatitis.

Prostate biopsy is commonly performed under ultrasound guidance to remove samples of tissue for pathologic analysis. MRI-guided biopsies or a hybrid of MRI images with ultrasound also can be used.

A **DNA probe** is a diagnostic test where a sample of the affected area is taken with a cotton swab. The sample is then analyzed for the presence of the DNA of bacteria *Chlamydia trachomatis* and/or *Neisseria gonorrhoeae.*

Therapeutic Procedures (LO 14.3 and 14.9)

Circumcision, the removal of the foreskin, can be indicated in an adult for pathological phimosis, **refractory** balanoposthitis, and chronic urinary tract infections. In many religions, circumcision is a ritual in the neonatal period or an elective procedure at varying ages before puberty. In the United States, 85% of all males are circumcised in the neonatal period. In Europe, only about 10% are circumcised.

Orchiopexy is a **surgical** procedure to move an undescended testicle (cryptorchid) from the abdomen into the scrotum and permanently fix it there.

Orchiectomy (orchidectomy) is the removal of one or both testicles performed for testicular cancer, sex reassignment surgery for transgender women and advanced prostate cancer to stop the production of testosterone.

Urethrotomy is incision of the urethra to relieve stricture caused by injury or infection.

Transurethral resection of the prostate (TURP) surgically treats benign prostatic hypertrophy (BPH). This procedure utilizes a **resectoscope,** which is inserted through the penile urethra to remove prostate tissue obstructing the urethra; **transurethral incision of the prostate (TUIP),** widens the urethra by incision in the neck of the bladder and in the prostate gland; laser surgery, which removes prostate tissue by **ablation** (melting) or **enucleation** (cutting) through insertion of a scope through the penile urethra; or open simple **prostatectomy,** in which the portion of the prostate gland blocking urine flow is removed through incisions or **laparoscopy** in the abdomen.

Cancer of the prostate can be treated with **active surveillance** for early-stage, asymptomatic, slow-growing lesions; external beam **radiation therapy** or **brachytherapy,** in which many rice-sized radioactive seeds are implanted in the prostate; **cryosurgery,** in which small needles containing a very cold gas are inserted in the cancer using ultrasound images as guidance; **radical prostatectomy,** to remove the prostate gland, surrounding tissue, and lymph nodes surgically; and **chemotherapy.**

In a **vasectomy,** performed under local anesthesia, the ductus deferens is pulled through a small incision in the scrotum and cut in two places, a 1-centimeter segment is removed, and the ends are cauterized and tied *(Figure 14.12).* The procedure to reverse (repair) a vasectomy is called a **vasovasostomy.**

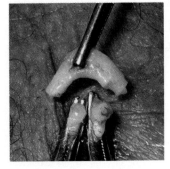

▲ **FIGURE 14.12**
Vasectomy Being Performed.

SPL/Science Source

Pharmacology (LO 14.3 and 14.9)

BPH can be treated medically with **alpha blockers** to relax the bladder neck muscles and muscle fibers in the prostate gland and/or **5-alpha reductase inhibitors,** which block hormones that spur the growth of the gland.

- **Prostate cancer** can be treated with **hormone therapy** using medications that stop the body from producing testosterone, which prostate cancer cells need to grow, or **anti-androgens** that block testosterone from reaching the cancer cells.

- Antibiotics are indicated to treat **prostatitis**, which is usually a bacterial infection and requires treatment with appropriate **antibiotics**.

Treatment of the underlying cause of **erectile dysfunction** can relieve the difficulty of achieving or maintaining an erection, and phosphodiesterase type 5 inhibitors **(PDE5)** such as *Viagra* and *Cialis* are now in common use. Less common treatments are a penile prosthesis or a penile pump.

Abbreviation

PDE5   phosphodiesterase type 5 inhibitor

Treatment for STDs (LO 14.3 and 14.8)

- **Antibiotic therapy** treats chlamydia, syphilis, trichomoniasis, and gonorrhea. A vaccine is available that can prevent lasting infections with strains that cause cervical cancers and genital warts. The vaccine can be given to females aged 9 to 26, before they are sexually active. The vaccine can be given to males aged 9 to 26 years to reduce the likelihood of acquiring genital warts.

- **Antiviral** medications can provide a clinical benefit by limiting the **replication** of the herpes virus.

- **HIV AIDS** There is no cure for HIV or AIDS, but combinations of anti-HIV medications can be taken to stop the replication of the virus in the cells of the body, and to slow the progression of the disease. However, a person may develop resistance to the medications.

WORD	PRONUNCIATION		ELEMENTS	DEFINITION
ablation	ab-**LAY**-shun	S/ P/ R/	**-ion** *action* **ab-** *away from* **-lat-** *to take*	Removal of tissue to destroy its function
brachytherapy	brah-kee-**THAIR**-ah-pee	P/ R/CF	**brachy-** *short* **-therapy** *treatment*	Radiation therapy in which the source of irradiation is implanted in the tissue to be treated
circumcision	ser-kum-**SIZH**-un	S/ P/ R/	**-ion** *process, action* **circum-** *around* **-cis-** *to cut*	To remove part or all of the prepuce
cryosurgery	cry-oh-**SUR**-jer-ee	S/ R/CF R/	**-ery** *process of* **cry/o-** *icy cold* **-surg-** *operate*	Use of liquid nitrogen or argon gas to freeze and kill abnormal tissue
digital	**DIJ**-ih-tal	S/ R/	**-al** *pertaining to* **digit-** *finger or toe*	Pertaining to a finger or toe
enucleation	ee-**NEW**-klee-**AY**-shun	S/ P/ R/	**-ation** *process* **e-** *out of, from* **-nucle-** *kernel*	Removal of an entire structure without rupture
laparoscope	**LAP**-ah-roh-skope	S/ R/CF	**-scope** *instrument for viewing* **lapar/o** *abdomen*	Endoscope to view the contents of the abdomen
laparoscopy	lap-ah-**ROS**-koh-pee	S/	**-scopy** *to view*	Endoscopic examination of the contents of the abdomen
orchiectomy (orchidectomy)	or-kee-**ECK**-toh-mee	S/ R/	**-ectomy** *surgical excision* **orchi-** *testicle*	Removal of one testis or both testes
orchiopexy	**OR**-kee-oh-**PEK**-see	S/ R/CF	**-pexy** *surgical fixation* **orchi/o-** *testicle*	Surgical fixation of a testis in the scrotum
prostatectomy	pross-tah-**TEK**-toh-mee	S/ R/	**-ectomy** *surgical excision* **prostat-** *prostate*	Surgical removal of the prostate
radical surgery	**RAD**-ih-kal **SUR**-jeh-ree	 S/ R/	**radical** Latin *root* **-ery** *condition, process of* **surg-** *operate*	Surgical procedure in which the affected organ is removed along with the blood and lymph supply to that organ.
replication	rep-lih-**KAY**-shun	S/ R/	**-ation** *process of* **replic-** *reply*	Reproduction to produce an exact copy
resection	ree-**SEK**-shun	S/ P/ R/	**-ion** *action* **re-** *back* **-sect-** *cut off*	Removal of a specific part of an organ or structure
resectoscope	ree-**SEK**-toe-skope	S/ R/CF	**-scope** *instrument for viewing* **resect/o-** *cut off*	Endoscope for the transurethral removal of lesions
surgical	**SUR**-jih-kal	S/ R/	**-ical** *pertaining to* **surg-** *operate*	Relating to surgery
urethrotomy	you-ree-**THROT**-oh-mee	S/ R/CF	**-tomy** *surgical incision* **urethr/o-** *urethra*	Incision of a stricture of the urethra
vasectomy	vah-**SEK**-toh-mee	S/ R/	**-ectomy** *surgical excision* **vas-** *duct*	Excision of a segment of the ductus (vas) deferens
vasovasostomy (also called vasectomy reversal)	**VAY**-soh-vay-**SOS**-toh-mee	S/ R/CF	**-stomy** *new opening* **vas/o-** *duct*	Reanastomosis of the ductus deferens to restore the flow of sperm

EXERCISES

A. Language of urology: *Refine your knowledge of urological terminology by selecting the correct term to complete the statement. Select the best choice. Be precise, and watch the spelling!* **LO 14.4 and 14.9**

1. Condition in which a retracted prepuce cannot be pulled forward to cover the glans:

   a. hypospadias   **b.** phimosis   **c.** spongiosum   **d.** paraphimosis

2. To remove all or part of the prepuce:

   a. circumcision   **b.** circumscion   **c.** circummcision   **d.** circumsion

3. Skin that covers the glans penis:

    a. forskin   **b.** fourskin   **c.** forksin   **d.** foreskin

4. Fold of mucous membrane:

    a. frennulum   **b.** freeulum   **c.** freenulum   **d.** frenulum

5. Abbreviation for the procedure in which a finger is inserted into the rectum to evaluate the prostate gland:

    a. DRE   **b.** BEP   **c.** BPH   **d.** TSE

B. Construct medical terms. *Fill in the blanks.* **LO 14.1, 14.2, and 14.9**

1. Use of liquid nitrogen to freeze abnormal tissue.   _____ /surgery

2. Removal of a specific part of an organ or tissue.   re/_____ /ion

3. Excision of a section of the ductus deferens.   vas/_____

4. Surgical fixation of a testis in the scrotum.   _____ /pexy

5. Pertaining to a finger or toe.   _____ /al

6. Removal of tissue to destroy its function.   _____ /lat/ion

7. Removal of entire structure without rupture.   e/_____ /ation

8. Radiation therapy for which the source of radiation is implanted into the tissue to be treated.   _____ /therapy

C. Pronunciation is important whether you are saying the word or listening to a word from a coworker. Identify the proper pronunciation of the following medical terms. **LO 14.2**

1. The correct pronunciation for varicose veins of the spermatic cord

    a. high-**DROH**-seal   **c.** **TOR**-shun

    b. **VAIR**-ih-koh-seal   **d.** **KRIP**-tork-ism

Correctly spell the term: _____

2. The correct pronunciation for the coiled tub attached to the testis

    a. **SKROH**-tal   **c.** epi-**DID**-uh-muss

    b. **SKROHT**-um   **d.** **EP**-ih-**DID**-ih-miss

Correctly spell the term: _____

3. The correct pronunciation for a condition in which the urethral opening is on the dorsum of the penis.

    a. ep-ih-**SPAY**-dee-as   **c.** **HIGH**-poh-spay-**DEE**-ass

    b. **EPEE**-spay-**DIH**-as   **d.** high-poh-**SPAY**-dee-as

Correctly spell the term: _____

4. The correct pronunciation for the removal of an entire structure without rupture.

    a. **EE**-nuh-klee-**AY**-shun   **c.** **VAY**-soh-**SOS**-toh-mee

    b. ee-**NEW**-klee-**AY**-shun   **d.** **VAY**-soh-saws-**TOH**-mee

Correctly spell the term: _____

5. The correct pronunciation for the fold of mucous membrane between the glans and the prepuce

    a. **PREE**-puce   **c.** **FREN**-you-lum

    b. preep-**UCE**   **d.** fren-**YULE**-um

Correctly spell the term: _____

Additional exercises available in **connect**

Chapter Review exercises, along with additional practice items, are available in Connect!

The Female Reproductive System

The Essentials of the Languages of Gynecology and Obstetrics

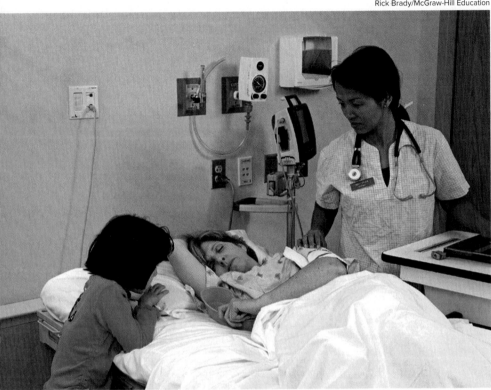

Rick Brady/McGraw-Hill Education

Learning Outcomes

As a health care professional in the area of **gynecology** and **obstetrics,** it is essential that you become familiar not only with the functions and structures of the female reproductive system but also with its associated medical terminology. To provide patients with the best possible care, you will need to be able to:

LO 15.1 Use roots, combining forms, suffixes, and prefixes to construct and analyze (deconstruct) medical terms related to the female reproductive system.

LO 15.2 Spell and pronounce correctly medical terms related to the female reproductive system in order to communicate them with accuracy and precision in any health care setting.

LO 15.3 Define accepted abbreviations related to the female reproductive system.

LO 15.4 Relate the anatomy and physiology of the female reproductive system.

LO 15.5 Identify and describe disorders and pathological conditions related to the female reproductive system.

LO 15.6 Identify gynecologic diagnostic and therapeutic procedures and pharmacologic agents used for gynecologic disorders.

LO 15.7 Describe conception and development during pregnancy and the perinatal period.

LO 15.8 Identify and describe disorders and pathological conditions related to obstetrics.

LO 15.9 Identify diagnostic and therapeutic procedures and pharmacologic agents used in treating obstetric disorders.

LO 15.10 Relate the structure of the breast to its disorders and to the development of lactation.

LO 15.11 Define diagnostic and therapeutic procedures and pharmacology for disorders of the breast.

LO 15.12 Identify health professionals involved in the care of patients with gynecologic and obstetrical disorders.

LO 15.13 Apply your knowledge of medical terms relating to the female reproductive system to documentation, medical records, and medical reports.

LO 15.14 Translate the medical terms relating to the female reproductive system into everyday language in order to communicate clearly with patients and their families.

The health professionals involved in the diagnosis and treatment of problems with the female reproductive system include:

- **Gynecologists** (GYN) are physicians who are specialists in diseases of the female reproductive tract.
- **Obstetricians** (OB) are physicians who are specialists in the care of women during pregnancy and childbirth.
- **Neonatologists** are physicians who are pediatric subspecialists in disorders of the newborn, particularly ill or premature infants.
- **Perinatologists** are physicians who are obstetric subspecialists in the care of the mother and fetus who are at higher-than-normal risk for prebirth complications.
- **Certified midwives/nurse-midwives** (CNM) are independent practitioners who provide care to mothers during pregnancy, delivery, and birth, and to mothers and newborn infants for 6 weeks after birth.
- **Obstetrical–gynecological nurse practitioners** (GNP) are registered nurses with at least a master's degree and specialized training who have acquired skills in the management of health and illness for women throughout their life cycle.

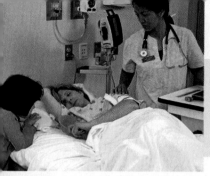

Rick Brady/McGraw-Hill Education

Section 15.1

Female Reproductive System

External Genitalia (LO 15.4)

Vulva (LO 15.4)

The female external genitalia occupy most of the perineum and are collectively called the **vulva**. The structures of the vulva *(Figure 15.1a)* include the:

• **Mons pubis,** a mound of skin and adipose or fatty tissue overlying the symphysis pubis.

• **Labia majora,** a pair of thick folds of skin, connective tissue, and adipose tissue.

• **Labia minora,** a pair of thin folds of hairless skin immediately internal to the labia majora. Anteriorly, the labia minora join together to form the prepuce (hood) of the **clitoris**. The clitoris is a small erectile body capped with a glans. Posteriorly, these structures merge with the labia majora.

• **Vestibule**, the area enclosed by the labia minora. It contains the urinary and vaginal openings.

Deep into the labia majora on each side of the vaginal **orifice** (opening) is a pea-sized **greater vestibular (Bartholin)** gland *(Figure 15.1b)*. These glands secrete mucus to lubricate the vulva and vagina, and this secretion increases during sexual stimulation.

▶ **FIGURE 15.1** Female Perineum and Vulva.
(a) Surface anatomy.
(b) Subcutaneous structures.

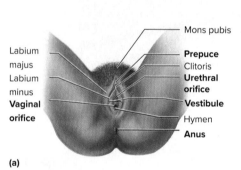

(a)

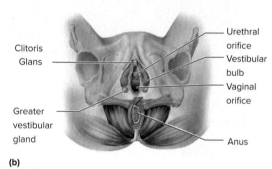

(b)

Word Analysis and Definition

S = Suffix   P = Prefix   R = Root   R/CF = Combining Form

WORD	PRONUNCIATION		ELEMENTS	DEFINITION
clitoris	**KLIT**-oh-ris		Greek *clitoris*	Erectile organ of the vulva
labium labia (pl)	**LAY**-bee-um **LAY**-bee-ah		Greek *lip*	Fold of the vulva
majus majora (pl)	**MAY**-jus mah-**JOR**-ah		Latin *greater*	Bigger or greater; e.g., the labia majora
minus minora (pl)	**MY**-nus mih-**NOR**-ah		Latin *smaller*	Smaller or lesser; e.g., the labia minora
mons pubis	MONZ **PYU**-bis		mons, Latin *mountain* pubis Latin *pubic bone*	Fleshy pad with pubic hair, overlying the pubic bone
orifice	**OR**-ih-fis		Latin *an opening*	Any opening or aperture
vestibule vestibular (adj) vestibular bulb	**VES**-tih-byul ves-**TIB**-you-lar ves-**TIB**-you-lar BULB	S/ R/	Latin *entrance* **-ar** *pertaining to* **vestibul-** *vestibule* Latin *bulb, onion*	Space at the entrance of a canal Pertaining to the vestibule Structure on each side of the entrance to the vagina
vulva vulvar (adj)	**VUL**-vah **VUL**-var	S/ R/	Latin *a wrapper or covering* **-ar** *pertaining to* **vulv-** *vulva*	Female external genitalia Pertaining to the vulva

Female Reproductive Tract (LO 15.4)

Ovaries (LO 15.4)

The primary female sex organs are the **ovaries**. The related internal accessory organs include a pair of **uterine tubes**, a **uterus**, and a vagina. Women are born with all the eggs (**ova**) that they will release in their lifetimes, but it is not until puberty that the eggs mature and start to leave the ovary.

Each **ovary** is an almond-shaped organ about 1 inch long and ½ inch in diameter. The ovaries are held in place by ligaments that attach them to the pelvic wall and uterus *(Figure 15.2)*. The ovaries' main functions are to:

- produce and release eggs; and
- secrete hormones that affect puberty, menstruation, and pregnancy.

Uterine (Fallopian) Tubes (LO 15.4)

Each **uterine (fallopian) tube** is a canal about 4 inches long that extends from the uterus and opens to the abdominal cavity near an ovary. At the ovarian end, the outer third of the tube flares out into finger-like folds, each of which is called a **fimbria**. At **ovulation**, the **fimbriae** enclose the ovary *(Figure 15.3)* and sweep the ovum into the uterine tube. Each tube's main function is to enable sperm and eggs to meet and fertilize.

Uterus (LO 15.4)

The **uterus** is a thick-walled, muscular organ in the pelvic cavity. The main functions of the uterus are to cradle and nourish the fetus from conception to birth and to produce a woman's monthly menstrual flow (period). Anatomically, the uterus is divided into these three regions:

- The **fundus** is the broad, curved upper region between the lateral attachments of the uterine (fallopian) tubes;
- The **body** is the midportion; and
- The **cervix** is the cylindrical inferior portion that projects into the vagina.

The cavity of the uterus is triangular, with its upper two corners receiving the openings of the uterine tubes. Its lower end communicates with the vagina through the cervical canal, which has an **internal os** (opening) from the lumen and an **external os** into the vagina *(see Figure 15.3)*. The uterus is supported by the muscular floor of the pelvic outlet and by ligaments that extend to the pelvic wall from the uterus and cervix.

The wall of the uterus has three layers. Starting at the outside layer, these are the:

- **Perimetrium**—a thin layer of connective tissue.
- **Myometrium**—a thick layer of smooth muscle.
- **Endometrium**—the lining that sheds in menstruation.

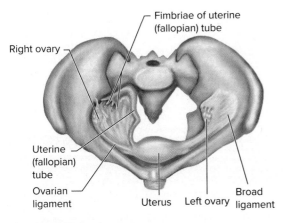

▲ **FIGURE 15.2** Ovaries.
The ovaries are located on each side of the pelvis against the lateral walls of the pelvic cavity. The right uterine (fallopian) tube is retracted to reveal the ovarian ligament.

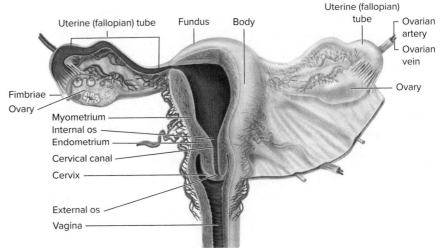

▲ **FIGURE 15.3** Female Reproductive Tract.

Vagina (LO 15.4)

The **vagina,** or birth canal, is a fibromuscular tube that measures 4 to 5 inches long. It connects the vulva with the uterus *(Figure 15.4)* and has three main functions:

- To discharge menstrual fluid;
- To receive the penis and semen; and
- To deliver a baby.

The vagina is located between the rectum and the urethra. The urethra is embedded in the anterior wall of the vagina.

At its posterior end, the vagina extends beyond the **cervix** of the uterus and forms arch-shaped blind spaces called the anterior and posterior **fornices.** The lower end of the vagina contains numerous crosswise folds.

These folds project into the vaginal opening to form the hymen, which stretches across the opening. The **hymen** contains one or two openings to allow menstrual fluid to escape.

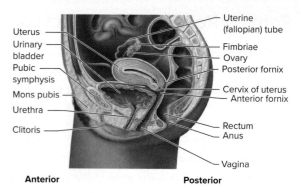

▲ FIGURE 15.4 Female Reproductive Organs.

Word Analysis and Definition

S = Suffix   P = Prefix   R = Root   R/CF = Combining Form

WORD	PRONUNCIATION	ELEMENTS		DEFINITION
cervix cervical (adj) (Note: *This term also means* pertaining to the neck region.)	**SER**-viks **SER**-vih-kal	S/ R/	Latin *neck* -al *pertaining to* **cervic-** *neck*	Lower part of the uterus Pertaining to the cervix
endometrium endometrial (adj)	en-doh-**ME**-tree-um en-doh-**ME**-tree-al	S/ P/ R/CF S/	-um *tissue* endo- *within, inside* -metr/i- *uterus* -al *pertaining to*	Inner lining of the uterus Pertaining to the inner lining of the uterus
fimbria fimbriae (pl)	**FIM**-bree-ah **FIM**-bree-ee		Latin *fringe*	Fringelike structure
fornix fornices (pl)	**FOR**-niks **FOR**-nih-seez		Latin *a vault*	Arch-shaped, blind-ended part of the vagina behind and around the cervix
fundus	**FUN**-dus		Latin *bottom*	The upper, rounded top of the uterus above the openings of the uterine tubes
hymen	**HIGH**-men		Greek *membrane*	Thin membrane partly occluding the vaginal orifice
myometrium	my-oh-**MEE**-tree-um	S/ R/CF R/CF	-um *tissue* my/o- *muscle* -metr/i- *uterus*	Muscle wall of the uterus
os	**OS**		Latin *mouth*	Opening into a canal; e.g., the cervix
ovary ovaries (pl) ovarian (adj)	**OH**-vah-ree **OH**-vah-reez oh-**VAIR**-ee-an	 S/ R/	Latin *egg* -an *pertaining to* ovari- *ovary*	One of the paired female reproductive glands Pertaining to the ovary(ies)
ovulation ovulate (verb)	**OV**-you-**LAY**-shun **OV**-you-late	S/ R/ S/	-ation *process* ovul- *egg* -ate *composed of, pertaining to*	Release of an oocyte from a follicle To release an oocyte from a follicle
ovum ova (pl)	**OH**-vum **OH**-vah		Latin *egg*	Egg
perimetrium	**PAIR**-ih-**MEE**-tree-um	S/ P/ R/CF	-um *structure* peri- *around* -metr/i- *uterus*	The covering of the uterus; part of the peritoneum
uterus uterine (adj) uterine tubes (also called fallopian tubes)	**YOU**-ter-us **YOU**-ter-in **YOU**-ter-ine TUBES fah-**LOH**-pee-an-**TUBES**	S/ R/	Latin *womb* -ine *pertaining to* uter- *uterus* Gabrielle Falloppio, Italian anatomist, 1523–1562	Organ in which an egg develops into a fetus Pertaining to the uterus Tubes connected from the uterus to the abdominal cavity. Carry the ovum from the ovary to the uterus.
vagina vaginal (adj)	vah-**JIE**-nah **VAJ**-ih-nal	 S/ R/	Latin *sheath* -al *pertaining to* vagin- *vagina*	The female genital canal extending from the uterus to the vulva Pertaining to the vagina

Ovarian Hormones (LO 15.4)

The ovaries of the sexually mature female secrete the hormones estrogen and progesterone.

Estrogens are produced in the ovarian follicles and their sexual functions are to:

1. Convert girls into sexually mature women through **thelarche**, **pubarche**, and **menarche**;

2. Regulate the menstrual cycle; and

3. Be involved in pregnancy when it occurs.

Progesterone is produced by the ovary's corpus luteum and also by the adrenal glands *(see Chapter 12)*. Its sexual functions are to:

1. Prepare the lining (endometrium) of the uterus for implantation of the egg *(Figure 15.3)*;

2. Inhibit lactation during pregnancy; and

3. Produce menstrual bleeding if pregnancy does not occur.

The ovaries also secrete small amounts of androgens, which are male hormones.

Uterine (Menstrual) Cycle (LO 15.4)

The **menstrual** cycle averages 28 days in length. Physiologists recognize the beginning of the sexual cycle as **menstruation**, which occurs for the first 3 to 5 days. After menstruation, developing ovarian follicles mature, and one of them releases an **oocyte** around day 14. After this ovulation, the lining of the uterus hypertrophies, and the residual ovarian **follicle** becomes a secretory gland, which then **involutes** around day 26 to form an inactive scar called a **corpus luteum**. At this time, the arteries supplying the lining of the uterus contract. This leads to ischemia, tissue necrosis, and the start of menstruation.

Word Analysis and Definition

S = Suffix   P = Prefix   **R = Root   R/CF = Combining Form**

WORD	PRONUNCIATION		ELEMENTS	DEFINITION
corpus luteum	**KOR**-puss **LOO**-tee-um		corpus Latin *body* luteum Latin *yellow*	Yellow structure formed at the site of a ruptured ovarian follicle
estrogen	**ES**-troh-jen	S/ **R/CF**	-gen *produce* **estr/o-** *woman*	Generic term for hormones that stimulate female secondary sex characteristics
follicle	**FOLL**-ih-kull		Latin *small sac*	Spherical mass of cells containing a cavity, such as a hair follicle
involution involute (verb)	in-voh-**LOO**-shun in-voh-**LOOT**	S/ P/ R/	-ion *process* in- *in* -volut- *shrink*	A decrease in size.
menarche	meh-**NAR**-key	S/ R/	-arche *beginning* **men-** *month*	First menstrual period
menses (noun) menstruation (noun)	**MEN**-seez men-stru-**AY**-shun	S/ R/	Latin *month* -ation *process* **menstru-** *menses*	Monthly uterine bleeding Same as *menses*
menstruate (verb) menstrual (adj)	**MEN**-stru-ate **MEN**-stru-al	S/ S/	-ate *composed of, pertaining to* -al *pertaining to*	Act of menstruation Pertaining to menstruation
oocyte	**OH**-oh-site	S/ R/	-cyte *cell* **oo-** *egg*	Female egg cell
progesterone (**Note:** *Two suffixes*)	pro-**JESS**-ter-own	S/ S/ P/ R/	-one *hormone, chemical substance* -er- *agent, one who does* pro- *before* **-gest-** *pregnancy*	Hormone that prepares the uterus for pregnancy
pubarche	pyu-**BAR**-key	S/ R/	-arche *beginning* **pub-** *pubis*	Onset of development of pubic and axillary hair
thelarche	thee-**LAR**-key	S/ R/	-arche *beginning* **thel-** *breast, nipple*	Onset of breast development

EXERCISES

A. Some Latin and Greek terms cannot be further deconstructed into prefix, root, or suffix. *Match the meaning in the first column with the correct medical term in the second column.* **LO 15.4**

_____	1. a covering or wrapper	a. labium
_____	2. a vault	b. vulva
_____	3. lesser	c. vagina
_____	4. lip	d. fornix
_____	5. pubic bone	e. pubis
_____	6. sheath	f. minora

B. Identify *the meanings of the word elements and terms related to the structures of the female reproductive system. Select the correct answer.* **LO 15.1 and 15.4**

1. Which term has an element meaning *menses?*

   a. menstruate   b. fallopian   c. ova

2. Which term refers to *egg?*

   a. menses   b. fallopian   c. ova

3. What other term means the same thing as *menses?*

   a. uterine   b. fallopian   c. menstruation

4. The plural of ovum is

   a. oval   b. oveas   c. ova

5. What is another name for the fallopian tubes?

   a. urinary tubes   b. uterine tubes   c. ureteral tubes

C. Meet lesson and chapter objectives *with the language of the female reproductive system. Fill in the blanks.* **LO 15.2 and 15.4**

1. Which body cavity contains the uterus? _____

2. What is the main function of the uterine tubes? _____

3. What two functions does the uterus have? _____

4. In the female reproductive system, where does the os open into? _____

5. What hormone is released by the ovarian follicles? _____

6. What is the medical term that means the *first* menstrual period? _____

D. Select *the correct pair of terms related to the question.* **LO 15.2 and 15.4**

1. Which two terms are structures inside the uterus?

   a. myocardium and pericardium   d. myometrium and endometrium

   b. perineum and periosteum   e. sphincter and meatus

   c. endocardium and myocardium

2. Name the regions of the uterus:

   a. fundus and os   c. fundus, cervix, and body

   b. fundus, os, and body   d. hypogastric, cervical, and fundus

3. Which pair of terms is associated with the production of progesterone?

   a. pubarche and menarche   d. fornix and myometrium

   b. fundus and cervix   e. fimbriae and urethra

   c. adrenal glands and corpus luteum

Section 15.2

Disorders of the Female Reproductive Tract

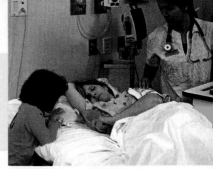

Rick Brady/McGraw-Hill Education

Disorders of the Vulva and Vagina (LO 15.5)

Bacterial vaginosis is the most common cause of **vaginitis** in women of childbearing age. The main symptom is an abnormal vaginal discharge with a fishlike odor. With bacterial vaginosis, different types of invading bacteria outnumber the vagina's normal bacteria. This disorder is diagnosed by a lab examination of a vaginal swab specimen, and it is treated with antibiotics.

Toxic shock syndrome (TSS) is a life-threatening illness caused by **toxins** (poisons) circulating in the bloodstream. It is theorized that bacteria in the vagina are encouraged to grow by the presence of a superabsorbent **tampon** that is not changed frequently *(see Case Report 15.1).* These bacteria produce toxins that are absorbed into the bloodstream. Other risk factors for TSS include skin wounds and surgery.

Vulvovaginal candidiasis, also known as yeast infection, is a common cause of genital itching or burning with a "cottage-cheese" vaginal discharge. It is caused by an overgrowth of the yeast fungus *Candida* and can occur after taking antibiotics.

Vulvovaginitis *(Figure 15.5)* describes vaginal inflammation and can be caused by allergic and irritative agents found in vaginal hygiene products, spermicides, detergents, and synthetic underwear.

Vulvodynia is a chronic, severe pain around the vaginal orifice, which causes a raw sensation. Painful intercourse (**dyspareunia**) is common. The vulva may look normal or be slightly swollen. The etiology (cause) is unknown.

Disorders of the Ovaries (LO 15.4 and 15.5)

Ovarian Cysts (LO 15.4 and 15.5)

Ovarian cysts are fluid-filled sacs that can form, often during ovulation. They are usually benign and symptom-free unless they bleed or rupture, or an ovary becomes twisted.

Polycystic ovarian syndrome (PCOS), describes the formation of multiple follicular cysts in both ovaries *(Figure 15.6).* The repeated cyst formation prevents any eggs from maturing or being released, so ovulation does not occur and progesterone is not produced. Without progesterone, a female's menstrual cycle is irregular or absent.

Ovarian cysts produce androgens, which prevent ovulation and produce acne, a male-pattern hair loss from the front of the scalp, and weight gain. Women with PCOS are also at increased risk for endometrial cancer, type 2 diabetes, high blood cholesterol, hypertension, and heart disease.

> **Keynotes**
>
> - Bacterial vaginosis is associated with increased risk of gonorrhea and HIV infection.
> - Of all adult women, 75% have at least one genital yeast infection in their lifetimes.
> - Ten million office visits annually are for vulvodynia.

> **Abbreviations**
>
> PCOS   polycystic ovarian syndrome
>
> TSS   toxic shock syndrome

▼ **FIGURE 15.6**
Polycystic Ovary.

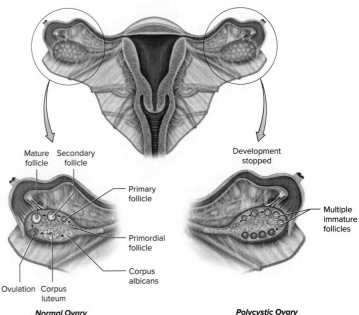

Vulvovaginitis

Mature follicle   Secondary follicle

Primary follicle

Primordial follicle

Corpus albicans

Ovulation   Corpus luteum

Normal Ovary

Development stopped

Multiple immature follicles

Polycystic Ovary

▶ **FIGURE 15.5**
Patient with
Vulvovaginitis.

Dr P. Marazzi/Science Source

Section 15.2 Disorders of the Female Reproductive Tract   403

Abbreviations

PID	pelvic inflammatory disease
PMS	premenstrual syndrome disease
STD	sexually transmitted disease

Keynotes

- In postmenopausal women, the risk of heart disease becomes almost the same as that of men.
- Oral contraceptives are 80% to 90% effective in relieving symptoms of PMS.
- The peak incidence of ovarian cancer is in the 50- and 60-year age groups.

Disorders of the Uterine Tubes (LO 15.3, 15.4, and 15.5)

Salpingitis is an inflammation of the uterine (fallopian) tubes and is part of pelvic inflammatory disease (**PID**). A bacterial infection, often from a sexually transmitted disease (**STD**), spreads from the vagina through the cervix and uterus. Symptoms are lower abdominal pain, fever, and a vaginal discharge.

Menstrual Disorders (LO 15.4 and 15.5)

Disorders of menstruation have many causes and are not simply disorders of the ovaries or uterus.

Primary amenorrhea occurs when a girl has not menstruated by age 16. This can occur with or without other signs of puberty.

Causes of primary amenorrhea include: drastic weight loss from malnutrition, dieting, bulimia, or anorexia nervosa; extreme exercise, as in some young gymnasts; extreme obesity; and chronic illness. Treatment is directed at the basic cause.

Secondary amenorrhea occurs when a woman who has menstruated normally misses three or more periods in a row and she is not pregnant or in her **menopause**.

The causes of secondary amenorrhea include: ovarian disorders, such as polycystic ovarian syndrome; excessive weight loss, low body fat percentage (e.g., as in athletes), or excessive exercise (e.g., as in marathon runners); and certain drugs, including antidepressants.

Primary dysmenorrhea, or **premenstrual syndrome (PMS),** refers to pain or discomfort associated with menstruation. The pain often begins 1 or 2 days before menses, peaks on the first day, and then slowly subsides.

Secondary dysmenorrhea is pain associated with disorders such as infection in the genital tract or endometriosis.

Menopause (LO 15.5)

Menopause is diagnosed when a woman has not menstruated for a year and is not pregnant. In this normal, natural, biological process of reproductive aging, levels of estrogen and progesterone start to decline around the age of 40, and most women stop menstruating between the ages of 45 and 55.

Without estrogen and progesterone, the uterus, vagina, and breasts atrophy, and more bone is lost than is replaced. Blood vessels constrict and dilate in response to changing hormone levels and can cause the characteristic menopausal "hot flashes."

WORD	PRONUNCIATION	ELEMENTS		DEFINITION
amenorrhea	a-men-oh-**REE**-ah	S/ P/ R/CF	-rrhea *flow, discharge* a- *without* -men/o- *menses*	Absence or abnormal cessation of menstrual flow
dysmenorrhea	dis-men-oh-**REE**-ah	S/ P/ R/CF	-rrhea *flow, discharge* dys- *painful or difficult* -men/o- *menses*	Painful and difficult menstruation
dyspareunia	dis-pah-**RUE**-nee-ah	S/ P/ R/	-ia *condition* dys- *painful* -pareun- *lying beside, sexual intercourse*	Pain during sexual intercourse
menopause (**Note:** *This term has no suffix, only a combining form and root.*)	**MEN**-oh-paws	R/ R/CF	-pause *cessation* men/o- *menses*	Permanent ending of menstrual periods
menopausal (adj)	**MEN**-oh-paws-al	S/	-al *pertaining to*	Pertaining to the menopause
polycystic	pol-ee-**SIS**-tik	S/ P/ R/	-ic *pertaining to* poly- *many* -cyst- *sac*	Composed of many cysts
premenstrual	pree-**MEN**-stru-al	S/ P/ R/	-al *pertaining to* pre- *before* -menstru- *menses*	Pertaining to the time immediately before the menses
primary	**PRY**-mair-ee		Latin *first*	The first disease or symptom, after which others may occur as complications
salpingitis	sal-pin-**JIE**-tis	S/ R/	-itis *inflammation* salping- *tube*	Inflammation of the uterine (fallopian) tube
secondary	**SEK**-ond-air-ee		Latin *following or second*	Diseases or symptoms following a primary disease or symptom
tampon	**TAM**-pon		French *plug*	Plug or pack in a cavity to absorb or stop bleeding
toxin toxic (adj)	**TOK**-sin **TOK**-sick	S/ R/	Greek *poison* -ic *pertaining to* tox- *poison*	Poisonous substance formed by a cell or organism Pertaining to a toxin
vaginosis	vah-jih-**NOH**-sis	S/ R/	-osis *condition* vagin- *vagina*	A disease of the vagina
vaginitis	vah-jih-**NIE**-tis	S/	-itis *inflammation*	Inflammation of the vagina
vulvodynia	vul-voh-**DIN**-ee-uh	S/ R/CF	-dynia *pain* vulv/o- *vulva*	Chronic vulvar pain
vulvovaginal	**VUL**-voh-**VAJ**-ih-nal	S/ R/CF R/	-al *pertaining to* vulv/o- *vulva* -vagin- *vagina*	Pertaining to the vulva and vagina
vulvovaginitis	**VUL**-voh-vaj-ih-**NIE**-tis	S/	-itis *inflammation*	Inflammation of the vulva and vagina

Disorders of the Uterus (LO 15.3, 15.4, and 15.5)

Endometriosis is said to affect 1 in 10 American women of childbearing age. Here, the endometrium becomes implanted outside the uterus on the uterine tubes, the ovaries, and the pelvic peritoneum. The displaced endometrium continues to go through its monthly cycle. It thickens and bleeds, leads to cysts and scar tissue, and produces pain. The cause of endometriosis is unknown.

Salpingitis is an inflammation of the uterine (fallopian) tubes and is part of pelvic inflammatory disease (**PID**). A bacterial infection, often from a sexually transmitted disease (**STD**), spreads from the vagina through the cervix and uterus. Symptoms are lower abdominal pain, fever, and a vaginal discharge.

Uterine Prolapse (LO 15.4 and 15.5)

The uterus is normally supported by the pelvic floor's muscles, ligaments, and connective tissue. However, a difficult childbirth, aging, obesity, lack of exercise, chronic coughing, and chronic constipation can weaken these tissues, causing the uterus to descend into the vaginal canal *(Figure 15.7)*. Uterine prolapse can be accompanied by **prolapse** of the bladder and anterior vaginal wall (**cystocele**), or by prolapse of the rectum and posterior wall of the vagina (**rectocele**).

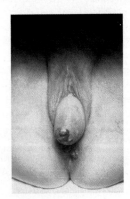

▲ **FIGURE 15.7**
Prolapsed Uterus
Protruding from the
Vagina.

BSIP/UIG/Getty Images

Retroversion of the uterus is a common variation, found in 20% of women. In retroversion, the body of the uterus is tipped backward instead of forward (**anteversion**). It can also be caused by lax pelvic muscles and ligaments, pelvic adhesions (scar tissue in the pelvis following salpingitis), or pelvic inflammatory disease. Retroversion by itself does not cause symptoms, and treatment is not usually necessary.

Uterine Fibroids (LO 15.4 and 15.5)

Uterine **fibroids** are noncancerous growths that appear during childbearing years. Three out of four women have them, but only one out of four women experiences their symptoms, which include **menorrhagia**, **metrorrhagia**, **polymenorrhea**, lower back pain, and pelvic pain.

Fibroids are also called **fibromyomas**, **leiomyomas**, or **myomas** *(Figure 15.8)*. They arise in the **myometrium** and produce a pale, firm, rubbery mass separate from the surrounding tissue. They vary in size from seedlings to large masses that distort the uterus. They can protrude into the uterine cavity, causing menorrhagia, or project outside the uterus and press on the bladder or rectum, thereby producing symptoms.

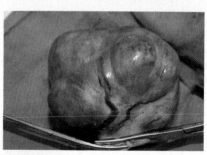

◀ **FIGURE 15.8** Large Tri-fold Fibroid in the Uterus.

Universal Images Group North America LLC/ Alamy Stock Photo

Word Analysis and Definition

S = Suffix   P = Prefix   R = Root   R/CF = Combining Form

WORD	PRONUNCIATION		ELEMENTS	DEFINITION
anteversion	an-teh-**VER**-shun	S/ P/ R/	-ion *action, condition* ante- *forward* -vers- *turn*	Forward displacement or tilting of a structure (in this case, the uterus)
cystocele	**SIS**-toh-seal	S/ R/CF	-cele *hernia* cyst/o- *bladder*	Hernia of the bladder into the anterior wall of the vagina
endometriosis	**EN**-doh-me-tree-**OH**-sis	S/ P/ R/CF	-osis *condition* endo- *within, inside* -metr/i- *uterus*	Endometrial tissue that functions outside the uterus
fibroid	**FIE**-broyd	S/ R/	-oid *resembling* fibr- *fiber*	Uterine tumor resembling fibrous tissue
fibromyoma	**FIE**-broh-my-**OH**-mah	S/ R/CF R/	-oma *tumor, mass* fibr/o- *fiber* -my- *muscle*	Benign neoplasm derived from smooth muscle and containing fibrous tissue
leiomyoma (also called *fibroid*)	**LIE**-oh-my-**OH**-mah	S/ R/CF R/	-oma *tumor, mass* lei/o- *smooth* -my- *muscle*	Benign neoplasm derived from smooth muscle
menorrhagia	men-oh-**RAY**-jee-ah	S/ R/CF	-rrhagia *flow, discharge* men/o- *menses*	Excessive menstrual bleeding
metrorrhagia	**MEH**-troh-**RAY**-jee-ah	S/ R/CF	-rrhagia *flow, discharge* metr/o- *uterus*	Irregular uterine bleeding between menses
myoma	my-**OH**-mah	S/ R/	-oma *tumor, mass* my- *muscle*	Benign tumor of muscle
polymenorrhea	**POL**-ee-men-oh-**REE**-ah	S/ P/ R/CF	-rrhea *flow* poly- *many, excessive* -men/o- *menses*	More than normal frequency of menses
prolapse	proh-**LAPS**		Latin *a falling*	The falling or slipping of a body part from its normal position
rectocele	**REK**-toe-seal	S/ R/CF	-cele *hernia* rect/o- *rectum*	Hernia of the rectum into the vagina
retroversion	reh-troh-**VER**-shun	S/ P/ R/	-ion *process, condition* retro- *backward* -vers- *turned*	The tipping backward of the uterus
retroverted	reh-troh-**VERT**-ed	S/	-ed *pertaining to*	Tilted backward

Endometrial Cancer (LO 15.5)

Ovarian cancer is the second most common gynecologic cancer after endometrial cancer. However, ovarian cancer accounts for more deaths than any other gynecologic cancer. Symptoms develop late in the disease process and are usually vague. Treatment is to surgically remove the tumor and administer chemotherapy. The 5-year survival rate depends on the location of the ovarian cancer but can be as high as over 90% in localized tumors.

Endometrial cancer is the fourth most common cancer in women, after lung, breast, and colon cancer. Each year, 40,000 new cases are diagnosed in the United States, mostly in women between ages 60 and 70. The most frequent symptom is vaginal bleeding after menopause.

Cervical cancer is less common than endometrial cancer, but 50% of cervical cancer cases occur between ages 35 and 55. Some 10,000 new cases are diagnosed in the United States each year. Early cervical cancer produces no symptoms. In the **precancerous** stage, abnormal cells (**dysplasia**) are found only in the outer layer of the cervix. Thirteen types of human papilloma virus (HPV) can convert these **dysplastic** cells to cancer cells.

Vaginal cancers are uncommon, comprising only 1% to 2% of gynecologic malignancies.

Other Causes of Abnormal Uterine Bleeding (LO 15.5)

Dysfunctional uterine bleeding is a term used when no cause can be found for a patient's menorrhagia.

Endometrial polyps are benign extensions of the endometrium that can cause irregular and heavy bleeding.

Female Infertility (LO 15.8)

Infertility is the inability to become pregnant after 1 year of unprotected intercourse. It affects 10% to 15% of all couples. The causes of infertility include:

- The female factor alone in 35% of cases.
- Male and female factors in 20% of cases.
- The male factor alone in 30% of cases.
- Unknown factors in 15% of cases.

Causes of female infertility include scarring of the uterine tubes, structural abnormalities of the uterus, and infrequent ovulation, all of which were addressed earlier in this chapter.

Word Analysis and Definition

S = Suffix   P = Prefix   R = Root   R/CF = Combining Form

WORD	PRONUNCIATION		ELEMENTS	DEFINITION
cancer	KAN-ser		Latin *crab*	General term for a malignant neoplasm
cancerous (adj)	KAN-ser-us	S/	-ous *pertaining to*	Pertaining to a malignant neoplasm
		R/	cancer- *cancer*	
precancerous (adj)	pree-KAN-ser-us	P/	pre- *before*	Lesion from which cancer can develop
dysfunctional	dis-FUNK-shun-al	S/	-al *pertaining to*	Difficulty in performing
		P/	dys- *painful, difficult*	
		R/	-function- *perform*	
dysplasia	dis-PLAY-zee-ah	S/	-ia *condition*	Abnormal tissue formation
		P/	dys- *painful, difficult*	
		R/	-plas- *development, formation*	
dysplastic (adj)	dis-PLAS-tik	S/	-tic *pertaining to*	Pertaining to or showing abnormal tissue formation
infertility	in-fer-TIL-ih-tee	S/	-ity *condition*	Inability to conceive over a long period of time
infertile (adj)	in-FER-tile	P/	in- *not*	
		R/	-fertil- *able to conceive*	
polyp	POL-ip		Latin *many feet*	Any mass of tissue that projects outward

Female Contraception (LO 15.4 and 15.6)

Contraception is the prevention of pregnancy. There are several common methods of contraception, including the approaches outlined below.

- **Behavioral methods:** These include **abstinence, coitus interruptus,** and the **rhythm method.** The latter two methods have a 20% failure rate.
- **Barrier methods:**

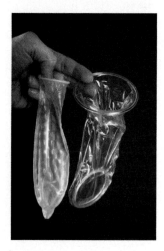

▲ **FIGURE 15.9** Male and Female Condoms.

Jill Braaten/McGraw-Hill Education

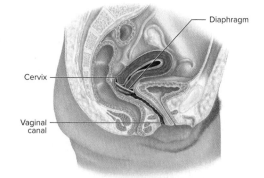

Diaphragm

Cervix

Vaginal canal

▲ **FIGURE 15.10** Diaphragm in Place.

- **Condoms** are available for males and females *(Figure 15.9)*. They have a 5% to 10% failure rate.
- **Diaphragms** *(Figure 15.10)* and **cervical caps** consist of a latex or rubber dome that is inserted into the vagina and placed over the cervix. When used with a spermicide, they have a 5% to 10% failure rate.
- **Spermicidal foams and gels** are inserted into the vagina. Used on their own, they have a 25% failure rate.
- **Intrauterine devices (IUDs)** are small plastic devices that are flexible and T-shaped and are placed high in the uterus. There are two types of IUDs: copper and hormonal.

The copper type is wrapped around the IUD *(ParaGard), which impairs the ability of sperm* to move, making it difficult for the sperm to reach the egg. It can be left in place for 5 to 10 years. Hormonal IUDs (Kileena, Liletta, Mirena, and Skyla) release progestin, which thickens cervical mucus making it difficult for sperm to enter the uterus and fertilize an egg. It can be left in place for 3 to 5 years.

Oral contraceptives usually contain the synthetic forms of the hormones progesterone (progestin) and estrogen (ethinyl estradiol). They work by (1) preventing ovulation, (2) thickening the cervical mucus to help prevent sperm from entering the uterus, and (3) making implantation in the uterine endometrium more difficult. They are taken for 3 weeks every month.

The **Minipill** contains only the synthetic progestin, and is taken every day, and functions in the same three ways as the oral contraceptives. It also stops the woman's menstrual period.

- **Hormonal methods:**
  - **Oral contraceptives** (birth control pills) utilize a mixture of estrogen and progesterone to prevent follicular development and ovulation. They have a 5% failure rate, usually due to inconsistent pill taking.
  - **Estrogen/progestin patches** deliver the hormones transdermally (through the skin). Their failure rate is below 1%.
    - **Injected progestins,** like Depo-Provera, are given by injection every 3 months. Their failure rate is below 1%.
    - **Implanted progestins**, like Norplant, are contained in porous silicone tubes that are inserted under the skin and slowly release the progestin for up to 5 years. Their failure rate is below 1%.
    - **Morning-after pills,** like Plan B, contain large doses of progestins to inhibit or delay ovulation. They are a backup when taken within 72 hours of unprotected intercourse. Their failure rate is around 10%.
    - **Mifepristone** (RU486), when taken with a prostaglandin, induces a miscarriage. It has an 8% failure rate.
    - **Tubal ligation** ("getting your tubes tied") is performed with laparoscopy. Both uterine (fallopian) tubes are cut, a segment is removed, and the ends are tied off and cauterized shut. The contraception failure rate is below 1%.

Word Analysis and Definition

S = Suffix   P = Prefix   R = Root   R/CF = Combining Form

WORD	PRONUNCIATION		ELEMENTS	DEFINITION
coitus postcoital (adj)	KOH-it-us post-KOH-ih-tal	S/ P/ R/	Latin *come together* -al *pertaining to* post- *after* -coit- *sexual intercourse*	Sexual intercourse After sexual intercourse
contraception	kon-trah-SEP-shun	S/ P/ R/	-ion *action, condition* contra- *against* -cept- *receive*	Prevention of pregnancy
contraceptive	kon-trah-SEP-tiv	S/	-ive *quality of*	An agent that prevents conception
diaphragm (Note: *Also the term for the muscle that separates the thoracic and abdominal cavities.*)	DIE-ah-fram		Greek *partition or wall*	A ring and dome-shaped material inserted into the vagina to prevent pregnancy
ligature ligate (verb) ligation (noun)	LIG-ah-chur LIE-gate lie-GAY-shun	 S/ S/ R/	Latin *band, tie* -ate *process* -tion *process* ligat- *tie up*	Thread or wire tied a tubal structure to close it Use of a tie to close a tube Tie off a structure, such as bleeding blood vessel
progestin	pro-JESS-tin	S/ P/ R/	-in *substance* pro- *before* -gest- *produce, gestation*	A synthetic form of progesterone

EXERCISES

Case Report 15.1

You are . . .

. . . a licensed practical nurse **(LPN)** working in the Emergency Department at Fulwood Medical Center.

You are communicating with . . .

. . . Ms. Lara Baker, a 32-year-old single mother who works in the billing department of the medical center. You have been asked to take her vital signs. For the past couple of days, she has had muscle aches and a general feeling of uneasiness that she thought was due to her heavy menstrual period. In the past 3 hours, she has developed a severe headache with nausea and vomiting. A diffuse rash over her trunk that looks like sunburn is now spreading to her upper arms and thighs. VS: T 104.2°F, P 120 and irregular, R 20, BP 86/50. As you took her VS, you noted that she did not seem to understand where she was. She was unable to pass a urine specimen. For this patient, the treatment she receives in the next few minutes is vital for her survival. You have your supervising nurse and the emergency physician come to see her immediately. As you participate in this patient's care, clear communication among the team members is essential.

Ms. Lara Baker presented to the Emergency Department with signs of toxic shock syndrome. Because of her heavy period, she was using a superabsorbent tampon.

She was admitted to intensive care. The tampon was removed and cultured. IV fluids and antibiotics were administered. Her kidney and liver functions were monitored. The causative organism was *Staphylococcus aureus*. She recovered well but had a second episode 6 months later.

A. Read *Case Report 15.1 and answer the following questions. Select the correct answer.* **LO 15.5**

1. What is Ms. Baker's diagnosis?

   a. vulvodynia   **b.** toxic shock syndrome   **c.** dyspareunia

2. The causative agent for her condition is:

   a. bacterial   **b.** viral

3. Antibiotics were given to her via:

   a. mouth   **b.** vagina   **c.** veins   **d.** arteries

Case Report 15.2

You are . . .

. . . a certified health education specialist **(CHES)** employed by Fulwood Medical Center.

You are communicating with . . .

. . . Ms. Claire Marcos, a 21-year-old student referred to you by Anna Rusak, MD, a gynecologist. Ms. Marcos has been diagnosed with polycystic ovarian syndrome **(PCOS),** and your task is to develop a program of self-care as part of her overall plan of therapy. From her medical record, you see that she presented with irregular, often-missed **menstrual** periods since the beginning of puberty; persistent acne; a loss of hair from the front of her scalp; and difficulty maintaining consistent bodyweight. She is 5 feet 4 inches tall and weighs 150 pounds. PCOS is a condition that is marked by uncontrollable weight gain. The pathophysiology of this condition is fat storage. Patient documentation includes height and weight. If the height and weight is average then the case report is not fat-shaming. You are expected to counsel her about her self-care program involving exercise, diet, and the use of birth control medications.

When Ms. Claire Marcos first presented in the gynecology clinic, Dr. Rusak examined her abdomen and pelvis. The doctor was able to palpate both enlarged ovaries on vaginal examination. A vaginal ultrasound scan showed multiple small cysts in each ovary. Dr. Rusack diagnosed Ms. Marcos with **polycystic ovarian syndrome,** and prescribed birth control pills because they contain estrogen and progesterone. The pills can correct the hormone imbalance, regulate Ms. Marcos' menses, and lower the level of testosterone to diminish her acne and hair loss problems.

B. Read *Case Report 15.2 along with the reading to fill in the blank with the correct answer to complete each statement.* **LO 15.4, 15.5, and 15.12**

1. In her past medical history, which symptom did Ms. Marcos have relating to her menstrual period?

_____ menstrual periods

2. What medication was prescribed for Ms. Marcos? _____

3. Give the abbreviation for the type of medical doctor that referred Ms. Marcos to you: _____

4. Ms. Marcos' acne and difficulty with weight control are likely due to (use the abbreviation): _____

C. Critical thinking. *Use Case Report 15.2 (continued) along with the reading to answer the following questions.* **LO 15.3, 15.4, and 15.5**

1. Ms. Marcos's ovaries were enlarged due to:

  a. cancer   **b.** endometriosis   **c.** cysts   **d.** testosterone

2. The abbreviation for her condition is:

  a. PMS   **b.** FSH   **c.** GnRH   **d.** PCOS

3. A consequence of her condition is that she does not:

  a. create oocytes   **b.** release oocytes   **c.** produce testosterone   **d.** have an appetite

4. Her condition is associated with what other condition?

  a. heart disease   **b.** peptic ulcer   **c.** decreased fat storage   **d.** hematuria

---

Case Report 15.3

You are ...

... a women's health nurse practitioner working with Anna Rusak, MD, a gynecologist at Fulwood Medical Center.

You are communicating with ...

... Mrs. Carol Isbell, a 29-year-old woman complains of severe **dysmenorrhea** since the age of 15. Mrs. Isbell has been unable to conceive after 2 years of unprotected intercourse. She experiences severe cramping and lower abdominal pain for 2 days before, during, and 2 days after her periods, which are very heavy. She also has lower abdominal pain on intercourse. Her physical examination is unremarkable except that her pelvic examination shows several tender masses on each side of a normal-sized uterus. Dr. Rusak has also examined her and agreed with your diagnosis of **endometriosis.** Mrs. Isbell is to have an ultrasound examination.

Study Hint

The combining form *metr/o* will be used to describe bleeding that is irregular. The combining form *men/o* will be used to describe bleeding that occurs at regular intervals.

D. Build the language of gynecology *by completing the medical term with the correct element.*
Fill in the blanks. **LO 15.1, 15.4, and 15.5**

1. Benign neoplasm derived from smooth muscle:

  leio/ _____ / _____

2. Irregular bleeding between menses: metro/_____

3. Permanent ending of menstrual periods: _____/pause

4. Uterine tumor resembling fibrous tissue: _____/oid

Note: *Although the suffix* **-oma** *means tumor (or mass), it is not necessarily a malignancy. Fibromyomas, leiomyomas, and myomas are all benign neoplasms or tumors.*

E. Deconstruct *medical terms related to disorders of the vulva and vagina. Fill in the chart.* **LO 15.1**

Medical Term	Suffix	Meaning of Suffix	Root/Combining Form	Meaning of Root/Combining Form
dyspareunia	1.	2.	3.	4.
vaginosis	5.	6.	7.	8.
salpingitis	9.	10.	11.	12.
toxic	13.	14.	15.	16.
vaginitis	17.	18.	19.	20.

F. Apply your knowledge *of the medical terminology for the female reproductive system by selecting the correct answer to each of the following questions. Select the best answer.* **LO 15.1, 15.4, and 15.5**

1. The permanent ending of menstrual periods is:

   a. menopause   **b.** dysmenorrhea   **c.** amenorrhea

2. *Premenstrual* happens:

   a. before menses   **b.** after menses   **c.** in the middle of menses

3. The gynecologic malignancy that accounts for the most deaths is:

   a. cervical cancer   **b.** breast cancer   **c.** ovarian cancer

4. Pick the term that contains a prefix, root, and suffix:

   a. menopause   **b.** secondary   **c.** premenstrual

5. In the medical term *dysmenorrhea,* the prefix *dys* means:

   a. without   **b.** first   **c.** painful

G. Deconstruct *the following medical terms into their elements with slashes. Then define the terms. Fill in the blanks.* **LO 15.1 and 15.5**

1. *menopause*   _____ / _____

   Definition: _____

2. *dysfunctional*   _____ / _____ / _____

   Definition: _____

3. *menopausal*   _____ / _____ / _____

   Definition: _____

4. *dysplastic*   _____ / _____ / _____

   Definition: _____

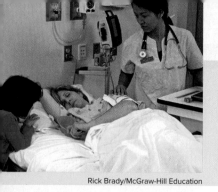
Rick Brady/McGraw-Hill Education

Section 15.3
Gynecologic Diagnostic and Therapeutic Procedures and Pharmacology

Abbreviations

D and C	dilation and curettage
GYN	gynecology
LEEP	loop electrosurgical excision procedure
CT	computed tomography
MRI	magnetic resonance imaging
WHNP	women's health nurse practitioner

Gynecologic Diagnostic Procedures (LO 15.6 and 15.12)

Gynecologists (GYN) are physicians who care for the female reproductive tract. A **Women's Health Nurse Practitioner (WHNP)** is a **nurse practitioner** caring for females from adolescence, annual Pap smear and breast exams and prenatal care. These professionals perform diagnostic and therapeutic procedures that diagnose and treat female reproductive tract disorders. **Palpation** (touching) and **visualization** are routinely used as diagnostic methods for the reproductive system. Visualization is a diagnostic component used to diagnose vaginitis, vulvovaginitis, discharges from sexually transmitted diseases, and vulvovaginal candidiasis. Swabs of the inflamed areas and discharges are sent to the lab for confirmation of condition.

Laparoscopy directly examines the uterus, fallopian tubes, and ovaries through a **laparoscope** inserted into the abdominal cavity through a small incision in the abdominal wall. Carbon dioxide can be pumped through the laparoscope to inflate the abdominal cavity so that the pelvic organs can be seen more clearly. It is used to diagnose uterine fibroids and is the gold standard for diagnosing endometriosis.

Procedures to view organs of the female reproductive tract:

A **speculum** is inserted into the vagina to visualize the tissue of the vaginal canal as well as take swabs or biopsies of these structures. These methods are used to diagnose vaginitis, vulvovaginitis, vulvovaginal candidiasis, and sexually transmitted diseases.

Colposcopy uses an instrument with a magnifying lens and a light called a **colposcope** to examine the lining of the vagina and cervical canal. Both colposcopy and cervical biopsy are often performed because a Pap test result was abnormal.

Hysteroscopy is the examination of the inside of the uterus using a thin, flexible, lighted tube called a **hysteroscope** to look for abnormalities of the cervical canal and endometrium.

Cervical biopsy is a procedure to remove tissue from the cervix for pathological testing for precancerous lesions or cervical cancer.

Endometrial biopsy—biopsy of the lining of the uterus—is performed to determine the cause of abnormal uterine bleeding and to check the effects of hormones on the endometrium. This procedure is useful to evaluate endometriosis, uterine fibroids, and polyps.

Dilation and **curettage** (D and C) is a surgical procedure in which the cervix is dilated so that the cervical canal and uterine endometrium can be scraped to remove abnormal tissues for pathological examination.

Loop electrosurgical excision procedure (LEEP) uses a wire loop heated by electricity to remove tissue from the vagina and cervix for pathological examination.

Conization is a procedure in which a cone-shaped piece of tissue is removed from the cervix with a laser, scalpel, or LEEP.

Radiologic procedures include **transabdominal ultrasound, transvaginal ultrasound, computed tomography (CT),** and **magnetic resonance imaging (MRI)** to scan and view pelvic organs, in particular uterine fibroids and polyps.

Pap Test (LO 15.3 and 15.5)

Pap test (also known as Pap smear) screens for cervical cancer. In a Pap test, the doctor brushes cells from the cervix *(Figure 15.11)*. The cells are smeared onto a slide or rinsed into a special liquid and sent to the laboratory for examination. This test enables abnormal cells (see *Figure 15.12*), precancerous or cancerous, to be detected. It is the most successful and accurate test for early detection of abnormalities. Current screening guidelines were last updated in April 2021 by the

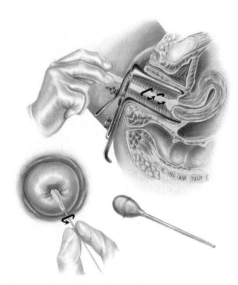

▲ **FIGURE 15.11**   Pap Smear Being Performed.

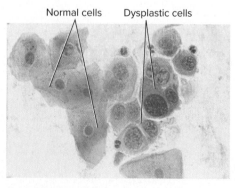
Normal cells   Dysplastic cells
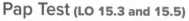

▲ **FIGURE 15.12**   Abnormal Pap Smear with Dysplastic Cells.

Parviz M. Pour/Science Source

American College of Obstetricians and Gynecologists. According to the guidelines, a Pap test should be scheduled as follows:

- **Initial Pap test**–at age 21.
- **Age 21 to 29**–every 3 years.
- **Age 30 to 65**–Pap and HPV cotesting every 5 years or Pap alone every 3 years.
- **Age 65 onward**–continue screening if risk factors are present including HIV infection, immunosuppression, previous treatment for precancerous cervical lesion or cervical cancer. Schedule individually with your doctor.
- **Any abnormal result** at any age mandates working out the best schedule for follow-up testing with your doctor.
- A Pap test is best performed 10 to 20 days after the first day of the **last menstrual period (LMP).**

More than 90% of abnormal **Papanicolaou (Pap)** smears are caused by HPV infections. A vaccine is now available that can prevent lasting infections from the two HPV strains that cause 70% of cervical cancers and another two strains that cause 90% of genital warts.

Infertility Testing (LO 15.3 and 15.5)

Diagnosing causes for infertility starts with a complete history and physical examination, including vagina and pelvic organs. Other diagnostic tools to determine the cause(s) for infertility include:

- **Hormone blood levels** of progesterone, estrogens, and FSH.
- **Ultrasound** of the abdomen, which can show the shape and size of the uterus, and vaginal ultrasound, which can show the shape and size of the ovaries.
- **Laparoscopy,** which allows inspection of the outside of the uterus and ovaries and removal of any scar tissue blocking tubes.
- **Postcoital testing,** in which the cervix is examined soon after unprotected intercourse to see if sperm can travel through into the uterus.
- **Hysterosalpingography** is a procedure in which X-rays (**hysterosalpingograms**) are taken after a radiopaque dye is injected through the cervix into the uterus through a slender catheter to outline the interior of the uterus and fallopian tubes *(Figure 15.13).* It can be used to help define the cause of female infertility or to confirm that a sterilization procedure to block the uterine tubes is successful.

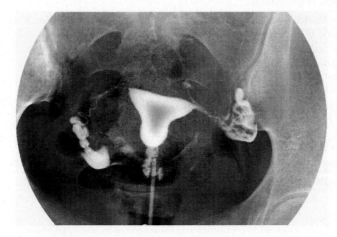

▲ **FIGURE 15.13**   Hysterosalpingogram of a Normal Uterus, Cervix, Uterine Tubes, and Ovaries.

Du Cane Medical Imaging Ltd/Science Source

WORD	PRONUNCIATION		ELEMENTS	DEFINITION
biopsy (Note: The "o" in the root *bio* is dropped from the spelling.)	BIE-op-see	S/ R/CF	-opsy *to view* bio- *life*	Removal of living tissue for laboratory examination
colposcopy	kol-POS-koh-pee	S/ R/CF	-scopy *to view* colp/o- *vagina*	Examination of vagina and cervix with an endoscope
colposcope	KOL-poh-scope	S/	-scope *instrument for viewing*	Endoscope to view the vagina and cervix
conization	koh-nih-ZAY-shun	S/ R/	-ation *process* coniz- *cone*	Surgical excision of a cone-shaped piece of tissue
curette curettage	kyu-RET kyu-reh-TAHZH	S/ R/	French *cleanse* -age *related to* curett- *to cleanse*	Instrument with sharpened edges for scraping Scraping of the interior of a cavity
dilation	die-LAY-shun		Latin *to spread out*	Artificial enlargement of an opening or hollow structure
excision	eck-SIZH-un	S/ R/	-ion *action* excis- *cut out*	Surgical removal of part or all of a structure
gynecology (GYN)	guy-nih-KOL-oh-jee	S/ R/CF	-logy *study of* gynec/o- *woman, female*	Medical specialty of diseases of the female reproductive tract
gynecologist	guy-nih-KOL-oh-jist	S/ S/	-logist *one who studies, specialist* -ic *pertaining to*	Specialist in gynecology
gynecologic (adj)	GUY-nih-koh-LOJ-ik	R/CF R/	gynec/o- *woman, female* -log- *to study*	Pertaining to gynecology
hysterosalpingogram	HIS-ter-oh-sal-PING-oh-gram	S/ R/CF R/CF	-gram *a record* hyster/o- *uterus* -salping/o- *uterine tube*	Radiograph of uterus and uterine tubes after injection of contrast material
hysteroscope hysteroscopy	HIS-ter-oh-skope his-ter-OS-koh-pee	S/ R/CF S/	-scope *instrument for viewing* hyster/o- *uterus* -scopy *to view*	Endoscope to visually examine the uterine cavity Visual examination of the uterine cavity
laparoscope	LAP-ah-roh-skope	S/ R/CF	-scope *instrument for viewing* lapar/o- *abdomen*	Endoscope to view the contents of the abdomen
laparoscopy	lap-ah-ROS-koh-pee	S/	-scopy *to view*	Endoscopic examination of the contents of the abdomen
palpate (verb) palpation (noun)	PAL-pate pal-PAY-shun	S/ R/	Latin *to touch* -ion *process, action* palpat- *touch, stroke*	To examine with the fingers and hands Examination using the fingers and hands
Pap test	PAP TEST		George Papanicolaou 1883–1962, Greek-U.S. physician and cytologist	Examination of cells taken from the cervix
postcoital	post-KOH-ih-tal	S/ P/ R/	-al *pertaining to* post- *after* -coit- *sexual intercourse*	After sexual intercourse
speculum specula (pl)	SPECK-you-lum SPECK-you-lah		Latin *a mirror*	An instrument inserted into a body orifice to enlarge its canal or cavity for inspection
swab	SWOB		Old English *to sweep*	Wad of cotton used to remove or apply something from/to a surface
ultrasound	ULL-trah-sound	P/ R/	ultra- *higher* -sound *noise*	Very high frequency sound waves

Abbreviation

LEEP   loop electrosurgical excision procedure

Gynecologic Therapeutic Procedures (LO 15.6)

Gynecologic surgical procedures can take place in the office or an operating room.

In-office procedures include those for cervical cancer. Treatment for cervical cancer depends on the stage of the cancer. In preinvasive cancer, when it is only in the outer layer of the lining of the cervix, treatment can include:

- **Conization.** A cone-shaped piece of tissue from around the abnormality is removed with a scalpel.
- **Loop electrosurgical excision procedure (LEEP).** A wire loop carries an electrical current to slice off cells from the mouth of the cervix.

- **Laser surgery.** A laser beam is used to kill precancerous and cancerous cells.
- **Cryosurgery.** Freezing is used to kill the precancerous and cancerous cells.

Dilation and curettage (D&C) involves dilating the entrance to the uterus through the cervix so that a thin instrument can be inserted to scrape or suction away the lining of the uterus.

Endometrial ablation is a heat-generating tool or a laser that removes or destroys the lining of the uterus and prevents or reduces menstruation. Endometrial ablation is used only in women who do not plan to have children.

Gynecologic surgeries performed in an operating room can be approached via the abdomen, vagina, or laparoscopically. **Robot-assisted laparoscopic** surgery uses sophisticated robotic surgical tools through a laparoscope.

Hysterectomy—removal of the uterus—is performed because of uterine fibroids, uterine cancer, and endometriosis.

- **Radical hysterectomy** removes the whole uterus, the cervix, and the top of the vagina; ovaries also may be removed.
- **Total hysterectomy** is removal of the whole uterus and cervix.
- **Subtotal hysterectomy** is removal of the upper uterus, leaving the cervix in place.

Treatment of rectocele, cystocele and prolapse of other pelvic organs depends on the severity of symptoms. Nonsurgical options include:

Physical therapy is directed at strengthening pelvic floor muscles.

Vaginal pessary is an individually fitted device inserted into the vagina, which supports pelvic organs.

Surgical options:

Sacral colpopexy surgery treats pelvic organ prolapse by suspending the vaginal vault to the sacral promontory using a graft or surgical mesh.

Colporrhaphy is surgical repair of a vaginal wall because of a cystocele (protrusion of the urinary bladder into the vagina) or a rectocele (protrusion of the rectum into the vagina).

Other gynecologic surgeries:

Oophorectomy is surgical removal of one or both ovaries.

A **salpingectomy** may be necessary in a woman who has salpingitis that has developed into a pelvic abscess.

Vestibulectomy is an option to treat vulvodynia.

Tubal ligation prevents future pregnancies.

Treatment options for fibroids are numerous and include:

- **Expectant management,** or watchful waiting.
- **Myomectomy,** removal of the fibroids surgically, leaving the uterus in place.
- **Hormone therapy,** which uses **GnRH agonists** to cause estrogen and progesterone levels to fall so that menstruation stops and fibroids shrink.
- **Hysterectomy,** major surgery that is performed by many gynecologists as a last resort.

Endometrial cancer is staged at the time of any surgical procedure into four groups, depending on its localization to the uterus or its spread outside. Surgery is the most common treatment. If the cancer has spread to other parts of the body, **progesterone therapy, radiation therapy,** and **chemotherapy** are used.

Infertility treatment is directed at the underlying cause. If the cause of infertility is infrequent ovulation, the patient can be treated with hormones to stimulate release of the egg. These hormones include clomiphene citrate and injectable forms of FSH, LH, and GnRH.

Surgical procedures to initiate pregnancy include:

- **Intrauterine insemination.** Sperm are inserted directly into the uterus via a special catheter.
- **In vitro fertilization (IVF).** Eggs and sperm are combined in a laboratory dish, and two resulting embryos are placed inside the uterus. This can result in twins.

Keynotes

- The success rate for IVF is approximately 30% for each egg retrieval.
- More than 600,000 hysterectomies are performed each year in the United States.

Abbreviations

IVF   in vitro fertilization

Word Analysis and Definition

S = Suffix   P = Prefix   R = Root   R/CF = Combining Form

WORD	PRONUNCIATION	ELEMENTS		DEFINITION
ablation	ab-**LAY**-shun	S/ P/ R/	-ion *action* ab- *away from* -lat- *to take*	Removal of tissue to destroy its function
agonist	**AG**-on-ist		Greek *contest*	Agent that combines with receptors on cells to initiate drug actions
colpopexy	**KOL**-poh-pek-see	S/ R/CF	-pexy *surgical fixation* colp/o- *vagina*	Surgical fixation of the vagina
colporrhaphy	kol-**POR**-ah-fee	R	-rrhaphy *suture*	Suture of a rupture of the vagina
cryosurgery	cry-oh-**SUR**-jer-ee	S/ R/CF R/	-ery *process of* cry/o- *icy, cold* -surg- *operate*	Use of liquid nitrogen or argon gas to freeze and kill tissue
estrogen	**ES**-troh-jen	S/ R/CF	-gen *create* estr/o- *woman*	Generic term for hormones that stimulate secondary sex characteristics
hysterectomy	his-ter-**EK**-toh-mee	S/ R/	-ectomy *surgical excision* hyster- *uterus*	Surgical removal of the uterus
inseminate (verb)	in-**SEM**-ih-nate	S/ P/ R/	-ation *process* in- *in* -semin- *scatter seed*	To introduce semen into the vagina
insemination	in-sem-ih-**NAY**-shun			Introduction of semen into the vagina
in vitro fertilization (IVF)	IN **VEE**-troh **FER**-til-eye-**ZAY**-shun	S/ R/	in vitro *Latin in glass* -ization *process of creating* fertil- *able to conceive*	Process of combining sperm and egg in a laboratory dish and placing the resulting embryos inside the uterus
myomectomy	my-oh-**MEK**-toh-mee	S/ R/ S/	-ectomy *surgical excision* my- *muscle* -om- *tumor*	Surgical removal of a fibroid
oophorectomy	**OH**-oh-for-**EK**-toh-mee	S/ R/	-ectomy *surgical excision* oophor- *ovary*	Surgical removal of the ovary(ies)
pessary	**PESS**-ah-ree		Greek *an oval stone*	Appliance inserted into the vagina to support the uterus
salpingectomy	sal-pin-**JEK**-toh-mee	S/ R/	-ectomy *surgical excision* salping- *uterine tube*	Surgical removal of uterine tube(s)
vestibulectomy	vess-tib-you-**LEK**-toe-me	S/ R/	-ectomy *surgical excision* vestibul- *entrance*	Surgical excision of the vulva

Abbreviation

HRT	hormone replacement therapy

Gynecologic Pharmacology (LO 15.6)

Hormone replacement therapy (HRT)—medications to relieve menopausal symptoms by replacement of diminished circulating estrogen and progesterone hormones—must be given in effective forms.

Synthetic estradiol is a more effective **bioidentical** estrogen with fewer side effects when used **transdermally** as a patch, gel, or vaginal pessary.

Micronized bioidentical progesterone is more effective and has fewer side effects than synthetic **progestin.** However, long-term **hormone therapy,** as it is now called, is no longer routinely recommended. When taken for more than a few years, it increases the risk of breast cancer.

Depo-Provera is also a progestin-only drug given by intramuscular injection every 3 months.

Bacterial vaginosis is treated with antibiotics such as clindamycin. **Vulvovaginal candidiasis** can be treated by applying miconazole (*Monistat*) or clotrimazole (*Desenex*) vaginally, and, if necessary, taking fluconazole (*Diflucan*) orally.

Treatment for **vulvodynia** varies from local anesthetics and creams to biofeedback therapy with exercises to the muscles of the pelvic floor.

Clomiphene (Clomid) is an oral medication used for stimulating ovulation by causing production of **gonadotrophins** by the pituitary gland (*see Chapter 12).*

Treatment for STDs (LO 15.6)

- **Trichomoniasis** infection of the vagina can be treated with a single oral dose of metronidazole (*Flagyl*). Because it is a "ping-pong" infection between partners, both individuals should be treated.

- Treatment for **chlamydia** is with oral antibiotics such as doxycycline, erythromycin, or azithromycin.

- **Gonorrhea** can be treated with a single dose of an antibiotic such as cefixime, but is otherwise resistant to antibiotics.

- Antibiotics such as azithromycin and ceftriaxone are effective in the treatment of **chancroid.**

- The lesions of **molluscum contagiosum** are treated with podophyllin ointment, or liquid nitrogen and laser surgery can be used.

Surgical removal of the affected area (vestibulectomy) has been tried with variable results.

There is no cure for genital herpes. Three antiviral medications can provide clinical benefit by limiting the **replication** of the virus. These are acyclovir (*Zovirax*), valacyclovir (*Valtrex*), and famcyclovir (*Famvir*). In people who have recurrent outbreaks, medication taken every day can reduce the recurrences by 70% to 80%.

The HPV vaccine (*Gardasil*) is offered to girls and women aged 9 to 26 and to boys and men of the same age group.

There is no cure for HIV or AIDS, but combinations of anti-HIV medications are taken to stop the replication of the virus in the cells of the body and stop the progression of the disease. Development of resistance to the drugs is a problem.

Word Analysis and Definition

S = Suffix   P = Prefix   R = Root   R/CF = Combining Form

WORD	PRONUNCIATION	ELEMENTS		DEFINITION
estradiol	ess-trah-**DIE**-ol	S/ R/	-diol *chemical name* estra- *woman*	The most potent natural estrogen
synthetic	sin-**THET**-ik	S/ P/ R/	-ic *pertaining to* syn- *together* -thet- *arrange*	Built up or put together from simpler compounds
transdermal	trans-**DER**-mal	S/ P/ R/	-al *pertaining to* trans- *across* -derm- *skin*	Going across or through the skin

EXERCISES

A. You are reviewing a patient chart at a gynecologic clinic for a follow-up appointment regarding her lab results. *Select a medical term below to correctly complete each sentence. Each term will be used only once, but not all terms will be used.* **LO 15.2, 15.4, 15.5, and 15.13**

dysfunction	dysplasia	dysplastic	menopause	menopausal

Mrs. Volinsky has not menstruated in 11 years and therefore is in (1) _____ This is appropriate for her age of 68 years. The pathology report notes that she has (2) _____ cells obtained from a swab of her cervix. During her last visit, she was prescribed hormones to treat her (3) _____ symptoms. Today, the nurse practitioner will discuss further diagnostic tests to confirm a diagnosis of cervical cell (4) _____.

B. Define gynecologic diagnostic procedures. *Select the correct answer to complete each statement.* **LO 15.6**

1. The term **palpate** means to:

a. visualize   b. touch   c. excise   d. incise

2. A diagnostic test for infertility in which the cervix is viewed after unprotected sexual intercourse:

a. hysteroscopy   b. biopsy   c. postcoital testing   d. ultrasound

3. The injection of dye followed by an X-ray of the uterus and uterine tubes is termed:

a. hysterosalpingography   b. postcoital testing   c. mammography   d. endometrial biopsy

4. A **colposcope** is used to:

a. view the vagina and cervical canal   b. X-ray the uterus   c. view the internal os of the cervix   d. remove cells from the uterus

C. Test your understanding *of the Pap test by answering these questions. Select the correct answer for each question.* **LO 15.3 and 15.5**

1. How often should a 30 to 40-year-old woman have a Pap test?

a. annually   b. biannually   c. every three years   d. every five years

2. What causes the majority of abnormal Pap smears?

a. improper specimen collection   b. poor hygiene   c. infection by the human papilloma virus   d. overgrowth of yeast in vagina

3. The optimal time to perform a Pap smear is _____ days after the last menstrual period.

a. 2–3   b. 4–6   c. 8–12   d. 10–20

D. Construct medical terms. *Complete medical terms related to gynecologic diagnostic procedures. Be precise. Fill in the blanks.* **LO 15.1, 15.6, 15.9, and 15.12**

1. Use of very high frequency sound waves   _____ /sound

2. Specialist in the study of the anatomy, physiology, and pathology of the cell   cyto/ _____

3. Visual inspection of the uterine cavity using an endoscope   hystero/ _____

E. Apply your knowledge of the language of gynecology. *Match the word element in the first column with its correct meaning in the second column.* **LO 15.1 and 15.6**

	Term		Meaning
_____	**1.** *oophor-*		**a.** to cleanse
_____	**2.** *-ectomy*		**b.** uterine tube
_____	**3.** *hyster/o*		**c.** ovary
_____	**4.** *-pexy*		**d.** uterus
_____	**5.** *salping/o*		**e.** surgical removal
_____	**6.** *semin-*		**f.** surgical fixation
_____	**7.** *curette-*		**g.** scatter seed
_____	**8.** *colp/o*		**h.** vagina

F. Demonstrate your knowledge of gynecologic pharmacology. *Select the correct answer that completes the sentence or answers the question.* **LO 15.4 and 15.6**

1. A pharmacologic method to treat vulvodynia is:

a. transdermal estradiol   b. micronized bioidentical progesterone   c. topical anesthetic cream   d. *Gardasil* injection

2. A medication used to promote ovulation:

a. clomiphene   b. podophyllin ointment   c. Minipill   d. acyclovir

3. Miconazole and clotrimazole are used to treat:

a. chlamydia   b. vulvodynia   c. infertility   d. fungal infections

4. An increased risk of breast cancer is seen with which type of long-term pharmacologic therapy?

a. pessary   b. antibiotic   c. hormone   d. antiviral

5. Which type of medication is used to reduce, not cure, herpes outbreaks?

a. metronidazole   b. liquid nitrogen   c. valacyclovir   d. Gardasil

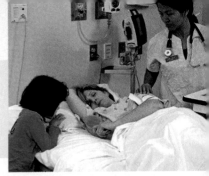

Conception and Development (LO 15.7)

Conception (LO 15.7)

When released from the ovary, an egg takes 72 hours to travel to the uterus—but it must be fertilized within 12 to 24 hours to survive. Therefore, **fertilization** must take place in the distal third of the uterine tube.

During unprotected intercourse, with male ejaculation, between 200 and 600 million sperm are deposited in the vagina near the cervix. The journey through the uterus into the uterine tube takes about an hour. Some 2,000 to 3,000 sperm reach the egg. Several of these sperm penetrate the outer layers of the egg to clear the path for the one sperm that will penetrate all the way into the egg to **fertilize** it (*Figure 15.14*). Once fertilized, the egg becomes a **zygote**.

Implantation (LO 15.7)

While still in the uterine tube, the zygote divides; a fluid-filled cavity develops, and the zygote becomes a **blastocyst** (its first 2 weeks as a developing **embryo**). A week after fertilization, the blastocyst enters the uterine cavity and burrows into the endometrium, and **implantation** occurs. A group of cells in the blastocyst differentiate into the embryo. Other cells from the blastocyst, together with endometrial cells, form the **placenta**.

Placenta (LO 15.7)

The placenta is a disc of tissue that increases in size as pregnancy proceeds *(Figure 15.15)*. The surface facing the **fetus** is smooth and gives rise to the **umbilical cord.** The surface attached to the uterine wall consists of treelike structures called **chorionic villi.** The cells of the villi keep the maternal and fetal circulations separate, but they are very thin and allow the exchange of gases, nutrients, and waste products.

The functions of the placenta are to:

- **Transport** nutrients and oxygen from the mother to the fetus;

- **Transport** nitrogenous wastes and carbon dioxide from the fetus to the mother, who can excrete them;

- **Transport** maternal antibodies and hormones to the fetus; and

- **Secrete** hormones like estrogen and progesterone.

Unfortunately, some undesirable matter and many medications can cross the placenta. These include: the HIV and rubella viruses; bacteria that cause syphilis; alcohol; nicotine and carbon monoxide from smoking; and drugs ranging from aspirin to heroin and cocaine. All of these can have detrimental effects on the fetus.

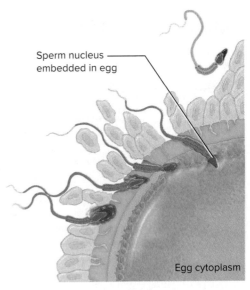

Sperm nucleus embedded in egg

Egg cytoplasm

▲ **FIGURE 15.14** Fertilization.

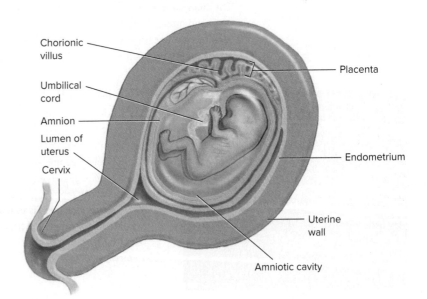

Chorionic villus

Umbilical cord

Amnion

Lumen of uterus

Cervix

Placenta

Endometrium

Uterine wall

Amniotic cavity

▲ **FIGURE 15.15** Embryo and Placenta at 13 Weeks.

WORD	PRONUNCIATION	ELEMENTS		DEFINITION
blastocyst	BLAS-toe-sist	S/ R/CF	-cyst *cyst, bladder* blast/o- *germ or immature cell*	First 2 weeks of the developing embryo
chorion chorionic (adj) chorionic villus	KOH-ree-on koh-ree-ON-ik VILL-us	S/ R/	Greek *membrane* -ic *pertaining to* chorion- *chorion* villus, Latin *shaggy hair*	The fetal membrane that forms the placenta Pertaining to the chorion Vascular process of the embryonic chorion to form the placenta
conception	kon-SEP-shun		Latin *something received*	Fertilization of the egg by sperm to form a zygote
embryo embryonic (adj)	EM-bree-oh em-bree-ON-ic	 S/ R/	Greek *a young one* -ic *pertaining to* embryon- *embryo*	Developing organism from conception until the end of the second month Pertaining to the embryo
fertilize (verb) fertilization (noun)	FER-til-ize FER-til-ih-ZAY-shun	 S/ R/	Latin *make fruitful* -ation *process* fertiliz- *make fruitful*	Penetration of the oocyte (ovum) by sperm Union of a male sperm and a female egg
fetus fetal (adj)	FEE-tus FEE-tal	 S/ R/	Latin *offspring* -al *pertaining to* fet- *fetus*	Human organism from the end of the eighth week after conception to birth Pertaining to the fetus
implantation	im-plan-TAY-shun	S/ P/ R/	-ation *process* im- *in* -plant- *to plant, insert*	Attachment of a fertilized egg to the endometrium
placenta	plah-SEN-tah		Latin *a cake*	Organ that allows metabolic exchange between the mother and the fetus
umbilicus umbilical (adj)	um-BIL-ih-kus um-BIL-ih-kal	 S/ R/	Latin *navel* -al *pertaining to* umbilic- *umbilicus*	Pit in the abdomen where the umbilical cord entered the fetus Pertaining to the umbilicus or the center of the abdomen
zygote	ZIGH-goat		Greek *joined together*	Cell resulting from the union of the sperm and egg

Development of Embryo and Fetus (LO 15.7)

Embryo (LO 15.7)

The **embryonic period** occurs from week 2 until week 8. During this time, most of the embryo's external structures and internal organs are formed, together with the placenta, umbilical cord, amnion (the amniotic fluid-filled membrane around the fetus), and **chorion**. The **amnion** grows to envelop the embryo. At the eighth week, all the embryo's organ systems are present, the embryo is just over 1 inch long, and is now officially a **fetus**.

Fetus (LO 15.7)

The fetal period lasts from the eighth week until birth. By week 8, the heart is beating. By the week 12, the bones have begun to calcify, and the external genitalia can be differentiated as male or female. In the fourth month, downy hair called **lanugo** appears on the body. In the fifth month, skeletal muscles become active, and the baby's movements are felt between 16 and 22 weeks of **gestation** *(Figure 15.16)*. A protective creamy substance called **vernix caseosa** covers the skin. In the sixth and seventh months, there is an increase in weight gain and body fat is deposited.

At 38 weeks, the baby is considered full-term and ready for birth.

Gestation is divided into **trimesters:**

The first trimester is up to week 12; the second from week 13 to 24; and the third from week 25 to birth.

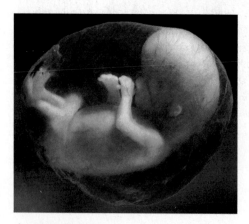

▲ **FIGURE 15.16**   Developing Fetus at 20 Weeks.

Steve Allen/Stockbyte/Getty Images

WORD	PRONUNCIATION	ELEMENTS		DEFINITION
amnion amniotic (adj)	AM-nee-on am-nee-OT-ik	S/ R/CF	Greek *membrane around fetus* -tic *pertaining to* amni/o- *amnion, fetal membrane*	Membrane around the fetus that contains amniotic fluid Pertaining to the amnion
gestation gestational (adj)	jes-TAY-shun jes-TAY-shun-al	S/ R/ S/	-ion *action, condition* gestat- *pregnancy* -al *pertaining to*	From conception to birth Pertaining to gestation
lanugo	la-NYU-go		Latin *wool*	Fine, soft hair on the fetal body
trimester	TRY-mes-ter		Latin *of 3 months' duration*	One-third of the length of a full-term pregnancy
vernix caseosa	VER-nicks kay-see-OH-sah		vernix, Latin *varnish* caseosa, *Latin cheese*	Cheesy substance covering the skin of the fetus

Labor and Childbirth (LO 15.7)

Labor contractions begin about 30 minutes apart. They have to be intermittent because each contraction decreases the maternal blood supply to the placenta and to the fetus. Labor pains are due to ischemia of the uterine muscle during contractions.

Labor is divided into three stages *(Figure 15.17)* each of which is usually longer in a **primipara** (one birth) than in a **multipara** (more than one birth). Another term for pregnant is **gravid**, and a pregnant woman can be called **gravida**. A woman in her first pregnancy is called a **primigravida**.

First Stage—Dilation of the Cervix (LO 15.7)

This is the longest stage of labor. It can be a few minutes in a multipara to more than 1 day in a primipara. **Dilation** is the widening of the cervical canal to the same diameter as that of the baby's head *(Figure 15.17b)*. At the same time that dilation occurs, the wall of the cervix becomes thinner—a process called **effacement**. During dilation, the fetal membranes rupture, and the "water breaks" as amniotic fluid is released.

Second Stage—Expulsion of the Fetus (LO 15.7)

While the uterus continues to contract, the baby's head generates additional pain as it stretches the cervix and vagina. When the head reaches the vaginal opening and stretches the vulva, the head is said to be **crowning** and the baby can be delivered *(Figure 15.18)*. Sometimes, this process can be helped by performing an **episiotomy** and making an incision in the perineum.

After the baby is delivered, the umbilical cord is clamped in two places and cut between the two clamps.

Third Stage—Expulsion of the Placenta (LO 15.7)

After the baby is delivered, the uterus continues to contract. It pushes the placenta off the uterine wall and expels it from the vagina *(Figure 15.17d)*.

Puerperium (LO 15.7)

The 6 weeks **postpartum** (after the birth) are called the **puerperium**. The uterus shrinks (**involution**) through self-digestion (**autolysis**) of uterine cells by their own enzymes. This generates a vaginal discharge called lochia that lasts about 10 days.

The **neonatal** time period is from birth to 1 month, while the **perinatal** time period lasts up to 18 to 24 months after the birth of the child.

A child is a **neonate** from birth up to 4 weeks and then is an **infant,** up to 1 year of age.

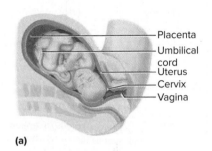

(a)

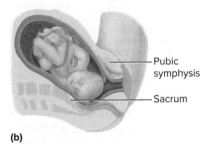

— Placenta
— Umbilical cord
— Uterus
— Cervix
— Vagina

— Pubic symphysis
— Sacrum

(b)

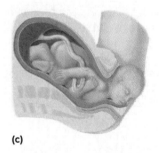

(c)

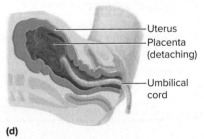

— Uterus
— Placenta (detaching)
— Umbilical cord

(d)

▲ **FIGURE 15.17** The Stages of Childbirth.
(a) First stage: Early dilation.
(b) First stage: Late dilation.
(c) Second stage: Expulsion of the fetus. (d) Third stage: Expulsion of the placenta.

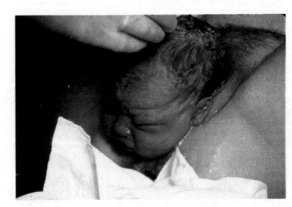

▲ **FIGURE 15.18** Delivery of the Head.

Petit Format/Science Source

Word Analysis and Definition

S = Suffix P = Prefix R = Root R/CF = Combining Form

WORD	PRONUNCIATION	ELEMENTS		DEFINITION
autolysis	awe-**TOL**-ih-sis	P/ R/	auto- *self, same* -lysis *destruction*	Destruction of cells by enzymes within the cells
dilation	die-**LAY**-shun	S/ R/	-ion *process* dilat- *open out*	Stretching or enlarging an opening
effacement	ee-**FACE**-ment	S/ R/	-ment *resulting state* efface- *wipe out*	Thinning of the cervix in relation to labor
episiotomy	eh-piz-ee-**OT**-oh-me	S/ R/CF	-tomy *surgical incision* episi/o- *vulva*	Surgical incision of the vulva
gravid gravida	**GRAV**-id **GRAV**-ih-dah		Latin *pregnant* Latin *pregnant woman*	Pregnant A pregnant woman
infant infantile (adj)	**IN**-fant **IN**-fan-tile	 S/ R/	Latin *not speaking* -ile *pertaining to* infant- *infant*	Child in the first year of life Pertaining to an infant
involution involute (verb)	in-voh-**LOO**-shun in-voh-**LUTE**	S/ P/ R/	-ion *action, condition* in- *in* -volut- *roll up, shrink*	Decrease in size
labor	**LAY**-bore		Latin *toil, suffering*	Process of expulsion of the fetus
lochia	**LOW**-kee-uh		Greek *relating to childbirth*	Vaginal discharge following childbirth
multipara	mul-**TIP**-ah-ruh	P/ R/	multi- *many* para *to bring forth*	Woman who has given birth to two or more children
neonate neonatal (adj) (**Note:** *The "e" in the root is dropped because of the following vowel.*)	**NEE**-oh-nate **NEE**-oh-**NAY**-tal	R/CF R/ S/	neo- *new* -nate *born* -al *pertaining to*	A newborn infant Pertaining to the newborn infant or the newborn period
perinatal	**PAIR**-ih-**NAY**-tal	S/ P/ R/	-al *pertaining to* peri- *around* -nat- *birth*	Around the time of birth
postpartum	post-**PAR**-tum	P/ R/	post- *after* -partum *childbirth, to bring forth*	After childbirth
primigravida	pree-mih-**GRAV**-ih-dah	P/ R/	primi- *first* -gravida *pregnancy*	A woman in her first pregnancy
primipara	pry-**MIP**-ah-ruh	P/ R/	primi- *first* -para *to bring forth*	Woman giving birth for the first time
puerperium (**Note:** *This term is composed of roots only.*)	pyu-er-**PEE**-ree-um	R/ R/	puer- *child* -perium *a bringing forth*	Six-week period after birth in which the uterus involutes

EXERCISES

A. Tracing the pathway of embryo implantation. *You are given the terminology—put it in the correct order according to the implantation process. Fill in the blanks.* **LO 15.2 and 15.7**

embryo   fertilization   blastocyst   zygote   egg

1. _____

2. _____

3. _____

4. _____

5. _____

B. Describe *conception and implantation. Select the correct answer to complete each statement.* **LO 15.7**

1. Fertilization occurs when a(n)

   a. ovum travels down the uterine tube

   b. blastocyst implants into the placenta

   c. sperm penetrates all the way into the egg

   d. blastocyst enters the uterine cavity

2. Implantation occurs when a(n)

   a. ovum travels down the uterine tube

   b. blastocyst burrows into the endometrium

   c. sperm penetrates all the way into the egg

   d. blastocyst enters the uterine cavity

C. Deconstruct *medical terms into their elements. Fill in the blanks.* **LO 15.1 and 15.7**

1. **embryonic:** _____ / _____

2. **blastocyst:** _____ / _____

3. **implantation:** _____ / _____ / _____

D. Precision in documentation *includes using the correct form (noun, verb, adjective) of the medical term. Fill in the blanks.* **LO 15.2, 15.7, and 15.13**

1. embryo   embryonic

   In the _____ stage of gestation, the _____ forms in the first 8 weeks of human development.

2. chorionic   chorion

   The _____ villi keep the maternal and fetal circulations separate. The _____ is the fetal membrane that forms the placenta.

E. Functions of the placenta. *Fill in each blank with either the term fetus or mother.* **LO 15.2 and 15.7**

1. Transportation of nitrogenous wastes and carbon dioxide moves from the _____ (a) to the _____ (b).

2. Transportation of maternal antibodies goes from the _____ (a) to the _____ (b).

3. Transportation of nutrients and oxygen goes from the _____ (a) to the _____ (b).

F. Challenge your knowledge *of the developing embryo and fetus. Fill in the blanks.* **LO 15.2, 15.8, and 15.14**

1. Where does the umbilical cord originate? _____

2. To what structure are the chorionic villi attached in the reproductive system? _____

3. The structure that keeps the maternal and fetal circulations separate: _____

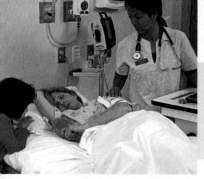

Section 15.5

Disorders of Pregnancy and Childbirth

Disorders of Pregnancy (LO 15.8)

The paragraphs below explain the disorders in pregnancy that you will need to be familiar with when caring for a pregnant patient.

Ectopic Pregnancy (LO 15.8)

In an **ectopic pregnancy**, there is an obstruction in the uterine tube. As a result, the fertilized egg will be prevented from moving into the uterus. Instead, the egg will continue its development in the uterine tube. Tubal disorders that cause ectopic pregnancy include previous salpingitis, pelvic inflammatory disease (PID), and endometriosis.

Preeclampsia and Eclampsia (LO 15.8)

Preeclampsia is a sudden, abnormal increase in maternal blood pressure after the 20th week of pregnancy, with edema (swelling) of the face, hands, and feet. It is commonly accompanied by proteinuria (protein in the urine). Severe preeclampsia can lead to stroke, bleeding disorders, and death of the mother and/or fetus.

Eclampsia is a life-threatening condition, characterized by the signs and symptoms of preeclampsia, but with more severe symptoms such as convulsions or resulting in coma. Management involves immediate admission to the hospital and control of the mother's blood pressure. The baby is delivered as soon as the mother is stabilized, regardless of its gestational age.

Amniotic Fluid Abnormalities (LO 15.8)

Amniotic fluid abnormalities occur in the second trimester, when the fetus breathes in and swallows amniotic fluid. This promotes development of the gastrointestinal tract and lungs. In the third trimester, the total amount of amniotic fluid is about 1 quart and is mostly fetal urine.

Oligohydramnios is a condition involving too little amniotic fluid. It is associated with an increase in the risk of birth defects and poor fetal growth. Its etiology is unknown.

Polyhydramnios is the opposite of oligohydramnios, and involves too much amniotic fluid. It causes abdominal discomfort and breathing difficulties for the mother. It is associated with **preterm delivery,** placental problems, and poor fetal growth.

Gestational Diabetes Mellitus (GDM) (LO 15.8)

In some pregnant women, the amount of insulin they can produce decreases and this leads to hyperglycemia. For the mother, **gestational diabetes mellitus (GDM)** increases the risk of preeclampsia and future type 2 diabetes. For the neonate (newborn child), it increases the risk of perinatal mortality, birth trauma, and neonatal hypoglycemia. Later in life, both mother and child are at increased risk for developing type 2 diabetes and obesity.

Hyperemesis Gravidarum (LO 15.8)

Eighty percent of pregnant women experience some degree of "morning sickness." It is at its worst between 2 and 12 weeks of pregnancy and usually resolves in the second trimester. For a few women, nausea is persistent, and vomiting is extreme and can lead to dehydration. This condition is called **hyperemesis gravidarum.** Severe cases may require hospital admission for IV fluids.

Teratogenesis (LO 15.8)

Teratogenesis is the production of fetal abnormalities—**congenital malformations**—by a chemical agent affecting the mother during the early development of the fetus, while organs and structures are being formed. All medications readily cross the placenta. **Teratogens** include alcohol, isotretinoin (acne medication), valproic acid (an anticonvulsant), and the rubella virus.

WORD	PRONUNCIATION	ELEMENTS		DEFINITION
eclampsia preeclampsia	eh-**KLAMP**-see-uh pree-eh-**KLAMP**-see-uh	S/ P/ R/	Greek *a shining forth* -ia *condition* pre- *before,* -eclamps- *shining forth*	Convulsions in a patient with preeclampsia Hypertension, edema, and proteinuria during pregnancy
ectopic	ek-**TOP**-ik	S/ R/	-ic *pertaining to* ectop- *on the outside, displaced*	Out of place, not in a normal position
oligohydramnios	**OL**-ih-goh-high-**DRAM**-nee-os	P/ R/ R/	oligo- *scanty, too little* -hydr- *water* -amnios *amnion*	Too little amniotic fluid
polyhydramnios	**POL**-ee-high-**DRAM**-nee-os	P/	poly- *many, excessive*	Too much amniotic fluid
preterm (*same as* premature)	pree-**TERM**	P/ R/	pre- *before* -term *limit, end*	Baby delivered before 37 weeks of gestation
hyperemesis	high-per-**EM**-eh-sis	P/ R/	hyper- *excessive* -emesis *vomiting*	Excessive vomiting
hyperemesis gravidarum	high-per-**EM**-eh-sis gray-vee-**DAY**-rum		Latin *associated with pregnant women*	Excessive nausea and vomiting during pregnancy
teratogen	**TER**-ah-toe-jen	S/ R/CF	-gen *create, produce* terat/o- *monster, malformed fetus*	Agent that produces fetal deformities
teratogenic (adj) teratogenesis	**TER**-ah-toe-**JEN**-ik **TER**-ah-toe-**JEN**-eh-sis	S/ S/	-ic *pertaining to* -esis *condition*	Capable of producing fetal deformities Process involved in producing fetal deformities

Disorders of Childbirth (LO 15.8)

Fetal distress, due to lack of oxygen, is a potential complication of labor, and it is detrimental if not recognized.

An **abnormal position of the fetus** occurs at the beginning of labor if the baby is not a head-first **(vertex)** presentation facing rearward. Abnormal positions include:

- **Breech:** The buttocks present first *(Figure 15.19).*
- **Face:** The face, instead of the top of the head, presents first.
- **Shoulder:** The shoulder and upper back are trying to exit the uterus first.

If the baby cannot be turned into a vertex presentation, a C-section is usually performed.

In addition, other conditions can occur involving an abnormal placement of the baby's umbilical cord.

In **prolapsed umbilical cord,** the cord precedes the baby down the birth canal. Pressure on the cord can cut off the baby's blood supply, which, until after birth, is still being provided through the umbilical arteries.

In **nuchal cord**, the cord is wrapped around the baby's neck during delivery. This occurs in about 20% of deliveries.

Premature rupture of the membranes occurs in 10% of normal pregnancies and increases the risk of infection of the uterus and fetus.

Gestational Classification (LO 15.7 and 15.8)

Prematurity occurs in about 10% of newborns. The earlier the baby is born, the more life-threatening problems occur.

Because their lungs are underdeveloped, premature babies can develop **respiratory distress syndrome (RDS),** also called **hyaline membrane disease (HMD).** Their lungs are not mature enough to produce **surfactant**, a mixture of lipids and proteins that keeps the alveoli from collapsing. As a result, this prevents the respiratory exchange of oxygen and carbon dioxide.

An immature liver can impair the excretion of bilirubin (yellowish bile pigment) *(see Chapter 9),* and premature babies often become jaundiced. High levels of bilirubin can produce **kernicterus**, in which deposits of bilirubin in the brain cause brain damage.

Abbreviations

HMD	hyaline membrane disease
RDS	respiratory distress syndrome

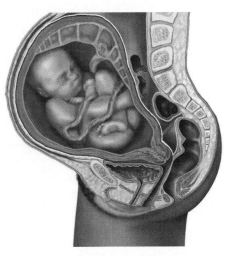

▲ **FIGURE 15.19**   Breech Presentation.

Postmaturity is much less common than prematurity. Its etiology is unknown, but the placenta begins to shrink, making it difficult to supply sufficient nutrients to the baby. For the baby, this leads to: hypoglycemia; loss of subcutaneous fat; dry, peeling skin; and, if oxygen is lacking, fetal distress. The baby can pass stools **(meconium)** into the amniotic fluid. In its distress, the baby can take deep gasping breaths and inhale the meconium fluid. This leads to **meconium aspiration syndrome (MAS)** and respiratory difficulty at birth.

An **abortion** is the expulsion of an embryo or fetus from the uterus before the 20th week of gestation. Spontaneous abortion, also known as miscarriage, describes an unplanned process where the fetus is lost to natural causes prior to 20 weeks, gestation.

Abbreviation

PPH   postpartum hemorrhage

Placental Disorders (LO 15.8)

Placenta abruption is the separation of the placenta from the uterine wall before delivery of the baby. The baby's oxygen supply is cut off, and fetal distress appears quickly. It is an **obstetric (OB)** emergency, and usually a **C-section** is performed.

Placenta previa is a low-lying placenta between the baby's head and the internal os of the cervix. It can cause severe bleeding during labor, and a C-section may be necessary.

In a **retained placenta,** all or part of the placenta and/ or membranes remain behind in the uterus 30 minutes to an hour after the baby has been delivered. The result of a retained placenta is heavy uterine bleeding called **postpartum hemorrhage (PPH).** Manual removal of the retained placenta may be necessary under spinal, epidural, or general anesthesia *(Figure 15.20).*

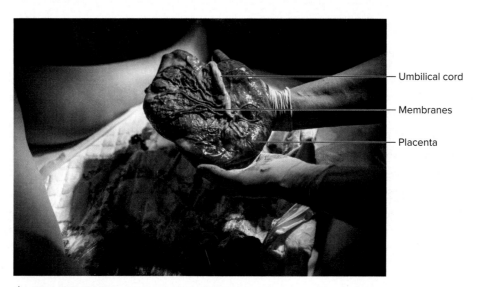

Umbilical cord

Membranes

Placenta

▲ **FIGURE 15.20** Placenta (Afterbirth).

AzmanL/E+/Getty Images

Word Analysis and Definition

S = Suffix   P = Prefix   R = Root   R/CF = Combining Form

WORD	PRONUNCIATION		ELEMENTS	DEFINITION
abortion	ah-**BOR**-shun	S/ R/	**-ion** *action* **abort-** *fail at onset*	Spontaneous or induced expulsion of the embryo or fetus from the uterus at 20 weeks or less
breech	**BREECH**		Old English *trousers*	Buttocks-first presentation of the fetus at delivery
hyaline membrane disease	**HIGH**-ah-line **MEM**-brain diz-**EEZ**	 P/ R/	**hyaline** Greek *glassy* **membrane** Latin *a skin* **dis-** *without* **-ease** *comfort*	Respiratory distress syndrome of the newborn
kernicterus	ker-**NICK**-ter-us	R/ R/	**kern-** *nucleus* **-icterus** *jaundice*	Bilirubin staining of the basal nuclei of the brain
meconium	meh-**KOH**-nee-um		Greek *a little poppy*	The first bowel movement of the newborn
nuchal cord	**NYU**-kul KORD		nuchal, French *the back (nape) of the neck*	Loop(s) of umbilical cord around the fetal neck
placenta abruption	plah-**SEN**-tah ab-**RUP**-shun	 S/	abruptio, Latin *to break off* **-ion** *action, condition*	The premature detachment of the placenta
placenta previa	plah-**SEN**-tah **PREE**-vee-ah	P/ R/	**pre-** *before, in front of* **-via** *the way*	Condition in which the placenta is positioned between the fetus and the cervix
postmature	post-mah-**TYUR**	P/ R/	**post-** *after* **-mature** *ripe, ready*	Infant born after 42 weeks of gestation
postmaturity	post-mah-**TYUR**-ih-tee	S/	**-ity** *condition, state*	Condition of being postmature
premature (slang term "preemie")	pree-mah-**TYUR**	P/ R/	**pre-** *before* **-mature** *ripe, ready*	Occurring before the expected time
prematurity (same as *preterm*)	pree-mah-**TYUR**-ih-tee	S/	**-ity** *condition, state*	Condition of being premature
surfactant	sir-**FAK**-tant		surface *active agent*	A protein and fat compound that creates surface tension to hold the lung alveolar walls apart
vertex	**VER**-teks		Latin *whorl*	Topmost point of the vault of the skull

EXERCISES

 Case Report 15.4

You are ...

. . . an obstetric medical assistant employed by Garry Joiner, MD, an obstetrician at Fulwood Medical Center.

You are communicating with ...

Mrs. Gloria Maggay, a 29-year-old housekeeper. Her last menstrual period was 8 weeks ago, and she has a positive home **pregnancy** test. This is her first pregnancy. She has breast tenderness and mild nausea. For the past 2 days, she has had some cramping, right-sided, lower abdominal pain and this morning had vaginal spotting. Her VS are T 99°F, P 80, R 14, BP 130/70. While you are waiting for Dr. Joiner to come and examine her, Mrs. Maggay complains of feeling faint and has a sharp, severe pain in the right side of her lower abdomen. Her pulse rate has increased to 105. You need to recognize what is happening and to use the correct medical terminology as you talk with Dr. Joiner.

Mrs. Gloria Maggay's symptoms are indicative of an **ectopic** pregnancy. The sudden increase in pain and the rise in pulse rate can signal that the tube has ruptured and is hemorrhaging into the abdominal cavity. The gynecologist should see Mrs. Maggay immediately and the patient be taken to the operating room **(OR)** for laparoscopic surgery to stop the bleeding and evacuate the **products of conception (POC).**

A. **After reading Case Report 15.4** *answer the following questions. Select the best answer.*   **LO 15.8, 15.11, and 15.12**

1. Which of the following symptoms did Mrs. Maggay develop while she was in the office?

   a. decreased pulse rate   c. severe right-sided abdominal pain

   b. vaginal spotting   d. mild nausea

2. Mrs. Maggay is most likely suffering from:

   a. fertilized egg implanted in a uterine tube   c. prolapsed uterus

   b. endometrial tissue occurring outside of the uterus   d. rupture of the appendix

3. The event that has elevated Mrs. Maggay's condition to an emergency is:

   a. large amount of blood entering the abdomen   c. labor has begun

   b. increased and irregular heart rate   d. intense nausea and vomiting

B. **Define the meaning of the word elements.** *Select the correct answer that completes each statement.*   **LO 15.1**

1. The word element that means **scanty**:

   a. poly-   b. hyper-   c. oligo-   d. ectop-   e. -amnios

2. The word element **ectop-** means:

   a. limit   b. pertaining to   c. amnion   d. on the outside   e. shining forth

3. The word element **-eclamps** means:

   a. cheese   b. shining forth   c. tension   d. bleeding   e. nausea

C. **Elements:** *Several of these elements you have seen before, and you will certainly see them again in other terms. Learn an element once, and recognize it all the time. Select the best answer to each question.*   **LO 15.1 and 15.7**

1. The term that contains the prefix meaning *many* is:

   a. primipara   b. lochia   c. multipara

2. The term that contains the suffix meaning *incision* is:

   a. episiotomy   b. effacement   c. dilation

3. The term that contains the root meaning *destruction* is:

   a. autolysis   b. involution   c. effacement

4. The term that contains the root meaning *child* is:

   a. gravid   b. multipara   c. puerperium

D. **Elements.** Real familiarity with obstetrical and reproductive terms means you can look at an element and identify it as either a prefix (P), root (R), or suffix (S). *Identify each element by inserting its type and meaning in the appropriate columns. The first one is done for you. Fill in the blanks.*   **LO 15.1 and 15.8**

Element	Type	Meaning of the Element
post-	P	after
-ity	1.	2.
kern	3.	4.
via	5.	6.
mature	7.	8.
pre-	9.	10.
abort	11.	12.

E. **Describe the disorders of childbirth.** *Match the disorder in the first column with its correct description in the second column. Fill in the blanks.*   **LO 15.8**

Term Meaning

_____   1. prolapsed umbilical cord   a. cord is wrapped around the baby's neck during delivery

_____   2. placenta previa   b. cord comes before the baby during delivery

_____   3. kernicterus   c. brain damage due to bilirubin deposits

_____   4. nuchal cord   d. separation of the placenta from the uterine wall before delivery

_____   5. placenta abruption   e. placenta is positioned over the internal os of the cervix

Obstetrical Diagnostic and Therapeutic Procedures

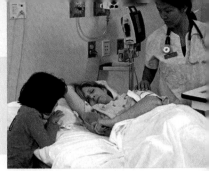

Rick Brady/McGraw-Hill Education

Obstetrical Diagnostic Procedures (LO 15.9)

Prenatal Screening Tests (LO 15.9 and 15.12)

Obstetricians (OB) are physicians who specialize in the treatment of pregnant women. Certified midwives are independent practitioners. Care begins in the prenatal period and typically ends 6 weeks after the birth of the baby. Certain diagnostic tests are integrated as part of prenatal care. These tests can help determine if the pregnancy is at a higher risk for the baby to have a specific problem; the test does not diagnose a problem, only whether it is more or less likely. These tests do not increase risk of miscarriage.

    First trimester screening is done between the 11th and 13th weeks of pregnancy. It combines **maternal** blood testing for **human chorionic gonadotropin (hCG)** (the pregnancy hormone) and **pregnancy-associated plasma protein A (PAPP-A)** with an ultrasound measurement of the back of the baby's neck (**nuchal translucency—NT**). Women with higher than average NT measurements and/or higher or lower than average hCG or PAPP-A values *might* be at risk for having a baby with Down Syndrome or with another rare chromosomal problem, Trisomy 18.

    Chorionic villus sampling (CVS) also uses ultrasound guidance to insert a needle through the abdomen or a catheter through the cervix to obtain a sample of placental tissue that can be tested for fetal chromosomal abnormalities. The main advantage of CVS is that it can be performed between 9 and 13 weeks of pregnancy, earlier than amniocentesis (*see below*).

    Second trimester screening is done between the 15th and 18th weeks of gestation. Called the **quad screen,** it measures the levels of four substances in a pregnant woman's blood: **alpha-fetoprotein (AFP), hCG, unconjugated estriol,** and **dimeric inhibin.** These chemicals are made by the placenta and fetus. Women with high or low levels of these substances *may* be at risk for having a baby with Down Syndrome, Trisomy 18, a **neural tube defect** such as **spina bifida,** or an abdominal wall defect in which abdominal contents protrude through the abdominal wall.

    Cystic fibrosis screening is a blood test to determine the presence of the gene that causes cystic fibrosis (*see Chapter 8*). Both parents have to be carriers of the gene for the baby to be at risk for cystic fibrosis.

    Ultrasound can be used to show most of the organs and bones of the baby in utero. In addition to the screenings described above, ultrasound can be used between 18 and 20 weeks of pregnancy to provide a detailed picture of the baby's anatomy, its size, and growth. Ultrasound carries no known risks and is the most frequently used method of prenatal screening.

Diagnostic Tests (LO 15.9)

Diagnostic tests, slightly different from screening tests, can confirm the presence of the congenital anomaly suggested by the screening test.

    Amniocentesis uses ultrasound guidance to insert a thin needle through the abdominal wall into the amniotic sac around the baby to remove a small amount of amniotic fluid. This fluid contains fetal skin fibroblasts that can be tested for abnormalities. Amniocentesis is performed between 15 and 20 weeks to diagnose chromosome abnormalities and neural tube defects.

Therapeutic Procedures (LO 15.9)

During labor, there is electronic fetal heart monitoring to determine whether the baby is in distress. Treatment is to give the mother oxygen or increase IV fluids. If distress persists, the baby is delivered as quickly as possible by **forceps extraction**, vacuum extractor, or **cesarean section (C-section).**

    An abortion describes the process of ending pregnancy and can be divided into various categories. Medical abortion is typically performed deliberately to end a pregnancy and usually involves the administration of hormones or other medications causing the elimination of growth and development during the early stages after conception. Invasive surgical procedures can also be utilized to remove a fetus at later stages of development.

Abbreviations

AFP	alpha-fetoprotein
C-section	cesarean section
CVS	chorionic villus sampling
hCG	human chorionic gonadotropin
NT	nuchal translucency
OB	obstetrician
PAPP-A	pregnancy-associated plasma protein A

Word Analysis and Definition

S = Suffix P = Prefix R = Root R/CF = Combining Form

WORD	PRONUNCIATION		ELEMENTS	DEFINITION
amniocentesis	AM-nee-oh-sen TEE-sis	S/ R/CF	-centesis *puncture* amni/o- *amnion*	Removal of amniotic fluid for diagnostic purposes
cesarean section (C-section) (syn)	seh-ZAH-ree-an SEK-shun		Roman law under the Caesars required that pregnant women who died be cut open and the fetus extracted	Extraction of the fetus through an incision in the abdomen and uterine wall
diagnostic	die-ag-NOS-tik	S/ P/ R/	-tic *pertaining to* dia- *complete* -gnos- *recognize an abnormal condition*	Pertaining to establishing the cause of a disease
estriol	ESS-tree-ol	S/ R/CF	-ol *chemical name* estr/i- *woman*	One of the three main estrogens
forceps extraction	FOR-seps ek-STRAK-shun		forceps Latin *a pair of tongs* extraction Latin *to draw out*	Assisted delivery of the baby by an instrument that grasps the head of the baby
gonadotropin	GO-nad-oh-TROH-pin	S/ R/CF	-tropin *nourishing* gonad/o- *gonad*	Hormone capable of promoting gonad function
maternal	mah-TER-nal	S/ R/	-al *pertaining to* matern- *mother*	Pertaining to, or derived from, the mother
neural neural tube	NYU-ral NYU-ral TYUB	S/ R/	-al *pertaining to* neur- *nerve*	Pertaining to any structure composed of nerve cells Embryologic tubelike structure that forms the brain and spinal cord
nuchal	NYU-kul		French *the back (nape) of the neck*	The back (nape) of the neck
obstetrics (OB) obstetrician	ob-STET-riks ob-steh-TRISH- un	S/ R/	Latin *a midwife* -ician *expert, specialist* obstetr- *midwifery*	Medical specialty for the care of women during pregnancy and the postpartum period Medical specialist in obstetrics
screen screening	SKREEN SKREEN-ing	S/ R/	Middle English *screne* -ing *process* screen- *a system for separating*	A test to determine the presence or absence of a disease. A testing process that determines the presence or absence of a disease
translucent	tranz-LOO-sent	S/ P/ R/	-ent *pertaining to* trans- *across, through* -luc- *light*	Allowing light to pass through

EXERCISES

A. Describe the meaning of abbreviations related to obstetrical screening tests. *Given the abbreviation, select its correct description.*   **LO 15.3 and 15.11**

1. PAPP-A is used to screen for:

   a. spina bifida   **b.** fetal alcohol syndrome   **c.** Down Syndrome   **d.** cystic fibrosis

2. Amniocentesis at 15 and 20 weeks is used to test for:

   a. nuchal translucency   **b.** neural tube defects   **c.** fetal alcohol syndrome   **d.** cystic fibrosis

3. How is NT measured?

   a. maternal blood testing   **b.** fetal blood testing   **c.** amniocentesis   **d.** ultrasound

B. Construct medical terms related to obstetrics. *Given the definition, complete the described medical terms by inputting the correct word element.*   **LO 15.1 and 15.11**

1. Hormone capable of promoting gonad function: gonado/_____

2. To puncture the amniotic sac: amnio/_____

3. Pertaining to the mother: _____/al

4. Allowing light to pass through: _____/luc/ent

5. Pertaining to a nerve: _____/al

Lesson 15.7

The Female Breast

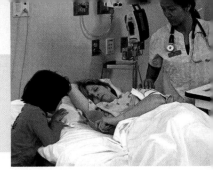

Rick Brady/McGraw-Hill Education

Until the introduction of bottle feeding with cow's milk or formula, the milk produced by the female breast was essential for the survival of the human species. Nourishment of the infant remains the breast's major function.

The Breast (LO 15.4 and 15.7)

Anatomy of the Breast (LO 15.14)

Female breasts provide all required nourishment for an infant after childbirth. Each adult female breast has a **body** located over the pectoralis major muscle and an **axillary tail** extending toward the armpit. The **nipple** projects from the breast and contains multiple openings of the main milk ducts. The reddish-brown **areola** surrounds the **nipple**. The small bumps on its surface are called **areolar glands.** These are sebaceous glands whose secretions prevent chapping and cracking during breastfeeding.

The **nonlactating breast** consists mostly of adipose and connective tissues. It has a system of ducts that branch through the connective tissue and converge on the nipple.

Mammary Gland (LO 15.4 and 15.7)

When the **mammary** gland develops during pregnancy, it is divided into 15 to 20 lobes that contain the secretory **alveoli** that produce milk. The main milk ducts, called **lactiferous ducts** (*Figure 15.21*) drain each lobe immediately before opening onto the nipple.

Lactation (LO 15.4 and 15.7)

In late pregnancy, the secretory alveoli and lactiferous ducts contain **colostrum**. This is the first secretion from the breasts during pregnancy. Colostrum contains more protein but less fat than human milk. It also contains high levels of **immunoglobulins** *(see Chapter 7)* that give the infant protection from infections. Colostrum begins to be replaced by milk 2 or 3 days after the baby's birth, and this replacement is complete by day 5.

The essential stimulus to milk production is the baby's sucking. This stimulates the pituitary gland to produce **prolactin**, which in turn stimulates milk production, and **oxytocin** *(see Chapter 12),* which causes milk to be ejected from the alveoli into the duct system.

After **lactation** completely stops, involution of the mammary gland occurs. The epithelial cells of the alveoli are lost through **apoptosis** (programmed cell death), the ducts shrink in size, and adipose and connective tissues return to be the major breast tissues.

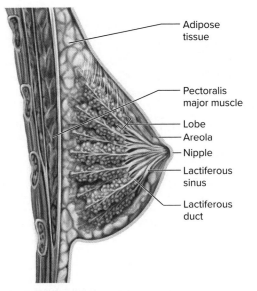

▲ **FIGURE 15.21** Anatomy of the Lactating Breast.

- Adipose tissue
- Pectoralis major muscle
- Lobe
- Areola
- Nipple
- Lactiferous sinus
- Lactiferous duct

Keynote

- There is no relation between breast size and the ability to breastfeed.

WORD	PRONUNCIATION		ELEMENTS	DEFINITION
apoptosis	AP-op-**TOE**-sis	P/ R/	apo- *separation from* -ptosis *drooping*	Programmed normal cell death
areola areolar (adj)	ah-**REE**-oh-lah ah-**REE**-oh-lar	 S/ R/	Latin *small area* -ar *pertaining to* areol- *areola*	Circular reddish area surrounding the nipple Pertaining to the areola
axilla axillae (pl) axillary (adj)	**AK**-sill-ah **AK**-sill-ee **AK**-sill-air-ee	 S/ R/	Latin *armpit* -ary *pertaining to* axill- *armpit*	Medical term for the armpit Pertaining to the armpit
colostrum	koh-**LOSS**-trum		Latin *foremilk*	The first breast secretion at the end of pregnancy
immunoglobulin	IM-you-noh-**GLOB**-you-lin	S/ R/CF R/	-in *chemical compound, substance* immun/o- *immune* -globul- *globular, protein*	Specific protein evoked by an antigen. All antibodies are immunoglobulins
lactation (noun) lactate (verb) lactiferous (adj)	lak-**TAY**-shun **LAK**-tate lak-**TIF**-er-us	S/ R/ S/ S/ R/	-ation *action, process of* lact- *milk* -ate *composed of, pertaining to* -ous *pertaining to* -ifer- *to bear, carry*	Production of milk To produce milk Pertaining to or yielding milk
mammary	**MAM**-ah-ree	S/ R/	-ary *pertaining to* mamm- *breast*	Pertaining to the lactating breast
nipple	**NIP**-el		Old English *small nose*	Projection from the breast into which the lactiferous ducts open
oxytocin	**OCK**-see-**TOE**-sin	S/ R/ R/	-in *substance* oxy- *oxygen* -toc- *labor*	Pituitary hormone that stimulates the uterus to contract
prolactin	pro-**LAK**-tin	S/ P/ R/	-in *substance* pro- *before* -lact- *milk*	Pituitary hormone that stimulates the production of milk

EXERCISES

A. Find the false statements in the following choices. *Choose T if the statement is True. Choose F if the statement is False.*   **LO 15.4 and 15.7**

1. The lactiferous ducts produce milk.   T   F

2. In late pregnancy, the breast secretory alveoli and lactiferous ducts contain colostrum.   T   F

3. High levels of immunoglobulins are in breast milk.   T   F

4. The essential stimulus for milk production is suckling of the breast.   T   F

5. The suckling of the nipple produces estrogen.   T   F

6. Milk flows from the lactiferous duct to the lactiferous sinus to the nipple. T   F

B. Spelling *your documentation correctly is a mark of an educated professional. Read the following statements, and insert the correctly spelled term in the blanks.*   **LO 15.2, 15.4, and 15.7**

1. The circular, reddish area surrounding the nipple is the *(aireola/areola)* _____.

2. After complete cessation of lactation, involution of the *(mamery/mammary)* _____ gland occurs.

3. Programmed cell death is known as *(apotosis/apoptosis)* _____.

4. The first breast secretion at the end of pregnancy is known as *(colestrium/colostrum)* _____.

C. Construct *medical terms related to the breast. Fill in the blanks with the correct word element.*   **LO 15.1, 15.4, and 15.7**

1. Pituitary hormone that stimulates the uterus to contract: _____ / _____ / _____

2. Programmed natural cell death: _____ / _____

3. Pituitary hormone that stimulates the production of milk: _____ / _____ / _____

4. Pertaining to or yielding milk: _____ / _____ / _____

5. Establishing the cause of disease: _____ / _____ / _____

Disorders of the Breast

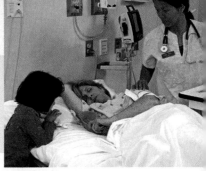

Rick Brady/McGraw-Hill Education

Disorders of the Breast (LO 15.10)

Mastitis, an inflammation of the breast, can occur in association with breastfeeding if the nipple or areola is cracked or traumatized. **Mastalgia** (breast pain) is the most common benign breast disorder. This pain may be associated with breast tenderness or premenstrual syndrome (PMS).

Paget disease of the nipple presents as a scaling, crusting lesion of the nipple, sometimes with a discharge from the nipple (*Figure 15.22*). It is indicative of an underlying cancer that must be the focus of diagnosis and treatment.

Nipple discharge, particularly if it is bloody and only from one breast, is an indication of an underlying disorder like breast cancer and should be investigated.

Fibroadenomas are confined, small, benign tumors that can be either cystic or solid, and can be multiple. These tumors can be surgically removed.

Fibrocystic breast disease presents as a dense, irregular, cobblestone consistency of the breast, often with intermittent breast discomfort. It occurs in over 60% of all women and is considered by many doctors as a normal condition since these changes in the breast are noncancerous.

Breast cancer affects one in eight women in their lifetimes. Risk factors include: a family history, particularly if a woman carries either the **BRCA1 or BRCA2 gene;** the use of postmenopausal estrogen therapy; and an early menarche and late menopause.

Galactorrhea occurs when a woman produces milk when she's not breastfeeding. This can occur in association with hormone therapy, antidepressants, a pituitary gland tumor, and the use of opioids in addition to certain herbal supplements. In most cases, the milk production ceases with time.

Gynecomastia is an enlargement of the breast that can be unilateral or bilateral. It can occur in both sexes and is usually associated with liver disease, marijuana use, or drug therapy involving estrogens, calcium channel blockers, and **antineoplastic** drugs. Gynecomastia sometimes remits or disappears after the drug is withdrawn. Occasionally, cosmetic surgery is needed.

Keynote

- There is some disagreement whether routine mammograms should begin at age 40 or 50 and whether they should be performed annually or every 2 years.

Abbreviations

BRCA1, breast cancer genes
BRCA2

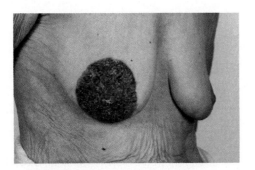

▲ **FIGURE 15.22** Paget Disease of the Nipple Is Associated with Breast Cancer.

Clinical Photography, Central Manchester University Hospitals NHS Foundation Trust, UK/Science Source

WORD	PRONUNCIATION	ELEMENTS		DEFINITION
antineoplastic	AN-tee-nee-oh-PLAS-tik	S/ P/ R/CF R/	-tic *pertaining to* anti- *against* -ne/o- *new* -plas- *growth*	Pertaining to the prevention of the growth and spread of cancer cells
fibroadenoma	FIE-broh-ad-en-OH-muh	S/ R/CF R/	-oma *tumor* fibr/o- *fiber* -aden- *gland*	Benign tumor containing much fibrous tissue
fibrocystic disease	fie-broh-SIS-tik diz-EEZ	S/ R/CF R/	-ic *pertaining to* fibr/o- *fiber* -cyst- *cyst*	Benign breast disease with multiple tiny lumps and cysts
galactorrhea	gah-LAK-toe-REE-ah	S/ R/CF	-rrhea *flow* galact/o- *milk*	Abnormal flow of milk from the breasts
gene genetics geneticist (**Note:** *Two suffixes*)	JEEN jeh-NET-iks jeh-NET-ih-sist	 S/ R/ S/	Greek *origin, birth* -ics *knowledge* genet- *origin* -ist *specialist*	Functional segment of DNA molecule Science of the inheritance of characteristics A specialist in genetics
gynecomastia	GUY-nih-koh-MAS-tee-ah	S/ R/CF R/	-ia *condition* gynec/o- *female* -mast- *breast*	Enlargement of the breast
mastalgia	mass-TAL-jee-uh	S/ R/	-algia *pain* mast- *breast*	Pain in the breast
mastitis	mass-TIE-tis	S/ R/	-itis *inflammation* mast- *breast*	Inflammation of the breast
Paget disease	PAJ-et diz-EEZ		Sir James Paget, 1814–1899, English surgeon	Scaling, crusting lesion of the nipple, often associated with an underlying cancer of the breast

EXERCISES

Case Report 15.5

You are . . .

. . . a surgical technologist working with Charles Walsh, MD, a surgeon at Fulwood Medical Center.

You are communicating with . . .

. . . Mrs. Victoria Post, a 62-year-old woman who has discovered a lump in her right breast. Mrs. Post found the lump in her right breast together with some lumps in her right armpit on self-examination. She had last examined her breasts about 6 months ago. She began her menopause at age 52. Her mother and a sister died of breast cancer. Physical examination shows a 2-cm firm, painless lesion in the upper outer quadrant of her right breast, and several small, painless lymph nodes in her right axilla. Dr. Walsh has scheduled her for a biopsy of the breast lesion and for DNA testing.

Mrs. Victoria Post's biopsy confirmed that the lump was cancerous. DNA testing showed the presence of the **BRCA1 gene,** which explained the occurrence of breast cancer in her mother and sister. Mrs. Post is to attend a consultation with her surgeon, Dr. Walsh, and her **geneticist,** Ingrid Hughes, MD, PhD, to determine what treatment should be undertaken. For example, because of her high risk of cancer, should she have her left breast, currently cancer-free, removed as a precaution? With BRCA1, there is also a 20% to 40% risk of ovarian cancer. Therefore, should her ovaries also be removed?

A. **Review** *the terms related to disorders of the breast. Insert the term that is being described. Fill in the blanks.*   LO 15.2 and 15.10

1. Pain in the breast: _____

2. Inflammation of the breast: _____

3. A small, benign tumor of the breast: _____

4. Enlargement of the breast: _____

5. Benign breast disease with multiple tiny bumps and cysts: _____

B. **Deconstruct medical terms to understand their meanings.** *Fill in the blanks with the correct definition.*   LO 15.1 and 15.10

1. The suffix in the term **galactorrhea** means: _____

2. The root in the term **mastalgia** means: _____

3. The combining form in the term **galactorrhea** means: _____

4. The suffix in the term **mastitis** means: _____

5. The suffix in the term **gynecomastia** means: _____

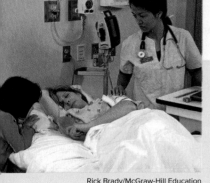

Section 15.9

Diagnostic and Therapeutic Procedures and Pharmacology of the Breast

Abbreviation

BSE   breast self-examination

Diagnostic Procedures (LO 15.11)

Breast self-examination (**BSE**) on a monthly basis has been shown to be of questionable value. It is recommended by the American College of Obstetricians and Gynecologists (**ACOG**) and the American Medical Association (**AMA**) but neither recommended nor discouraged by the American Cancer Society (**ACS**), the National Cancer Institute (**NCI**), and other organizations.

However, many breast cancers are discovered as a lump by the patient during a self-examination. Another 40% are discovered on routine **mammogram** *(Figure 15.23)*. Routine **mammography** reduces breast cancer mortality by 25% to 30%. However, it has a false positive rate of 7% and a false negative rate of 10%.

- **2-D mammography** takes two images of the breast, one from the side and one from the top.

- **3-D mammography** takes multiple x-ray images that are taken when the camera moves in an arc over the breast. A computer combines the images to recreate a 3-D image of the breast. As of 2020, the ACS does not recommend a 3-D mammogram over a 2-D mammogram.

- Ultrasound, magnetic resonance imaging (MRI), and positron emission mammography (PEM) are adjuncts to routine 2-D or 3-D mammography for further evaluation of suspicious lesions.

The pathology report on breast cancer cells will include results of a hormone receptor assay. A breast cancer is called **estrogen-receptor-positive (ER-positive)** if its cells have receptors for estrogen that promote their growth. A breast cancer is called **progesterone-receptor-positive** if its cells have receptors for progesterone that can promote their growth. Approximately two-thirds of breast cancers test positive for hormone receptors. The pathology report also will tell if the breast cancer cells have too many copies of the **gene HER2.** If the breast cancer cells are negative for both hormone receptors and HER2, it is called a **triple negative** breast cancer.

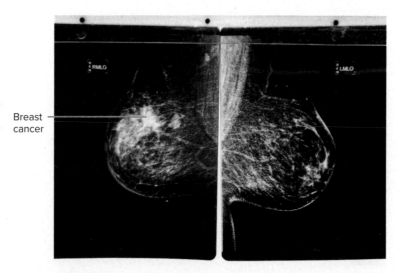

Breast cancer

▲ **FIGURE 15.23** Mammogram Showing Breast Cancer and a Normal Breast.

Alan Nissa/Shutterstock

Stereotactic biopsy, a needle biopsy performed during mammography, and excisional biopsy, surgical removal of a tumor with a surrounding margin of normal breast tissue, provide material for a pathological diagnosis.

Staging of breast cancer (TNM) is based on the size of the tumor in the breast (T), the status of the lymph nodes in the axilla (N), and the metastatic spread to distant sites (M).

Therapeutic Procedures (LO 15.11)

Surgical treatments for breast cancer include the following:

- Lumpectomy and quadrantectomy are breast-conserving surgical procedures.

- Simple mastectomy removes the whole breast.

- Modified radical mastectomy removes the whole breast and the axillary lymph nodes, but the muscle is left intact.

- Radical mastectomy is complete removal of all breast tissue, the underlying pectoralis major muscle, and all associated lymph nodes.

Radiation therapy uses high energy rays or particles to destroy cancer cells. External beam radiation is delivered from a machine outside the body. Internal radiation (brachytherapy) uses radioactive seeds or pellets placed inside the body for a short time at the site of the lesion.

Suction lipectomy (liposuction) is the insertion of a metal tube into an incision of the skin, and then suction is applied and fat tissue is aspirated and removed. This technique is used to treat excess breast tissue in gynecomastia. It also is used for other areas of the body not related to disorders of the breast.

Pharmacology (LO 15.11)

Chemotherapy is a systemic therapy affecting the whole body by going through the bloodstream to destroy any cancer cells; unfortunately it also affects other body cells, producing side effects. There are numerous chemotherapy drugs that are used to treat breast cancer which are often used in combination. Examples of these medications include but are not limited to 5-fluorouracil (5-FU), capecitabine, carboplatin (Paraplatin), cyclophosphamide (Cytoxan), docetaxel (Taxotere), doxorubicin (Adriamycin), methotrexate sodium, paclitaxel (Taxol), and pertuzumab.

In 2019, the U.S. FDA approved the first immunotherapy treatment. It is a combination of atezolizumab (Tecentriq) and nab-paclitaxel (Abraxane) for people with advanced triple negative breast cancer. Women with stage IV cancers are treated with chemotherapy and other types of medications including hormone therapy (tamoxifen) and target therapy such as ribociclib (Kisquali). Numerous standard chemotherapy regimens use combinations of the drugs.

Selective estrogen receptor modulator (SERM) medications include tamoxifen (Soltamox or Novaldex), raloxifene (Evista), and toremifene (Fareston). These medications block estrogen from attaching to the estrogen receptors of ER-positive breast cancer cells, either slowing the growth of or killing the cancer cells.

For breast cancer cells that produce excessive amounts of HER2, Herceptin blocks this production, causing the cancer cells to die.

Word Analysis and Definition

S = Suffix P = Prefix R = Root R/CF = Combining Form

WORD	PRONUNCIATION	ELEMENTS		DEFINITION
assay	**ASS**-ay		French *to try*	Analysis of concentration of drugs or other biological markers
brachytherapy	brack-ee-**THAIR**-ah-pee	P/ R/	**brachy-** *short* **-therapy** *treatment*	Radiation therapy in which the source of irradiation is implanted in the tissue to be treated
chemotherapy	**KEE**-moh-**THAIR**-ah-pee	R/CF R/	**chem/o-** *chemical* **-therapy** *treatment*	Treatment using chemical agents
lipectomy	lip-**EK**-toh-mee	S/ R/	**-ectomy** *surgical excision* **lip-** *fatty tissue*	Surgical removal of adipose tissue
lumpectomy	lump-**EK**-toh-mee	S/ R/	**-ectomy** *surgical excision* **lump-** *piece*	Removal of a lesion with preservation of surrounding tissue
mammogram	**MAM**-oh-gram	S/ R/CF	**-gram** *a record* **mamm/o-** *breast*	The record produced by x-ray imaging of the breast
mammography	mah-**MOG**-rah-fee	S/	**-graphy** *process of recording*	Process of X-ray imaging of the breast
mastectomy	mass-**TEK**-toh-mee	S/ R/	**-ectomy** *surgical excision* **mast-** *breast*	Surgical excision of the breast
quadrantectomy	kwad-ran-**TEK**-toh-mee	S/ R/	**-ectomy** *surgical excision* **quadrant-** *quarter*	Surgical excision of a quadrant of the breast
radiation	ray-dee-**AY**-shun	S/ R/	**-ation** *process* **radi-** *radiation*	The sending forth of X-rays or other rays for treatment or diagnosis
radical	**RAD**-ih-kal		Latin *root*	Extensive or thorough
stereotactic	**STAIR**-ee-oh-**TAK**-tik	S/ R/CF R/	**-ic** *pertaining to* **stere/o-** *three-dimensional* **-tact-** *orderly arrangement*	Pertaining to a precise three-dimensional method to locate a lesion

EXERCISES

A. As a health care professional, you must know the proper use of each medical term. *Use the words provided below to correctly complete each sentence. Fill in the blanks.* **LO 15.11**

mammography   mammogram   mastectomy

1. Mrs. Rivera makes a yearly checkup with her gynecologist to include a _____ .

2. This year, the radiologist responsible for evaluating Mrs. Rivera's _____ tests noted an abnormal area in her right breast.

3. The pathologist reported her findings and the surgeon deemed it necessary to remove Mrs. Rivera's entire right breast along with the pectoralis major muscle and associated lymph nodes. Mrs. Rivera was advised to have a radical _____ .

B. Pronunciation is important whether you are saying the word or listening to a word from a coworker. Identify the proper pronunciation of the following medical terms.   **LO 15.2, 15.5, 15.7, 15.8, 15.9, and 15.12**

1. The correct pronunciation for a condition of pain during sexual intercourse

   a. DIS-pair-you-nee-ah

   b. dis-pah-**RUE**-nee-ah

   c. dis-**YOU**-ree-ah

   d. DIS-your-**EE**-ah

   Correctly spell the term: _____

2. The correct pronunciation for the human organism from the end of the eighth week after conception to birth

   a. nee-oh-**NATE**

   b. **EM**-bree-oh

   c. **ZIE**-goht

   d. **FEE**-tus

Correctly spell the term: _____

3. The correct pronunciation for an endoscope to view the vagina and cervix

   a. **KOL**-poh-scope

   b. col-**POR**-ah-fee

   c. kyu-**REH**-rahzh

   d. **KOH**-nih-**ZAY**-shun

Correctly spell the term: _____

4. The correct pronunciation for the specialist that cares for pregnant woman

   a. **OHB**-steht-ri-**SHUN**

   b. ob-steh-**TRISH**-un

   c. guy-nih-**KOL**-oh-jist

   d. **GUY**-nigh-**KOL**-ohj-ist

Correctly spell the term: _____

5. The correct pronunciation for the first bowel movement of the newborn

   a. **KERN**-ict-er-us

   b. ker-**NIK**-ter-us

   c. meh-**KOH**-nee-um

   d. meek-**OH**-nee-yum

Correctly spell the term: _____

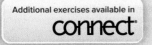
Additional exercises available in
connect
**Chapter Review exercises, along with additional practice items,
are available in Connect!**

Infancy to Old Age

The Languages of Pediatrics and Geriatrics

Learning Outcomes

Immediately after birth and in the whole neonatal period, dramatic and rapid changes occur in the growth and development of cells, tissues, and body systems. These changes slow down through infancy, childhood, adolescence and young adulthood until maturity, all of which occur at different ages for each body system. In general, biological maturity occurs in the late twenties. Eventually and inevitably, different physiological changes in cells, tissues, and body systems lead to a progressive deterioration and decline in function. This process is called **senescence** and is manifested as the changes that occur in aging and eventually in death. To communicate with your colleagues and patients about this process, you will need to:

LO 16.1 Use roots, combining forms, suffixes, and prefixes to construct and analyze (deconstruct) medical terms related to pediatrics and geriatrics.

LO 16.2 Spell and pronounce correctly medical terms related to pediatrics and geriatrics to communicate them with accuracy and precision in any health care setting.

LO 16.3 Define accepted abbreviations related to pediatrics and geriatrics.

LO 16.4 Relate the adaptations of each body system that occur in the neonatal period to their functions.

LO 16.5 Relate the structures of the body systems to their changes of aging, senescence, and death.

LO 16.6 Identify and describe developmental disorders of childhood and adolescence.

LO 16.7 Identify and describe disorders and pathological conditions related to aging and senescence.

LO 16.8 Identify the diagnostic and therapeutic procedures and pharmacologic agents used for developmental disorders of childhood and adolescence and for aging, senescence, and death.

LO 16.9 Identify health professionals involved in the care of neonatal and geriatric patients.

LO 16.10 Apply your knowledge of medical terms relating to pediatrics and geriatrics to documentation, medical records, and medical reports.

LO 16.11 Translate the medical terms relating to pediatrics and geriatrics into everyday language in order to communicate clearly with patients and their families.

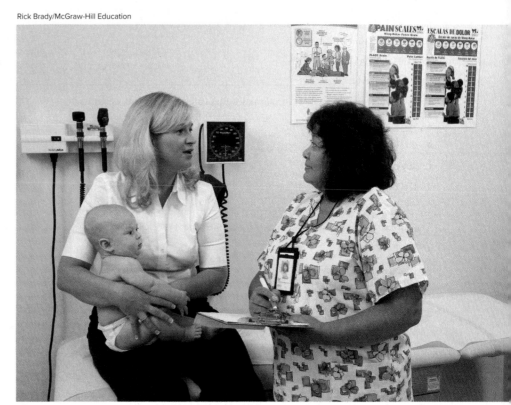

Rick Brady/McGraw-Hill Education

The health professionals involved in the treatment of children and the elderly include:

- **Neonatologists** are physicians who are subspecialists in disorders of the newborn, particularly ill, or premature infants.
- **Pediatricians** are physicians who are specialists in disorders of childhood and adolescence.
- **Geriatricians** are physicians who are specialists in the process of and problems of aging.
- **Gerontologists** are professionals who are specially trained in the process of and general problems of aging.
- **Geriatric nurse practitioners** are nurses with at least a master's degree and special training in the care of the elderly.
- **Social workers, nutritionists, and physical and occupational therapists** are members of the geriatric care team as needs for their services arise.

Neonatal Period

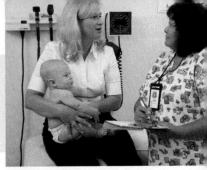

Rick Brady/McGraw-Hill Education

Neonatal Adaptations (LO 16.1, 16.3, 16.4, and 16.9)

Fetal life is a preparation for birth, and at the end of the first 8 weeks, all the fetus' organ systems are in place *(Figure 16.1)*. From then until birth, the organs grow and acquire the functional capabilities to support life outside the mother. Sometimes, a part of this process may fail, causing a developmental abnormality in the **fetus**.

At birth, normal organ development is not yet complete, but the **neonate** *(Figure 16.2)* or newborn infant suddenly has to **adapt** to a totally different environment: life outside the womb. Each of the neonate's organ systems has to adapt to this new environment, and go on to complete its development during childhood. This developmental process is why children are not just "little adults," and why **pediatricians** are needed to practice the specialty of **pediatrics**.

Immediately after birth, the neonate is evaluated and given an **Apgar score** at 1 minute and again at 5 minutes of life, occasionally again at 10 minutes. This score gives health care providers an immediate assessment of the baby's condition at birth. The five measurements of **A**ctivity, **P**ulse, **G**rimace, **A**ppearance, and **R**espiration are each scored on a 3-point scale: 0 (poor), 1, or 2 (normal). The total score obtainable is between 0 and 10. A score of 7 or above is normal. A score below 7 indicates the baby needs special immediate care, including oxygen and other potential life support measures. The Apgar score does not necessarily predict long-term health, intellectual status, or outcome.

Abbreviations

APGAR	activity, pulse, grimace, appearance, respiration

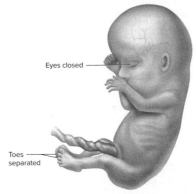

Eyes closed

Toes separated

▲ **FIGURE 16.1**
Fetus at 8 Weeks (56 Days).

McGraw-Hill Education

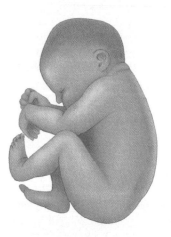

▲ **FIGURE 16.2**
Full-Term Infant (38 Weeks).

McGraw-Hill Education

Word Analysis and Definition

S = Suffix   P = Prefix   R = Root   R/CF = Combining Form

WORD	PRONUNCIATION	ELEMENTS		DEFINITION
adaptation adapt (verb)	ad-ap-**TAY**-shun a-**DAPT**	S/ R/	-ation *process* adapt- *to adjust*	Change in the function or structure of an organ or organism to meet new conditions
anomaly anomalies (pl)	ah-**NOM**-ah-lee		Greek *irregularity*	Structural abnormality present at birth
Apgar score	**AP**-gar SKOR		Virginia Apgar, U.S. anesthesiologist, 1909–1974	Evaluation of a newborn's status
fetus fetal (adj)	**FEE**-tus **FEE**-tal	 S/ R/	Latin *offspring* -al *pertaining to* fet- *fetus*	Human organism from the end of the eighth week after conception to birth Pertaining to the fetus
neonate neonatal (adj) (Note: The "e" is dropped as it is followed by another vowel, "a.")	**NEE**-oh-nate **NEE**-oh-**NAY**-tal	R/CF R/CF S/ R/	neo- *new* -nat/e *born* -al *pertaining to* -nat- *born*	A newborn infant Pertaining to the newborn infant or the newborn period
neonatologist	**NEE**-oh-nay-**TOL**-oh-jist	S/	-logist *one who studies, specialist*	Medical specialist in disorders of the newborn
pediatrics	pee-dee-**AT**-riks	S/ R/ R/	-ics *knowledge* -iatr- *medical treatment* ped- *child*	Medical specialty of treating children during development from birth through adolescence
pediatrician	**PEE**-dee-ah-**TRISH**-an	S/	-ician *expert*	Medical specialist in disorders of childhood and adolescence

ASD	atrial septal defect
PDA	patent ductus arteriosus
TOF	tetralogy of Fallot
VSD	ventricular septal defect

Cardiovascular System (CVS) Adaptations (LO 16.1, 16.3, and 16.5)

In utero (when the fetus is still in the uterus), the fetus is dependent on the placenta and umbilical cord to provide oxygen and nutrients, and to remove carbon dioxide and fetal wastes. At birth, the two major divisions of the cardiovascular system—the pulmonary and systemic circulations *(see Chapter 6)*—become separate and operational.

Congenital (meaning inherited or existing at birth) cardiovascular defects are present in about 1% of births. Before birth, a **patent** (open) vessel called the ductus arteriosus connects the aorta and pulmonary artery. Normally, this closes within a few hours of birth. However, when it does not close, the **patent ductus arteriosus (PDA)** allows blood that should normally flow through the aorta and nourish the body to be shunted to the lungs. Children with a PDA grow slowly, tire easily, and are at higher risk for developing lung infections. A small PDA can close spontaneously, or a ductus can be closed with medication, by surgically tying it, or by inserting a plug.

Septal defects occur when the baby is born with an opening ("hole in the heart") in the **septum** (wall) that separates the right and left sides of the heart. An opening between the two upper chambers is called an **atrial septal defect (ASD)**. An opening between the two lower chambers is called a **ventricular septal defect (VSD)**. Small defects often close on their own during the first year of life; if not, they can be closed surgically.

Cyanosis occurs when the body lacks oxygen either because the right heart fails to pump a sufficient amount of blood to the lungs or the left heart fails to deliver adequate oxygen to the rest of the body. If the tissues are extremely low in oxygen, a bluish grey discoloration (cyanosis) will occur. Neonates with cyanosis are called "blue babies" because of their **cyanotic** blue skin *(Figure 16.3)*. One type of cyanotic heart disease is the **tetralogy of Fallot (TOF)**, in which four heart defects prevent adequate blood flow to the lungs. Children with TOF are slow to grow, are **dyspneic**, and require open-heart surgery to correct the defects.

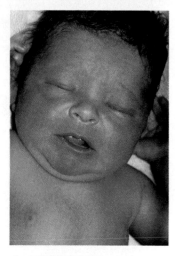

▲ **FIGURE 16.3**
Cyanotic ("Blue") Baby.

St Bartholomew's Hospital, London/
Science Source

Word Analysis and Definition

S = Suffix P = Prefix R = Root R/CF = Combining Form

WORD	PRONUNCIATION		ELEMENTS	DEFINITION
atrium atria (pl) atrial (adj)	A-tree-um A-tree-ah A-tree-al	S/ R/ S/	-um *structure* atri- *entrance, atrium* -al *pertaining to*	Chamber where blood enters the heart on both the right and left sides Pertaining to the atrium
congenital	kon-**JEN**-ih-tal	S/ P/ R/	-al *pertaining to* con- *together, with* -genit- *bring forth*	Present at birth, either inherited or due to an event during gestation up to the moment of birth
cyanosis cyanotic (adj)	sigh-ah-**NO**-sis sigh-ah-**NOT**-ik	S/ R/ S/ R/CF	-osis *condition* cyan- *blue* -tic *pertaining to* cyan/o- *blue*	Blue discoloration of skin, lips, and nail beds due to low levels of oxygen in the blood Pertaining to or marked by cyanosis
defect	**DEE**-fect		Latin *to lack*	An absence, malformation, or imperfection
dyspnea dyspneic (adj)	disp-**NEE**-ah disp-**NEE**-ik	P/ R/ S/	dys- *bad, difficult* -pnea *breathe* -ic *pertaining to*	Difficulty breathing Pertaining to or suffering from difficulty in breathing
in utero	IN **YOU**-ter-oh	R/CF	uter/o *uterus*	Within the womb; not yet born
patent patent ductus arteriosus (PDA)	**PAY**-tent **PAY**-tent **DUK**-tus ar-**TEER**-ee-oh-sus		Latin *lie open* ductus Latin *leading* arteriosus Latin *like an artery*	Open An open, direct channel between the aorta and the pulmonary artery
septum septa (pl)	**SEP**-tum **SEP**-tah		Latin *partition*	A thin wall dividing two cavities
tetralogy of fallot (TOF)	teh-**TRAL**-oh-jee OV fah-**LOH**	S/ P/	-logy *study of* tetra- *four* Etienne-Louis Fallot, 1850–1911, French physician	Set of four congenital heart defects occurring together
ventricle	**VEN**-trih-kel		Latin *small belly*	Chamber of the heart (pumps blood) or a cavity in the brain (produces cerebrospinal fluid)

Respiratory Adaptations (LO 16.1, 16.3, and 16.5)

Respiratory adaptations occur immediately at birth when the baby takes its first breath spontaneously, unless the baby's respiratory function is depressed by too much sedation or anesthesia in the mother.

The development of the chemical **surfactant** is necessary for the growth of fully functioning lungs. When surfactant is deficient, the lung alveoli collapse and are difficult to re-expand; this prevents a normal exchange of respiratory gases. This deficiency occurs in **premature** infants born before the 35th week of gestation and produces **respiratory distress syndrome (RDS),** previously called **hyaline membrane disease (HMD)**. The more premature the baby, the greater its risk of developing RDS. Infants with RDS are at risk for cerebral ischemia, hemorrhage, and neonatal death.

Meconium aspiration syndrome (MAS) occurs in newborns who are stressed in utero or at the time of delivery, most common in full-term or postterm babies. The distress causes the fetus to expel **meconium** into the amniotic fluid. Deep gasping for breath by the distressed fetus causes the **aspiration** (or inhalation) of meconium into the lungs. This is treated using **intubation** and **suction** to remove the meconium-stained fluid from the lungs.

Transient tachypnea of the newborn (TTN) occurs most often in C-sections and **precipitate** (unduly rapid) vaginal deliveries. With TTN, amniotic fluid remains in the infant's lungs and causes a self-limiting respiratory distress.

Sudden infant death syndrome (SIDS) may be caused by a failure of cardiorespiratory control mechanisms to **mature.** It is the sudden death of an infant with no identifiable cause found after a thorough investigation and autopsy. It occurs during sleep and peaks between 2 and 3 months, and can be prevented by placing infants on their backs to sleep *(Figure 16.4)*.

Keynote

• Meconium is the first stool a baby passes.

Abbreviations

HMD	hyaline membrane disease
MAS	meconium aspiration syndrome
RDS	respiratory distress syndrome
SIDS	sudden infant death syndrome
TTN	transient tachypnea of the newborn

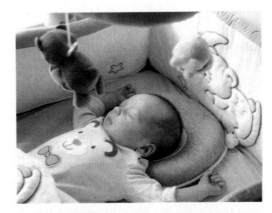

▲ **FIGURE 16.4**   Infant Sleeping on Back.

DigitalMammoth/Shutterstock

Word Analysis and Definition

S = Suffix   P = Prefix   R = Root   R/CF = Combining Form

WORD	PRONUNCIATION		ELEMENTS	DEFINITION
aspiration	as-pih-**RAY**-shun	S/ R/	-ion *process* aspirat- *to breathe on*	Removal by suction of fluid or gas from a body cavity
hyaline membrane disease	**HIGH**-ah-line **MEM**-brain diz-**EEZ**	S/ R/ R/ P/ R/	-ine *pertaining to* hyal- *glass* membrane *cover* dis- *apart from* -ease *normal function*	Respiratory distress syndrome of the newborn
intubation	**IN**-tyu-**BAY**-shun	S/ P/ R/	-ation *a process* in- *in* -tub- *tube*	Insertion of a tube into the trachea
mature maturity	mah-**CHUR** mah-**CHUR**-ih-tee	S/ R/	Latin *mature* -ity *condition, state* matur- *ripe, ready*	Fully developed A state of full development or growth
premature	pree-mah-**TYUR**	P/	pre- *before*	Baby delivered before 37 weeks of gestation
meconium	meh-**KOH**-nee-um		Greek a *little poppy*	The first bowel movement of the newborn
precipitate labor	pree-**SIP**-ih-tate **LAY**-bore		precipitate, Latin *to throw down* labor, Latin toil *suffering*	A very rapid labor and delivery
respiratory distress syndrome	**RES**-pih-rah-tor-ee dis-**TRESS SIN**-drome	S/ R/ P/ R/	-atory *pertaining to* respir- *to breathe* Latin *to draw apart* syn- *together* -drome *running*	A condition of premature infants caused by lack of surfactant characterized by increased respiratory rate and dyspnea
surfactant	sir-**FAK**-tant		surface, *active agent*	A protein and fat compound that creates surface tension to hold the lung alveolar walls apart
suction	**SUK**-shun		Latin *sucking*	Use of a catheter to clear the upper airway or other tubes
transient	**TRAN**-see-ent		Latin *to pass*	Not permanent

Thermoregulation Adaptations (LO 16.3 and 16.5)

Thermoregulation simply means the body's ability to maintain a steady temperature. This is especially important for newborns. Because an infant has a larger ratio of surface area to body volume than an adult, it loses heat more easily. This is particularly true if the infant's body surface is wet, and is the reason that a newborn is dried, wrapped, and placed in a warmer soon after birth. **Hypothermia** (very low body temperature) is more likely to occur in premature or small for gestational age (**SGA**) neonates.

Brain and Neurologic Adaptations (LO 16.4)

A newborn baby's brain is one-quarter of its adult size. A pediatrician monitors the growth of the baby's brain by charting increases in the baby's head circumference. At birth, only the spinal cord and brainstem are well developed. The cortex is primitive. All of the newborn's kicking, grasping, **rooting reflex** (searching for the nipple), and crying behaviors are functions of the brainstem, which is why they are involuntary and/or not well coordinated.

Congenital Neurologic Abnormalities (LO 16.4 and 16.6)

There are some congenital neurologic abnormalities that can severely affect the neonate's quality of life, and its ability to carry on living.

Anencephaly is the absence of the cerebral hemispheres, which is incompatible with life.

Microcephaly is characterized by small cerebral hemispheres, leading to motor and mental retardation.

An **encephalocele** is a protrusion of nervous tissue and meninges through a defect in the skull.

Hydrocephalus is an enlargement of the ventricles with excessive cerebrospinal fluid (**CSF**), and is the most common cause of a visibly large head in the neonate *(see Chapter 10)*.

Spina bifida is a failure of the vertebral column to close over the spinal cord in the lumbar and sacral regions. **Spina bifida occulta** occurs when the vertebral arches fail to unite and there is no neurologic involvement *(see Chapter 10)*. When the vertebral defect is more open, nervous tissue can protrude through the arch in a sac. In **spina bifida cystica** *(Figure 16.5)*, the sac can contain meninges **(meningocele),** part of the spinal cord **(myelocele),** or both **(myelomeningocele)** *(see Chapter 10)*.

Neonatal seizures are a common and sometimes serious neonatal disorder. These seizures can be primary—caused by an intracranial process like meningitis or a cerebral hemorrhage from a difficult birth—or secondary, caused by a systemic or metabolic problem like hypoxia, hypoglycemia, or hypocalcemia. Treatment is directed to the underlying condition.

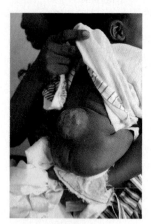

▲ **FIGURE 16.5**
Child with Spina Bifida Cystica.

Photo By BSIP/UIG Via Getty Images

Skeletal Adaptations (LO 16.4 and 16.6)

The skeletal system can fail in utero and produce congenital abnormalities in different parts of the newborn's body.

Craniofacial malformations most often present in the form of **cleft lip** and **cleft palate**, which occur once in 800 births *(Figure 16.6)*. A cleft palate interferes with feeding and speech development. The end treatment is surgical closure.

Developmental dysplasia of the hip (congenital dislocation of the hip) occurs more commonly in female infants and following a breech delivery. A hip ultrasound can confirm this diagnosis. Treatment is with padded diapers to keep the affected femur pulled back and stabilized. Surgery may be necessary.

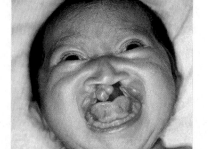

▲ **FIGURE 16.6**
Infant with Cleft Lip and Palate.

Scott Camazine/Alamy Stock Photo

Word Analysis and Definition

WORD	PRONUNCIATION		ELEMENTS	DEFINITION
anencephaly	AN-en-SEF-ah-lee	P/ R/	an- *without* -encephaly *condition of the brain*	Born without cerebral hemispheres
cleft lip cleft palate	KLEFT LIP KLEFT PAL-at		cleft, Latin *fissure, separation of parts*	Congenital defect of the upper lip Congenital defect of the palate
craniofacial	KRAY-nee-oh-FAY-shal	S/ R/CF R/	-al *pertaining to* crani/o- *cranium* -faci- *face*	Pertaining to both the face and the cranium
dysplasia	dis-PLAY-zee-ah	S/ P/ R/	-ia *condition* dys- *bad, difficult* -plas- *molding, formation*	Abnormal tissue formation
dysplastic (adj)	dis-PLAS-tik	S/	-tic *pertaining to*	Pertaining to or showing abnormal tissue formation
encephalocele	en-SEF-ah-loh-seal	S/ R/CF	-cele *swelling, hernia* encephal/o- *brain*	Congenital defect of the cranium with herniation of brain tissue
hydrocephalus	high-droh-SEF-ah-lus	P/ R/	hydro- *water* -cephalus *head*	Enlarged head due to excess CSF in the cerebral ventricles
hypothermia	high-poh-THER-me-ah	P/ S/ R/	hypo- *below* -ia *condition* -therm- *heat*	Very low core body temperature
meningocele	meh-NING-oh-seal	S/ R/CF	-cele *hernia* -mening/o- *meninges*	Protrusion of the meninges from the spinal cord or brain through a defect in the vertebral column or cranium
microcephaly	MY-kroh-SEF-ah-lee	P/ R/	micro- *small* -cephaly *condition of the head*	Small head
microcephalic (adj)	MY-kroh-seh-FAL	S/	-ic *pertaining to*	Pertaining to or suffering from a small head
myelocele	MY-eh-low-seal	S/ R/CF	-cele *hernia, swelling* myel/o- *spinal cord*	Protrusion of the spinal cord through a defect in the vertebral arch
myelomeningocele (Note: also referred to as meningomyelocele)	MY-eh-low-meh-NING-oh-seal	R/CF	-mening/o- *meninges*	Protrusion of the spinal cord and meninges through a defect in the vertebral arch of one or more vertebrae
rooting reflex	RUE-ting REE-fleks		Latin *root* Latin *bend back*	A neonatal reflex to turn toward the nipple and open the mouth when a nipple is placed on the cheek
spina bifida	SPY-nah BIH-fih-dah	R/CF P/ R/	spin/a *spine* bi- *two* -fida *split*	Failure of one or more vertebral arches to close during fetal development
spina bifida cystica	SIS-tik-ah	S/ R/	-ica *pertaining to* cyst- *cyst*	Meninges and spinal cord protruding through the absent vertebral arch and having the appearance of a cyst
spina bifida occulta	OH-kul-tah	R/CF	occult/a *hidden*	The deformity of the vertebral arch is not apparent from the surface

Abbreviations

FAS   fetal alcohol syndrome
FTT   failure to thrive
SGA   small for gestational age

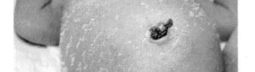

▲ **FIGURE 16.7**
Premature Baby.

Susan Leavines/Science Source

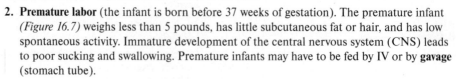

▲ **FIGURE 16.8**
Postmature Infant with Skin Changes.

Vipada Kanajod/Shutterstock

Growth Adaptations (LO 16.1, 16.3, and 16.6)

The neonate's failure to grow fully in the uterus has two main causes:

1. **Inadequate nutrition** (caused by poor placental function). Here, the newborn is below the 10th percentile of babies of the same gestational age. This is called **small for gestational age (SGA).** Good nutrition after delivery will enable the neonate's growth to accelerate to normal.

2. **Premature labor** (the infant is born before 37 weeks of gestation). The premature infant *(Figure 16.7)* weighs less than 5 pounds, has little subcutaneous fat or hair, and has low spontaneous activity. Immature development of the central nervous system (CNS) leads to poor sucking and swallowing. Premature infants may have to be fed by IV or by **gavage** (stomach tube).

Occasionally, labor does not start until after 42 weeks' gestation and produces a **postmature infant**, also known as postterm. *(Figure 16.8).* When birth is delayed beyond term, the placenta atrophies and may calcify, so the fetus receives insufficient nutrition in the days after term. As a result, postterm infants have decreased subcutaneous fat and dry, peeling skin *(Figure 16.8).*

Failure to thrive (FTT) is the term used for an infant or young child who is not growing and developing as expected. There are two main reasons for the failure:

1. **Organic disorders,** like chronic illness (e.g., **celiac disease**), genetic (e.g., Down syndrome), metabolic (e.g., **fetal alcohol syndrome FAS**), and hormone disorders (e.g., pituitary dwarfism).

2. **Psychosocial disorders,** including poverty, lack of education about feeding, neglect or abuse, and parental mental illness or substance abuse.

Urinary System Adaptations (LO 16.1 and 16.6)

Congenital urinary tract disorders include the following conditions:

• Renal **agenesis,** in which one or both kidneys are absent;

• Blockage of urinary flow in utero, causing hydronephrosis of the kidneys;

• **Polycystic kidney disease,** one of the most common genetic disorders; and

• **Hypospadias of the penis,** in which the urethra does not extend to the end of the penis and instead, opens along its underside *(see Chapter 13).*

Digestive System Adaptations (LO 16.1 and 16.6)

Until 6 months of age, the baby needs only breast milk or commercially prepared formula. Around 1 month of age, a feeding routine will usually be established.

Esophageal **atresia**—incomplete formation of the esophagus—is often associated with a **fistula** (abnormal passage) between the esophagus and the trachea. This leads to feeding difficulties and respiratory distress in the neonate's first few days of life.

An immature digestive system may be the cause of **colic,** in which the neonate cries for hours at a time and is difficult to console. About 25% of all infants have colic, which begins between the 3rd and 6th weeks, and usually disappears by the 12th week. There is no known treatment.

Food intolerance, which is totally different from a food allergy *(see Immunological Adaptations),* is an adverse digestive system reaction to food that does not involve the immune system. It can be a metabolic reaction to a digestive enzyme deficiency like **lactase deficiency** *(see Chapter 9),* causing an intolerance to cows' milk.

Hematologic Adaptations (LO 16.1 and 16.6)

The newborn infant has an excess of red blood cells (RBCs). When RBCs are broken down, bilirubin is produced *(see Chapter 7).* Because the neonate's liver is immature and cannot process bilirubin quickly, excess bilirubin is deposited in the tissues, producing jaundice. In the first 3 days after birth, neonatal jaundice affects 50% to 60% of full-term infants and a higher portion of premature infants. In most infants, no specific treatment is needed. More severe cases respond to **phototherapy,** which employs blue wavelengths of light to convert bilirubin to less toxic chemicals that can be excreted in bile or urine.

Hearing Adaptations (LO 16.1, 16.4, and 16.6)

The fetus begins to hear loud noises around the beginning of the third trimester (24 weeks). By the seventh month of pregnancy, the fetus can hear **maternal** speech and, after birth, remember what is heard. **Congenital malformations** of the external auditory canal and middle ear can result in a conductive hearing loss *(see Chapter 11)*. Congenital malformations of the inner ear can result in a sensorineural hearing loss *(see Chapter 11)*.

Visual Adaptations (LO 16.4 and 16.6)

At birth, a non-anesthetized baby is able to see and focus on an object between 8 and 12 inches away. This distance probably relates to the distance between the mother's and baby's faces during breastfeeding *(Figure 16.9)*. For color vision, the baby will see only very brightly colored objects. Full color vision is developed between 3 and 4 months of age.

Immunologic Adaptations (LO 16.1, 16.4, and 16.6)

The baby is born with immunoglobulin G (IgG) levels *(see Chapter 7)* near those of an adult, having acquired them from the mother through the placenta. These levels of antibody molecules remain high enough in the first 6 months to protect the baby against some infectious diseases, but not against others, like **whooping cough (pertussis)** and **diphtheria**. This is why immunization against these diseases takes place in the first 6 months of life.

In **food allergies,** the body's immune system reacts as though a particular food is harmful (an allergen) and creates immunoglobulin E (IgE) antibodies to it *(see Chapter 7)*. This process generates chemicals like histamine that produce the symptoms of a runny nose, itchy skin rash, swelling of the lips, or wheezing. The most common allergens in the neonate are milk, eggs, wheat, soy, and peanuts.

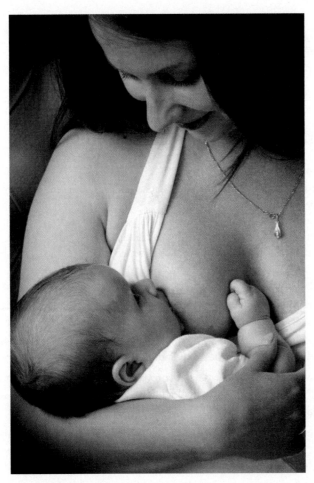

▲ **FIGURE 16.9**
One-Month-Old Baby Breastfeeds and Interacts with Mother.

Tetiana Mandziuk/Shutterstock

WORD	PRONUNCIATION	ELEMENTS		DEFINITION
agenesis	a-**JEN**-eh-sis	P/ R/	a- *without* -genesis *creation, production*	Failure to develop any organ or any part
atresia	a-**TREE**-zee-ah	P/ R/	a- *without* -tresia *a hole*	Congenital absence of a normal opening or lumen
colic	**KOL**-ik	S/ R/	-ic *pertaining to* col- *colon*	Spasmodic, crampy pains in the abdomen
diphtheria	dif-**THEER**-ee-ah		Greek *leather*	Disease with a thick (leathery) coating of the pharynx
fistula	**FIS**-tyu-lah		Latin *pipe, tube*	Abnormal passage
gavage	guh-**VAHZH**		French *to force-feed geese (to make pate de foie gras)*	To feed by a stomach tube
intolerance	in-**TOL**-er-ance		Latin *impatient*	Inability of the small intestine to digest and dispose of a particular dietary substance
lactase	**LAK**-tase	S/ R/	-ase *enzyme* lact- *milk*	Enzyme that breaks down lactose (milk sugar) to glucose and galactose
malformation	**MAL**-for-**MAY**-shun	S/ P/ R/	-ion *condition* mal- *bad* -format- *to form*	Failure of proper or normal development
maternal	mah-**TER**-nal	S/ R/	-al *pertaining to* matern- *mother*	Pertaining to or derived from the mother
pertussis (also known as whooping cough)	per-**TUSS**-is **WHO**-ping KOFF	P/ R/	per- *intense* -tussis *cough*	Infectious disease with a spasmodic, intense cough ending with a whoop
phototherapy	foh-toe-**THAIR**-ah-pee	S/ R/CF	-therapy *treatment* phot/o- *light*	Treatment using light rays
psychosocial	**SIGH**-koh-**SOH**-shal	S/ R/CF R/	-al *pertaining to* -psycho- *mind* -soci/o- *society, social*	Involving both the mind and various social and community aspects of life

Developmental Disorders of Childhood and Adolescence (LO 16.1 and 16.6)

Certain developmental disorders can occur during childhood and/or **adolescence.** The most common of these conditions are outlined below.

Enuresis, also known as bedwetting, occurs in the child who is dry by day, but wets the bed at night without waking up. Fifteen percent of children aged 5 have this condition.

Encopresis is a persistent fecal soiling beyond the age at which toilet training should be complete (i.e., at 3 to 4 years of age).

Eating disorders in early childhood are part of the syndrome **failure to thrive,** and these can include the following:

- **Pica** is the persistent ingestion of nonnutritive substances like paper or soil, and is associated with certain nutritional deficiencies, medical conditions, or mental health conditions and can cause a developmental delay.

- **Rumination** disorder occurs between 3 and 12 months and is characterized by the persistent **regurgitation** and re-chewing of food after feeding. It goes away spontaneously.

- **Feeding disorder of infancy** occurs when a child under 6 years refuses to eat adequately and fails to gain the expected weight. There is no physical explanation found.

Eating disorders in adolescence include the following:

- **Anorexia nervosa** is a condition in which the perception of body image is skewed. This eating disorder entails a refusal to maintain a normal body weight and occurs more frequently in **adolescent** females. Those who suffer from this condition have an inaccurate perception of their body size, weight, and shape.

- **Bulimia (bulimia nervosa)** occurs more frequently in females than males. A person demonstrating bulimic behavior will "binge eat" two or three times per week and then make themselves throw up (**purge**). They tend to **fast** (not eat) between the binges.

- **Binge-eating disorder** is characterized by binge eating two or three times per week with no compensatory vomiting.

Treatment for adolescent eating disorders requires nutritional support and intense psychiatric care.

Keynote

- 90% of adolescent eating disorders occur in females.

S = Suffix   P = Prefix   R = Root   R/CF = Combining Form

WORD	PRONUNCIATION	ELEMENTS		DEFINITION
adolescence (state of)	ad-oh-**LESS**-ents	S/ R/	-ence *state of, quality of* adolesc- *beginning of adulthood*	Stage that begins with puberty and ends with physical maturity
adolescent (person)	ad-oh-**LESS**-ent	S/	-ent *end result, pertaining to*	Pertaining to adolescence or a person in that stage
anorexia nervosa	an-oh-**RECK**-see-ah ner-**VOH**-suh	S/ P/ R/	-ia *condition* an- *without* -orex- *appetite*	An aversion to food due to fear of becoming obese
binge eating	BINJ **EE**-ting		binge, Old English *to soak*	Eating with periods of excessive intake
bulimia	buh-**LEEM**-ee-ah		Greek *hunger*	Episodic bouts of excessive eating with compensatory throwing up
encopresis	en-koh-**PREE**-sis		Greek *full of manure*	Repeated soiling with feces
enuresis	en-you-**REE**-sis	S/ R/	-esis *condition* enur- *urinate*	Involuntary bedwetting
fast (n)	FAST		Old English *hold firm*	The act of eating little or no food
pica	**PIE**-kah		Latin *magpie*	Eating substances not considered to be food
purge	PURJ		Latin *to cleanse*	Consciously throw up or cause bowel evacuation
regurgitation	ree-gur-jih-**TAY**-shun	S/ P/ R/	-ation *process* re- *back, backward* -gurgit- *flood*	Expel contents of the stomach into the mouth, short of vomiting
rumination	**ROO**-min-ay-shun	S/ R/	-ation *process* rumin- *throat*	To bring back food into the mouth to chew over and over

Attention deficit hyperactivity disorder (ADHD) affects almost 10% of school-age children, boys more than twice as often as girls. ADHD has three major components:

1. **Inattention**, with an inability to pay attention to details, carelessness, distractibility, and problems with organization;
2. **Hyperactivity**, shown by fidgeting, squirming, always being on the go, and talking excessively; and
3. **Impulsiveness,** shown by interrupting, intruding, and acting inappropriately.

The etiology is unknown, but some areas of the brain are known to be smaller in patients with ADHD. There is no evidence that parenting plays any role in the development of ADHD. Treatment is with **stimulants**, like *Ritalin* (methylphenidate HCl), or antidepressants, like *Prozac* (fluoxetine), in combination with special educational interventions, parent training to support the child, and **cognitive behavioral therapy (CBT)**. This form of therapy identifies the thinking that is causing unwanted feelings and behaviors, and tries to replace this thinking with thoughts that lead to more desirable behaviors.

Learning disability refers to a group of disorders with difficulties in the acquisition and use of listening, speaking, reading, writing, and reasoning abilities. Learning disability is not associated with obvious problems like bad eyesight and lack of intellectual ability, but instead refers to a discrepancy between a child's capacity to learn and level of achievement. The term **dyslexia** is used for a learning disability characterized primarily by a difficulty with reading and spelling.

Oppositional defiant disorder (ODD) shows a persistent pattern of defiance, disobedience, and hostility to parents and teachers. Children with ODD blame others for their mistakes and frequently lose their tempers.

Conduct disorder occurs between 9 and 17 years and is expressed by fighting, bullying, cruelty, and early substance abuse. Running away from home is also common. Of all children with conduct disorder, up to 50% become antisocial adults.

Therapy for these disruptive disorders is difficult. Behavioral therapy and psychotherapy can help patients express and control their anger. The only two therapeutic programs shown to be effective each involve parent training to help their children.

Obsessive compulsive disorder (OCD) is an anxiety disorder with recurrent unwanted thoughts **(obsessions)** and repetitive behaviors **(compulsions** or **rituals)** like hand washing, counting, and cleaning. Treatment involves finding the right medication (from the many anti-anxiety and antidepressant options) and using CBT.

An **autism spectrum disorder (ASD)** is characterized by varying degrees of impairment in social interactions and communication skills. These disorders are associated with repetitive and **stereotyped** patterns of behavior. Asperger syndrome and pervasive developmental disorder, not otherwise specified (PPD_NOS) are no longer used and instead are included as a part of ASD.

Keynote

- Autism spectrum disorder is a complex range of symptoms with a highly variable clinical presentation.

Abbreviations

ADHD	attention deficit hyperactivity disorder
ASD	autism spectrum disorder
CBT	cognitive behavioral therapy
OCD	obsessive compulsive disorder
ODD	oppositional defiant disorder

WORD	PRONUNCIATION	ELEMENTS		DEFINITION
autism	AWE-tizm		Greek *self*	Developmental disorder of children
cognitive behavioral therapy	KOG-nih-tiv be-HAYV-yur-al THAIR-ah-pee	S/ R/ S/ S/ R/	-ive *quality of* cognit- *thinking* -al *pertaining to* -ior- *pertaining to* behav- *mental or motor activity* Greek *medical treatment*	Psychotherapy that emphasizes thoughts and attitudes in one's behavior
compulsion	kom-PUL-shun	S/ R/	-ion *action, condition* compuls- *to drive, compel*	Uncontrollable impulses to perform an act repetitively
compulsive (adj)	kom-PUL-siv	S/	-ive *quality of*	Possessing uncontrollable impulses to perform an act repetitively
dyslexia (noun)	dis-LEK-see-ah	S/ P/ R/	-ia *condition* dys- *difficult, painful* -lex- *word*	Impaired reading and writing ability below the person's level of intelligence
dyslexic (adj)	dis-LEK-sik	S/	-ic *pertaining to*	Pertaining to or suffering from dyslexia
hyperactivity	HIGH-per-ac-TIV-ih-tee	S/ P/ R/	-ity *state, condition* hyper- *excessive* -activ- *movement*	Excessive restlessness and movement
impulsive	im-PUL-siv	S/ P/ R/	-ive *quality of* im- *not* -puls- *to drive*	Unable to resist performing inappropriate actions
inattention	IN-ah-TEN-shun	S/ P/ R/	-ion *condition* in- *not* -attent- *awareness*	Lack of concentration and direction
obsession (noun)	ob-SESH-un		Latin *to besiege*	Persistent, recurrent, uncontrollable thoughts or impulses
obsessive (adj)	ob-SES-iv	S/ R/	-ive *quality of* obsess- *besieged by thoughts*	Possessing persistent, recurrent, uncontrollable thoughts or impulses
ritual	RICH-oo-al		Latin, *rite*	In psychiatry or psychology, repeated set of actions to relieve or prevent anxiety
stereotype	STER-ee-oh-tipe	S/ R/CF	-type *particular kind, model* stere/o- *three-dimensional*	An image held in common by members of a group
stimulus stimuli (pl)	STIM-you-lus STIM-you-lie		Latin *goad, incite*	Something that excites or strengthens the functional activity of an organ or part
stimulant	STIM-you-lant	S/ R/	-ant *forming* stimul- *excite, strengthen*	An agent that excites or strengthens

EXERCISES

 Case Report 16.1

You are . . .

. . . a pediatric medical assistant employed by Sandra Mendes, MD, a **pediatrician** at Fulwood Medical Center. You are working in her Well-Baby Clinic.

You are communicating with . . .

. . . Mrs. Anna Hotteling, a 35-year-old mother, who has brought her 10-week-old daughter, Caroline, to the Well-Baby Clinic. Caroline, Mrs. Hotteling's first baby, was born via a normal vaginal delivery at term. She weighed 7 pounds 2 ounces. She had normal **Apgar** scores. Carol had persistent jaundice when seen at 2 weeks of age. She is being breastfed. You ask Mrs. Hotteling if she has any concerns.

Mrs. Anna Hotteling, the mother, has several areas of concern. A friend's baby recently died of **SIDS** (sudden infant death syndrome). How can Mrs. Hotteling prevent this from happening to her child? Caroline wants to feed every 2 to 3 hours day and night, and Mrs. Hotteling is exhausted. How long will this go on, and for how long should she continue breastfeeding? Mrs. Hotteling also wants to know what her baby can see and how she should communicate with her.

A. Demonstrate *your understanding of medical professionals. Insert the medical professional being described. Fill in the blanks.* **LO 16.9**

1. Physician that specializes in the process and problems of aging: _____

2. Physician specializing in disorders of the newborn: _____

3. Nurses with special training in the care of the elderly: _____

4. Physician specializing in the care of children and adolescents: _____

B. Match *the meaning in the first column with the correct element in the second column. The elements are ones you will see in terms throughout this chapter. Knowledge of these elements will help to increase your medical vocabulary. Fill in the blanks.* **LO 16.1**

_____ 1. new   **a.** -nate

_____ 2. expert   **b.** -ics

_____ 3. medical treatment   **c.** -ped

_____ 4. knowledge   **d.** -ician

_____ 5. to adjust   **e.** neo-

_____ 6. child   **f.** -al

_____ 7. born   **g.** -iatr

_____ 8. pertaining to   **h.** -ation

_____ 9. process   **i.** adapt-

C. Construct *medical terms that relate to the neonatal period. Fill in the blanks with the correct word element.* **LO 16.1 and 16.2**

1. Pertaining to the fetus: _____/_____

2. Medical specialty of treating children during development from birth through adolescence: _____/_____/_____

3. Change in function of an organ to meet new conditions: _____/_____

📁 Case Report 16.2

You are ...

A singer in a Master Chorale during her seventh and eighth months of pregnancy was in rehearsal for Handel's ***Messiah*** for a Christmas concert. At home, she frequently practiced her solo, which began, "I know that my redeemer liveth." When her daughter was 6 months old, the mother was changing the baby's diaper and started to sing, "I know that my . . ." The child turned her head and chimed in, "redeemer." Now, at 10 years old, the daughter has absolute pitch—the rare ability to replicate any musical note made on the piano.

D. Review *hearing and visual adaptations of the newborn. Fill in the blanks with the correct answer to each question or to complete each statement.* **LO 16.2, 16.4, 16.6, and 16.11**

1. Newborns are able to see at a distance of _____ to _____ inches.

2. In which trimester can the fetus hear loud noises? _____

3. What type of hearing loss results from congenital malformations of the external auditory canal and middle ear? _____

_____

4. What type of diagnostic test should all newborns have before they leave the hospital? _____

5. Congenital malformation of the inner ear can result in _____ hearing loss.

6. By the seventh month of pregnancy, the fetus can hear maternal _____.

E. Meet chapter and section objectives *by correctly answering the following questions.* **LO 16.2, 16.3, 16.6, and 16.11**

1. The baby's Ig levels are acquired through the _____.

2. Write a brief definition for *congenital*. _____

3. In the first 6 months of life, a child needs immunizations against _____ and _____.

4. What immunoglobulin is created in response to a food allergen? _____

F. Abbreviations: *Incorporate your knowledge of abbreviations from this lesson into the following patient documentation. Fill in the blanks, using the choices below; there are more choices than answers.* **LO 16.3 and 16.6**

RDS   ASD   SIDS   TOF   TTN   VSD   PDA

1. Diagnostic testing confirms _____, an opening between the two lower chambers of the infant's heart. Patient will be scheduled for open-heart surgery early next week.

2. Due to a precipitate delivery, and amniotic fluid remaining in the lungs, this infant has _____.

3. Because this infant's cardiorespiratory mechanisms have failed to mature, he is at great risk for _____.

4. The septal defect in this infant has been confirmed on testing as being between the two upper heart chambers. _____

5. One type of cyanotic heart disease is _____.

G. These terms *are related to cardiovascular and respiratory adaptations of the newborn. Fill in the blanks with the appropriate explanations.* **LO 16.2 and 16.11**

1. patent _____

2. in utero _____

3. dyspnea _____

4. meconium _____

5. precipitate (delivery) _____

H. Construct *the correct medical term based on the statement given. Insert the element on the line to construct the term.* **LO 16.1, 16.2, and 16.6**

1. pertaining to both the face and the cranium: _____ / _____ / _____

2. small head: _____ / _____ / _____

3. very low core body temperature: _____ / _____ / _____

4. congenital defect of the cranium with herniation of brain tissue: _____ / _____

I. Use the language *of pediatrics to answer the following questions. Select the correct answer to complete each statement or answer each question.* **LO 16.1 and 16.6**

1. Which term means "absence of cerebral hemispheres" :
   a. microcephaly   b. anencephaly   c. myelocele

2. Which element means *spinal cord?*
   a. micro   b. an   c. cele   d. myel/o

3. The element *cephaly* means:
   a. condition of the brain   b. condition of the head   c. spinal cord   d. cranium

4. Which of these two terms is *incompatible with life?*
   a. microcephaly   b. anencephaly

J. Documentation: *Use the terminology and the abbreviations related to neonatal adaptations to correctly fill in the following patient documentation.* **LO 16.6, 16.10, and 16.11**

1. This infant's mother has been an alcoholic for the past year and a half. Infant was born suffering from (use the abbreviation)_____.

2. This preemie falls below the 10th percentile and is (use the abbreviation)_____.

3. Because of difficulty in swallowing, this infant is being fed by _____.

4. Patient was born with only the right kidney present. Diagnosis: renal _____.

5. Because of jaundice, this infant will receive 8 hours of _____ each day until discharge.

K. Assess *the information in the following statements. Fill in the blanks with the medical term to correctly complete each sentence.* **LO 16.2 and 16.6**

1. Inadequate nutrition of the fetus can be caused by poor _____ function.

2. Premature infants may have to be fed by IV or _____.

3. Renal agenesis occurs when one or more of the _____ is absent at birth.

L. Match *the element in the first column to its meaning in the second column.*   **LO 16.1**

1. _____ -tresia   **a.** creation

2. _____ -genesis   **b.** milk

3. _____ col-   **c.** light

4. _____ lact-   **d.** a hole

5. _____ photo-   **e.** colon

M. Eating disorders in early childhood. *Select the answer that correctly completes each statement.*   **LO 16.6**

1. Eating substances that are considered as nonnutritive:

   a. rumination

   b. pica

   c. regurgitation

   d. bulimia

2. Persistent fecal soiling beyond the age of toilet training:

   a. rumination

   b. enuresis

   c. anorexia nervosa

   d. encopresis

3. Eating disorders can be a part of the syndrome:

   a. failure to thrive

   b. encopresis

   c. enuresis

N. Match *the element in the first column to its meaning in the second column.*   **LO 16.1**

1. _____ rumin-   **a.** appetite

2. _____ re-   **b.** flood

3. _____ enur-   **c.** condition

4. _____ -orex   **d.** back

5. _____ -gurgit   **e.** urinate

6. _____ -esis   **f.** throat

O. Use *what you have just learned in this chapter and match the description in the first column to the abbreviation in the second column.*   **LO 16.3 and 16.6**

1. _____ varying degrees of impairment in social and communication skills   **a.** ODD

2. _____ generalized inattentiveness and impulsivity   **b.** OCD

3. _____ persistent pattern of defiance, disobedience, and hostility   **c.** ASD

4. _____ anxiety disorder with recurrent unwanted thoughts and repetitive behaviors   **d.** ADHD

P. Use medical terms *related to developmental disorders of children and adolescents. Fill in the blanks with the term being described.*   **LO 16.2, 16.6, and 16.11**

1. An agent that excites or strengthens: _____

2. Unable to resist performing inappropriate actions: _____

3. Uncontrollable impulses to perform an act repetitively: _____

4. Excessive restlessness and movement: _____

5. Lack of concentration and direction: _____

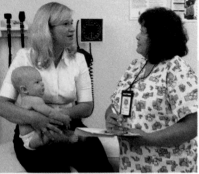

Rick Brady/McGraw-Hill Education

Section 16.2

Aging, Senescence, and Death

Aging (LO 16.7 and 16.8)

Aging consists of the gradual, spontaneous changes resulting in maturation through childhood, adolescence, and young adulthood and causing a decline in function (rather than maturation) through late adulthood and old age.

Senile is a term used to refer to the characteristics of old age, and **senility** is the general term used when referring to a person who demonstrates a variety of conditions of mental disorders occurring in old age.

Gerontology is the study of the social, mental, and physical aspects of aging. Professionals from diverse fields call themselves **gerontologists**. The medical field that involves the study, care, and treatment of the elderly *(Figure 16.10)* is called **geriatrics**, and a medical specialist in geriatrics is called a **geriatrician**.

- **Life expectancy** is the average length of life for any given population.
- **Life span** is the age to which individuals aspire to live and the process of getting there.
- **Longevity** is living beyond the normal life expectancy.
- **Senescence** is the loss over time of the ability of cells to divide, grow, and function—a process that terminates in death. It is sometimes used interchangeably with the term aging.

Senescence of Organ Systems (LO 16.5)

Organ systems begin to show signs of senescence at very different ages and do not degenerate at the same speed. Most physiologic studies show general peak physical performance in the twenties.

Integumentary system changes in our bodies begin in our forties. The cells that produce melanin called melanocytes *(see Chapter 3)* die, and our hair becomes gray and thinner. Our skin gets paper-thin, loses its elasticity, hangs loose, and wrinkles *(Figure 16.11)*. Flat brown-black spots, **senile lentigines** (age spots), appear on the backs of our hands and other areas exposed to sunlight.

Our special senses start to decline in our twenties, including our visual acuity. In our forties, presbyopia *(see Chapter 11)* appears, and many people develop cataracts in old age. Hearing loss occurs as the ossicles become stiffer and the number of cochlear hair cells declines *(see Chapter 11)*. Our ability to taste and smell is blunted late in life, as taste cells and olfactory buds decline in number.

Skeletal system changes appear in our thirties, when osteoblasts become less active than osteoclasts. This results in osteopenia, which goes on to become osteoporosis, particularly in postmenopausal women. Joints in the older age groups have less synovial fluid and thinner articular cartilage, leading to osteoarthritis *(see Chapter 4)*.

Muscular system *(see Chapter 5)* changes occur with age as we lose muscle mass and strength **(sarcopenia).** As muscle **atrophies** (shrinks and weakens), we have fewer muscle fibers to do the work and the available blood supply to these muscles is decreased.

Nervous system changes begin around age 30, when our brain weighs twice as much as it does at age 75. Motor coordination, balance, intellectual function, and short-term memory decline more quickly than long-term memory and language skills.

Dementia is an overall term for diseases characterized by a decline in memory and **cognitive** (thinking) skills. All dementias are caused by damage inside and around the brain's neurons.

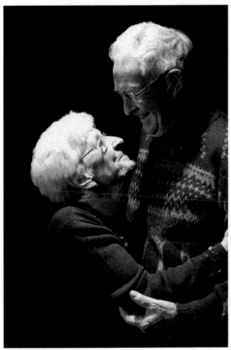

▲ **FIGURE 16.10**
Elderly Couple.

Darren Greenwood/Design Pics

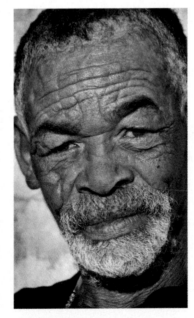

▲ **FIGURE 16.11**
Senescence of the Skin. An elderly Black man.

Tish1/Shutterstock

Cardiovascular systems may show coronary artery atherosclerosis from an early age. As a result, when aging myocardial cells die, our heart wall gets thinner and weaker and cardiac output declines. This causes the decline in physical capabilities with aging. The atherosclerotic plaques narrow arteries and trigger thrombosis, leading to strokes and heart attacks *(see Chapter 6)*. In veins, valves become weaker and blood flows back and pools in the legs, leading to poor venous return to the heart and heart failure.

Respiratory system changes may be noticeable in our thirties, when pulmonary ventilation declines (a factor in the gradual loss of stamina). Our rib cage becomes less flexible; our lungs, less elastic, with declining efficiency in alveoli. With advanced age, our respiratory health deteriorates and hypoxic **degenerative** changes occur in all the other organ systems.

Urinary system changes begin in our twenties, when the number of nephrons starts to decline. Later in life, many of the remaining glomeruli become atherosclerotic, and our kidneys become less efficient. This causes drug doses in the elderly need to be reduced because drugs cannot be cleared from the blood as rapidly.

Immune system function declines in the elderly as the amounts of lymphatic tissue and red bone marrow decrease with age. This leads to a reduction in both cellular and humoral (antibody) immunity. This means that the elderly have less protection against infectious diseases and cancer. Because of lowered immunity, vaccinations against **influenza** and other seasonal infections are recommended for the elderly.

Word Analysis and Definition

S = Suffix   P = Prefix   R = Root   R/CF = Combining Form

WORD	PRONUNCIATION		ELEMENTS	DEFINITION
aging aged	A-jing A-jid		Latin *aging*	The decline in function through late adulthood and old age Having lived to advanced age
atrophy	A-troh-fee	P/ R/	a- *without* -trophy *nourishment*	The wasting away or diminished volume of tissue, an organ, or a body part Increase in size, but not in number, of an individual tissue element
cognitive	KOG-nih-tiv	S/ R/	-ive *quality of* cognit- *thinking*	Pertaining to the mental activities of thinking and learning
degenerative	dee-JEN-er-a-tiv	S/ R/	-ive *quality of* degenerat- *deteriorate*	Relating to the deterioration of a structure
dementia	da-MEN-sha	S/ P/ R/	-ia *condition* de- *removal, take away* -ment- *mind*	Chronic, progressive, irreversible loss of cognitive and intellectual functions
geriatrics (**Note:** This term contains two roots.) geriatrician	jer-ee-AT-riks jer-ee-ah-TRISH-an	S/ R/ R/ S/	-ics *knowledge of* ger- *old age* -iatr- *medical treatment* -ician *one who does*	Medical specialty that deals with the problems of old age Medical specialist in the process and problems of aging
gerontology gerontologist	jer-on-TOL-oh-jee jer-on-TOL-oh-jist	S/ R/CF S/	-logy *study of* geront/o- *old age* -logist *specialist*	Study of the process and general problems of aging Specialist in the process and general problems of aging
influenza	in-flew-EN-zah		Latin *caused by the influence of the heavenly bodies*	Acute viral infection of upper and lower respiratory tracts
lentigo lentigines (pl)	len-TIE-go len-TIHJ-ih-neez		Greek *lentil*	Age spot; small, flat, brown-black spot in the skin of older people
life expectancy life span	LIFE ek-SPEK-tan-see LIFE SPAN	S/ R/	-ancy *state of* expect- *await* life Old *English life* span Old English *reach or stretch*	Statistical determination of the number of years an individual is expected to live The age that a person reaches.
longevity	lon-JEV-ih-tee	S/ R/	-ity *condition* longev- *long life*	Duration of life beyond the normal expectation
sarcopenia	sar-koh-PEE-nee-ah	S/ R/CF	-penia *deficiency* sarc/o- *flesh*	Progressive loss of muscle mass and strength in aging
senescence senescent	seh-NES-ens seh-NES-ent	 S/ S/ R/	 -ence *the quality of* -ent *end result, pertaining to* senesc- *growing old* Latin *to grow old*	The changes in cells and tissues leading to the decline of function in old age and death Growing old
senile senility	SEE-nile seh-NIL-ih-tee	S/ R/ S/ R/	-ile *pertaining to* sen- *old age* -ity *condition* senil- *senile*	Characteristic of old age Mental disorders occurring in old age

Abbreviations

MCS minimally conscious state
PVS persistent vegetative
     state

Dying and Death (LO 16.3, 16.7, and 16.8)

Death is unavoidable. Just as fetal life in the womb is a preparation for birth, living and aging are a preparation for death. The process of dying, rather than death itself, is of concern to most elderly people. Dying should be dignified and free from physical and emotional pain.

A **hospice** provides comfort care at the end of life when death is imminent to include support for the emotional and spiritual needs of terminally ill patients and their loved ones at an in-patient facility or in the patient's home. **Palliative care** is designed to provide pain and symptom management at any stage of a disease to maintain the highest quality of life for as long as life remains.

There is no universally accepted moment of biological death. In most states in the United States, death is now defined in terms of **brain death,** in which there is no cerebral or brainstem activity and the EEG is flat for a specific length of time *(Figure 16.12)*. The two other conditions involving brain damage and loss of brain function that cause medical difficulty are:

1. **Persistent vegetative state (PVS)** occurs in people who suffer enough brain damage (usually from trauma) that they are unaware of themselves or their surroundings, although their eyes remain open. They still have certain reflexes and can breathe and maintain heart functions because the brainstem still functions. With medical care and artificial feeding, these patients can survive for decades, but there is no measureable quality of life.

2. **Minimally conscious state (MCS)** is a condition of severely altered **consciousness** in which minimal, inconsistent evidence of awareness of self or surroundings is demonstrated. PET scans of MCS patients show cortical function, for example, when the patients' loved ones speak to them. They are more likely to improve than are PVS patients. Trauma to the brain is a common cause of MCS.

PVS and MCS differ from **coma,** in which the person is unresponsive and his or her eyes are closed.
If the cause of death is uncertain or a crime is suspected, an **autopsy** (**postmortem**) may be performed.

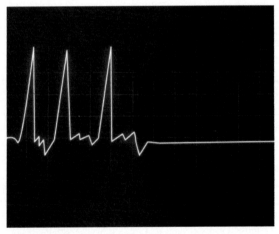

▲ **FIGURE 16.12**
Electroencephalogram Demonstrating
Brain Death.

argus/Shutterstock

Word Analysis and Definition

WORD	PRONUNCIATION		ELEMENTS	DEFINITION
autopsy (same as **postmortem**)	AWE-top-see		Greek *see with one's own eyes*	Examination of the body and organs of a dead person to determine the cause of death
postmortem	post-**MOR**-tem	S/ P/ R/	-em *condition* post- *after* -mort- *death*	
coma	KOH-mah		Greek *deep sleep*	State of deep unconsciousness
consciousness	KON-shus-ness	S/ R/	-ness *quality, state* conscious- *to be aware*	The state of being aware of and responsive to the environment
conscious	KON-shus		Latin *to be aware*	Having present knowledge of oneself and one's surroundings
unconscious	un-KON-shus	P/	un- *not*	Not conscious, lacking awareness
death	DETH		Old English *to die*	Total and permanent cessation of all vital body functions
hospice	HOS-pis		Latin *lodging*	Provides supportive and palliative care
palliative care	PAL-ee-ah-tiv KAIR	S/ R/ R/	-ive *quality of* palliat- *reduce suffering* care *be responsible for*	To relieve symptoms and pain without curing
vegetative	VEJ-eh-tay-tiv	S/ R/	-ive *quality of* vegetat- *growth*	Functioning unconsciously, as plant life is assumed to do

EXERCISES

Case Report 16.3

You are . . .

. . . a medical assistant working in the **Geriatric** Clinic at Fulwood Medical Center.

You are communicating with . . .

. . . 85-year-old Mr. Mathew Hickman, who has an early **dementia**. Mr. Hickman also has a slow-growing prostate cancer, for which he has opted to have no treatment. With the help of his two daughters and his day care providers, he is struggling to stay at home. His daughter, Sandra Hotteling, is with him.

Mr. Hickman: "I'm still here, you know, somewhere inside this frail old body. I can remember yesteryear, though I'm a bit hazy about today. I can't hear like I used to. But I can still put my own socks on and tie my shoes. I'm not frightened of death, but the process of getting there scares the heck out of me. I've lived my life with dignity. I want to live my death the same way, you know, and leave in peace."

A. Senescence *of the organ system. Insert the correct answer that completes each statement. Fill in the blanks.*   **LO 16.2, 16.5, and 16.7**

1. The plural form of lentigo: _____

2. Progressive loss of muscle mass and strength: _____

3. Chronic, progressive, irreversible loss of the mind's cognitive and intellectual functions: _____

4. Mental disorders occurring in old age: _____

B. Review *of elements will make them easier to remember and apply to medical terms. Match the element to its definition.*   **LO 16.1**

1. _____ sen-   **a.** growing old

2. _____ -ile   **b.** deficiency

3. _____ de-   **c.** pertaining to

4. _____ senesc-   **d.** old age

5. _____ -penia   **e.** removal, take away

C. Differentiate between medical terms associated with death and dying. *Match the term in the first column with its correct definition in the second column.*
 LO 16.7 and 16.8

_____ 1. hospice   **a.** cessation of life

_____ 2. minimally conscious state   **b.** patient is completely unaware of surroundings

_____ 3. palliative care   **c.** facility to provide care for dying patients and their families

_____ 4. vegetative state   **d.** patient that has minimal awareness of self or surroundings

_____ 5. death   **e.** care that treats but does not cure

D. Abbreviations *for terms related to death and dying. Insert the abbreviation that the statement is describing.* **LO 16.3 and 16.7**

1. Person inconsistently displays evidence of awareness of self or surroundings: _____

2. Person is unaware of themselves or their surroundings: _____

3. Person lacks cerebral and brainstem activity: _____

E. Review *the terms related to death and dying. Insert the correct medical term that answers each question.* **LO 16.7 and 16.11**

1. What is another term for autopsy? _____

2. What condition is described as a state of deep unconsciousness? _____

3. What is the medical term for an acute viral infection of the upper and lower respiratory tracts? _____

F. Pronunciation is important whether you are saying the word or listening to a word from a coworker. Identify the proper pronunciation of the following
 medical terms. Correctly spell the term. **LO 16.2, 16.6, 16.7, 16.8, and 16.9**

1. The correct pronunciation for the specialist in the process and general problems of aging
 a. gur-rhee-uh-**TRISH**-un   **b.** gur-eehn-**TOL**-uh-jus   **c.** jer-ee-ah-**TRISH**-an   **d.** jer-on-**TOL**-oh-jist
 Correctly spell the term: _____

2. The correct pronunciation for multiple small, flat, brown-black spots on the skin of older people
 a. **LOW**-ee **BOD**-ee   **b.** **LOO**-ee **BOD**-ee   **c.** lent-ih-**JIHN**-ez   **d.** len-**TIHJ**-ih-neez
 Correctly spell the term: _____

3. The correct pronunciation for an abnormal blue color of skin
 a. sigh-**AN**-oh-sik   **b.** **SIGH**-an-ot-**IK**   **c.** sigh-ah-**NOT**-ik   **d.** sigh-**NOS**-tik
 Correctly spell the term: _____

4. The correct pronunciation for an acute altered state of consciousness with agitation and disorientation; condition is reversible
 a. dee-**MEN**-she-ah   **b.** duh-men-**SHE**-ah   **c.** deh-**LIR**-ee-um   **d.** duh-**LEER**-ee-um
 Correctly spell the term: _____

5. The correct pronunciation for the state of being old
 a. seh-**NES**-ens   **b.** sigh-**NES**-ens   **c.** **SEE**-nile   **d.** **SIGHN**-ile
 Correctly spell the term: _____

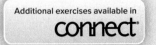
Additional exercises available in
connect

**Chapter Review exercises, along with additional practice items,
are available in Connect!**

Word Parts and Abbreviations

Note: For easy identification, the word parts in this appendix appear in the same colors as in the Word Analysis and Definition boxes: suffix, prefix, root, root/combining form. Any term that is used in the text in both root and combining form is shown only in this appendix as a combining form.

S = Suffix   P = Prefix   R = Root   R/CF = Combining Form

Word Part	Definition
a-	not, without
a-	variant of ad
ab-	away from
abdomin/o	abdomen
ability	competence
ablat	take away
-able	capable
abort	fail at onset, expel nonviable fetus
abras	scrape off
absorpt	to swallow, take in
ac-	toward
-ac	pertaining to
acid/o	acid, low pH
acin	grape
acous	hearing
acr/o	peak, topmost, extremity, highest point
acromi/o	acromion
act	to do, perform, performance
activ	movement
acu	needle
acu-	sharp
acumin	to sharpen
ad-	to, toward, into
adapt	to adjust
-ade	process
aden/o	gland
adenoid	adenoid
adip	fat
adjust	alter
adjuv	give help
adolesc	beginning of adulthood
adren/o	adrenal gland
aer/o	air, gas

Word Part	Definition
affer	move toward the center
ag-	to
-age	pertaining to
agglutin	sticking together, clumping
-ago	disease
agon	to fight
-agon	to fight
agor/a	marketplace
-agra	severe pain
-al	pertaining to
alanine	an amino acid, protein synthesized in muscle
albicans	white
albin/o	white
albumin	albumin
ald/o	organic compound
-ale	pertaining to
alges	sensation of pain
-algia	pain, painful condition
aliment	nourishment
-alis	pertaining to
alkal	base
all/o	strange, other
allo-	strange, other
alopec-	baldness, mange
alpha-	first letter in the Greek alphabet
alveol	alveolus, air sac
-aly	condition
ambly-	dull
ambulat	to walk, walking
amin/o	nitrogen containing
-amine	nitrogen-containing substance
ammon	ammonia
amni/o	amnion, fetal membrane

Word Part	Definition
amnios	amnion
amph-	around
ampull	bottle-shaped
amput	to prune, cut off
amyl	starch
an-	not, lack of, without
-an	pertaining to
an/o	anus
ana-	away from, excessive
anabol	build up
analysis	process to study whole in terms of its parts
analyst	one who separates
anastom	provide a mouth
-ance	condition, state of
-ancy	state of
andr/o	male, masculine
aneurysm	dilation
angi/o	blood vessel, lymph vessel
angina	sore throat, chest pain radiating to throat
ankyl	stiff
-ant	forming, pertaining to
ant-	against
ante-	before, forward, in front of
anter	before, front part
anthrac	coal
anti-	against
aort	aorta
apo-	different from, separation from
appendic	appendix
apse	clasp
aqu-	water
-ar	pertaining to
arachn	cobweb, spider
-arche	beginning
areol	areola, small area
aria	air
-arian	one who is
-aris	pertaining to
aroma	smell, sweet herb
array	place in order
arter	artery
arteri/o	artery
arteriosus	like an artery

Word Part	Definition
arthr/o	joint
articul	joint
-ary	pertaining to
asbest	asbestos
ascit	fluid in the belly
-ase	enzyme
aspartate	an amino acid
aspergill	aspergillus
aspirat	to breathe on
assay	evaluate
assist	aid, help
asthm	asthma
astr/o	star
-ata	action, place, use
-ate	composed of, pertaining to
-ated	pertaining to a condition
atel	incomplete
ather/o	porridge, gruel, fatty substance
athet	without position, uncontrolled
-atic	pertaining to
-ation	a process
-ative	pertaining to, quality of
-ator	agent, instrument, person or thing that does something
-atory	pertaining to
atri/o	entrance, atrium
-atric	treatment
attent	awareness
attenu	to weaken
audi/o	hearing
audit	hearing
aur-	ear
auscult	listen to
auto-	self, same
avail	useful
axill	armpit, axilla
ayur-	life
azot	nitrogen
-back	back, toward the starting point
bacteri/o	bacteria
balan	glans penis
bar	pressure
bari	weight
bas/o	base, opposite of acid

Word Part	Definition
basal	deepest part
basil	base, support
be	life
behav	mental or motor activity
beta	second letter of Greek alphabet
bi-	two, twice, double
bi/o	life
-bil	able
bil/i	bile
bis-	twice
-blast	germ cell, immature cell
blast/o	germ cell, immature cell
blephar/o	eyelid
body	body, mass, substance
bov	cattle
brachi/o	arm
brachii	of the arm
brachy-	short
brady-	slow
bride	rubbish, rubble
bronch/i	bronchus
bronch/o	bronchus
brucell	pathologist David Bruce
buccinat	cheek
bulb/o	bulb
burs	bursa
calc/i	calcium
calcan	calcaneous
calcul	stone, little stone
callos	thickening
calor	heat
canal	duct or channel
cancer	cancer
candid	Candida
capill	hairlike, capillary
capit	head
capn	carbon dioxide
caps	box, cover, shell
capsul	box
carb/o	carbon
carboxy	group of organic compounds
carcin/o	cancer
card	heart
cardi/o	heart

Word Part	Definition
care	be responsible for
carotene	yellow-red pigment
carotid	large neck artery
carp/o	bones of the wrist
cartilag	cartilage
cata-	down
catabol	break down
catechol	tyrosine-containing
catheter	insert, catheter
caud	tail
cav	hollow space
cava	cave
cavern	cave
cec	cecum
-cele	cave, hernia, swelling
celi	abdomen
cellul	cell, small cell
cent-	hundred
-centesis	to puncture
centr/o	central
ceph	head
cephal/o	head
-cephalus	head
cephaly	condition of the head
ceps	head
cept	to receive
cerebell	little brain, cerebellum
cerebr/o	brain
cerumin	cerumen
cervic	neck
cess	going forward
chancr	chancre
chem/o	chemical
chemic	chemical
-chete	hair
-chezia	pass a stool
chir/o	hand
chlor	green
chol/e	bile
cholangi	bile duct
cholecyst	gallbladder
choledoch/o	common bile duct
chondr/o	cartilage, rib, granule
chorion	chorion, membrane

Word Part	Definition
chrom/o	color
chromat	color
chron/o	time
chym/o	juice
-cidal	pertaining to killing
cide	to kill
cili	hairlike structure
circulat	circular route
circum-	around
cirrh	yellow
cis	to cut
cit/i	cell
-clast	break, break down
claudic	limp
claustr/o-	confined space
clav	clavicle
clave	lock
clavicul	clavicle
-cle	small
clitor	clitoris
clon	cutting used for propagation, tumult
-clonus	violent action
co-	with, together
coagul/o	clot, clump
coarct	press together, narrow
cobal	cobalt
cocc	round bacterium
coccus	berry, spherical bacterium
cochle	cochlear
code	information system
cognit	thinking
coit	sexual intercourse
col-	with, together
col	colon
coll	collect, glue
coll/a	glue
colon/o	colon
coloniz	form a colony
colp/o	vagina
com	take care of
com-	with, together
comat	coma
combin	combine

Word Part	Definition
comminut	break into pieces
commodat	adjust
compat	tolerate
compet	strive together
complex	woven together
compli	fulfill
compress	press together
compuls	drive, compel
con-	with, together
concav	arched, hollow
concept	become pregnant
concuss	shake or jar violently
condyl	knuckle
confus	bewildered
congest	accumulation of fluid
coni	dust
coniz	cone
conjunctiv	conjunctiva
connect	join together
conscious	awareness
constip	press together
constrict	to narrow
contagi/o	transmissible by contact
contaminat/o	to corrupt, make unclean
contin	hold together
contra-	against
contract	draw together, pull together
contus	bruise
convalesc	recover
cor	heart
core	pupil
cori	skin
corne/o	cornea
coron	crown, coronary
corpor/e	body
corpus	body
cortic/o	cortex, cortisone
cortis	cortisone
cost	rib
crani/o	cranium, skull
crease	groove
creat	flesh
creatin	creatine

Word Part	Definition
crete	to separate
cretin	cretin
crimin	distinguish
crine	secrete
crista	crest
-crit	to separate
cry/o	cold
crypt-	hidden
cub	cube
cubit	elbow
cubitus	elbow, ulna
cune/i	wedge
cur	cleanse, cure
curat	to care for
curett	to cleanse
cursor	run
cusp	point
cutan/e	skin
cyan/o	dark blue
-cyst	cyst, bladder
cyst/o	bladder, sac, cyst
cysteine	an amino acid
cyt/o	cell
-cyte	cell
cyte	cell
dacry/o	tears, lacrimal duct
dai	day
de-	without, out of, removal from
defec	clear out waste
defici	failure, lacking, inadequate
degenerat	deteriorate
deglutit	to swallow
del	visible
deliri	confusion, disorientation
delt	triangle
delus	deceive
dem	the people
demi-	half
dendr/o	treelike
dent	tooth
depend	rely on
depress	press down
derm/a	skin

Word Part	Definition
-derma	skin
dermat/o	skin
dermis	skin
-desis	bind together, fixation of bone or joint
di-	two
dia-	complete
diabet	diabetes
diagnost	decision
dialectic	argument
dialy	separate
diaphor	sweat
diaphragm/a	diaphragm
diastol	diastole, relaxation
dict	consent, surrender
didym/o	testis
didymis	testis
diet	a way of life
different	not identical
digest	to break down food
digit	finger or toe
dilat	open up, expand, widen
dips	thirst
dis-	apart, away from
discipl	understand
disciplin	disciple, instruction
dist	away from the center
-dium	appearance
diuret	increase urine output
diverticul	byroad
dorm	sleep
dors	back
dorsi	of the back
drome	running
drop	liquid globule
duce	to lead
ducer	to lead, leader
duct	to lead, lead
ductus	leading
duoden	twelve, duodenum
dur	dura
dura	hard
dwarf	miniature
dynam/o	power

Word Part	Definition
-dynia	pain
dys-	bad, difficult, painful
e-	out of, from
-eal	pertaining to
ease	normal function, freedom from pain
ec-	out, outside
ech/o	sound wave
echin	hedgehog
eclamps	shining forth
eco-	environment
-ectasis	dilation
-ectomy	excision, surgical excision
ectop	on the outside, displaced
eczem/a	eczema
-ed	pertaining to
edema	edema, swelling
-ee	person who is the object of an action
efface	wipe out
effer	move out from the center
effus	pour out
ejacul	shoot out
ejaculat	shoot out
elasma	plate
elect	choice
electr/o	electric, electricity
elimin	throw away, expel
-elle	small
-em	condition
em-	in, into
-ema	quality of, quantity of
emac/i	make thin
embol	plug
embryon	embryo, fertilized egg
emesis	vomiting
-emesis	to vomit, vomiting
emet	to vomit
emia	a blood condition
-emia	a blood condition
-emic	pertaining to a blood condition
emmetr-	measure
emuls	suspend in a liquid
en-	in
-ence	forming, quality of, state of

Word Part	Definition
enceph	brain
encephal/o	brain
encephaly	condition of the brain
-ency	condition, state of, quality of
end-	inside, within
endo-	inside, within
-ent	end result, pertaining to
enter/o	intestine
entery	condition of the intestine
enur	urinate
environ	surroundings
-eon	one who does
eosin/o	dawn
ependym	lining membrane
epi-	above, upon, over
epilept	seizure
epiphys/i	growth
episi/o	vulva
equi-	equal
equin	horse
equip	to fit out
-er	agent, one who does
erect	straight, to set up
erg/o	work
-ergy	process of working
-ery	process of
erysi-	red
erythemat	redness
erythr/o	red
-escent	process
-esis	condition
eso-	inward
esophag/e	esophagus
essent	existence
esthes	sensation, perception
esthet	sensation, perception
estr/o	woman
ethm	sieve
eti/o	cause
-etic	pertaining to
-etics	pertaining to
-ette	little
eu-	good, normal

Word Part	Definition
ex-	away from, out, out of
exacerbat	increase, aggravate
examin	test, examine
excis	cut out
excret	separate, discharge
exo-	outside, outward
expect	await
expir	breathe out
extra-	out of, outside
faci	face
factor	maker
farct	area of dead tissue
fasc/i	fascia
febr	fever
fec	feces
feed	to give food, nourish
femor	femur
fer	to bear, to carry
ferrit	iron
fertil	able to conceive
fertiliz	to make fruitful
fet/o	fetus
fibr/o	fiber, fibrous
fibrill	small fiber
fibrin/o	fibrin
fibul	fibula
-fication	remove
fida	split
field	definite area
filar	roundworm
filtr	strain through
fiss	split
fistul	tube, pipe
flammat	flame
flat	flatus
flatul	excessive gas
flavin	yellow
flex	bend
fluid	flowing
fluo-	fluorine
fluor/o	flux, flow
flux	flow
foc	center, focus

Word Part	Definition
follicul	follicle
foramin	opening, foramen
fore-	in front
-form	appearance of, resembling
format	to form
fract	break
fraction	small amount
free	free
frequ	repeated, often
front	front, forehead
fructos	fruit sugar
function	perform
fund/o	fundus
fung/i	fungus
fusion	to pour
galact/o	milk
gall	bile
gastr/o	stomach
gastrin	stomach hormone
gastrocnem	calf of leg
gemin	twin, double
gen/o	produce, create
-gen	create, produce, form
gen-	birth
-gene	production, give birth
gener	create, produce
genesis	origin, creation, production
-genesis	creation, origin, formation, source
genet	origin
-genic	creation, producing
genit	bring forth, birth, primary male or female sex organ
genitor	offspring
ger	old age
geront/o	old age
gest	gestation, pregnancy, produce
gestat	gestation, pregnancy, to bear
gigant	giant
gingiv	gums
gland	gland
glauc	lens opacity, grey
gli/o	glue, supportive tissue of nervous system
-glia	glue, supportive tissue of nervous system
globin/o	protein

Word Part	Definition
globul	globular, protein
glomerul/o	glomerulus
gloss/o	tongue
glott	mouth of windpipe
glottis	mouth of windpipe
gluc/o	glucose, sugar
glut	buttocks
glutin	glue, stick
glyc/o	glycogen, glucose, sugar
glycer	glycerol, sweet
gnath	jaw
gnose	use knowledge
gnosis	knowledge
gomph	bolt, nail
gon/o	seed
gonad/o	gonads, testes, or ovaries
gong	daily practice
-grade	going
graft	splice, transplant
-graft	tissue for transplant
graine	head pain
-gram	a record, recording
grand-	big
grand	big
granul/o	granule, small grain
-graph	to record, write
-grapher	one who records
-graphy	process of recording
gravida	pregnant
gravis	serious
gru	to move
guan	dung
gurgit	flood
gynec/o	woman, female
habilitat	restore
hale	breathe
halit	breath
hallucin	imagination
hallux	big toe
hem/o	blood
hemangi/o	blood vessel
hemat/o	blood
heme	red iron-containing pigment

Word Part	Definition
hemi-	half
-hemia	blood condition
hepar	liver
hepat/o	liver
herb/i	plant
herni/o	hernia, rupture
herp	blister
hetero-	different
hiat	opening
hidr/o	sweat
hist	derived from histidine
hist/o	tissue
holist	entire, whole
hom/i	man
home/o	the same
homo-	same, alike
hormon	chemical messenger, hormone
human	human being
humor	fluid
hyal	glass
hydr/o	water
hyp-	below
hyper-	above, beyond, excess, excessive
hypn/o	sleep
hypo-	below, deficient, smaller, low, under
hyster/o	uterus
-ia	condition
-iac	pertaining to
-ial	pertaining to
-ian	one who does, specialist
-ias	condition
-iasis	abnormal condition
iatr	medical treatment, physician
-iatric	relating to medicine, medical knowledge
iatrics	medical knowledge
-iatrist	practitioner, one who treats
-iatry	treatment, field of medicine
-ibility	able to do
-ible	can do, able to
-ic	pertaining to
-ica	pertaining to
-ical	pertaining to
-ician	expert

Word Part	Definition
-ics	knowledge
ict	seizure
icterus	jaundice
-id	having a particular quality, pertaining to
-ide	having a particular quality
idi/o	unknown, personal
ifer	to bear, carry
-ify	to become
-il	a thing
-ile	pertaining to
ile/o	ileum
ili/o	ilium (hip bone)
im-	in, not
imag	likeness
immun/o	immune, immune response, immunity
immune	protected from
immuniz	make immune
impair	worsen
impede	obstruct
-imus	most
-in	substance, chemical compound
in-	not, into, in
incis	cut into
incub	sit on, lie on, hatch
index	to declare
-ine	pertaining to
infant	infant
infect	internal invasion, infection
infer	below, beneath
infest	invade, attack
inflammat	set on fire
inflat	blow up
infra-	below, beneath
-ing	quality of, doing
ingest	carry in
inguin	groin
inhal	breathe in
inhibit	repress
inject	force in
ino	sinew
insect/i	insect
insert	put together
inspir	breathe in

Word Part	Definition
insul	island
integr	whole
integument	covering of the body
inter-	between
interstiti	space between tissues
intestin	gut, intestine
intra-	inside, within
intrins	on the inside
intus-	within
iod	violet, iodine
-ion	action, condition
-ior	pertaining to
-iosum	pertaining to
-ious	pertaining to
irrig	to water
-is	belonging to, pertaining to
isch	to block
ischi	ischium
-ism	condition, process
-ismus	take action
iso-	equal
-ist	agent, specialist
-istic	pertaining to
-isy	inflammation
-ites	associated with
-ition	process
-itis	inflammation, infection
-ity	condition, state
-ium	structure
-ius	pertaining to
-ive	nature of, quality of, pertaining to
-iz	subject to
-ization	process of inserting or creating
-ize	action, affect in a specific way, policy
-ized	affected in a specific way
-izer	affects in a particular way, line of action
jejun	jejunum
jugul	throat
junct	joining together
juxta-	beside, near, close to
kal	potassium
kary/o	nucleus
kel/o	tumor

Word Part	Definition
kerat	keratin, hard protein
kerat/o	cornea
kern	nucleus
ket/o	ketone
keton	ketone
ketone	organic compound
kin	motion
kinase	enzyme
kinesi/o	movement
kinet	motion
-kinin	move in
klept/o	to steal
kyph/o	bent, humpback
labi	lip
labyrinth	inner ear
lacer	to tear
lacrim	tears, tear duct
lact	milk
lactat	secrete milk
lapar/o	abdomen in general
lapse	clasp, fall together
-lapse	fall together, slide
laryng/o	larynx
lash	end of whip
lat	to take
lateral	at the side
latiss	wide
-le	small
lei/o	smooth
-lemma	covering
-lepsy	seizure
lept	thin, small
-let	small
leuk/o	white
lex	word
librium	balance
ligament	ligament
ligat	tie up, tie off
lign	line
-ling	small
lingu	tongue
lip/o	fat
lipid	fat

Word Part	Definition
lith/o	stone
liv	life, live
load	to carry
lob	lobe
locat	a place
log	to study
-logist	one who studies, specialist
logous	relation
logy	study of
-logy	study of
longev	long life
lord/o	curve, swayback
lubric	make slippery
lucid	bright, clear
lumb	lower back, loin
lump	piece
lun	moon
lupus	wolf
-lus	small
lute	yellow
luxat	dislocate
ly	break down, separate
-ly	every
lymph/o	lymph, lymphatic system
lymphaden/o	lymph node
lymphangi/o	lymphatic vessels
lys/o	decompose, dissolve
lysis	destruction
-lysis	destruction, dissolve, separation
lyt	dissolve, destroy
-lyte	soluble
-lytic	relating to destruction
lyze	destruct, dissolve
macro-	large
macul	spot
magnet	magnet
mak	makes
-maker	one who makes
mal	bad, difficult, inadequate
mal-	bad, difficult
-malacia	abnormal softness
malign	harmful, bad
malleol	small hammer, malleolus

Word Part	Definition
mamm/o	breast
man	frenzy, madness
man/o	pressure
mandibul	mandible
-mania	frenzy, madness
manic	affected by frenzy
manipul	handful, use of hands
marker	sign
mast	breast
mastic	chew
mastoid	mastoid process
mater	mother
matern	mother
matur(e)	ripe, ready, fully developed
maxilla	maxilla
medi	middle
media	middle
mediastin/o	mediastinum
medic	medicine
medulla	middle
mega-	enormous
megal/o	large
-megaly	enlargement
mei	lessening
mela	black
melan/o	melanin, black pigment
mellit	sweetened with honey
membran/o	cover, skin
men/o	menses, monthly, month
mening/o	meninges, membranes
menisc	crescent, meniscus
menstr/u	menses, occurring monthly
ment	mind, chin
-ment	action, state, resulting state
mere	part
mero-	partial
meso-	middle
meta-	after, beyond, subsequent to
metabol	change
-meter	measure, instrument to measure
metr/o	uterus
-metric	pertaining to measurement
-metrist	skilled in measurement

Word Part	Definition
-metry	process of measuring
mi-	derived from *hemi*, half
micro-	small
mictur	pass urine
mid-	middle
mileusis	lathe
milli	one-thousandth
miner	mines
mineral/o	inorganic material
miss	send
mit	thread
mito-	thread
mitr	having two points
mitt	send
mod	nature, form, method
molec	mass
mollusc	soft
mon	single
monas	single unit
monil	type of fungus
mono-	one, single
morbid	disease
morph/o	shape
mort	death
mot	move
motiv	move
muc/o	mucus, mucous membrane
mucosa	lining of a cavity
multi-	many
mune	in service
muscul/o	muscle
mut	silent
muta	genetic change
mutil	to maim
my/o	muscle
myc/o	fungus
myel/o	spinal cord, bone marrow
myelin	in the spinal cord, myelin
myo-	to blink
myop	to blink
myos	muscle
myring/o	tympanic membrane, eardrum
myx-	mucus

Word Part	Definition
narc/o	stupor
nas	nose
nat	born, birth
nate	born, birth
natr/i	sodium
natur/o	nature
ne/o	new
nebul	cloud
necr/o	death
neo-	new
nephr/o	kidney
nerv	nerve
-ness	quality, state
neur/o	nerve, nervous tissue
neutr/o	neutral
nici	lethal
nitr/o	nitrogen
noct-	night
noia	to think
nom	law
non-	no, not
nor-	normal
norm-	normal
nos/o	disease
nucle/o	nucleus
nucleol	small nucleus
nutri	nourish
nutrit	nourishment
o/o	egg
oblong	elongated
obsess	besieged by thoughts
obstetr	pregnancy and childbirth
occipit	back of head
occulta	hidden
ocul/o	eye
-ode	way, road, path
odont	tooth
odyn/o	pain
-oid	resembling
-ol	alcohol, chemical, substance
-ola	small
-ole	small
olfact	smell

Word Part	Definition
oligo-	scanty, too little
om/o	body, tumor
-oma	tumor, mass
onc/o	tumor
-one	chemical substance, hormone
onych/o	nail
ophthalm/o	eye
ophthalmos	eye
-opia	sight
opportun	take advantage of
-opsis	vision
-opsy	to view
opt/o	vision
optic	eye
-or	a doer, one who does, that which does something
or/o	mouth
orbit	orbit
orchi/o	testicle
ordin	arrange
orex	appetite
organ	organ, tool, instrument
orth/o	straight
orthot	correct
-orum	function of
-ory	having the function of
os	mouth
-osa	full of, like
-ose	full of
-osis	abnormal condition
osmo	push
osmol	concentration
oss/e	bone
oste/o	bone
-osus	condition
ot/o	ear
-otomy	incision
-ous	pertaining to
ov/i	egg
ovari	ovary
ovul	ovum, egg
ox	oxygen
-oxia	oxygen condition
oxid	oxidize

Word Part	Definition
oxy	oxygen
pace	step
palat	palate
palliat	reduce suffering
palm	palm
palpat	touch, stroke
palpit	throb
pan-	all
pancreat	pancreas
panto-	entire
papill/o	pimple
par-	abnormal, beside
para	to bring forth
para-	adjacent to, alongside, beside, abnormal
parasit	parasite
paresis	weakness
pareun	lying beside, sexual intercourse
pariet	wall
paroxysm	irritate; sudden, sharp attack
particul	little piece
partum	childbirth, to bring forth
pat	lie open
patell	patella
patent	lie open
-path	disease
path/o	disease
pathet	suffering
-pathic	pertaining to a disease
pathy	disease, emotion
-pathy	disease
paus	cessation
pause	cessation
pector	chest
ped	child, foot
pedicul	louse
pelas	skin
pelv	pelvis
pen	penis
-penia	deficient, deficiency
peps	digestion
pepsin/o	pepsin
pept	digest
per-	through, intense

Word Part	Definition
perforat	bore through
perfus	to pour
peri-	around
perine	perineum
peripher	external boundary, outer part, outer edge
periton/e	stretch over, peritoneum
perium	a bringing forth
perm/e	pass through
pes	foot
pesti	pest
petit	small
petit-	small
-pexy	fixation, surgical fixation
phaco-	lens
phag/o	to eat
phage	to eat
-phage	to eat
phagia	swallowing
-phagia	swallowing, eating
phalang/e	phalanx, finger, toe
pharmac/o	drug
pharyng/o	pharynx
pharynx	pharynx, throat
phenol	benzene derivative
phenyl	chemical group
pheo-	gray
pher/o	to carry
-pheresis	removal
-phil	attraction
-phile	attraction
-philia	attraction
phim	muzzle
phleb/o	vein
phob	fear
-phobia	fear
phon/o	sound, voice
phor	bear, carry
phosphat	phosphorus
phot/o	light
phren	mind
phylac	protect
phylaxis	protection
-phyll	leaf

Word Part	Definition
physema	blowing
physi/o	body
physis	growth
phyt/o	plant
pia	delicate
pituit	pituitary
pituitar	pituitary
plak	plate, plaque
plant	insert, plant
planus	flat surface
plas	molding, formation, growth
-plasia	formation
-plasm	something formed
plasm/o	to form
-plasty	formation, repair, surgical repair
plate	flat
pleg	paralysis
plete	filled
pleur	pleura
plexy	stroke
-pnea	breathe
pneum/o	air, lung
pneumat	structure filled with air
pneumon	air, lung
pod	foot
-poiesis	to make
-poiet	the making
-poietin	the maker
poikilo-	irregular
point	to pierce
pol	pole
polio	gray matter
pollut	unclean
poly-	excessive, many, much
polyp	polyp
poplit/e	ham, back of knee
por/o	opening
post-	after
poster	back part
pract	efficient, practical
prand/i	breakfast
pre-	before, in front of
precis	accurate

Word Part	Definition
pregn	with child, pregnant
presby	old person
press	press close, press down, squeeze
prevent	prevent
primi-	first
pro-	before, in front, projecting forward
proct/o	anus and rectum
product	lead forth
prolifer	bear offspring
pronat	bend down
prosta	prostate
prosthet	artificial part
prot/e	protein
protein	protein
proto-	first
provision	provide
proxim	nearest to the center
prurit	itch
pseudo-	false
psych/o	mind, soul
psyche	mind, soul
pteryg	wing
ptosis	drooping, falling
-ptosis	drooping
ptysis	spit
pub	pubis
puer	child
pulmon/o	lung
puls	to drive
pump	pump
punct	puncture
pupill-	pupil
pur	pus
purul	pus
py/o	pus
pyel/o	renal pelvis
pylor	gate, pylorus
pyr/o	fire, heat
pyrex	fever
pyrid	heat
quadrant	quadrant
quadri-	four
radi/o	radius, X-ray, radiation

Word Part	Definition
radic	root
re-	again, back, backward
recept	receive
rect/o	rectum
reflex	bend back
refract	bend
regul	to rule, control
remiss	send back, give up
ren	kidney
replic	reply
rescein	resin
resect/o	cut off
resid/u	left over, what is left over
resist	to withstand
respire/a	to breathe
restor	renew
resuscit	revive from apparent death
reticul	fine net, network
retin/o	retina
retinacul	hold back
retro-	backward
rhabd/o	rod shaped, striated
rheumat	a flow, rheumatism
rhin/o	nose
rhythm	rhythm
rib/o	like a rib
ribo	a sugar, pentose
ribo-	from ribose, a sugar
rigid	stiff
rose	rose
rotat	rotate
-rrhagia	excessive flow, discharge
-rrhaphy	suture
rrhea	flow, discharge
-rrhoid	flow
rrhyth	rhythm
rrhythm	rhythm
-rubin	rust colored
rumin	throat
sacchar	sugar
sacr/o	sacrum
sagitt	arrow
saliv	saliva

Word Part	Definition
salping/o	fallopian tube, uterine tube
salpinx	trumpet
san	sound, healthy
sanit	health
sapon	soap
sarc/o	flesh, muscle, sarcoma
satur	to fill
scapul	scapula
schiz/o	to split, cleave
scintill	spark
scler/o	hardness, white of eye
scoli/o	crooked
scope	instrument for viewing
-scope	instrument for viewing, instrument to examine
-scopy	to examine, to view
scorb	scurvy
scrot	scrotum
seb/o	sebum
sebac/e	wax
sebum	wax
secret	secrete, produce, separate
sect	cut off
sedat	to calm
sedent	sitting
segment	section
seiz	to grab
self	me, own individual
semi-	half
semin/i	semen
seminat	scatter seed
sen	old age
senesc	growing old
senil	senile
sens	feel
sensitiv	feeling
sensor/i	sensation, sensory
separat	move apart
seps	decay, infection
sept/o	septum, partition
ser/o	serum
serum	serum
sib	relative
-side	glycoside

Word Part	Definition
sigm	Greek letter "S"
silic	silicon, glass
simi	ape, monkey
simul	imitate
sin/o	sinus
sinus	sinus
sipid	flavor
-sis	abnormal condition, process
sit/u	place
skelet	skeleton
smear	spread
soc	partner
soci/o	society, social
soma	body
somat/o	body
-some	body
somn/o	sleep
son/o	sound
sorbit	fruit of a tree
sorpt	swallow
spad	tear or cut
spasm	spasm, sudden involuntary tightening
spast	tight
specif	species
sperm/i	sperm
spermat/o	sperm
sphen	wedge
spher/o	sphere
sphygm/o	pulse
spin/a	spine
spin/o	spine, spinal cord
spir/o	to breathe
spirat	breathe
spirit/u	spirit
spiro-	spiral, coil
splen/o	spleen
spongios	sponge
spor	spore
stable	steady
stag	standing place
stalsis	constrict, constriction
staphyl/o	bunch of grapes
stasis	stagnate, to stand still

Word Part	Definition
-stasis	stop, stand still, control
stat	stationary
-static	stopped, standing still
-statin	inhibit
stax	fall in drops
steat	fat
stein	stone
sten/o	narrow, contract
ster	solid, steroid
stere/o	three-dimensional
steril	sterile, make sterile
stern	chest, breastbone
-steroid	steroid
-sterol	steroid
-sterone	steroid
steth/o	chest
sthen	strength
stigmat	focus
stimul	excite, strengthen
stin	partition
stip	press
stiti	space
stoma	mouth
-stomy	new opening
stone	stone, pebble
storm	crisis
strab	squint
strat	layer
strept/o	twisted
strict	narrow
study	inquiry
su/i	self
sub-	below, under, underneath
suct	suck
suffic/i	enough
sulf	sulfur
super	above, excessive
super-	above, excessive
supinat	bend backward
supplement	supply to remedy a deficiency
suppress	pressed under, push under
supra-	above
surfact	surface

Word Part	Definition
surg	operate
suscept	to take up
-sylated	linked
sym-	together
symptomat	collection of symptoms
syn-	together
syndesm	bind together
synov	synovial membrane
syring/o	tube, pipe
system	the body as a whole
systol/e	contraction, systole
tachy-	rapid
tact	orderly arrangement
tag	touch
tain	hold
talip	ankle bone
tamin	touch
tampon	plug
tangent	touch
tars	ankle
tax	coordination
tempor/o	time, temple
ten/o	tendon
tendin	tendon
tens	pressure
-tensin	tense, taut
terat/o	monster, malformed fetus
term	limit, end
test/o	testis, testicle
testicul	testicle, testis
tetra-	four
thalam	thalamus
thalamus	thalamus
thalass	sea
thel	breast, nipple
then	motion
thenar	palm
therap/o	healing, treatment
therapeut	healing, treatment
-therapist	one who treats
therapy	treatment
-therapy	treatment
therm/o	heat

Word Part	Definition
thesis	arrange, place, organize
thet	arrange, place, organize
thi	sulfur
thora	chest
thorac/o	chest
thorax	chest
thromb/o	blood clot, clot
thym	thymus gland
thyr/o	thyroid
tibi	tibia
-tic	pertaining to
-tion	process, being
-tiz	pertaining to
toc	labor, birth
toler	endure
tom/o	cut, slice, layer
-tome	instrument to cut
-tomy	surgical incision
ton/o	pressure, tension
tonsil	tonsil
tonsill/o	tonsil
tope	part, location
topic	local
-tous	pertaining to
tox	poison
-toxic	able to kill
toxic/o	poison
trache/o	trachea, windpipe
tract	draw, pull
tranquil	calm
trans-	across, through
traumat	wound, injury
tresia	a hole
tri-	three
trich/o	hair
-tripsy	crushing
-tripter	crusher
trochle	pulley
trop	turn, turning
troph	development, nourishment
trophy	development, nourishment
-tropic	a turning, change
-tropin	nourishing, stimulation

Word Part	Definition
tryps	friction
tub	tube
tubercul	swelling, nodule, tuberculosis
tubul	small tube
tussis	cough
tympan/o	eardrum, tympanic membrane
-type	model, particular kind
typh	typhus
ulcer	a sore
-ule	little, small
-ulent	abounding in
uln	ulnar
ultra-	higher, beyond
-um	tissue, structure
umbilic	navel, umbilicus
un	one
un-	not
uni-	one
ur/o	urine, urinary system
-ure	process, result of
uresis	to urinate
uret	ureter, urine, urination
ureter/o	ureter
urethr/o	urethra
-uria	urine
urin	urine
-us	pertaining to
uter/o	uterus
uve	uvea
uvul	uvula
vaccin	vaccine, giving a vaccine
vag	vagus nerve
vagin	sheath, vagina
valgus	turn out
valv	valve
varic/o	varicosity; dilated, tortuous vein
vas/o	blood vessel, duct
vascul	blood vessel
ved	knowledge

Word Part	Definition
veget	plants
vegetat	growth
ven/a	vein
ven/o	vein
ventil	wind
ventr	belly
ventricul	ventricle
vers	turn
-version	change
vert	to turn
vertebr	vertebra
vesic	sac containing fluid
vestibul/o	vestibule, entrance
via	the way
violet	bluish purple
viril	masculine
virus	poison
viscer	internal organs
viscos	viscous, sticky
visu	sight
vita	life
voc	voice
vol	volume
volunt	willing
volut	shrink, roll up
-volut	rolled up
vuls	tear, pull
vulv/o	vulva
whip	to swing
xanth	yellow
xeno-	foreign
-xis	condition
-yl	substance
zea-	to live
-zoa	animal
zyg	zygote
zygomat	cheekbone
zyme	fermenting, enzyme, transform

Abbreviations

ABBREVIATION	DEFINITION
μg	microgram; one-millionth of a gram
Ab	antibody
ABG	arterial blood gas
ABO	agents of biologic origin
ABO	blood group system
ABR	auditory brainstem response
AC	acromioclavicular
ACE	angiotensin-converting enzyme
ACL	anterior cruciate ligament
ACLS	advanced cardiac life support
ACTH	adrenocorticotropic hormone
AD	right ear (Latin **a**uris **d**extra)
ADD	attention deficit disorder
ADH	antidiuretic hormone
ADHD	attention deficit hyperactivity disorder
ADL	activity of daily living
AED	automatic external defibrillator
Afib	atrial fibrillation
AFP	alpha-fetoprotein
Ag	antigen
AIDS	acquired immunodeficiency syndrome
AKA	above-knee amputation
ALL	acute lymphocytic leukemia
ALS	amyotrophic lateral sclerosis
ALT	alanine transaminase
AMI	acute myocardial infarction
AMS	altered mental state
ANS	autonomic nervous system
AOM	acute otitis media
AP	anteroposterior
APGAR	activity, pulse, grimace, appearance, respiration
ARDS	adult respiratory distress syndrome
ARF	acute renal failure
ARF	acute respiratory failure
AROM	active range of motion
AS	left ear (Latin **a**uris **s**inistra)
ASD	atrial septal defect

ABBREVIATION	DEFINITION
ASD	autism spectrum disorder
AST	asparate aminotransferase
AU	both ears (Latin **a**uris **u**terque)
AuD	Doctor of audiology
AV	atrioventricular
AVM	arteriovenous malformation
BBB	blood brain barrier
BEP	benign enlargement of the prostate
BKA	below-knee amputation
BM	bowel movement
BMD	bone mineral density
BMR	basal metabolic rate
BP	blood pressure
BPD	borderline personality disorder
BPH	benign prostatic hyperplasia
BPPV	benign paroxysmal positional vertigo
BRCA1	genetic mutation responsible for breast and ovarian cancer (**br**east **ca**ncer 1)
BRCA2	genetic mutation responsible for breast cancer (**br**east **ca**ncer 2)
BSE	bovine spongiform encephalopathy
BSE	breast self-examination
BUN	blood urea nitrogen
Bx	biopsy
C1	first cervical vertebra
C5	fifth cervical vertebra or nerve
C6	6th cervical vertebra
C7	seventh cervical vertebra
CA	cancer
Ca	calcium
CABG	coronary artery bypass graft
CAD	coronary artery disease
CAPD	continuous ambulatory peritoneal dialysis
CAT	computer-aided tomography
CBC	complete blood count
CBT	cognitive-behavioral therapy
CCPD	continuous cycling peritoneal dialysis
CD	conduct disorder

ABBREVIATION	DEFINITION
CDC	Centers for Disease Control and Prevention
CF	cystic fibrosis
CHD	congenital heart disease
CHES	certified health education specialist
CHF	congestive heart failure
CJD	Creutzfeldt–Jakob disease
CK	creatine kinase
CKD	chronic kidney disease
CMA	certified medical assistant
CMV	cytomegalovirus
CNA	certified nurse assistant
CNS	central nervous system
CNM	certified nurse midwife
c/o	complains of
c/o	complained/complaining of
CO_2	carbon dioxide
COPD	chronic obstructive pulmonary disease
COT	certified occupational therapist
COTA	certified occupational therapist assistant
COX	cyclooxygenase
CP	cerebral palsy
CPAP	continuous positive airway pressure
CPR	cardiopulmonary resuscitation
CPT	cognitive processing therapy
CPT	chest physical (physio) therapy
CRE	carbapenem-resistant Enterobacteriaoaceae
CRF	chronic renal failure
CRH	corticoreleasing hormone
CRP	C-reactive protein
C-section	cesarean section
CSF	cerebrospinal fluid
CT	computed tomography
CTS	carpal tunnel syndrome
CVA	cerebrovascular accident
CVP	central venous pressure
CVS	cardiovascular system
CVS	chorionic villus sampling
CVT	cardiovascular technologist
CXR	chest X-ray
D and C	dilation and curettage
DASH	dietary approaches to stop hypertension
DC	doctor of chiropractic
DEXA	dual-energy X-ray absorptiometry
DI	diabetes insipidus

ABBREVIATION	DEFINITION
DIC	disseminated intravascular coagulation
DID	dissociative identity disorder
DIFF	differential white blood cell count
DJD	degenerative joint disease
DKA	diabetic ketoacidosis
dL	deciliter; one-tenth of a liter
DM	diabetes mellitus
DMARD	disease-modifying antirheumatic drug
DMD	Duchenne muscular dystrophy
DNA	deoxyribonucleic acid
DNR	do not resuscitate
DO	Doctor of Osteopathy
DRE	digital rectal examination
DSM-5	*Diagnostic and Statistical Manual of Mental Disorders,* Fifth Edition
DTaP	diphtheria, tetanus, and pertussis vaccine
DVT	deep vein thrombosis
EBV	Epstein–Barr virus
ECG	electrocardiogram
ECOG	electrocochleography
ECT	electroconvulsive therapy
ED	emergency department
ED	erectile dysfunction
EEG	electroencephalogram
EKG	electrocardiogram
ELISA	enzyme-linked immunosorbent assay
EMG	electromyography
EMT	emergency medical technician
EMT-P	emergency medical technician-paramedic
ENG	electronystagmography
ENT	ear, nose throat
EPCA-2	early prostate cancer antigen-2
ER	emergency room
ERCP	endoscopic retrograde cholangiopancreatography
ERT	estrogen replacement therapy
ESR	erythrocyte sedimentation rate
ESRD	end-stage renal disease
ESWL	extracorporeal shock wave lithotripsy
EUS	endoscopic ultrasound
FAS	fetal alcohol syndrome
FDA	U.S. Food and Drug Administration
FEV1	forced expiratory volume in 1 second
FSH	follicle-stimulating hormone
FTD	fronto-temporal dementia

ABBREVIATION	DEFINITION
FTT	failure to thrive
FUS	focused ultrasound surgery
FVC	forced vital capacity
Fx	fracture
g	gram
GAD	generalized anxiety disorder
GB	galbladder
GDM	gestational diabetes mellitus
GERD	gastroesophageal reflux disease
GFR	glomerular filtration rate
GGT	gamma-glutamyl transferase test
GH	growth hormone, somatotrophin
GHRH	growth hormone-releasing hormone
GI	gastrointestinal
GI	glycemic index
GnRH	gonadotrophin-releasing hormone
GTT	glucose tolerance test
GYN	gynecology; gynecologist
HAV	hepatitis A virus
Hb A1c	glycosylated hemoglobin A-one-C
Hb, Hgb	hemoglobin
HBOT	hyperbaric oxygen therapy
HBV	hepatitis B virus
hCG	human chorionic gonadotropin
HCl	hydrochloric acid
Hct	hematocrit
HCV	hepatitis C virus
HDL	high-density lipoprotein
HDN	hemolytic disease of the newborn
Hep B	hepatitis type B
Hgb	hemoglobin
HIPAA	Health Insurance Portability and Accountability Act
Hib	haemophilus influenzae type B
HIV	human immunodeficiency virus
HMD	hyaline membrane disease
HPI	history of present illness
HPV	human papilloma virus
HRT	hormone replacement therapy
HSV	herpes simplex virus
HSV-1	herpes simplex virus, type 1
HsV2	herpes simplex virus 2
HTN	hypertension
HUS	hemolytic uremic syndrome

ABBREVIATION	DEFINITION
IADL	instrumental activities of daily living
IBD	inflammatory bowel disease
IBS	irritable bowel syndrome
ICD	implantable cardioverter/defibrillator
ICU	intensive care unit
IDDM	insulin-dependent diabetes mellitus
Ig	immunoglobulin
IgA	immunoglobulin A
IgD	immunoglobulin D
IgE	immunoglobulin E
IGF-1	insulin-like growth factor 1
IgG	immunoglobulin G
ILEA	International League Against Epilepsy
IgM	immunoglobulin M
IM	intramuscular
INR	International Normalized Ratio
IPV	inactivated polio virus
IRDS	infant respiratory distress syndrome
ITP	idiopathic (immunologic) thrombocytopenic purpura
IU	international unit(s)
IUD	intrauterine device
IV	intravenous
IVC	inferior vena cava
IVF	in vitro fertilization
IVP	intravenous pyelogram
JRA	juvenile rheumatoid arthritis
K	potassium
KUB	X-ray of abdomen to show **k**idneys, **u**reters, and **b**ladder
LADA	latent autoimmune diabetes in adults
LASER	**l**ight **a**mplification by **s**timulated **e**mission of **r**adiation
LASIK	laser-assisted in situ keratomileusis
LCL	lateral collateral ligament
LD	learning disability
LDL	low-density lipoprotein
LEEP	loop electrosurgical excision procedure
LFT	liver function test
LH	luteinizing hormone
LLQ	left lower quadrant
LMP	last menstrual period
LOC	loss of consciousness
LP	lumbar puncture

ABBREVIATION	DEFINITION
LPC	licensed professional counselor
LPN	licensed practical nurse
LSD	lysergic acid diethylamide
LUQ	left upper quadrant
LVN	licensed vocational nurse
MA	medical assistant
MAOI	monoamine oxidase inhibitors
mcg	microgram; one-millionth of a gram
MCL	medial collateral ligament
MCP	metacarpophalangeal
MCS	minimally conscious state
MCV	mean corpuscular volume
MD	Doctor of Medicine
MDMA	methhylenedioxymethamphetamine
Mg	magnesium
mg	milligram
MI	myocardial infarction
mL	milliliter
mm³	cubic millimeter
MMR	measles, mumps, rubella vaccine
MOAB	monoclonal antibody
MODY	mature onset diabetes of the young
MONA	morphine, oxygen, nitroglycerine, and aspirin
MPD	multiple personality disorder
MRA	magnetic resonance angiography
MRI	magnetic resonance imaging
mRNA	messenger RNA
MRSA	methicillin-resistant *Staphylococcus aureus*
MS	multiple sclerosis
MSA	myositis specific antibody
MVD	microvascular decompression
Na	sodium
NCI	National Cancer Institute
NIDDM	non-insulin-dependent diabetes mellitus
NIH	National Institutes of Health
NKA	no known allergies
NO	nitric oxide
NRDS	neonatal respiratory distress syndrome
NSAID	nonsteroidal anti-inflammatory drug
NT	nuchal translucency
O₂	oxygen
OA	obstetric assistant
OA	osteoarthritis

ABBREVIATION	DEFINITION
OB	obstetrics; obstetrician
OCD	obsessive compulsive disorder
OD	Doctor of Osteopathy
OD	right eye (Latin **o**culus **d**exter)
ODD	oppositional defiant disorder
OGTT	oral glucose tolerance test
OI	osteogenesis imperfecta
OME	otitis media with effusion
OR	operating room
OS	left eye (Latin **o**culus **s**inister)
OSHA	Occupational Safety and Health Administration
OT	occupational therapy; occupational therapist
OT	ophthalmic technician
OT	oxytocin
OTC	over the counter
OU	both eyes (Latin **o**culus **u**terque)
P	pulse rate
PA	pernicious anemia
PA	posteroanterior
PA	physician assistant
PAPP-A	pregnancy-associated plasma protein A
PaO₂	partial pressure of arterial oxygen
Pap	Papanicolaou (Pap test, Pap smear)
PAT	paroxysmal atrial tachycardia
PCL	posterior cruciate ligament
PCOS	polycystic ovarian syndrome
PCP	phenylcyclohexyl piperidine
PCV	pneumococcal conjugate vaccine
PDA	patent ductus arteriosus
PDD-NOS	pervasive developmental disorder, not otherwise specified
PDT	postural drainage therapy
PE (tube)	pressure equalization
PEEP	positive end-expiratory pressure
PEFR	peak expiratory flow rate
PERRLA	pupils equal, round, reactive to light, and accommodation
PET	positron emission tomography
PFTs	pulmonary function tests
pH	hydrogen ion concentration
PhD	Doctor of Philosophy
PID	pelvic inflammatory disease
PIP	proximal interphalangeal
PKD	polycystic kidney disease

ABBREVIATION	DEFINITION
PMDD	premenstrual dysphoric disorder
PMNL	polymorphonuclear leukocyte
PM&R	physical medicine and rehabilitation
PMS	premenstrual syndrome
PNS	peripheral nervous system
PO	by mouth (Latin **p**er **o**s)
POC	products of conception
polio	poliomyelitis
PPH	postpartum hemorrhage
PPS	postpolio syndrome
PPI	proton-pump inhibitor
p.r.n, PRN	when necessary (Latin **p**ro **re** **n**ata)
PRK	photoreactive keratectomy
PRL	prolactin
PSA	prostate-specific antigen
PT	physical therapy, physical therapist
PT	physiotherapy
PT	prothrombin time
PTA	physical therapy assistant
PTCA	percutaneous transluminal coronary angioplasty
PTH	parathyroid hormone
PTSD	posttraumatic stress disorder
PTT	partial thromboplastin time
PVC	premature ventricular contractions
PVD	peripheral vascular disease
PVS	persistent vegetative state
q.4.h.	every 4 hours
q.i.d.	four times each day
R	respiration rate
RA	rheumatoid arthritis
RAST	radioallergosorbent test
RBC	red blood cell
RDA	recommended dietary allowance
RDS	respiratory distress syndrome
Rh	Rhesus
Rho-GAM	Rhesus immune globulin
RICE	rest, ice, compression, and elevation
RLQ	right lower quadrant
RN	registered nurse
RNA	ribonucleic acid
ROM	range of motion
RT	respiratory therapy; respiratory therapist
RRT	registered respiratory therapist

ABBREVIATION	DEFINITION
RUQ	right upper quadrant
SA	sinoatrial
SAD	seasonal affective disorder
SARS	severe acute respiratory syndrome
SBS	shaken baby syndrome
SC	subcutaneous
SCI	spinal cord injury
SET	self-examination of the testes
SERM	selective estrogen receptor modulator
SG	specific gravity
SGA	small for gestational age
SGPT	serum glutamic-pyruvic transaminase
SI	sacroiliac
SIDS	sudden infant death syndrome
SLE	systemic lupus erythematosus
SNRI	serotonin and norepinephrine reuptake inhibitor
SOB	short(ness) of breath
SP	standard precautions
SSD	somatic symptom disorder
SSRI	selective serotonin reuptake inhibitor
STAT	immediately
STD	sexually transmitted disease
SVC	superior vena cava
T	temperature
T1	first thoracic vertebra or nerve
T3	triiodothyronine
T4	tetraiodothyronine (thyroxine)
TB	tuberculosis
TBI	traumatic brain injury
TCA	tricyclic antidepressant
TENS	transcutaneous electrical nerve stimulation
THC	tetrahydrocannabinol
THR	total hip replacement
TIA	transient ischemic attack
t.i.d.	(Latin *ter in die*) three times a day
TNF	tumor necrosis factor
TMJ	temporomandibular joint
TN	trigeminal neuralgia
TNM	**t**umor-**n**ode-**m**etastasis staging system for cancer
TOF	tetralogy of Fallot
tPA	tissue plasminogen activator
TRH	thyrotrophin-releasing hormone
TSE	testicular self exam

ABBREVIATION	DEFINITION
TSH	thyroid-stimulating hormone
TTM	trichotillomania
TTN	transient tachypnea of the newborn
TTP	thrombotic thrombocytopenic purpura
TUIP	transurethral incision of the prostate
TURP	transurethral resection of the prostate
UA	urinalysis
UP	universal precautions
URI	upper respiratory infection
UTI	urinary tract infection
UV	ultraviolet
VCUG	voiding cystourethrogram
VEP	visual evoked potential

ABBREVIATION	DEFINITION
Vfib	ventricular fibrillation
VNG	videonystagmography
VS	vital signs
VSD	ventricular septal defect
V-tach	ventricular tachycardia
vWD	von Willebrand disease
vWF	von Willebrand factor
WAD	Word Analysis and Definition (box)
WBC	white blood cell; white blood (cell) count
WHO	World Health Organization
WNL	within normal limits
WNV	West Nile virus

Diagnostic and Therapeutic Procedures

A compilation of the diagnostic and therapeutic procedural terms used in this book.

A

abdominoplasty Esthetic operation on the abdominal wall (tummy tuck).

ablation Removal of tissue to destroy its function.

activated partial thromboplastin time (APTT) Blood test used to monitor the dose of heparin, an anticoagulant.

adenoidectomy Surgical removal of the adenoid tissue.

alignment Process of bringing the ends of a fractured bone at the break back opposite each other so that they fit together as they did in the original bone.

ambulatory Surgery or any other care provided without an overnight stay in a medical facility.

ambulatory blood pressure monitor Device that provides a record of blood pressure readings over a 24-hour period as patients go about their daily activities.

amniocentesis Removal of amniotic fluid for diagnostic purposes.

amputation Process of removing a limb, part of a limb, a breast, or other projecting part.

anastomosis Surgically made union between two tubular structures.

angiogram Radiographic image of arteries or veins after injection of contrast material.

angiography The process of obtaining an angiogram.

angioplasty Reopening of a blood vessel by surgery.

anoscopy Examination of the anus and lower rectum with a rigid instrument.

Apgar score Evaluation of a newborn's status.

appendectomy Surgical removal of the appendix.

arterial blood gases The measurement of the levels of oxygen and carbon dioxide in the blood—a good indicator of respiratory function.

arteriography X-ray visualization of an artery after injection of contrast material.

arthrocentesis Aspiration of fluid from a joint; used to establish a diagnosis by laboratory examination of the fluid, drain off infected fluid, or insert medication such as local corticosteroids.

arthrodesis Fixation or stiffening of a joint by surgery.

arthrography X-ray of a joint after injection of a contrast medium into the joint to make the inside details of the joint visible.

arthroplasty Replacement of a joint with a prosthesis.

arthroscopy Procedure performed using an arthroscope to examine the internal compartments of a joint or perform a surgical procedure such as debridement, removal of damaged tissue, or repair of torn ligaments.

aspiration Removal by suction of fluid or gas from a body cavity.

atherectomy Surgical removal of atheroma from a blood vessel.

audiometer Electronic device that generates sounds in different frequencies and intensities to test for hearing loss.

auscultation Diagnostic method of listening to body sounds with a stethoscope.

autograft Graft removed from the patient's skin.

automatic external defibrillator (AED) Device that sends an electric shock to the heart to stop the heart and allow a normal contraction rhythm to resume.

B

bariatric surgery Surgical treatment of obesity.

barium meal Ingestion of barium sulfate to study the distal esophagus, stomach, and duodenum on X-ray.

barium swallow Ingestion of barium sulfate, a contrast material, to show details of the pharynx and esophagus on X-ray.

biopsy Removal of tissue from a living person for laboratory examination.

blepharoplasty Correction of defects in the eyelids.

bone marrow aspiration or biopsy Use of a needle to remove bone marrow cells.

bone mineral density (BMD) Screening test for osteoporosis using a dual-energy X-ray absorptiometry (DEXA) scan.

brace Appliance to support a part of the body in its correct position.

brachytherapy Radiation therapy in which the source of irradiation is implanted in the tissue to be treated.

bronchoscopy Examination of the interior of the tracheobronchial tree with an endoscope.

C

cannula Tube inserted into a blood vessel or cavity as a channel for fluid or gas.

cardiac catheterization Procedure that detects patterns of pressures and blood flows in the heart. A thin tube is guided into the heart under X-ray guidance after being inserted into a vein or artery.

cardiac stress testing Exercise tolerance test that raises the heart rate and monitors the effect on cardiac function.

cardiopulmonary resuscitation Attempt to restore cardiac and pulmonary function.

cardioversion Restoration of a normal heart rhythm by electrical shock. Also called *defibrillation*.

catheterization Introduction of a catheter.

cerebral angiography Injection of a radiopaque dye into the blood vessels of the neck and brain to detect blood vessels that are partially or completely blocked, aneurysms, or arteriovenous malformations.

cerebral arteriography Procedure used to determine the site of bleeding in hemorrhagic strokes, enabling surgery to be performed to stop the bleed or to clip off the aneurysm.

chest X-ray Radiograph image of the chest that can be taken in anteroposterior (AP), posteroanterior (PA), lateral, and sometimes oblique and lateral decubitus positions.

cholangiography Use of a contrast medium to radiographically visualize the bile ducts.

cholecystectomy Surgical removal of the gallbladder.

cholelithotomy Surgical removal of a gallstone(s).

circumcision Removal of part or all of the prepuce of the penis.

clean-catch, midstream urine specimen Sample collected after the external urethral meatus is cleaned. The first part of the urine stream is not collected, and the sterile collecting vessel is introduced into the urinary stream to collect the last part.

clot-busting drugs Drugs injected within a few hours of an MI or thrombotic stroke to dissolve the thrombus. Also called *thrombolytic drugs.*

cognitive behavioral therapy (CBT) A form of psychotherapy that emphasizes the role of thoughts and attitudes in one's feelings and behaviors.

cognitive processing therapy (CPT) Uses a variety of techniques in psychotherapy such as self-discovery and self-instruction.

colonoscopy Examination of the inside of the colon by endoscopy.

colostomy Artificial opening from the colon to the outside of the body.

colpopexy Surgical fixation of a relaxed and prolapsed vagina to the anterior abdominal wall.

computed tomography (CT) Scan in which images of sections of the body are generated by a computer synthesis of X-rays obtained in many different directions in a given plane.

conization Surgical excision of a cone-shaped piece of tissue, for example, from the outer lining of the cervix.

constant positive airway pressure (CPAP) Attempt to keep alveoli open by maintaining a positive pressure in the airways. A mask is fitted over the nose and mouth and attached to a ventilator.

continuous ambulatory peritoneal dialysis (CAPD) Dialysis performed by the patient at home through an implanted peritoneal catheter, usually 4 times a day, 7 days a week.

continuous cycling peritoneal dialysis Use of a machine to automatically infuse dialysis solution into and out of the abdominal cavity through a peritoneal catheter during sleep.

coronary angiogram Injection of a contrast dye during cardiac catheterization to identify coronary artery blockages.

coronary artery bypass graft surgery (CABG) Procedure in which healthy blood vessels harvested as a graft from the leg, chest, or arm are used to bypass (detour) the blood around blocked coronary arteries.

cryosurgery Use of liquid nitrogen or argon gas in a probe to freeze and kill abnormal tissue.

curetteage process of using a scoop-shaped instrument for scraping or removing new growths (or earwax).

cystoscopy Insertion of a pencil-thin, flexible, tubelike telescope through the urethra into the bladder to examine directly the lining of the bladder and to take a biopsy if needed.

cystourethrogram X-ray image during voiding to show the structure and function of the bladder and urethra.

D

debridement Removal of injured or necrotic tissue.

defibrillation Restoration of uncontrolled twitching of cardiac muscle fibers to a normal rhythm.

dermabrasion Removal of upper layers of the skin using a high-powered rotating brush.

dermascope An instrument that shines a light on the skin and magnifies a lesion for better diagnostic viewing.

dialysis Artificial method of removing waste materials and excess fluid from blood.

digital rectal examination (DRE) Palpation of the rectum and prostate gland with an index finger.

dilation and curettage (D & C) Dilation of the cervix so that a thin instrument can be inserted to scrape away the lining of the uterus and take tissue samples.

dipstick Plastic strip bearing paper squares of reagent—the most cost-effective method of screening urine. After the stick is dipped in the urine specimen, the color change in each segment of the dipstick is compared to a color chart on the container. Dipsticks can screen for pH, specific gravity, protein, blood, glucose, ketones, bilirubin, nitrite, and leukocyte esterase.

Doppler ultrasound Diagnostic instrument that sends an ultrasonic beam into the body.

E

early morning urine collection Process used to determine the ability of the kidneys to concentrate urine following overnight dehydration.

echocardiography Ultrasound recording of heart function.

echoencephalography Use of ultrasound in the diagnosis of intracranial lesions.

electrocardiogram Record of the electrical signals of the heart.

electrocardiography Interpretation of electrocardiograms.

electroconvulsive therapy (ECT) Passage of electric current through the brain to produce convulsions and treat persistent depression.

electroencephalography Recording of the electrical activity of the brain.

electromyography Recording of electrical activity in muscle.

endarterectomy Surgical removal of plaque from an artery.

endometrial ablation Use of a heat-generating tool or a laser to remove or destroy the lining of the uterus and prevent or reduce menstruation.

endoscope An instrument for the examination of the interior of a hollow or tubular organ.

endoscopy Use of an endoscope to examine the interior of a tubular or hollow organ and perform a biopsy, remove polyps (polypectomy), and coagulate bleeding lesions.

enema Injection of fluid into the rectum and lower bowel.

enteroscopy Examination of the lining of the digestive tract.

episiotomy Surgical incision in the perineum to dilate the opening of the vagina.

evoked responses Use of stimuli for vision, sound, and touch to activate specific areas of the brain and measure their responses with EEG.

excision Surgical removal of part or all of a structure or organ.

excisional biopsy Removal of a tumor with a surrounding margin of normal tissue.

external fixation Method of maintaining the alignment of a fractured bone by immobilizing the bone through the use of plaster casts, splints, traction, and external fixators such as steel rods and pins.

extracorporeal shock wave lithotripsy (ESWL) Process in which a machine called a *lithotripter* produces shock waves that crumble renal or ureteral stones into small pieces that can pass down the ureter.

F

fasciectomy Surgical removal of fascia.

fecal occult blood test Diagnostic procedure that detects the presence of blood not visible to the naked eye. Trade name: *Hemoccult* test.

fistulectomy Surgical excision of a fistula.

fistulotomy Surgical enlargement or opening up of a fistula.

flexible endoscopy Use of a flexible, slim fiber-optic instrument that transmits light and sends back images to the observer.

forceps extraction Assisted delivery of a baby by an instrument that grasps the head of the baby.

fundoscopy Examination of the retina with an ophthalmoscope.

G

gamma knife A minimally invasive radiosurgical system.

gastroscopy Endoscopic examination of the inside of the stomach.

gavage To feed by a stomach tube.

gingivectomy Surgical removal of diseased gum tissue.

H

heart transplant Surgery in which the heart of a recently deceased person (donor) is transplanted to the recipient after the recipient's diseased heart has been removed.

Hemoccult test Trade name for *fecal occult blood test.*

hemodialysis Process that filters blood through an artificial kidney machine (dialyzer).

hemorrhoidectomy Surgical removal of hemorrhoids.

herniorrhaphy Surgical repair of a hernia.

heterograft Graft from a nonhuman species. Also called *xenograft.*

Holter monitor Continuous ECG recorded on a tape cassette for at least 24 hours as a person works, plays, and rests.

homocysteine Amino acid in the blood. Elevated levels are related to a higher risk of CAD, stroke, and peripheral vascular disease.

homograft Skin graft from another person or a cadaver. Also called *allograft.*

hysterectomy Surgical removal of the uterus.

I

ileostomy Artificial opening from the ileum to the outside of the body.

implantable cardioverter/defibrillator (ICD) Implanted device that senses abnormal rhythms and gives the heart a small electrical shock to return the rhythm to normal.

incision Cut or surgical wound.

internal fixation Use of tissue-compatible materials such as stainless steel and titanium to stabilize fractured bony parts, enabling the patient to return to function more quickly and reducing the incidence of nonunion and malunion (improper healing). The types of internal fixation are wires used as sutures to "sew" the bone fragments together; plates that extend along both or all fragments of bone and are held in place by screws; rods inserted through the medullary cavity of both fragments to align the bones; and screws that can be used on their own as well as with plates.

intradermal injection Introduction of a short, thin needle into the epidermis, thus raising a small wheal. This site is used for allergy and tuberculosis (TB) testing.

intramuscular (IM) injection Use of a long needle that penetrates the epidermis, dermis, and hypodermis to reach into the muscles underneath. Some antibiotics and immunizations are given by this route.

intrauterine insemination Insertion of sperm directly into the uterus via a special catheter to initiate pregnancy.

intravenous pyelogram (IVP) Procedure in which a contrast material containing iodine is injected intravenously and its progress through the urinary tract is then recorded on a series of rapid radiological images.

intubation Insertion of a tube into a canal, hollow organ, or cavity, for example, into the trachea for anesthesia or control of ventilation.

in vitro fertilization (IVF) Process of combining sperm and egg in a laboratory dish and placing the resulting embryos inside the uterus.

Ishihara color system Test for color vision defects.

J

Jaeger reading card Chart containing type in different sizes of print for testing near vision.

K

keratomileusis Procedure that cuts and shapes the cornea.

keratoplasty Corneal graft or transplant.

keratotomy Incision through the cornea.

kidney transplant Surgery in which the kidney of a donor is transplanted to a recipient; provides a better quality of life than kidney dialysis, if a suitable donor can be found.

KUB X-ray of the abdomen to show **k**idneys, **u**reters, and **b**ladder.

L

laparoscopy Examination of the contents of the abdomen using an endoscope, which can also be used to perform surgery and take samples for biopsy.

laryngoscopy Use of a hollow tube with a light and camera to visualize or operate on the larynx.

laser surgery Use of a concentrated, intense narrow beam of electromagnetic radiation for surgery. (*laser:* light amplification by simulated emission of radiation)

LASIK Acronym for laser-assisted in situ keratomileusis.

lipectomy Surgical removal of fatty tissue.

lipid profile Group of blood tests that help determine the risk of CAD and comprise total cholesterol; high-density lipoprotein (HDL), or "good cholesterol"; low-density lipoprotein (LDL), or "bad cholesterol"; and triglycerides.

liposuction Surgical removal of fatty tissue using suction.

lobectomy Surgical removal of a lobe of a structure, for example, a lobe of a lung.

lumbar puncture Use of a hollow needle to remove CSF so that it can be examined in the laboratory. Also called *spinal tap*.

lumpectomy Removal of a lesion with preservation of surrounding tissue.

lymphadenectomy Surgical removal of a lymph gland(s).

lymphangiogram Radiographic images of lymph vessels and nodes following injection of contrast material.

M

magnetic resonance angiography (MRA) Method of visualizing vessels that contain flowing structures by producing a contrast between them and stationary structures.

magnetic resonance imaging (MRI) Diagnostic technique that creates detailed images of structures and tissues in various planes without exposing patients to radiation as in conventional radiography or computed tomography.

mammogram Record produced by X-ray imaging of the breast.

mammoplasty Surgical reshaping of the breasts.

mastectomy Surgical excision of the breast.

mechanical ventilation Process by which gases are moved into and out of the lungs via a ventilator that is set to meet the respiratory requirements of the patient.

mediastinoscopy Examination of the mediastinum using an endoscope inserted through an incision in the suprasternal notch.

myomectomy Surgical removal of a uterine myoma (fibroid).

myringotomy Incision through the tympanic membrane; for example, for the placement of pressure equalization (PE) tubes to allow an effusion to drain.

N

nebulizer Device used to deliver liquid medicine in a fine mist to be inhaled.

nephrectomy Surgical removal of a kidney.

nephrolithotomy Incision into the kidney for removal of a stone.

nephroscopy Examination of the pelvis of the kidney.

nerve conduction studies Studies that measure the speed at which motor or sensory nerves conduct impulses.

nuclear imaging of the heart Use of an injection of a radioactive substance in association with a cardiac stress test to assess cardiac function.

O

ophthalmoscopy Examination of the retina using an ophthalmoscope.

orchiopexy Surgical fixation of a testis in the scrotum.

ostomy Artificial opening into a tubular structure, for example, ileostomy and colostomy.

otoscopy Examination of the ear using an otoscope.

P

pacemaker Device that regulates cardiac electrical activity. The device generates electronic signals carried along thin, insulated wires to the heart muscle.

palpation Examination with the fingers and hands.

panendoscopy Visual examination of the inside of the esophagus, stomach, and upper duodenum using a flexible fiber-optic endoscope.

Pap test Examination of cells taken from the cervix.

parathyroidectomy Surgical removal of the parathyroid glands.

peak flow meter Instrument used to record the greatest flow of air that can be sustained for 10 milliseconds on forced expiration, the peak expiratory flow rate (PEFR). It is of value in following the course of asthma and in postoperative care to monitor the return of lung function after anesthesia.

percutaneous nephrolithotomy Insertion of a nephroscope through the skin to locate and remove a renal pelvic or ureteral stone.

percutaneous transluminal coronary angioplasty (PTCA) Procedure in which a balloon-tipped catheter is guided to the site of the blockage and inflated to expand the artery from the inside by compressing the plaque against the walls of the artery.

percutaneous transthoracic needle aspiration Insertion of a needle with a cutting chamber through an intercostal space to hook a specimen of parietal pleura for laboratory examination.

peritoneal dialysis Procedure in which a dialysis solution is infused into and drained out of the abdominal cavity through a small, flexible, implanted catheter.

phacoemulsification To break down and remove the lens of the eye using an ultrasound needle.

phlebotomy Process of taking blood from a vein.

photocoagulation Use of a laser beam to form a clot or destroy abnormal capillaries. In the eye, this slows the pace of the visual loss in macular degeneration.

phototherapy Treatment using light rays.

pneumonectomy Surgical removal of a lung.

polypectomy Excision or removal of a polyp.

polysomnography Test to monitor brain waves, muscle tension, eye movement, and oxygen levels in the blood as the patient sleeps.

positive end expiratory pressure (PEEP) Technique in ventilation to keep the alveoli from collapsing in adult and neonatal respiratory distress syndromes.

positron emission tomography (PET) Scan that shows the uptake and distribution of substances such as sugar in tissues to locate abnormal, often malignant, structures.

postural drainage therapy (PDT) Treatment that involves positioning and tilting the patient so that gravity promotes drainage of secretions from lung segments. Chest percussion (tapping) on the chest wall can help loosen, mobilize, and drain the retained secretions.

proctoscopy Examination of the inside of the anus and rectum by endoscopy.

prostatectomy Surgical removal of part or all of the prostate.

prosthesis Manufactured substitute for a missing part of the body.

prothrombin time (PT) Test used to monitor the dose of Coumadin, an anticoagulant. It is reported as an *international normalized ratio (INR)* instead of in seconds.

psychotherapy Treatment of psychiatric disorders based on verbal and nonverbal interventions with the patient.

pulmonary rehabilitation Therapeutic restoration of lung function that includes education, breathing exercises and retraining, exercises for the upper and lower extremities, and psychosocial support.

pulse oximeter Sensor placed on the finger to measure the oxygen saturation of the blood.

pyelogram X-ray image of the renal pelvis and ureters.

Q

quadrantectomy Surgical excision of a quadrant of the breast.

R

radical hysterectomy Surgical removal of the fallopian tubes and ovaries as well as the uterus.

radical mastectomy Complete surgical removal of all breast tissue, the pectoralis major muscle, and associated lymph nodes.

radical prostatectomy Complete surgical removal of the prostate and surrounding tissues.

random urine collection Process in which a sample is taken with no precautions regarding contamination. It is often used for collecting samples for drug testing. "Pee into a cup."

reduction Procedure in which the distal segment of a fractured bone is pulled back into alignment with the proximal segment. Anesthesia may be used.

rehabilitation Therapeutic restoration of an ability to function as before after disease, illness, or injury.

renal angiogram X-ray with contrast material used to assess blood flow to the kidneys.

resection Removal of a specific part of an organ or structure.

retrograde pyelogram Injection of contrast material through a urinary catheter into the ureters to locate stones and other obstructions.

rhinoplasty Surgical procedure to alter the size or shape of the nose.

Rinne test Test for a conductive hearing loss.

S

salpingectomy Surgical removal of a fallopian tube.

sclerotherapy Injection of a solution into a vein to thrombose it.

segmentectomy Surgical excision of a segment of a tissue or organ.

sigmoidoscopy Endoscopic examination of the sigmoid colon.

Snellen letter chart Test for acuity of distant vision.

sphygmomanometer Instrument for measuring arterial blood pressure.

spinal tap Placement of a needle through an intervertebral space into the subarachnoid space to withdraw CSF.

spirometer Device used to measure the volume of air that a patient moves in and out of the respiratory system.

splenectomy Surgical removal of the spleen.

staging Process of determining the extent of the distribution of a neoplasm. The TNM (tumor-node-metastasis) staging system can be used.

stent placement Procedure in which a wire mesh tube, or stent, is placed inside the vessel to reduce the likelihood that an occluded artery will close up again. Some stents (drug-eluting stents) are covered with a special medication to help keep the artery open.

sterilization Process of making sterile.

stethoscope Instrument for listening to cardiac, respiratory, and other sounds.

stoma Artificial opening.

subcutaneous (SC) injection Injection in which a needle pierces the epidermis and dermis to reach the hypodermis (subcutaneous) layer. This site is used for insulin injections and for some immunizations.

suprapubic transabdominal needle aspiration of the bladder Procedure used with newborns and small infants to obtain a pure sample of urine.

suture Process or material that brings together the edges of a wound to enhance tissue healing. Also, a form of fibrous joint to unite two bones.

T

thoracentesis Insertion of a needle through an intercostal space to remove fluid from a pleural effusion for laboratory study or to relieve pressure. Also called *pleural tap*.

thoracoscopy Examination of the pleural cavity with an endoscope.

thoracotomy Incision through the chest wall.

thymectomy Surgical removal of the thymus gland.

thyroidectomy Surgical removal of the thyroid gland.

tomography Radiographic image of a selected slice of tissue.

tonometry Measurement of intraocular pressure.

tonsillectomy Surgical removal of the tonsils.

tracheal aspiration Procedure in which a soft catheter is passed into the trachea to allow brushings and washings to remove cells and secretions from the trachea and main bronchi for diagnostic study.

tracheostomy Insertion of a tube into the windpipe to assist breathing.

tracheotomy The process of making an incision into the trachea.

traction Gentle but continuous application of a pulling force that can align a fracture, reduce muscle spasm, and relieve pain.

transdermal application Administration of some medications through the skin by an adhesive transdermal patch that is applied to the skin. The medication diffuses across the epidermis and enters the blood vessels in the dermis. Contraceptive hormones, analgesics, and antinausea/seasickness medications are examples.

transplant The tissue or organ used or the transfer of tissue from one person to another.

transthoracic Going through the chest wall.

tubal ligation Surgery, using laparoscopy, in which both fallopian tubes are cut, a segment is removed, and the ends are tied off and cauterized shut.

24-hour urine collection Process that determines the amount of protein being excreted daily and estimates the kidneys' filtration ability.

tympanostomy Surgically created new opening in the tympanic membrane to allow fluid to drain from the middle ear.

U

ultrasonography Delineation of deep structures using sound waves.

ureteroscopy Examination of the ureter. A small flexible ureteroscope is passed through the urethra and bladder into the ureter. Devices can be passed through the endoscope to remove or fragment stones.

urinalysis (microscopic) Analysis of the solids deposited by centrifuging a specimen of urine. It can reveal RBCs, WBCs, and renal tubular epithelial cells stuck together to form casts (cylindrical molds of cells) in nephrotic syndrome.

urinalysis (U/A) Examination of urine to separate it into its elements and define their kind and/or quantity. A routine urinalysis in the laboratory can include tests for color, clarity, pH, specific gravity, protein, glucose, ketones, and leukocyte esterase (indicator of infection).

urine culture Culture taken from a clean-catch urine specimen. It is the definitive test for a urinary tract infection.

V

vasectomy Excision of a segment of the ductus deferens to interrupt the flow of sperm.

vasovasostomy Microsurgical procedure to suture back together the cut ends of the ductus deferens to restore the flow of sperm. Also called *vasectomy reversal.*

venogram Radiograph of veins after injection of radiopaque contrast material.

vestibulectomy Surgical excision of the vulva.

visual evoked response (VEP) Detects damage to the optic nerve, a condition associated with multiple sclerosis (MS).

voiding cystourethrogram (VCUG) Imaging in which a contrast material is inserted into the bladder through a catheter and X-rays are taken during voiding.

W

Weber test Test for sensorineural hearing loss.

X

xenograft Graft from a nonhuman species. Also called *heterograft.*

Pharmacology

A compilation of pharmacologic terms used in this book.

A

acetaminophen Analgesic (reduces response to pain) and antipyretic (reduces fever).

adrenaline (1) Hormone produced by the adrenal medulla that boosts the supply of oxygen and glucose to the brain and increases heart rate and output. (2) Drug used to treat cardiac arrest and dysrhythmias and relieve bronchospasm in asthma. Also called *epinephrine.*

allergen Substance producing a hypersensitivity (allergic) reaction. Examples are animal fur and dander, penicillins, and foods such as eggs, milk, and wheat.

alpha-glucosidase inhibitors Block the breakdown of starches in the intestine.

analgesic Substance that reduces or relieves the response to pain without producing loss of consciousness. Examples are aspirin and other NSAIDs, acetaminophen, and codeine.

androgen Hormone that promotes masculine characteristics. An example is testosterone.

anesthetic Agent that causes absence of feeling or sensation. Examples of local anesthetics are lidocaine and novocaine; examples of general anesthetics are nitrous oxide, thiopental, and ketamine.

antacid Agent that neutralizes the acidity of stomach contents. Examples are aluminum hydroxide, magnesium hydroxide, and calcium carbonate.

antiarrhythmic Agents that restore normal heart rate and rhythm.

antibiotic Substance that has the capacity to inhibit the growth of or destroy bacteria and other microorganisms. Examples are penicillin, erythromycin, cefotaxime, and flucloxacillin.

anticholinergics Agents antagonistic to parasympathetic nerve fibers.

anticoagulant Substance that prevents clotting. Examples are heparin and Coumadin (warfarin).

antidepressants A class of drugs that alleviate the symptoms of depression.

antidiabetic drugs Medications used to treat diabetes. Those given orally include metformin, acarbose, and thiazolidinediones, such as troglitazone. Insulin is given by injection or inhaled.

antidiuretic Agent that decreases urine production. Examples are vasopressin, amiloride, and chlorpropamide.

antiepileptic Agent capable of preventing or arresting epilepsy. Examples are phenobarbitol, phenytoin, and valproate.

antifungal agents Agents used to prevent and arrest fungal infections. Examples are the topical applications 1% clotrimazole (Lomotrin, Mycelex) and 1% terbinafine (Lamisol), which are available without prescriptions.

antihistamine Agent used to treat allergic symptoms because of its action antagonistic to histamine. Examples are benadryl, diphenhydramine, and cimetidine.

anti-inflammatory Agent that reduces inflammation by acting on the body's responses, without affecting the causative agent. Examples are corticosteroids and aspirin.

antimicrobial Agent used to destroy or prevent multiplication of organisms. (See *antibiotic.*)

antineoplastic Agent that prevents the growth and spread of cancer cells. Examples are methotrexate, fluorouracil, and cyclophosphamide.

antipruritic Medication against itching. Examples are calamine lotion, hydrocortisone cream applied topically, and diphenhydramine (Benadryl) taken orally.

antipyretic Agent that reduces fever. Examples are aspirin and acetaminophen.

antiseptic Agent that reduces the number of microorganisms in different situations. Examples are alcohol, chlorhexidine, and providone-iodine.

anxiolytics Class of drugs that relieve the symptoms of anxiety.

atropine Agent used to dilate the pupils.

B

benzothiazide Diuretic that increases the excretion of sodium and potassium with an accompanying volume of water.

beta blocker Agent used in the treatment of a variety of cardiovascular diseases. Examples are propanalol and acebutolol.

biguanides Agents that decrease glucose production in the liver.

bronchodilator Agent that relaxes the smooth muscles of the bronchi and bronchioles. Examples are theophylline; beta-2 agonists, such as salbutamol and terbutaline; and anticholinergics, such as ipratropium bromide.

C

calcium channel blocker Agent that decreases the force of contraction of the myocardium, dilates coronary arteries, and reduces blood pressure. Examples are amlodipine and verapamil.

chemotherapy Treatment using chemical agents, usually in relation to neoplastic disease. Examples are platinum compounds such as cisplatin or paraplatin.

chronotropic Agents that alter the heart rate.

cleansing agents Soaps, shampoos, and detergents that are used to clean wounds and abrasions or to remove crusts and scales.

coagulant Substance that causes clotting. Thrombin and fibrin glue are used surgically to treat bleeding.

contraceptive Agent that prevents conception. Examples are condoms, diaphragms, and birth control pills using a mixture of estrogen and progesterone.

corticosteroids Hormones produced by the adrenal cortex. Examples are cortisol and aldosterone.

cortisol One of the glucocorticoids produced by the adrenal cortex; has anti-inflammatory effects. Also called *hydrocortisone.*

creams Water-based emulsions with a cooling and soothing effect that are cosmetically well tolerated.

D

decongestant An agent that reduces the swelling and fluid in the nose and sinuses. Examples are pseudoephedrine and phenylephrine.

depressant Substance that diminishes activity, sensation, or tone, particularly in relation to the nervous system. Examples are alcohol, barbiturates, and benzodiazepines.

disease-modifying drug Agent that has partial success in slowing down the accumulation of disabilities in a specific disease process. Examples in multiple sclerosis (MS) include interferons and mitoxantrone.

disinfectant Agent used to destroy pathogenic and other microorganisms on nonliving surfaces. Examples are alcohol, hydrogen peroxide, and hypochlorites.

diuretic Agent that increases urine output. Examples are furosemide, hydrochlorthiazide, spironolactone, and mannitol.

dopamine Chemical neurotransmitter in some specific areas of the brain.

E

epinephrine (1) Hormone produced by the adrenal medulla that boosts the supply of oxygen and glucose to the brain and increases heart rate and output. (2) Drug used to treat cardiac arrest and dysrhythmias and relieve bronchospasm in asthma. Also called *adrenaline*.

estrogen Generic term for hormones that stimulate female secondary sex characteristics.

F

fluorescein Dye that produces a vivid green color under a blue light; used to diagnose corneal abrasions and foreign bodies in the eye.

G

gels Jelly-like watery suspension using a chemical gelling agent for insoluble drugs such as corticosteroids and retinoids.

H

histamine Compound liberated in tissues as a result of injury or an immune response.

hydrocortisone Potent glucocorticoid with anti-inflammatory properties. Also called *cortisol*.

I

immunization Treatment with an agent designed to protect susceptible people from a communicable disease, such as agents that protect against the childhood diseases of measles, rubella, and pertussis.

inotropic Agents that change the force of ventricular contraction.

insulin Hormone produced by the islet cells of the pancreas that promotes glucose use. Injectable insulin preparations are classified by their speed of action.

L

lidocaine Ocular local anesthetic.

loop diuretic Promotes evacuation of urine in the kidney.

M

melatonin Hormone formed and secreted by the pineal gland during darkness. Serotonin is a precursor. It assists in the control of daily body rhythms, stimulates the immune system, and is an antioxidant.

morphine Derivative of opium used as an analgesic or sedative.

mucolytic Agent that attempts to break up mucus to allow it to be cleared more effectively from the airways. Examples are guaifenesin (common in over-the-counter cough medications), potassium iodide, and *N*-acetylcysteine (taken through a nebulizer).

mydriatic Agent that dilates the pupils of the eye.

N

narcotic Drug derived from opium. Examples are heroin, morphine, codeine, and demerol.

neurotransmitter Chemical that crosses a synapse to stimulate or inhibit another neuron or the cell of a muscle or gland. Examples are norepinephrine, serotonin, and dopamine.

O

ointments Agents that contain no water and are oil-based to provide an occlusive layer to retain water in the skin; they are used to treat chronic, dry, and scaly conditions.

opiate Drug derived from opium. Examples are morphine, codeine, heroin, and demerol.

osmotic diuretic Promotes evacuation of water and electrolytes in the kidney.

oxygen Gas given by nasal cannula or by mask and intubation to relieve hypoxia. Patients with severe, chronic COPD can be attached to a portable cylinder of oxygen.

P

pharmacist Person licensed by the state to prepare and dispense drugs.

pharmacology Science of the preparation, uses, and effects of drugs.

pharmacy Facility licensed to prepare and dispense drugs.

placebo Inert, medicinally inactive compound with no intrinsic therapeutic value.

pressor (PRESS-or) Producing increased blood pressure.

progesterone Hormone used to correct abnormalities of menstruation, and as a contraceptive.

prostaglandin Hormone present in many tissues; first isolated from the prostate gland.

psychedelic A class of drugs that enhance sensory experiences and consciousness.

psychoactive Agent able to alter mood, behavior, and/or cognition. Examples include narcotics, stimulants, antidepressants, and hallucinogens.

R

retinoids Keratolytic agents applied for psoriasis, acne, and photo damage.

S

saline Salt solution, usually sodium chloride.

selective serotonin reuptake inhibitors Class of drugs that prevent the reuptake of serotonin and are used in the treatment of depression.

somatotropin Hormone of the anterior pituitary gland that stimulates the growth of body tissues. Also called *growth hormone (GH)*.

spermicide Agent that destroys sperm. Examples are nonoxynol-9 and benzalkonium chloride.

sterilization Elimination of all microorganisms by high-pressure steam (autoclave), dry heat (oven), or radiation.

steroid Large family of chemical substances found in many drugs, hormones, and body components.

stimulant Agent that excites or strengthens. Examples include caffeine, nicotine, and cocaine.

sulfonylureas Agents that stimulate the beta cells of the pancreas to produce more insulin.

surfactant Protein and fat compound that creates surface tension to hold the lung alveolar walls apart.

T

teratogen Agent that produces fetal abnormalities—congenital malformations—while organs and structures are being formed. (All medications readily cross the placenta.) Examples include alcohol, isotretinoin (acne medication), valproic acid (anticonvulsant), and the rubella virus.

testosterone The major androgen that promotes development of male sex characteristics.

thrombolytic Agent injected within a few hours of a myocardial infarction (MI) or stroke to dissolve the thrombus causing the arterial blockage. Examples are streptokinase and tissue plasminogen activator (tPA). Also called *clot-busting drug*.

thyroxine Thyroid hormone T4, tetraiodothyronine.

topical Medication applied to the skin to obtain a local effect. Examples are ointments, creams, gels, lotions, patches, and sprays.

toxin Poisonous substance formed by a living cell or organism. Examples are venom from bee stings, snake bites, and jellyfish stings.

triamcinolone Synthetic corticosteroid.

V

vaccine Agent used to generate immunity and composed of the antigenic components of a killed or attenuated microorganism or its inactivated toxins. See *immunization*.

vasopressin Synthetic hormone causing contraction of smooth muscle.

vitamin Essential organic substance necessary in small amounts for normal cell function.

W

warfarin Anticoagulant; also used as rat poison. Trade name: *Coumadin*.

A

abdomen (AB-doh-men) Part of the trunk between the thorax and the pelvis.

abdominal (ab-DOM-in-al) Pertaining to the abdomen.

abdominopelvic (ab-DOM-ih-no-PEL-vik) Pertaining to the abdomen and pelvis.

abdominoplasty (ab-DOM-ih-noh-plas-tee) Surgical removal of excess subcutaneous fat from the abdominal wall (tummy tuck).

abduct (ab-DUKT) To move away from midline.

abduction (ab-DUCK-shun) Action of moving away from the midline.

abductor (ab-DUCK-tor) Muscle that moves a body part away from the midline.

ablation (ab-LAY-shun) Removal of tissue to destroy its function.

abortion (ah-BOR-shun) Spontaneous or induced expulsion of the fetus from the uterus at 20 weeks or less.

abrasion (ah-BRAY-zhun) Area of skin or mucous membrane that has been scraped off.

abruptio (ab-RUP-she-oh) Placenta abruptio is the premature detachment of the placenta.

abscess (AB-ses) A collection of pus surrounded by infected tissue that is swollen and inflamed.

absorb (ab-SORB) To take in.

absorption (ab-SORP-shun) Uptake of nutrients and water by cells in the GI tract.

abstinence (AB-stih-nens) Choosing to not participate in a behavior, in this case, sexual intercourse.

accessory (ak-SESS-oh-ree) A muscle, nerve or other structure that is a supplemental to a more major structure.

accommodate (ah-KOM-oh-date) To adapt to meet a need.

accommodation (ah-kom-oh-DAY-shun) The act of adjusting something to make it fit the needs; for example, the lens of the eye adjusts itself.

accommodative (ah-kom-oh-DAY-tiv) Pertaining to accommodation.

acetabulum (ass-eh-TAB-you-lum) The cup-shaped cavity of the hip bone that receives the head of the femur to form the hip joint.

acetaminophen (ah-seat-ah-MIN-oh-fen) Medication that is an analgesic and an antipyretic.

acetone (ASS-eh-tone) Ketone that is found in blood, urine, and breath when diabetes mellitus is out of control.

Achilles tendon (ah-KILL-eeze) A tendon formed from gastrocnemius and soleus muscles and inserted into the calcaneus bone. Also called *calcaneal tendon.*

achondroplasia (a-kon-droh-PLAY-zee-ah) Condition with abnormal conversion of cartilage into bone, leading to dwarfism.

acne (AK-nee) Inflammatory disease of sebaceous glands and hair follicles.

acoustic (ah-KYU-stik) Pertaining to hearing.

acquired immunodeficiency syndrome (AIDS) (ah-KWIRED IM-you-noh-dee-FISH-en-see SIN-drohm) Infection with the HIV.

acromegaly (ak-roe-MEG-ah-lee) Enlargement of the head, face, hands, and feet due to excess growth hormone in an adult.

acromioclavicular (AC) (ah-CROW-mee-oh-klah-VICK-you-lar) The joint between the acromion and the clavicle.

acromion (ah-CROW-mee-on) Lateral end of the scapula, extending over the shoulder joint.

actinic (ak-TIN-ik) Pertaining to the sun.

acrophobia (ak-roh-FOH-bee-ah) Pathologic fear of heights.

active (AK-tiv) Causing action or change.

activities of daily living (ADLs) (ak-TIV-ih-teez of DAY-lee LIV-ing) Daily routines for mobility, personal care, bathing, dressing, eating, and moving.

activity (ak-TIV-ih-tee) A goal-directed human action.

acute (ah-KYOUT) Having a rapid onset and duration.

adapt (a-DAPT) To adjust to different conditions.

adaptation (ad-ap-TAY-shun) Change in the function or structure of an organ to meet new conditions.

addict (ADD-ikt) One who cannot live without a substance or practice.

addiction (ah-DIK-shun) Habitual psychologic and physiologic dependence on a substance or practice.

Addison disease (ADD-ih-son diz-EEZ) An autoimmune disease leading to decreased production of adrenocortical steroids.

adduction (ah-DUCK-shun) Action of moving toward the midline.

adductor (ah-DUCK-tor) Muscle that moves a body part toward the midline.

adenocarcinoma (ADD-eh-noh-kar-sih-NOH-mah) A cancer arising from glandular epithelial cells.

adenoid (ADD-eh-noyd) Single mass of lymphoid tissue in the midline at the back of the throat.

adenoidectomy (ADD-eh-noy-DEK-toh-me) Surgical removal of the adenoid tissue.

adenoma (AD-eh-NOH-mah) Benign tumor that originates from glandular tissue.

adhere (add-HEER) To stick to something.

adherence (add-HEER-ents) The act of sticking to something.

adipose (ADD-ih-pose) Containing fat.

adolescence (ad-oh-LESS-ence) Stage that begins with puberty and ends with physical maturity.

adolescent (ad-oh-LESS-ent) Pertaining to adolescence or a person in that stage.

adrenal gland (ah-DREE-nal GLAND) The suprarenal gland on the upper pole of each kidney.

adrenaline (ah-DREN-ah-lin) One of the catecholamines. Also called *epinephrine.*

adrenocortical (ah-DREE-noh-KOR-tih-kal) Pertaining to the cortex of the adrenal gland.

adrenocorticotropic (ah-DREE-noh-KOR-tih-koh-TROH-pik) Hormone of the anterior pituitary that stimulates the cortex of the adrenal gland to produce its own hormones.

affect (AF-fekt) External display of feelings, thoughts, and emotions.

affective (af-FEK-tiv) Expressing emotion.

afferent (**AFF**-eh-rent) Moving toward a center; for example, nerve fibers conducting impulses to the spinal cord and brain.

aged (**A**-jid) Having lived to an advanced age.

agenesis (a-**JEN**-eh-sis) Failure to develop any organ or any part.

agglutinate (ah-**GLUE**-tin-ate) Stick together to form clumps.

agglutination (ah-glue-tih-**NAY**-shun) Process by which cells or other particles adhere to each other to form clumps.

aging (**A**-jing) The process of human maturation and decline.

agonist (**AG**-on-ist) Agent that combines with receptors to initiate drug actions.

agoraphobia (ah-gor-ah-**FOH**-bee-ah) Pathologic fear of being trapped in a public place.

agranulocyte (a-**GRAN**-you-loh-site) A white blood cell without any granules in its cytoplasm.

aldosterone (al-**DOS**-ter-own) Mineralocorticoid hormone of the adrenal cortex.

alignment (a-**LINE**-ment) Having a structure in its correct position relative to other structures.

alimentary (al-ih-**MEN**-tar-ee) Pertaining to the digestive tract.

alimentary canal (al-ih-**MEN**-tar-ee kah-**NAL**) Digestive tract.

alkylation (al-kih-**LAY**-shun) Introduction of a side chain into a compound.

allergen (**AL**-er-jen) Substance producing a hypersensitivity (allergic) reaction.

allergenic (al-er-**JEN**-ik) Pertaining to the capacity to produce an allergic reaction.

allergic (ah-**LER**-jik) Pertaining to or suffering from an allergy.

allergy (**AL**-er-jee) Hypersensitivity to an allergen.

allograft (**AL**-oh-graft) Skin graft from another person or a cadaver. Also called *homograft.*

alloimmune (**AL**-oh-im-**YUNE**) Immune reaction directed against foreign tissue.

alopecia (al-oh-**PEE**-shah) Partial or complete loss of hair, naturally or from medication.

alveolus (al-**VEE**-oh-lus) Terminal element of the respiratory tract where gas exchange occurs. Plural *alveoli.*

Alzheimer disease (**AWLZ**-high-mer diz-**EEZ**) Common form of dementia.

ambiguous (am-**BIG**-you-us) Uncertain.

amblyopia (am-blee-**OH**-pee-ah) Failure or incomplete development of the pathways of vision to the brain.

ambulatory (**AM**-byu-lah-tor-ee) Surgery or any other care provided without an overnight stay in a medical facility.

amenorrhea (a-men-oh-**REE**-ah) Absence or abnormal cessation of menstrual flow.

amino acid (ah-**ME**-no **ASS**-id) The basic building block for protein.

ammonia (ah-**MOAN**-ih-ah) Toxic breakdown product of amino acids (proteins).

amniocentesis (**AM**-nee-oh-sen-**TEE**-sis) Removal of amniotic fluid for diagnostic purposes.

amnion (**AM**-nee-on) Membrane around the fetus that contains amniotic fluid.

amniotic (am-nee-**OT**-ik) Pertaining to the amnion.

ampulla (am-**PULL**-ah) Dilated portion of a canal or duct.

amputation (am-pyu-**TAY**-shun) Process of removing a limb, a part of a limb, a breast, or some other projecting part. Verb *amputate.*

amputee (**AM**-pyu-tee) A person with an amputation.

amylase (**AM**-il-ase) One of a group of enzymes that breaks down starch.

amyotrophic (a-my-oh-**TROH**-fik) Pertaining to muscular atrophy.

anabolic steroid (an-ah-**BOL**-ik **STAIR**-oyd) Prescription drug used by some athletes to increase muscle mass.

anabolism (an-**AB**-oh-lizm) The buildup of complex substances in the cell from simpler ones as a part of metabolism.

anal (**A**-nal) Pertaining to the anus.

analog (**AN**-ah-log) A compound that resembles another in structure but not in function; *or* a means of the transmission of continuous information to our senses, in contrast with the digital transmission of only zeros and ones.

analgesia (an-al-**JEE**-zee-ah) State in which pain is reduced.

analgesic (an-al-**JEE**-zic) Substance that produces analgesia.

anaphylactic (**AN**-ah-fih-**LAK**-tik) Pertaining to anaphylaxis.

anaphylaxis (**AN**-ah-fih-**LAK**-sis) Immediate severe allergic response.

anastomosis (ah-**NAS**-toh-**MOH**-sis) A surgically made union between two tubular structures. Plural *anastomoses.*

anatomical (an-ah-**TOM**-ik-al) Pertaining to anatomy.

anatomy (ah-**NAT**-oh-mee) Study of the structures of the human body.

androgen (**AN**-droh-jen) Hormone that promotes masculine characteristics.

anemia (ah-**NEE**-me-ah) Decreased number of red blood cells.

anemic (ah-**NEE**-mik) Pertaining to or suffering from anemia.

anencephaly (**AN**-en-**SEF**-ah-lee) Born without cerebral hemispheres.

anesthesia (an-es-**THEE**-zee-ah) Complete loss of sensation.

anesthesiologist (**AN**-es-thee-zee-**OL**-oh-jist) Medical specialist in anesthesia.

anesthesiology (**AN**-es-thee-zee-**OL**-oh-jee) Medical specialty related to anesthesia.

anesthetic (an-es-**THET**-ik) Agent that causes absence of feeling or sensation.

aneurysm (**AN**-yur-izm) Circumscribed dilation of an artery or cardiac chamber.

angina pectoris (an-**JIH**-nuh **PEK**-tor-iss) Condition of severe pain in the chest due to coronary heart disease.

angiogram (**AN**-jee-oh-gram) Radiograph obtained after injection of radiopaque contrast material into blood vessels.

angiography (an-jee-**OG**-rah-fee) Radiography of vessels after injection of contrast material.

anisocoria (an-**EYE**-so-**KOR**-ee-ah) Unequal pupil size.

angioplasty (**AN**-jee-oh-**PLAS**-tee) Recanalization of a blood vessel by surgery.

anomaly (ah-**NOM**-ah-lee) Structural abnormality present at birth.

anorectal junction (**A**-no-**RECK**-tal **JUNK**-shun) Junction between the anus and the rectum.

anorexia (an-oh-**RECK**-see-ah) Without an appetite; *or* having an aversion to food.

anoscopy (**A**-nos-koh-pee) Endoscopic examination of the anus.

anoxia (an-**OCK**-see-ah) Without oxygen.

anoxic (an-**OCK**-sik) Pertaining to or suffering from a lack of oxygen.

antacid (ant-**ASS**-id) Agent that neutralizes the acidity of stomach contents.

antagonist (an-**TAG**-oh-nist) An opposing structure, agent, disease, or process.

antagonistic (an-**TAG**-oh-nist-ik) Having an opposite function.

antecubital (an-teh-**KYU**-bit-al) In front of the elbow.

anterior (an-**TEER**-ee-or) Front surface of body; situated in front.

anteversion (an-teh-**VER**-zhun) Forward displacement or tilting of a structure.

anthracosis (an-thra-**KOH**-sis) Lung disease caused by the inhalation of coal dust.

anthrax (**AN**-thraks) A severe, malignant infectious disease.

antiarrhythmic (**AN**-tee-a-**RITH**-mik) Pertaining to restoring a normal cardiac rhythm.

antibacterial (**AN**-tee-bak-**TEER**-ee-al) Destroying or preventing the growth of bacteria.

antibiotic (**AN**-tih-bye-**OT**-ik) A substance that has the capacity to inhibit growth of and destroy bacteria and other microorganisms.

antibody (**AN**-tee-bod-ee) Protein produced in response to an antigen. Plural *antibodies.*

anticholinergic (**AN**-tee-koh-lih-**NER**-jik) Antagonistic to parasympathetic nerve fibers.

anticoagulant (**AN**-tee-koh-**AG**-you-lant) Substance that prevents clotting.

antidepressant (**AN**-tee-dee-**PRESS**-ant) An agent used to counteract depression.

antidiarrheal (**AN**-tee-die-ah-**REE**-al) Drug that prevents abnormally frequent and loose stools.

antidiuretic (**AN**-tih-die-you-**RET**-ik) An agent that decreases urine production.

antidiuretic hormone (ADH) (**AN**-tih-die-you-**RET**-ik **HOR**-mohn) Posterior pituitary hormone that decreases urine output by acting on the kidney. Also called *vasopressin.*

antiemetic (**AN**-tee-eh-**MEH**-tik) Agent that prevents vomiting.

antiepileptic (**AN**-tih-epi-**LEP**-tik) A pharmacologic agent capable of preventing or arresting epilepsy.

antifungal Destroying or preventing the growth of a fungus.

anti-infective (**AN**-teh-in-**FEK**-tiv) Made incapable of transmitting an infection.

anti-inflammatory (**AN**-teh-in-**FLAM**-ah-toh-ree) Reducing, removing, or preventing inflammation.

antigen (**AN**-tee-jen) Substance capable of triggering an immune response.

antihistamine (**AN**-tih-**HISS**-tah-mean) Drug used to treat allergic symptoms because of its action antagonistic to histamine.

antimetabolite (**AN**-tee-meh-**TAB**-oh-lite) A substance that replaces or inhibits a specific part of a cell's normal metabolism.

antimuscarinic (**AN**-tee-**MUS**-ka-**RIN**-ik) Blocking the cholinergic and acetylcholine receptors.

antineoplastic (**AN**-tee-nee-oh-**PLAS**-tik) Pertaining to the prevention of the growth and spread of cancer cells.

antipruritic (**AN**-tee-pru-**RIT**-ik) Medication against itching.

antipyretic (**AN**-tee-pie-**RET**-ik) Agent that reduces fever.

antisepsis (an-tee-**SEP**-sis) Inhibiting the growth of infectious agents.

antiseptic (an-tee-**SEP**-tik) An agent or substance capable of affecting antisepsis.

antisocial personality disorder (**AN**-tee-**SOH**-shall per-son-**AL**-ih-tee dis-**OR**-der) Chronic violation of the rights of others.

antiviral (an-teh-**VIE**-ral) To weaken or abolish the action or replication of a virus.

antrum (**AN**-trum) A closed cavity.

anuria (an-**YOU**-ree-ah) Absence of urine production.

anus (**A**-nus) Terminal opening of the digestive tract through which feces are discharged.

anxiety (ang-**ZI**-eh-tee) Distress and dread caused by fear.

aorta (a-**OR**-tuh) Main trunk of the systemic arterial system.

aortic (a-**OR**-tik) Pertaining to the aorta.

apex (**A**-peks) Tip or end, for example, of a cone-shaped structure, such as the heart or lung.

Apgar score (**AP**-gar SKOR) Evaluation of a newborn's status.

aphthous (**AF**-thus) Painful small oral ulcers (canker sores).

aplastic anemia (a-**PLAS**-tik ah-**NEE**-me-ah) Condition in which the bone marrow is unable to produce sufficient red cells, white cells, and platelets.

apnea (**AP**-nee-ah) Absence of spontaneous respiration.

apoptosis (**AP**-op-**TOH**-sis) Programmed normal cell death.

appendectomy (ah-pen-**DEK**-toh-me) Surgical removal of the appendix.

appendicitis (ah-pen-dih-**SIGH**-tis) Inflammation of the appendix.

appendicular (**AP**-en-**DICK**-you-lar) Relating to the limbs, for example, the appendicular skeleton.

appendix (ah-**PEN**-dicks) Small blind projection from the pouch of the cecum.

aqueous humor (**AK**-we-us **HEW**-mor) Watery liquid in the anterior and posterior chambers of the eye.

arachnoid mater (ah-**RACK**-noyd **MAY**-ter) Weblike middle layer of the three meninges.

areola (ah-**REE**-oh-luh) Circular reddish area surrounding the nipple.

areolar (ah-**REE**-oh-lar) Pertaining to the areola.

argon laser (**AR**-gon **LAY**-zer) Laser used for ophthalmic procedures consisting of photons in the blue and/or green spectrum.

arrhythmia (a-**RITH**-me-ah) Condition when the heart rhythm is abnormal.

arteriography (ar-teer-ee-**OG**-rah-fee) X-ray visualization of an artery after injection of contrast material.

arteriole (ar-**TIER**-ee-ole) Small terminal artery leading into the capillary network.

arteriosclerosis (ar-**TIER**-ee-oh-skler-**OH**-sis) Hardening of the arteries.

arteriosclerotic (ar-**TIER**-ee-oh-skler-**OT**-ik) Pertaining to or suffering from arteriosclerosis.

artery (**AR**-ter-ee) Thick-walled blood vessel carrying blood away from the heart.

arthritis (ar-**THRI**-tis) Inflammation of a joint or joints.

arthrocentesis (**AR**-throh-sen-**TEE**-sis) Withdrawal of fluid from a joint through a needle.

arthrodesis (ar-**THROHD**-ee-sis) Fixation or stiffening of a joint by surgery.

arthrography (ar-**THROG**-rah-fee) X-ray of a joint taken after the injection of a contrast medium into the joint.

arthroplasty (**AR**-throh-plas-tee) Surgery to restore, as far as possible, the function of a joint.

arthroscope (**AR**-throh-skope) Endoscope used to examine the interior of a joint.

arthroscopy (ar-**THROS**-koh-pee) Visual examination of the interior of a joint.

articulate (ar-**TIK**-you-late) Two separate bones have formed a joint.

articulation (ar-tik-you-**LAY**-shun) A joint.

asbestosis (as-bes-**TOH**-sis) Lung disease caused by the inhalation of asbestos particles.

ascites (ah-**SIGH**-teez) Accumulation of fluid in the abdominal cavity.

asepsis (a-**SEP**-sis) Absence of living pathogenic organisms.

aspiration (**AS**-pih-**RAY**-shun) Removal by suction of fluid or gas from a body cavity. Verb *aspirate.*

assistive device (ah-**SIS**-tiv dee-**VICE**) Tool, software, or hardware to assist in performing daily activities.

asthma (**AZ**-mah) Episodes of breathing difficulty due to narrowed or obstructed airways.

asthmatic (az-**MAT**-ik) Suffering from or pertaining to asthma.

astigmatism (ah-**STIG**-maht-izm) Inability to focus light rays that enter the eye in different planes.

asymptomatic (**A**-simp-toh-**MAT**-ik) Without any symptoms experienced by the patient.

asystole (a-**SIS**-toh-lee) Absence of contractions of the heart.

ataxia (a-**TAK**-see-ah) Inability to coordinate muscle activity, leading to jerky movements.

ataxic (a-**TAK**-sik) Pertaining to or suffering from ataxia.

atelectasis (at-el-**ECK**-tah-sis) Collapse of part of a lung.

atherectomy (ath-er-**EK**-toh-me) Surgical removal of atheroma.

atheroma (**ATH**-er-**OH**-mah) Lipid deposit in the lining of an artery.

atherosclerosis (**ATH**-er-oh-skler-**OH**-sis) Atheroma in arteries.

athetoid (**ATH**-eh-toyd) Resembling or suffering from athetosis.

athetosis (ath-eh-**TOH**-sis) Slow, writhing involuntary movements.

atom (**AT**-om) A small unit of matter.

atonic (a-**TOHN**-ik) Without normal muscular tone.

atopic (a-**TOP**-ik) Pertaining to an allergy.

atopy (**AT**-oh-pee) State of hypersensitivity to an allergen—allergic.

atresia (a-**TREE**-zee-ah) Congenital absence of a normal opening or lumen.

atrial (**A**-tree-al) Pertaining to the atrium.

atrioventricular (AV) (**A**-tree-oh-ven-**TRICK**-you-lar) Pertaining to both the atrium and the ventricle.

atrium (**A**-tree-um) Chamber where blood enters the heart on both right and left sides. Plural *atria.*

atrophy (**A**-troh-fee) Wasting or diminished volume of a tissue or organ.

atropine (**AT**-ro-peen) Pharmacologic agent used to dilate pupils.

attenuate (ah-**TEN**-you-ate) Weaken the ability of an organism to produce disease.

audiologist (aw-dee-**OL**-oh-jist) Specialist in evaluation of hearing function.

audiology (aw-dee-**OL**-oh-jee) Study of hearing disorders.

audiometer (aw-dee-**OM**-eh-ter) Instrument to measure hearing.

audiometric (**AW**-dee-oh-**MET**-rik) Pertaining to the measurement of hearing.

audiometry (aw-dee-**OM**-eh-tree) The measurement of hearing.

auditory (**AW**-dih-tor-ee) Pertaining to the sense or the organs of hearing.

aura (**AWE**-rah) Sensory experience preceding an epileptic seizure or a migraine headache.

auricle (**AW**-ri-kul) The shell-like external ear.

auscultation (aws-kul-**TAY**-shun) Diagnostic method of listening to body sounds with a stethoscope.

autism (**AWE**-tizm) Developmental disorder of children.

autistic (awe-**TIS**-tik) Pertaining to autism.

autoantibody (awe-toh-**AN**-tee-bod-ee) Antibody produced in response to an antigen from the host's own tissue.

autograft (**AWE**-toh-graft) A graft using tissue taken from the same individual who is receiving the graft.

autoimmune (awe-toh-im-**YUNE**) Immune reaction directed against a person's own tissue.

autologous (awe-**TOL**-oh-gus) Blood transfusion with the same person as donor and recipient.

autolysis (awe-**TOL**-ih-sis) Destruction of cells by enzymes within the cells.

autonomic (awe-toh-**NOM**-ik) Self-governing visceral motor division of the peripheral nervous system.

autopsy (**AWE**-top-see) Examination of the body and organs of a dead person to determine the cause of death.

avascular (a-**VAS**-cue-lar) Without a blood supply.

axial (**AK**-see-al) Relating to the head and trunk, for example, the axial skeleton.

axilla (**AK**-sill-ah) Medical name for the armpit. Plural *axillae.*

axillary (**AK**-sill-air-ee) Pertaining to the armpit.

axon (**ACK**-son) Single process of a nerve cell carrying nervous impulses away from the cell body.

azoospermia (a-zoh-oh-**SPER**-me-ah) Absence of living sperm in the semen.

B

bacterial (bak-**TEER**-ee-al) Pertaining to bacteria.

bacterium (bak-**TEER**-ee-um) A unicellular (single-cell), simple, microscopic organism. Plural *bacteria.*

balanitis (bal-ah-**NIE**-tis) Inflammation of the glans and prepuce of the penis.

bariatric (bar-ee-**AT**-rik) Treatment of obesity.

barium sulfate (**BAIR**-ee-um **SUL**-fate or **BAR**-ee-um **SUL**-fate) A chalky, white radiopaque contrast substance used for radiologic view of the digestive tract.

base (BASE) Structurally, it is the lower part or bottom of a structure or the area opposite the apex. Referring to pH, it is a substance greater than 7.0.

basilar (BAS-ih-lar) Pertaining to the base of a structure.

basophil (BAY-so-fill) A basophil's granules attract basic blue stain in the laboratory.

Bell palsy (BELL PAWL-zee) Paresis, or paralysis, of one side of the face.

biceps brachii (BYE-sepz BRAY-key-eye) A muscle of the arm that has two heads or points of origin on the scapula.

bicuspid (by-KUSS-pid) Having two points. A bicuspid heart valve has two flaps; a bicuspid (premolar) tooth has two points.

bifid (BI-fid) Separated into two parts.

bilateral (by-LAT-er-al) On two sides; for example, in both ears.

bile (BILE) Fluid secreted by the liver into the duodenum.

bile acids (BILE AH-sids) Steroids synthesized from cholesterol.

biliary (BILL-ee-air-ree) Pertaining to bile or the biliary tract.

bilirubin (bill-ee-RU-bin) Bile pigment formed in the liver from hemoglobin.

binge eating (BINJ EE-ting) Eating with periods of excessive intake.

biofeedback (bie-oh-FEED-bak) Training techniques to achieve voluntary control of responses to stimuli.

biologic (BI-oh-LOJ-ik) Pertaining to the study of life and living organisms.

biopsy (BI-op-see) Removing tissue from a living person for laboratory examination.

bipolar disorder (bi-POH-lar dis-OR-der) A mood disorder with alternating episodes of depression and mania.

bladder (BLAD-er) Hollow sac that holds fluid, for example, urine or bile.

blastocyst (BLAS-toh-sist) First 2 weeks of the developing embryo.

blepharitis (blef-ah-RYE-tis) Inflammation of the eyelid.

blepharoplasty (BLEF-ah-roh-PLAS-tee) Surgical repair of the eyelid.

blepharoptosis (BLEF-ah-ROP-toh-sis) Drooping of the upper eyelid.

blood-brain barrier (BBB) (BLUD BRAYN BAIR-ee-er) A selective mechanism that protects the brain from toxins and infections.

bolus (BOH-lus) Single mass of a substance.

bone (BOHN) Hard connective tissue forming an organ of the skeletal system; or any distinct piece of the skeleton of the body.

bovine spongiform encephalopathy (BO-vine SPON-jee-form en-sef-ah-LOP-ah-thee) Disease of cattle that can be transmitted to humans, causing Creutzfeldt-Jakob disease. Also called *mad cow disease*.

bowel (BOUGH-el) Another name for *intestine*.

brace (BRACE) Appliance to support a part of the body in its correct position.

brachial (BRAY-kee-al) Pertaining to the arm.

brachialis (BRAY-kee-al-is) Muscle that lies underneath the biceps and is the strongest flexor of the forearm.

brachioradialis (BRAY-kee-oh-RAY-dee-al-is) Muscle that helps flex the forearm.

brachytherapy (brah-kee-THAIR-ah pee) Radiation therapy in which the source of radiation is implanted in the tissue to be treated.

bradycardia (brad-ee-KAR-dee-ah) Slow heart rate (below 60 beats per minute).

bradypnea (brad-ip-NEE-ah) Slow breathing.

brainstem (BRAYN-stem) Comprises the thalamus, pineal gland, pons, fourth ventricle, and medulla oblongata.

breech (BREECH) Buttocks-first presentation of the fetus at delivery.

broad-spectrum (broad-SPECK-trum) An antibiotic with a wide range of activity against a variety of organisms.

bronchiectasis (brong-key-ECK-tah-sis) Chronic dilation of the bronchi following inflammatory disease and obstruction.

bronchiole (BRONG-key-ole) Increasingly smaller subdivisions of bronchi.

bronchiolitis (brong-key-oh-LYE-tis) Inflammation of the small bronchioles.

bronchitis (bron-KI-tis) Inflammation of the bronchi.

bronchoconstriction (BRONG-koh-kon-STRIK-shun) Reduction in the diameter of a bronchus.

bronchodilator (BRONG-koh-die-LAY-tor) Agent that increases the diameter of a bronchus.

bronchogenic (BRONG-koh-JEN-ik) Arising from a bronchus.

bronchopneumonia (BRONG-koh-new-MOH-nee-ah) Acute inflammation of the walls of smaller bronchioles with spread to lung parenchyma.

bronchoscope (BRONG-koh-skope) Endoscope used for bronchoscopy.

bronchoscopy (brong-KOS-koh-pee) Examination of the interior of the tracheobronchial tree with an endoscope.

bronchus (BRONG-kuss) One of two subdivisions of the trachea. Plural *bronchi*.

bulbourethral (BUL-boh-you-REE-thral) Pertaining to the bulbous penis and urethra.

bulimia (buh-LEEM-ee-ah) Episodic bouts of excessive eating with compensatory throwing up.

bulla (BULL-ah) Bubble-like dilated structure. Plural *bullae*.

bunion (BUN-yun) A swelling at the base of the big toe.

bursa (BURR-sah) A closed sac containing synovial fluid. Plural *bursae*.

bursitis (burr-SIGH-tis) Inflammation of a bursa.

C

cachexia (kah-KEK-see-ah) A general weight loss and wasting of the body.

cadaver (kah-DAV-er) A dead body or corpse.

calcaneal (kal-KAY-knee-al) Pertaining to the calcaneus.

calcaneus (kal-KAY-knee-us) Bone of the tarsus that forms the heel.

calcitonin (kal-sih-TONE-in) Thyroid hormone that moves calcium from blood to bones.

calculus (KAL-kyu-lus) Small stone. Plural *calculi*.

callus (KAL-us) Bony tissue that forms at a fracture site early in healing.

calyx (KAY-licks) Funnel-shaped structure. Plural *calyces*.

cancellous (KAN-seh-lus) Bone that has a spongy or lattice-like structure.

cancer (KAN-ser) General term for a malignant neoplasm.

Candida (KAN-did-ah) A yeastlike fungus.

Candida albicans (KAN-did-ah AL-bih-kanz) The most common form of *Candida*.

candidiasis (can-dih-DIE-ah-sis) Infection with the yeastlike fungus *Candida*. Also called *thrush*.

canker (**KANG**-ker) Nonmedical term for an aphthous ulcer. Also called *mouth ulcer.*

cannabinoid (can-**AH**-bi-noyd) A group of chemical compounds, some of which increase appetite and others treat nausea and vomiting.

cannula (**KAN**-you-lah) Tube inserted into a blood vessel or cavity as a channel for fluid or gas.

capillary (**KAP**-ih-lair-ee) Minute blood vessel between the arterial and venous systems.

capitulum (kah-**PIT**-you-lum) A small head or rounded extremity of a bone.

capsular (**KAP**-syu-lar) Pertaining to a capsule.

capsule (**KAP**-syul) Fibrous tissue layer surrounding a joint or other structure.

carbohydrate (kar-boh-**HIGH**-drate) Group of organic food compounds that includes sugars, starch, glycogen, and cellulose.

carbuncle (**KAR**-bunk-ul) Infection of many furuncles in a small area, often on the back of the neck.

carcinogen (kar-**SIN**-oh-jen) Cancer-producing agent.

carcinogenesis (kar-**SIN**-oh-**JEN**-eh-sis) Origin and development of cancer.

carcinoma (kar-sih-**NOH**-mah) A malignant and invasive epithelial tumor.

carcinoma in situ (kar-sih-**NOH**-mah in **SIGH**-too) Carcinoma that has not invaded surrounding tissues.

cardiac (**KAR**-dee-ak) Pertaining to the heart.

cardiogenic (**KAR**-dee-oh-**JEN**-ik) Of cardiac origin.

cardiologist (**KAR**-dee-**OL**-oh-jist) A medical specialist in the diagnosis and treatment of disorders of the heart (cardiology).

cardiology (**KAR**-dee-**OL**-oh-jee) Medical specialty of diseases of the heart.

cardiomegaly (**KAR**-dee-oh-**MEG**-ah-lee) Enlargement of the heart.

cardiomyopathy (**KAR**-dee-oh-my-**OP**-ah-thee) Disease of the heart muscle, the myocardium.

cardiopulmonary resuscitation (**KAR**-dee-oh-**PUL**-moh-nary ree-sus-ih-**TAY**-shun) The attempt to restore cardiac and pulmonary function.

cardiovascular (**KAR**-dee-oh-**VAS**-kyu-lar) Pertaining to the heart and blood vessels.

cardioversion (**KAR**-dee-oh-**VER**-zhun) Restoration of a normal heart rhythm by electric shock. Also called *defibrillation.*

caries (**KARE**-eez) Bacterial destruction of teeth.

carotid (kah-**ROT**-id) Main artery of the neck.

carotid endarterectomy (kah-**ROT**-id **END**-ar-ter-**EK**-toh-me) Surgical removal of diseased lining from the carotid artery to leave a smooth lining and restore blood flow.

carpal (**KAR**-pal) Pertaining to the wrist.

carpus (**KAR**-pus) Collective term for the eight carpal bones of the wrist.

cartilage (**KAR**-tih-laj) Nonvascular, firm connective tissue found mostly in joints.

catabolism (kah-**TAB**-oh-lizm) Breakdown of complex substances into simpler ones as a part of metabolism.

cast (**KAST**) A cylindrical mold formed by materials in tubules; *or* a rigid encasement of a fractured bone to immobilize a fractured bone.

cataract (**KAT**-ah-ract) Complete or partial opacity of the lens.

catecholamine (kat-eh-**COAL**-ah-meen) Major element in the stress response; includes epinephrine and norepinephrine.

catheter (**KATH**-eh-ter) Hollow tube to allow passage of fluid into or out of a body cavity, organ, or vessel.

catheterization (**KATH**-eh-ter-ih-**ZAY**-shun) Introduction of a catheter.

catheterize (**KATH**-eh-teh-**RIZE**) To introduce a catheter.

caudal (**KAW**-dal) Pertaining to or nearer to the tailbone.

cauterization (**KAW**-ter-eye-**ZAY**-shun) The act of cauterizing.

cauterize (**KAW**-ter-ize) To apply a cautery.

cautery (**KAW**-ter-ee) Agent or device used to burn or scar a tissue.

cavernosa (kav-er-**NOH**-sah) Resembling a cave.

cavity (**KAV**-ih-tee) Hollow space or body compartment. Plural *cavities.*

cecal (**SEE**-kal) Pertaining to the cecum.

cecum (**SEE**-kum) Blind pouch that is the first part of the large intestine.

celiac (**SEE**-lee-ack) Relating to the abdominal cavity.

celiac disease (**SEE**-lee-ak diz-**EEZ**) Disease caused by sensitivity to gluten.

cell (**SELL**) The smallest unit of the body capable of independent existence.

cellular (**SELL**-you-lar) Pertaining to a cell.

cellulitis (**SELL**-you-**LIE**-tis) Infection of subcutaneous connective tissue.

Central canals (sen-**TRAHL** ka-**NALS**) Vascular canals in bone. Also called *Haversian canals.*

cephalic (seh-**FAL**-ik) Pertaining to or nearer to the head.

cerebellum (ser-eh-**BELL**-um) The most posterior area of the brain, located between the midbrain and the cerebral hemispheres.

cerebral (**SER**-ee-bral) Pertaining to the cerebral hemispheres or the brain.

cerebrospinal (**SER**-ee-broh-**SPY**-nal) Pertaining to the brain and spinal cord.

cerebrospinal fluid (CSF) (**SER**-ee-broh-**SPY**-nal **FLU**-id) Fluid formed in the ventricles of the brain that surrounds the brain and spinal cord.

cerebrum (**SER**-ee-brum) Cerebral hemispheres.

cerumen (seh-**ROO**-men) Waxy secretion of the ceruminous glands of the external ear.

ceruminous (seh-**ROO**-mih-nus) Pertaining to cerumen.

cervical (**SER**-vih-kal) Pertaining to the cervix or to the neck region.

cervix (**SER**-viks) The lower part of the uterus.

cesarean section (seh-**ZAH**-ree-an **SEK**-shun) Extraction of the fetus through an incision in the abdomen and uterine wall. Also called *C-section.*

chancre (**SHAN**-ker) Primary lesion of syphilis.

chemotherapy (**KEY**-moh-**THAIR**-ah-pee) Treatment using chemical agents.

chiasm (**KYE**-asm) X-shaped crossing of the two optic nerves at the base of the brain. Alternative term *chiasma.*

chickenpox (**CHICK**-en-pocks) Acute, contagious viral disease. Also called *varicella.*

chiropractic (kye-roh-**PRAK**-tik) Diagnosis, treatment, and prevention of mechanical disorders of the musculoskeletal system.

chiropractor (kye-roh-**PRAK**-tor) Practitioner of chiropractic.

chlamydia (klah-**MID**-ee-ah) An STD caused by an infection with *Chlamydia,* a species of bacteria.

cholangiography (**KOH**-lan-jee-**OG**-rah-fee) Use of a contrast medium to radiographically visualize the bile ducts.

cholecystectomy (**KOH**-leh-sis-**TECK**-toh-me) Surgical removal of the gallbladder.

cholecystitis (**KOH**-leh-sis-**TIE**-tis) Inflammation of the gallbladder.

choledocholithiasis (koh-**LED**-oh-koh-lih-**THIGH**-ah-sis) Presence of a gallstone in the common bile duct.

cholelithiasis (**KOH**-leh-lih-**THIGH**-ah-sis) Condition of having bile stones (gallstones).

cholelithotomy (**KOH**-leh-lih-**THOT**-oh-me) Surgical removal of a gallstone(s).

cholesteatoma (**KOH**-less-tee-ah-**TOH**-mah) Yellow, waxy tumor arising in the middle ear.

cholesterol (koh-**LESS**-ter-ol) Formed in liver cells; is the most abundant steroid in tissues and circulates in the plasma attached to proteins of different densities.

chondrosarcoma (**KON**-droh-sar-**KOH**-mah) Cancer arising from cartilage cells.

chorea (kor-**EE**-ah) Involuntary, irregular spasms of limb and facial muscles.

choreic (kor-**EE**-ik) Pertaining to or suffering from chorea.

chorion (**KOH**-ree-on) The fetal membrane that forms the placenta.

chorionic (koh-ree-**ON**-ik) Pertaining to the chorion.

chorionic villus (koh-ree-**ON**-ik **VILL**-us) Vascular process of the embryonic chorion to form the placenta.

choroid (**KOR**-oid) Region of the retina and uvea.

chromatin (**KROH**-ma-tin) Substance composed of DNA that forms chromosomes during cell division.

chromosomal (**KROH**-moh-**SO**-mal) Pertaining to a chromosome.

chromosome (**KROH**-moh-sohm) Body in the nucleus that contains DNA and genes.

chronic (**KRON**-ik) A persistent, long-term disease.

chyle (KYLE) A milky fluid that results from the digestion and absorption of fats in the small intestine.

chronotropic (**KRONE**-oh-**TROH**-pik) Affecting the heart rate.

chyme (KYME) Semifluid, partially digested food passed from the stomach into the duodenum.

cilium (**SILL**-ee-um) Hairlike motile projection from the surface of a cell. Plural *cilia*.

circulation (**SER**-kyu-**LAY**-shun) Continuous movement of blood through the heart and blood vessels.

circumcision (ser-kum-**SIZH**-un) To remove part or all of the prepuce.

circumduct (ser-kum-**DUCKT**) To move an extremity in a circular motion.

circumduction (ser-kum-**DUCK**-shun) Movement of an extremity in a circular motion.

cirrhosis (sir-**ROE**-sis) Extensive fibrotic liver disease.

claudication (klaw-dih-**KAY**-shun) Intermittent leg pain and limping.

claustrophobia (klaw-stroh-**FOH**-bee-ah) Pathologic fear of being trapped in a confined space.

clavicle (**KLAV**-ih-kul) Curved bone that forms the anterior part of the pectoral girdle.

clavicular (klah-**VICK**-you-lar) Pertaining to the clavicle.

cleft lip (KLEFT LIP) Congenital defect of the upper lip.

cleft palate (KLEFT **PAL**-ate) Congenital defect of the palate.

clitoris (**KLIT**-oh-ris) Erectile organ of the vulva.

clonic (**KLON**-ik) State of rapid successions of muscular contractions and relaxations.

closed fracture (KLOSD **FRAK**-chur) A bone is broken but the skin over it is intact.

Clostridium botulinum (klos-**TRID**-ee-um bot-you-**LIE**-num) Bacterium that causes food poisoning.

clot (KLOT) The mass of fibrin and cells that is produced in a wound.

coagulant (koh-**AG**-you-lant) Substance that causes clotting.

coagulate (koh-**AG**-you-late) Form a clot.

coagulation (koh-ag-you-**LAY**-shun) The process of blood clotting.

coagulopathy (koh-ag-you-**LOP**-ah-thee) Disorder of blood clotting. Plural *coagulopathies*.

coarctation (koh-ark-**TAY**-shun) Constriction, stenosis, particularly of the aorta.

coccyx (**KOK**-sicks) Small tailbone at the lower end of the vertebral column.

cochlea (**KOK**-lee-ah) An intricate combination of passages; used to describe the inner ear.

cochlear (**KOK**-lee-ar) Pertaining to the cochlea.

cognition (kog-**NIH**-shun) Process of acquiring knowledge through thinking, learning, and memory.

cognitive (**KOG**-nih-tiv) Pertaining to the mental activities of thinking and learning.

cognitive-behavioral therapy (CBT) (**KOG**-nih-tiv be-**HAYV**-yur-al **THAIR**-ah-pee) Psychotherapy that emphasizes thoughts and attitudes in one's behavior.

coitus (**KOH**-it-us) Sexual intercourse.

colic (**KOL**-ik) Spasmodic, crampy pains in the abdomen.

colitis (koh-**LIE**-tis) Inflammation of the colon.

collagen (**KOLL**-ah-jen) Major protein of connective tissue, cartilage, and bone.

collateral (koh-**LAT**-er-al) Situated at the side, often to bypass an obstruction.

Colles fracture (**KOL**-ez **FRAK**-chur) Fracture of the distal radius at the wrist.

colloid (**COLL**-oyd) Liquid containing suspended particles.

colon (**KOH**-lon) The large intestine, extending from the cecum to the rectum.

colostomy (koh-**LOSS**-toh-me) Artificial opening from the colon to the outside of the body.

colostrum (koh-**LOSS**-trum) The first breast secretion at the end of pregnancy.

colpopexy (**KOL**-poh-peck-see) Surgical fixation of the vagina.

colporrhaphy (col-**POR**-ah-fee) Suture of a rupture of the vagina.

colposcope (**KOL**-poh-scope) Endoscope to view the vagina and cervix.

colposcopy (kol-**POS**-koh-pee) Examination of vagina and cervix with an endoscope.

coma (**KOH**-mah) State of deep unconsciousness.

comatose (**KOH**-mah-tohs) In a state of coma.

comedo (**KOM**-ee-doh) A whitehead or blackhead caused by too much sebum and too many keratin cells blocking the hair follicle. Plural *comedones.*

comminuted fracture (**KOM**-ih-nyu-ted **FRAK**-chur) A fracture in which the bone is broken into small pieces.

competent (**KOM**-peh-tent) Capable of performing a task or function.

complement (**KOM**-pleh-ment) Group of proteins in the serum that finish off the work of antibodies to destroy bacteria and other cells.

complete fracture (kom-**PLEET FRAK**-chur) A bone is fractured into two separate pieces.

complex (**KOM**-pleks) A stable combination of two or more compounds in the body.

compliance (kom-**PLY**-ance) Measure of the capacity of a chamber or hollow viscus (e.g., the lungs) to expand; *or* consistency and accuracy with which a patient follows a treatment regimen.

compression (kom-**PRESH**-un) Squeeze together to increase density and/or decrease a dimension of a structure.

compression fracture (kom-**PRESH**-un **FRAK**-chur) Fracture of a vertebra causing loss of height of the vertebra.

compulsion (kom-**PUL**-shun) Uncontrollable impulses to perform an act repetitively.

compulsive (kom-**PUL**-siv) Possessing uncontrollable impulses to perform an act repetitively.

conception (kon-**SEP**-shun) Fertilization of the egg by sperm to form a zygote.

concha (**KON**-kah) Shell-shaped bone on the medial wall of the nasal cavity. Plural *conchae.*

concussion (kon-**KUSH**-un) Mild brain injury.

condom (**KON**-dom) A sheath or cover for the penis or vagina to prevent conception and infection.

conductive hearing loss (kon-**DUK**-tiv) Hearing loss caused by lesions in the outer ear or middle ear.

condyle (**KON**-dile) Large, smooth, rounded expansion of the end of a bone where it forms a joint with another bone.

confusion (kon-**FEW**-zhun) Mental state in which environmental stimuli are not processed appropriately.

congenital (kon-**JEN**-ih-tal) Present at birth, either inherited or due to an event during gestation up to the moment of birth.

congruent (**KONG**-roo-ent) Coinciding or agreeing with.

conization (koh-ni-**ZAY**-shun) Surgical excision of a cone-shaped piece of tissue.

conjunctiva (kon-junk-**TIE**-vah) Inner lining of the eyelids.

conjunctival (kon-junk-**TIE**-val) Pertaining to the conjunctiva.

conjunctivitis (kon-junk-tih-**VI**-tis) Inflammation of the conjunctiva.

conjugate (**KON**-joo-gate) To join together, usually in pairs.

connective tissue (koh-**NECK**-tiv **TISH**-you) The supporting tissue of the body.

conscious (**KON**-shus) Having present knowledge of oneself and one's surroundings.

consciousness (**KON**-shus-ness) The state of being aware of and responsive to the environment.

consolidate (v) (kon-**SOL**-i-date) Making firm or solid.

consolidated (adj) (kon-**SOL**-i-day-tid) An aerated tissue that has become firm or solid.

consolidation (kon-**SOL**-i-day-shun) Area of solid tissue that was once aerated.

constipation (kon-stih-**PAY**-shun) Hard, infrequent bowel movements.

constrict (kon-**STRIKT**) To become or make narrow.

constriction (kon-**STRIK**-shun) A narrowed portion of a structure.

contagious (kon-**TAY**-jus) Infection can be transmitted from person to person or from a person to a surface to a person.

contaminate (kon-**TAM**-in-ate) To cause the presence of an infectious agent to be on any surface or in any substance.

contamination (**KON**-tam-ih-**NAY**-shun) Presence of an infectious agent on a surface or in substances.

contraception (kon-trah-**SEP**-shun) Prevention of pregnancy.

contraceptive (kon-trah-**SEP**-tiv) An agent that prevents conception.

contract (kon-**TRAKT**) Draw together or shorten.

contracture (kon-**TRAK**-chur) Muscle shortening due to spasm or fibrosis.

contrecoup (**KON**-treh-koo) Injury to the brain at a point directly opposite the point of original contact.

contusion (kon-**TOO**-zhun) Hemorrhage into a tissue (bruising), including the brain.

convulsion (kon-**VUL**-shun) Alternative name for seizure.

cor pulmonale (**KOR** pul-moh-**NAH**-lee) Right-sided heart failure arising from chronic lung disease.

corpuscle (**KOR**-pus-ul) A red blood cell.

corpuscular (kor-**PUS**-kyu-lar) Pertaining to a red blood cell.

cornea (**KOR**-nee-ah) The central, transparent part of the outer coat of the eye covering the iris and pupil.

corneal (**KOR**-nee-al) Pertaining to the cornea.

coronal (**KOR**-oh-nal) Pertaining to the vertical plane dividing the body into anterior and posterior portions.

coronal plane (**KOR**-oh-nal **PLAIN**) Vertical plane dividing the body into anterior and posterior portions.

coronary circulation (**KOR**-oh-nair-ee **SER**-kyu-**LAY**-shun) Blood vessels supplying the heart.

corpus (**KOR**-pus) Major part of a structure. Plural *corpora.*

corpus albicans (**KOR**-pus **AL**-bih-kanz) An atrophied corpus luteum.

corpus callosum (**KOR**-pus kah-**LOW**-sum) Bridge of nerve fibers connecting the two cerebral hemispheres.

corpus luteum (**KOR**-pus **LOO**-teh-um) Yellow structure formed at the site of a ruptured ovarian follicle.

corpuscle (**KOR**-pus-ul) A blood cell.

cortex (**KOR**-teks) Outer portion of an organ, such as bone; gray covering of cerebral hemispheres. Plural *cortices.*

cortical (**KOR**-tih-cal) Pertaining to a cortex.

corticosteroid (**KOR**-tih-koh-**STAIR**-oyd) A hormone produced by the adrenal cortex.

corticotropin (**KOR**-tih-koh-**TROH**-pin) Pituitary hormone that stimulates the cortex of the adrenal gland to secrete corticosteroids.

cortisol (**KOR**-tih-sol) One of the glucocorticoids produced by the adrenal cortex; has anti-inflammatory effects. Also called *hydrocortisone.*

cortisone (**KOR**-tih-sohn) A corticosteroid produced in small amounts by the adrenal cortex.

coryza (koh-**RYE**-zah) Viral inflammation of the mucous membrane of the nose. Also called *acute rhinitis.*

cough (**KAWF**) Forceful expulsion of air from the lungs, occurring immediately after a closed glottis.

coup (**KOO**) Injury to the brain occurring directly under the skull at the point of contact.

coxa (**COCK**-sah) Hipbone. Plural *coxae.*

cranioplasty (**KRAY**-nee-oh-**PLASTY**) Repair of a bone defect in the skull.

craniotomy (**KRAY**-nee-**OT**-oh-mee) Surgical removal of part of a skull bone to expose the brain for surgery.

cranial (**KRAY**-nee-al) Pertaining to the skull.

craniofacial (**KRAY**-nee-oh-**FAY**-shal) Pertaining to both the face and the cranium.

cranial (**KRAY**-nee-um) The skull.

cranium (**KRAY**-nee-um) The skull.

creatine kinase (**KREE**-ah-teen **KIE**-naze) Enzyme elevated in plasma following heart muscle damage in myocardial infarction.

cretin (**KREH**-tin) A person with severe congenital hypothyroidism.

cretinism (**KREH**-tin-izm) Condition of severe congenital hypothyroidism.

Creutzfeldt-Jakob disease (**KROITS**-felt **YAK**-op diz-**EEZ**) Progressive incurable neurologic disease caused by infectious prions.

cricoid (**CRY**-koyd) Ring-shaped cartilage in the larynx.

crista ampullaris (**KRIS**-tah am-**PULL**-air-is) Mound of hair cells and gelatinous material in the ampulla of a semicircular canal.

Crohn disease (**KRONE** diz-**EEZ**) Narrowing and thickening of terminal small bowel. Also called *regional enteritis.*

croup (**KROOP**) Infection of the upper airways in children, characterized by a barking cough. Also called *laryngotracheobronchitis.*

cruciate (**KRU**-she-ate) Shaped like a cross.

cryosurgery (cry-oh-**SUR**-jer-ee) Use of liquid nitrogen or argon gas in a probe to freeze and kill abnormal tissue.

cryotherapy (**CRY**-oh-**THAIR**-ah-pee) The use of cold in the treatment of injury.

cryptorchidism (krip-**TOR**-kizm) Failure of one or both testes to descend into the scrotum.

curettage (kyu-reh-**TAHJ**) Scraping the interior of a cavity.

curette (kyu-**RET**) Scoop-shaped instrument for scraping the interior of a cavity or removing new growths.

Cushing syndrome (**KUSH**-ing **SIN**-drohm) Hypersecretion of cortisol (hydrocortisone) by the adrenal cortex.

cutaneous (kyu-**TAY**-nee-us) Pertaining to the skin.

cuticle (**KEW**-tih-cul) Nonliving epidermis at the base of the fingernails and toenails.

cyanosis (sigh-ah-**NO**-sis) Blue discoloration of the skin, lips, and nail beds due to low levels of oxygen in the blood.

cyanotic (sigh-ah-**NOT**-ik) Pertaining to or marked by cyanosis.

cyst (**SIST**) An abnormal, fluid-containing sac.

cystic (**SIS**-tik) Relating to a cyst.

cystic fibrosis (CF) (**SIS**-tik fie-**BROH**-sis) Genetic disease in which excessive viscid mucus obstructs passages, including bronchi.

cystitis (sis-**TIE**-tis) Inflammation of the urinary bladder.

cystocele (**SIS**-toh-seal) Hernia of the bladder into the vagina.

cystopexy (**SIS**-toh-pek-see) Surgical procedure to support the urinary bladder.

cystoscope (**SIS**-toh-skope) An endoscope inserted to view the inside of the bladder.

cystoscopy (sis-**TOS**-koh-pee) Using a cystoscope to examine the inside of the urinary bladder.

cystourethrogram (sis-toh-you-**REETH**-roe-gram) X-ray image during voiding to show the structure and function of the bladder and urethra.

cytogenetics (**SIGH**-toh-jeh-**NET**-iks) Study of chromosomal abnormalities in a cell.

cytokine (**SIGH**-toh-kine) Proteins produced by different cells that communicate with other cells in the immune system.

cytologist (sigh-**TOL**-oh-jist) Specialist in the structure, chemistry, and pathology of the cell.

cytology (sigh-**TOL**-oh-jee) Study of the cell.

cytoplasm (**SIGH**-toh-plazm) Clear, gelatinous substance that forms the substance of a cell except for the nucleus.

cytostatic (**SIGH**-toh-**STAT**-ik) Inhibiting cell division.

cytotoxic (sigh-toh-**TOX**-ik) Destructive to cells.

D

dandruff (**DAN**-druff) Scales in hair from shedding of the epidermis.

death (**DETH**) Total and permanent cessation of all vital functions.

debridement (day-**BREED**-mon) The removal of injured or necrotic tissue.

decongestant (dee-con-**JESS**-tant) Agent that reduces the swelling and fluid in the nose and sinuses.

decubitus ulcer (de-**KYU**-bit-us **UL**-ser) Sore caused by lying down for long periods of time.

defecation (def-eh-**KAY**-shun) Evacuation of feces from the rectum and anus.

defect (**DEE**-fect) An absence, malformation, or imperfection.

defective (dee-**FEK**-tiv) Imperfect.

defibrillation (de-fib-rih-**LAY**-shun) Restoration of uncontrolled twitching of cardiac muscle fibers to normal rhythm.

defibrillator (de-fib-rih-**LAY**-tor) Instrument for defibrillation.

deformity (de-**FOR**-mih-tee) A permanent structural deviation from the normal.

degenerative (dee-**JEN**-er-a-tiv) Relating to the deterioration of a structure.

deglutition (dee-glue-**TISH**-un) The act of swallowing.

dehydration (dee-high-**DRAY**-shun) Process of losing body water.

delirium (de-**LIR**-ee-um) Acute altered state of consciousness with agitation and disorientation; condition is reversible.

deltoid (**DEL**-toyd) Large, fan-shaped muscle connecting the scapula and clavicle to the humerus.

delusion (dee-**LOO**-zhun) Fixed, unyielding false belief held despite strong evidence to the contrary.

dementia (da-**MEN**-sha) Chronic, progressive, irreversible loss of intellectual and mental functions.

demyelination (dee-**MY**-eh-lin-**A**-shun) Process of losing the myelin sheath of a nerve fiber.

dendrite (**DEN**-dright) Branched extension of the nerve cell body that receives nervous stimuli.

dental (**DEN**-tal) Pertaining to the teeth.

dentine (**DEN**-tin) Dense, ivory-like substance located under the enamel in a tooth. (Also spelled *dentin.*)

dentist (**DEN**-tist) Legally qualified specialist in dentistry.

dentistry (**DEN**-tis-tree) Evaluation, diagnosis, prevention, and treatment of conditions of the oral cavity and associated structures.

deoxygenate (dee-**OCK**-se-je-nate) Remove oxygen from a liquid (blood).

deoxygenation (dee-**OCK**-se-je-**NAY**-shun) The removal of oxygen from a liquid (blood).

deoxyribonucleic acid (DNA) (dee-**OCK**-see-rye-boh-nyu-**KLEE**-ik **ASS**-id) Source of hereditary characteristics found in chromosomes.

dependence (dee-**PEN**-dense) The state of needing or relying on someone or something else.

dependent (dee-**PEN**-dent) Having to rely on someone else.

depressant (de-**PRESS**-ant) Substance that diminishes activity, sensation, or tone.

depression (de-**PRESS**-shun) Mental disorder with feelings of deep sadness and despair.

dermabrasion (der-mah-**BRAY**-zhun) Removal of upper layers of skin by rotary brush.

dermal (**DER**-mal) Pertaining to the skin.

dermascope (**DER**-mah-skope) Instrument that shines a light on the skin and magnifies a lesion.

dermatitis (der-mah-**TYE**-tis) Inflammation of the skin.

dermatologic (der-mah-toh-**LOJ**-ik) Pertaining to the skin and dermatology.

dermatologist (der-mah-**TOL**-oh-jist) Medical specialist in diseases of the skin.

dermatology (der-mah-**TOL**-oh-jee) Medical specialty concerned with disorders of the skin.

dermatomyositis (**DER**-mah-toh-my-oh-**SIGH**-tis) Inflammation of the skin and muscles.

dermis (**DER**-miss) Connective tissue layer of the skin beneath the epidermis.

desquamation (**DEES**-kwah-**MAY**-shun) The peeling of outer layer of skin; shedding of epidermis.

detoxification (dee-**TOKS**-ih-fih-**KAY**-shun) Remove poison from a tissue or substance.

deviate (**DEE**-vee-ate) Move away from normal place.

diabetes insipidus (dye-ah-**BEE**-teez in-**SIP**-ih-dus) Excretion of large amounts of dilute urine as a result of inadequate ADH production.

diabetes mellitus (dye-ah-**BEE**-teez **MEL**-ih-tus) Metabolic syndrome caused by absolute or relative insulin deficiency and/or insulin ineffectiveness.

diabetic (dye-ah-**BET**-ik) Pertaining to or suffering from diabetes.

diagnose (die-ag-**NOSE**) To make a diagnosis.

diagnosis (die-ag-**NO**-sis) The determination of the cause of a disease. Plural *diagnoses.*

diagnostic (die-ag-**NOS**-tik) Pertaining to or establishing a diagnosis.

dialysis (die-**AL**-ih-sis) An artificial method of filtration to remove excess waste materials and water from the body.

diaphoresis (**DIE**-ah-foh-**REE**-sis) Sweat or perspiration.

diaphoretic (**DIE**-ah-foh-**RET**-ic) Pertaining to sweat or perspiration.

diaphragm (**DIE**-ah-fram) A ring and dome-shaped material inserted into the vagina to prevent pregnancy; *or* the muscular sheet separating the abdominal and thoracic cavities.

diaphragmatic (**DIE**-ah-frag-**MAT**-ik) Pertaining to the diaphragm.

diaphysis (die-**AF**-ih-sis) The shaft of a long bone.

diarrhea (die-ah-**REE**-ah) Abnormally frequent and loose stools.

diastasis (die-**ASS**-tah-sis) Separation of normally joined parts.

diastole (die-**AS**-toh-lee) Dilation of heart cavities, during which they fill with blood.

diastolic (die-as-**TOL**-ik) Pertaining to diastole.

differential (dif-er-**EN**-shal) A differential white blood cell count lists percentages of the different leukocytes in a blood sample.

diffuse (di-**FUSE**) To disseminate or spread out.

diffusion (di-**FYU**-zhun) The means by which small particles move between tissues.

digestion (die-**JESS**-shun) Breakdown of food into elements suitable for cell metabolism.

digestive (die-**JEST**-iv) Pertaining to digestion.

digital (**DIJ**-ih-tal) Pertaining to a finger or toe.

digitize (**DIJ**-ih-tize) To change analog information into a numerical format to facilitate computer processing.

dilate (**DIE**-late) To perform or undergo dilation.

dilation (die-**LAY**-shun) Stretching or enlarging an opening or a structure.

diphtheria (dif-**THEER**-ee-ah) Disease with a thick, membranous (leathery) coating of the pharynx.

diplegia (die-**PLEE**-jee-ah) Paralysis of all four limbs, with the two legs affected most severely.

dipstick (**DIP**-stick) Strip of plastic or paper bearing squares of reagents that change color in the presence of abnormal chemicals in the urine.

disability (dis-ah-**BILL**-ih-tee) Diminished capacity to perform certain activities or functions.

disc (DISK) Flattened, round structure. In the skeletal system, a flattened round fibrocartilaginous structure between bones.

discipline (**DIS**-ih-plin) Training for proper conduct or action.

discrimination (**DIS**-krim-ih-**NAY**-shun) Ability to distinguish between different things.

disease (diz-**EEZ**) A disorder of body functions, systems, or organs.

disinfectant (dis-in-**FEK**-tant) Agent that disinfects.

disinfection (dis-in-**FEK**-shun) Process of destruction of microorganisms by chemical agents.

dislocation (dis-low-**KAY**-shun) Completely out of joint.

displaced fracture (dis-**PLAYSD FRAK**-chur) A fracture in which the fragments are separated and are not in alignment.

disseminate (dih-**SEM**-in-ate) Widely scattered throughout the body or an organ.

dissociative identity disorder (di-**SO**-see-ah-tiv eye-**DEN**-tih-tee dis-**OR**-der) Part of an individual's personality is separated from the rest, leading to multiple personalities.

distal (**DISS**-tal) Situated away from the center of the body.

diuresis (die-you-**REE**-sis) Excretion of large volumes of urine.

diuretic (die-you-**RET**-ik) Agent that increases urine output.

diverticulitis (**DIE**-ver-tick-you-**LIE**-tis) Inflammation of the diverticula.

diverticulosis (**DIE**-ver-tick-you-**LOW**-sis) Presence of a number of small pouches in the wall of the large intestine.

diverticulum (die-ver-**TICK**-you-lum) A pouchlike opening or sac from a tubular structure (e.g., gut). Plural *diverticula.*

dopamine (**DOH**-pah-meen) Neurotransmitter in specific small areas of the brain.

Doppler (**DOP**-ler) Diagnostic instrument that sends an ultrasonic beam into the body.

Doppler ultrasonography (**DOP**-ler **UL**-trah-soh-**NOG**-rah-fee) Detects direction, velocity, and turbulence of blood flow; used in workup of stroke patients.

dormant (**DOOR**-mant) Inactive.

dorsal (**DOOR**-sal) Pertaining to the back or situated behind.

dorsum (**DOOR**-sum) Upper, posterior, or back surface.

Down syndrome (**DOWN SIN**-drome) A syndrome with variable abnormalities associated with three copies of chromosome 21.

Duchenne muscular dystrophy (**DOO**-shen **MUSS**-kyu-lar **DISS**-troh-fee) Symmetrical weakness and wasting of pelvic, shoulder, and proximal limb muscles.

ductus arteriosus (**DUK**-tus ar-**TEER**-ih-**OH**-sus) Fetal vessel that connects the descending aorta with the left pulmonary artery.

ductus deferens (**DUK**-tus **DEH**-fuh-renz) Tube that receives sperm from the epididymis. Also known as *vas deferens.*

duodenal (du-oh-**DEE**-nal) Pertaining to the duodenum.

duodenum (du-oh-**DEE**-num) The first part of the small intestine; approximately 12 finger-breadths (9 to 10 inches) in length.

dura mater (**DYU**-rah **MAY**-ter) Hard, fibrous outer layer of the meninges.

dwarfism (**DWORF**-izm) Short stature due to underproduction of growth hormone.

dysentery (**DIS**-en-tare-ee) Disease with diarrhea, bowel spasms, fever, and dehydration.

dysfunctional (dis-**FUNK**-shun-al) Difficulty in functioning.

dyslexia (dis-**LEK**-see-ah) Impaired reading and writing ability below the person's level of intelligence.

dyslexic (dis-**LEK**-sik) Pertaining to or suffering from dyslexia.

dysmenorrhea (dis-men-oh-**REE**-ah) Painful and difficult menstruation.

dysmorphic (dis-**MOR**-fik) Possessing a developmental structural defect.

dysmorphology (dis-mor-**FOLL**-oh-jee) The study of developmental structural defects.

dyspareunia (dis-pah-**RUE**-nee-ah) Pain during sexual intercourse.

dyspepsia (dis-**PEP**-see-ah) "Upset stomach," epigastric pain, nausea, and gas.

dysphagia (dis-**FAY**-jee-ah) Difficulty in swallowing.

dysphoria (dis-**FOR**-ee-ah) Psychiatric mood disorder.

dysplasia (dis-**PLAY**-zee-ah) Abnormal tissue formation.

dysplastic (dis-**PLAS**-tik) Pertaining to or showing abnormal tissue formation.

dyspnea (disp-**NEE**-ah) Difficulty breathing.

dyspneic (disp-**NEE**-ik) Pertaining to or suffering from difficulty in breathing.

dysrhythmia (dis-**RITH**-me-ah) An abnormal heart rhythm.

dysuria (dis-**YOU**-ree-ah) Difficulty or pain with urination.

E

echocardiography (**EK**-oh-kar-dee-**OG**-rah-fee) Ultrasound recording of heart function.

echoencephalography (**EK**-oh-en-sef-ah-**LOG**-rah-fee) Use of ultrasound in the diagnosis of intracranial lesions.

ecchymosis (**EK**-i-**MO**-sis) Small hematoma resulting from a bruise.

eclampsia (ek-**LAMP**-see-uh) Convulsions in a patient with preeclampsia.

ectopic (ek-**TOP**-ik) Out of place, not in a normal position.

eczema (**EK**-zeh-mah) Inflammatory skin disease, often with a serous discharge.

eczematous (ek-**ZEM**-ah-tus) Pertaining to or marked by eczema.

edema (eh-**DEE**-mah) Excessive accumulation of fluid in cells and tissues.

edematous (ee-**DEM**-ah-tus) Pertaining to or marked by edema.

effacement (ee-**FACE**-ment) Thinning of the cervix in relation to labor.

efferent (**EFF**-eh-rent) Moving away from a center; for example, conducting nerve impulses away from the brain or spinal cord.

effusion (eh-**FYU**-zhun) Collection of fluid that has escaped from blood vessels into a cavity or tissues.

ejaculate (ee-**JACK**-you-late) To expel suddenly; *or* the semen expelled in ejaculation.

ejaculation (ee-**JACK**-you-**LAY**-shun) Process of expelling semen suddenly.

ejaculatory (ee-**JACK**-you-**LAY**-tor-ee) Pertaining to ejaculation.

elective (e-**LEK**-tiv) Surgery or a procedure that is not urgent or vital.

electrocardiogram (ECG or EKG) (ee-**LEK**-troh-**KAR**-dee-oh-gram) Record of the electrical signals of the heart.

electrocardiograph (ee-**LEK**-troh-**KAR**-dee-oh-graf) Machine that makes the electrocardiogram.

electrocardiography (ee-**LEK**-troh-kar-dee-**OG**-rah-fee) Interpretation of electrocardiograms.

electroconvulsive therapy (ECT) (ee-**LEK**-troh-kon-**VUL**-siv **THAIR**-ah-pee) Passage of electric current through the brain to produce convulsions and treat persistent depression.

electrode (ee-**LEK**-trode) A device for conducting electricity.

electroencephalogram (EEG) (ee-**LEK**-troh-en-**SEF**-ah-low-gram) Record of the electrical activity of the brain.

electroencephalograph (ee-**LEK**-troh-en-**SEF**-ah-low-graf) Device used to record the electrical activity of the brain.

electroencephalography (ee-**LEK**-troh-en-**SEF**-ah-**LOG**-rah-fee) The process of recording the electrical activity of the brain.

electrolyte (ee-**LEK**-troh-lite) Substance that, when dissolved in a suitable medium, forms electrically charged particles.

electromyogram (ee-**LEK**-troh-**MY**-oh-gram) Recording of electric currents associated with muscle action.

electromyography (ee-**LEK**-troh-my-**OG**-rah-fee) Recording of electrical activity in muscle.

electroneurodiagnostic (ee-**LEK**-troh-**NYUR**-oh-die-ag-**NOS**-tik) Pertaining to the use of electricity in the diagnosis of a neurologic disorder.

elimination (e-lim-ih-**NAY**-shun) Removal of waste material from the digestive tract.

emaciated (ee-**MAY**-see-**AY**-ted) Pertaining to or suffering from emaciation.

emaciation (ee-may-see-**AY**-shun) Abnormal thinness.

embolism (**EM**-boh-lizm) A plug of tissue or air from afar that obstructs a blood vessel.

embolus (**EM**-boh-lus) Detached piece of thrombus, a mass of bacteria, quantity of air, or foreign body that blocks a blood vessel.

embryo (**EM**-bree-oh) Developing organism from conception until the end of the second month.

embryology (em-bree-**OL**-oh-jee) Science of the origin and early development of an organism.

embryonic (em-bree-**ON**-ic) Pertaining to the embryo.

emesis (**EM**-eh-sis) Vomit.

emmetropia (emm-eh-**TROH**-pee-ah) Normal refractive condition of the eye.

empathy (**EM**-pah-thee) Ability to place yourself into the feelings, emotions, and reactions of another person.

emphysema (em-fih-**SEE**-mah) Dilation of respiratory bronchioles and alveoli.

empyema (**EM**-pie-**EE**-mah) Pus in a body cavity, particularly in the pleural cavity.

emulsify (ee-**MUL**-sih-fye) Break up into very small droplets to suspend in a solution (emulsion).

emulsion (ee-**MUL**-shun) The system that contains small droplets suspended in a liquid.

enamel (ee-**NAM**-el) Hard substance covering a tooth.

encephalitis (en-**SEF**-ah-**LIE**-tis) Inflammation of brain cells and tissues.

encephalocele (en-**SEF**-ah-loh-seal) Congenital defect of the cranium with herniation of brain tissue.

encephalomyelitis (en-**SEF**-ah-loh-**MY**-eh-**LIE**-tis) Inflammation of the brain and spinal cord.

encephalopathy (en-sef-ah-**LOP**-ah-thee) Any disorder of the brain.

encopresis (en-koh-**PREE**-sis) Repeated soiling with feces.

endarterectomy (**END**-ar-ter-**EK**-toh-me) Surgical removal of plaque from an artery.

endemic (en-**DEM**-ik) Pertaining to a disease always present in a community.

endocardial (en-doh-**KAR**-dee-al) Pertaining to the endocardium.

endocarditis (**EN**-doh-kar-**DIE**-tis) Inflammation of the lining of the heart.

endocardium (en-doh-**KAR**-dee-um) The inside lining of the heart.

endocrine (**EN**-doh-krin) A gland that produces an internal or hormonal substance.

endocrinologist (**EN**-doh-krih-**NOL**-oh-jist) A medical specialist in endocrinology.

endocrinology (**EN**-doh-krih-**NOL**-oh-jee) Medical specialty concerned with the production and effects of hormones.

endometrial (en-doh-**ME**-tree-al) Pertaining to the inner lining of the uterus.

endometriosis (**EN**-doh-me-tree-**OH**-sis) Endometrial tissue outside the uterus.

endometrium (en-doh-**ME**-tree-um) Inner lining of the uterus.

endoplasmic reticulum (**EN**-doh-**PLAZ**-mik reh-**TIC**-you-lum) Structure inside a cell that synthesizes steroids, detoxifies drugs, and manufactures cell membranes.

endorphin (en-**DOR**-fin) A natural substance in the brain that simulates opium.

endoscope (**EN**-doh-skope) Instrument to examine the inside of a tubular or hollow organ.

endoscopy (en-**DOS**-koh-pee) The use of an endoscope.

endotracheal (en-doh-**TRAY**-kee-al) Pertaining to being inside the trachea.

enema (**EN**-eh-mah) An injection of fluid into the rectum.

enteric (en-**TEHR**-ik) Pertaining to the intestine.

enteroscope (**EN**-ter-oh-**SKOPE**) Slender, tubular instrument with light source and camera to visualize the digestive tract.

enteroscopy (en-ter-**OSS**-koh-pee) The examination of the lining of the digestive tract.

enucleation (ee-nu-klee-**A**-shun) Removal of an entire structure without rupture.

enuresis (en-you-**REE**-sis) Bedwetting; urinary incontinence.

enzyme (**EN**-zime) Protein that induces changes in other substances.

eosinophil (ee-oh-**SIN**-oh-fill) An eosinophil's granules attract a rosy-red color on staining.

epicardial (ep-ih-**KAR**-dee-al) Pertaining to the epicardium.

epicardium (ep-ih-**KAR**-dee-um) The outer layer of the heart wall.

epicondyle (ep-ih-**KON**-dile) Projection above the condyle for attachment of a ligament or tendon.

epidemic (ep-ih-**DEM**-ik) Pertaining to an outbreak in a community of a disease or a health-related behavior.

epidermal (ep-ih-**DER**-mal) Pertaining to the epidermis.

epidermis (ep-ih-**DER**-miss) Top layer of the skin.

epididymis (ep-ih-**DID**-ih-miss) Coiled tube attached to the testis.

epididymitis (ep-ih-did-ih-**MY**-tis) Inflammation of the epididymis.

epididymoorchitis (ep-ih-**DID**-ih-moh-or-**KIE**-tis) Inflammation of the epididymis and testicle. Also called *orchitis*.

epidural (ep-ih-**DYU**-ral) Above the dura.

epidural space (ep-ih-**DYU**-ral SPASE) Space between the dura mater and the wall of the vertebral canal.

epigastric (ep-ih-**GAS**-trik) Pertaining to the abdominal region above the stomach.

epigastrium (**EP**-ih-**GAS**-tree-um) The abdominal region above the stomach.

epigenetics (**EP**-ih-jeh-**NET**-iks) The study of disorders produced by the effects of chemical compounds (e.g., pollutants) or environmental influences (such as diet) on genes.

epiglottis (ep-ih-**GLOT**-is) Leaf-shaped plate of cartilage that shuts off the larynx during swallowing.

epiglottitis (ep-ih-glot-**EYE**-tis) Inflammation of the epiglottis.

epilepsy (**EP**-ih-**LEP**-see) Chronic brain disorder due to paroxysmal excessive neuronal discharges.

epileptic (**EP**-ih-**LEP**-tik) Pertaining to or suffering from epilepsy.

epinephrine (ep-ih-**NEF**-rin) Main catecholamine produced by the adrenal medulla. Also called *adrenaline*.

epiphysial (ep-ih-**FIZ**-ee-al) Pertaining to an epiphysis. Also spelled *epiphyseal*.

epiphysial plate (ep-ih-**FIZ**-ee-al PLATE) Layer of cartilage between the epiphysis and the metaphysis where bone growth occurs. Also spelled *epiphyseal plate*.

epiphysis (eh-**PIF**-ih-sis) Expanded area at the proximal and distal ends of a long bone to provide increased surface area for attachment of ligaments and tendons.

episiotomy (eh-piz-ee-**OT**-oh-me) Surgical incision of the vulva.

epispadias (ep-ih-**SPAY**-dee-as) Condition in which the urethral opening is on the dorsum of the penis.

epistaxis (ep-ih-**STAK**-sis) Nosebleed.

epithelium (ep-ih-**THEE**-lee-um) Tissue that covers surfaces or lines cavities.

equilibrium (ee-kwi-**LIB**-ree-um) Being evenly balanced.

erectile (ee-**REK**-tile) Capable of erection or being distended with blood.

erection (ee-**REK**-shun) Distended and rigid state of an organ.

erosion (ee-**ROE**-zhun) Form a shallow ulcer in the lining of a structure.

erythroblast (eh-**RITH**-ro-blast) Precursor to a red blood cell.

erythroblastosis (eh-**RITH**-roh-blas-**TOH**-sis) Condition of many immature red cells in blood.

erythrocyte (eh-**RITH**-roh-site) A red blood cell.

erythropoiesis (eh-**RITH**-roh-poy-**EE**-sis) The formation of red blood cells.

erythropoietin (eh-**RITH**-roh-**POY**-ee-tin) Protein secreted by the kidney that stimulates red blood cell production.

eschar (**ESS**-kar) The burnt, dead tissue lying on top of third-degree burns.

Escherichia coli (esh-eh-**RIK**-ee-ah **KOH**-lie) Organism in the intestine; releases an exotoxin that can cause diarrhea.

esophageal (ee-**SOF**-ah-**JEE**-al) Pertaining to the esophagus.

esophagitis (ee-**SOF**-ah-**JI**-tis) Inflammation of the lining of the esophagus.

esophagus (ee-**SOF**-ah-gus) Tube linking the pharynx to the stomach.

esotropia (es-oh-**TROH**-pee-ah) Turning the eye inward toward the nose.

estradiol (ess-trah-**DIE**-ol) The most potent natural estrogen.

estriol (**ESS**-tree-ol) One of the three main estrogens.

estrogen (**ES**-troh-jen) Generic term for hormones that stimulate female secondary sex characteristics.

ethmoid (**ETH**-moyd) Bone that forms the back of the nose and encloses numerous air cells.

etiology (ee-tee-**OL**-oh-jee) The study of the causes of a disease.

eupnea (yoop-**NEE**-ah) Normal breathing.

eustachian tube (you-**STAY**-shun TYUB) Tube that connects the middle ear to the nasopharynx. Also called *auditory tube*.

euthyroid (you-**THIGH**-royd) Normal thyroid function.

eversion (ee-**VER**-zhun) Turning outward.

evert (ee-**VERT**) To turn outward.

evolve (ee-**VOLV**) To develop gradually.

Ewing sarcoma (**YOU**-ing sar-**KOH**-mah) A malignant neoplasm of bone.

exacerbation (ek-zas-er-**BAY**-shun) Period when there is an increase in the severity of a disease.

excision (ek-**SIZH**-un) Surgical removal of part or all of a structure.

excoriate (eks-**KOR**-ee-ate) To scratch.

excoriation (eks-**KOR**-ee-**AY**-shun) Scratch mark.

excrete (eks-**KREET**) To pass waste products of metabolism out of the body.

excretion (eks-**KREE**-shun) Removal of waste products of metabolism out of the body.

exhale (**EKS**-hail) Breathe out.

exocrine (**EK**-soh-krin) A gland that secretes substances outwardly through excretory ducts.

exophthalmos (ek-sof-**THAL**-mos) Protrusion of the eyeball.

exotropia (ek-soh-**TROH**-pee-ah) Turning the eye outward away from the nose.

expectorate (ek-**SPEK**-toh-rate) Cough up and spit out mucus from the respiratory tract.

expiration (**EKS**-pih-**RAY**-shun) Breathe out.

extension (eks-**TEN**-shun) Straighten a joint to increase its angle.

extracorporeal (**EKS**-tra-kor-**POH**-ree-al) Outside the body.

extrinsic (eks-**TRIN**-sik) Any muscle located entirely on the outside of the structure under consideration; for example, the eye.

exudate (**EKS**-you-date) Fluid that has passed out of a tissue or capillaries as a result of inflammation or injury.

F

facies (**FASH**-eez) Facial features and expressions.

fallopian tubes (fah-**LOW**-pee-an) Uterine tubes connected to the fundus of the uterus.

Fallot (fah-**LOW**) First described the tetralogy of congenital heart defects.

fascia (**FASH**-ee-ah) Sheet of fibrous connective tissue.

fasciectomy (fash-ee-**EK**-toh-me) Surgical removal of fascia.

fasciitis (fash-ee-**EYE**-tis) Inflammation of fascia.

fasciotomy (fash-ee-**OT**-oh-me) An incision through a band of fascia, usually to relieve pressure on underlying structures.

fast (FAST) The act of eating little or no food.

febrile (**FEB**-ril or **FEB**-rile) Pertaining to or suffering from fever.

fecal (**FEE**-kal) Pertaining to feces.

feces (**FEE**-seez) Undigested, waste material discharged from the bowel.

femoral (**FEM**-oh-ral) Pertaining to the femur.

femur (**FEE**-mur) The thigh bone.

fertilization (**FER**-til-eye-**ZAY**-shun) Union of a male sperm and a female egg.

fertilize (**FER**-til-ize) Penetration of the egg by sperm.

fetal (**FEE**-tal) Pertaining to the fetus.

fetalis (fee-**TAH**-lis) Erythroblastosis fetalis is a hemolytic disease of the newborn.

fetus (**FEE**-tus) Human organism from the end of the eighth week after conception to birth.

fever (**FEE**-ver) Increased body temperature that is a physiologic response to disease.

fiber (**FIE**-ber) Carbohydrate not digested by intestinal enzymes; or a strand or filament.

fibrillation (fi-brih-**LAY**-shun) Uncontrolled quivering or twitching of the heart muscle.

fibrin (**FIE**-brin) Stringy protein fiber that is a component of a blood clot.

fibrinogen (fie-**BRIN**-oh-jen) Precursor of fibrin in blood-clotting process.

fibroadenoma (**FIE**-broh-ad-en-**OH**-muh) Benign tumor containing much fibrous tissue.

fibroblast (**FIE**-broh-blast) Cell that forms collagen fibers.

fibrocystic disease (fie-broh-**SIS**-tik diz-**EEZ**) Benign breast disease with multiple tiny lumps and cysts.

fibroid (**FIE**-broyd) Uterine tumor resembling fibrous tissue.

fibromyalgia (fie-broh-my-**AL**-jee-ah) Pain in the muscle fibers.

fibromyoma (**FIE**-broh-my-**OH**-mah) Benign neoplasm derived from smooth muscle and containing fibrous tissue.

fibrosis (fie-**BROH**-sis) Repair of dead tissue cells by formation of fibrous tissue.

fibrotic (fie-**BROT**-ik) Pertaining to or affected by fibrosis.

fibula (**FIB**-you-lah) The smaller of the two bones of the lower leg.

fibular (**FIB**-you-lar) Pertaining to the fibula.

filter (**FIL**-ter) Porous substance used to separate liquids or gases from particulate matter; or to subject a substance to the action of a filter.

filtrate (**FIL**-trate) That which has passed through a filter.

filtration (fil-**TRAY**-shun) Process of passing liquid through a filter.

fimbria (**FIM**-bree-ah) A fringelike structure on the surface of a cell or microorganism. Plural *fimbriae.*

fissure (**FISH**-ur) Deep furrow or cleft. Plural *fissures.*

fistula (**FIS**-tyu-lah) Abnormal passage. Plural *fistulae* or *fistulas.*

fistulectomy (**FIS**-tyu-**LEK**-toh-mee) Surgical removal of a fistula.

fistulotomy (**FIS**-tyu-**LOT**-toh-mee) Incision of a fistula.

flank (**FLANK**) Side of the body between pelvis and ribs.

flatulence (**FLAT**-you-lence) Excessive amount of gas in the stomach and intestines.

flatus (**FLAY**-tus) Gas or air expelled through the anus.

flex (**FLEKS**) To bend a joint so that the two parts come together.

flexion (**FLEK**-shun) Bend a joint to decrease its angle.

flexor (**FLEK**-sor) Muscle or tendon that flexes a joint.

flexure (**FLEK**-shur) A bend in a structure.

flora (**FLO**-rah) Microorganisms covering the exterior and interior surfaces of a healthy animal.

fluorescein (flor-**ESS**-ee-in) Dye that produces a vivid green color under a blue light to diagnose corneal abrasions and foreign bodies.

follicle (**FOLL**-ih-kull) Spherical mass of cells containing a cavity; or a small cul-de-sac, such as a hair follicle.

follicular (fo-**LIK**-you-lar) Pertaining to a follicle.

foramen (fo-**RAY**-men) An opening through a structure. Plural *foramina.*

forceps extraction (**FOR**-seps ek-**STRAK**-shun) Assisted delivery of the baby by an instrument that grasps the head of the baby.

foreskin (**FOR**-skin) Skin that covers the glans penis.

fornix (**FOR**-niks) Arch-shaped, blind-ended part of the vagina behind and around the cervix. Plural *fornices.*

fovea centralis (**FOH**-vee-ah sen-**TRAH**-lis) Small pit in the center of the macula that has the highest visual acuity.

frenulum (**FREN**-you-lum) Fold of mucous membrane between the glans and the prepuce.

frontal (**FRON**-tal) Pertaining to the front; *or* vertical plane dividing the body into anterior and posterior portions; *or* pertaining to the frontal bone of the cranium.

frontal lobe (**FRON**-tal LOBE) Area of the brain behind the frontal bone.

function (**FUNK**-shun) The ability of an organ or tissue to perform its special work.

fundoscopic (fun-doh-**SKOP**-ik) Pertaining to fundoscopy.

fundoscopy (fun-**DOS**-koh-pee) Examination of the fundus (retina) of the eye.

fundus (**FUN**-dus) Part farthest from the opening of a hollow organ.

fungicide (**FUN**-ji-side) Agent to destroy fungi.

fungus (**FUN**-gus) General term used to describe yeasts and molds. Plural *fungi.*

G

galactorrhea (gah-**LAK**-toh-**REE**-ah) Abnormal flow of milk from the breasts.

gallbladder (**GAWL**-blad-er) Receptacle on the inferior surface of the liver for storing bile.

gallstone (**GAWL**-stone) Hard mass of cholesterol, calcium, and bilirubin that can be formed in the gallbladder and bile duct.

gamma knife (**GAM**-ah NIFE) A minimally invasive radiosurgical system.

ganglion (**GANG**-lee-on) Collection of nerve cells outside the brain and spinal cord; *or* a fluid-filled cyst. Plural *ganglia.*

gastric (**GAS**-trik) Pertaining to the stomach.

gastrin (**GAS**-trin) Hormone secreted in the stomach that stimulates secretion of HCl and increases gastric motility.

gastritis (gas-**TRY**-tis) Inflammation of the lining of the stomach.

gastrocnemius (gas-trok-**NEE**-me-us) Major muscle in back of the lower leg (the calf).

gastroenteritis (**GAS**-troh-en-ter-**I**-tis) Inflammation of the stomach and intestines.

gastroenterologist (**GAS**-troh-en-ter-**OL**-oh-jist) Medical specialist in gastroenterology.

gastroenterology (**GAS**-troh-en-ter-**OL**-oh-jee) Medical specialty of the stomach and intestines.

gastroesophageal (**GAS**-troh-ee-sof-ah-**JEE**-al) Pertaining to the stomach and esophagus.

gastrointestinal (GI) (**GAS**-troh-in-**TESS**-tin-al) Pertaining to the stomach and intestines.

gastroscope (**GAS**-troh-skope) Endoscope for examining the inside of the stomach.

gastroscopy (gas-**TROS**-koh-pee) Endoscopic examination of the stomach.

gavage (guh-**VAHZH**) To feed by a stomach tube.

gene (JEEN) Functional segment of DNA molecule.

geneticist (jeh-**NET**-ih-sist) A specialist in genetics.

genetics (jeh-**NET**-iks) Science of the inheritance of characteristics.

genital (**JEN**-ih-tal) Relating to reproduction or to the male or female sex organs.

genome (**JEE**-nome) A complete set of chromosomes.

genitalia (**JEN**-ih-**TAY**-lee-ah) External and internal organs of reproduction.

geriatrician (jai-ee-ah-**TRISH**-an) Medical specialist in the process and problems of aging.

geriatrics (jair-ee-**AT**-riks) Medical specialty that deals with the problems of aging.

gerontologist (jair-on-**TOL**-oh-jist) Medical specialist in the process and general problems of aging.

gerontology (jair-on-**TOL**-oh-jee) Study of the process and problems of aging.

gestation (jes-**TAY**-shun) From conception to birth.

gestational (jes-**TAY**-shun-al) Pertaining to gestation.

Giardia (jee-**AR**-dee-ah) Parasite in the small intestine.

gigantism (**JI**-gan-tizm) Abnormal height and size of the entire body.

gingiva (**JIN**-jih-vah) Tissue surrounding the teeth and covering the jaw.

gingival (**JIN**-jih-val) Pertaining to the gingiva.

gingivectomy (jin-jih-**VEC**-toh-me) Surgical removal of diseased gum tissue.

gingivitis (jin-jih-**VI**-tis) Inflammation of the gums.

glans (GLANZ) Head of the penis or clitoris.

glaucoma (glau-**KOH**-mah) Increased intraocular pressure.

glia (**GLEE**-ah) Connective tissue that holds a structure together.

glial (**GLEE**-al) Pertaining to glia or neuroglia.

glioma (gli-**OH**-mah) Tumor of a glial cell.

glomerulonephritis (glo-**MAIR**-you-low-nef-**RYE**-tis) Infection of the glomeruli of the kidney.

glomerulus (glo-**MAIR**-you-lus) Plexus of capillaries; part of a nephron. Plural *glomeruli.*

glossodynia (gloss-oh-**DIN**-ee-ah) Painful, burning tongue.

glossopharyngeal (**GLOSS**-oh-fah-**RIN**-jee-al) Ninth (IX) cranial nerve, supplying the tongue and pharynx.

glottis (**GLOT**-is) Vocal apparatus of the larynx.

glucagon (**GLU**-kah-gon) Pancreatic hormone that supports blood glucose levels.

glucocorticoid (glu-co-**KOR**-tih-koyd) Hormone of the adrenal cortex that helps regulate glucose metabolism.

gluconeogenesis (**GLU**-koh-nee-oh-**JEN**-eh-sis) Formation of glucose from noncarbohydrate sources.

glucose (**GLU**-kose) The final product of carbohydrate digestion and the main sugar in the blood.

gluteal (**GLU**-tee-al) Pertaining to the buttocks.

gluten (**GLU**-ten) Insoluble protein found in wheat, barley, and oats.

gluteus (**GLU**-tee-us) Refers to one of three muscles in the buttocks.

glycogen (**GLYE**-koh-jen) The body's principal carbohydrate reserve, stored in the liver and skeletal muscle.

glycogenolysis (**GLYE**-koh-jen-**OL**-ih-sis) Conversion of glycogen to glucose.

glycosuria (**GLYE**-koh-**SYU**-ree-ah) Presence of glucose in urine.

glycosylated hemoglobin (Hb A1c) (**GLYE**-koh-sih-lay-ted **HE**-moh-**GLOW**-bin) Hemoglobin A fraction linked to glucose; used as an index of glucose control.

goiter (**GOY**-ter) Enlargement of the thyroid gland.

gomphosis (gom-**FOE**-sis) Joint formed by a peg and socket. Plural *gomphoses.*

gonad (**GO**-nad) Testis or ovary. Plural *gonads.*

gonadal (go-**NAD**-al) Pertaining to the testis or ovary.

gonadotropin (**GO**-nad-oh-**TROH**-pin) Any hormone that stimulates gonad function.

gonorrhea (gon-oh-**REE**-ah) Specific contagious sexually transmitted infection

grade (GRAYD) In cancer pathology, a classification of the rate of growth of cancer cells.

graft (GRAFT) Transplantation of living tissue.

grand mal (GRAHN MAL) Old name for generalized tonic-clonic seizure.

granulation (gran-you-**LAY**-shun) New fibrous tissue formed during wound healing.

granulocyte (**GRAN**-you-loh-site) A white blood cell that contains multiple small granules in its cytoplasm.

granulosa cell (gran-you-**LOW**-sah SELL) Cell lining the ovarian follicle.

Graves disease (GRAVZ diz-**EEZ**) Hyperthyroidism with toxic goiter.

gravid (**GRAV**-id) Pregnant.

gravida (**GRAV**-ih-dah) A pregnant woman.

gray matter (GRAY **MATT**-er) Regions of the brain and spinal cord occupied by cell bodies and dendrites.

greenstick fracture (**GREEN**-stik **FRAK**-chur) A fracture in which one side of the bone is partially broken and the other side is bent. Occurs mostly in children.

groin (GROYN) Crease where the thigh joins the abdomen.

Guillain-Barré syndrome (**GEE**-yan bah-**RAY SIN**-drom) Disorder in which the body makes antibodies against myelin, disrupting nerve conduction.

gynecologic (**GUY**-nih-koh-**LOJ**-ik) Pertaining to gynecology.

gynecologist (guy-nih-**KOL**-oh-jist) Specialist in gynecology.

gynecology (guy-nih-**KOL**-oh-jee) Medical specialty of diseases of the female.

gynecomastia (**GUY**-nih-koh-**MAS**-tee-ah) Enlargement of the breast.

gyrus (**JI**-rus) Rounded elevation on the surface of the cerebral hemispheres. Plural *gyri.*

H

hairline fracture (**HAIR**-line **FRAK**-chur) A fracture without separation of the fragments.

halitosis (hal-ih-**TOH**-sis) Bad odor of the breath.

hallucination (hah-loo-sih-**NAY**-shun) Perception of an object or event when there is no such thing present.

hallux valgus (**HAL**-uks **VAL**-gus) Deviation of the big toe toward the lateral side of the foot.

hamstring (**HAM**-string) Group of three muscles on the posterior side of the thigh that join at the back of the knee.

Hashimoto disease (hah-shee-**MOH**-toh diz-**EEZ**) Autoimmune disease of the thyroid gland. Also called *Hashimoto thyroiditis.*

Haversian canals (hah-**VER**-shan ka-**NALS**) Vascular canals in bone. Also called *central canals.*

Heberden node (**HEH**-ber-den **NOHD**) Bony lump on the terminal phalanx of the fingers in osteoarthritis.

helix (**HEE**-liks) A line in the shape of a coil.

hemangioma (he-**MAN**-jee-oh-mah) Abnormal mass of proliferating blood vessels.

hematemesis (he-mah-**TEM**-eh-sis) Vomiting of red blood.

hematochezia (he-mat-oh-**KEY**-zee-ah) The passage of red, bloody stools.

hematocrit (Hct) (**HE**-mat-oh-krit) Percentage of red blood cells in the blood.

hematologist (he-mah-**TOL**-oh-jist) Specialist in hematology.

hematology (he-mah-**TOL**-oh-jee) Medical specialty of disorders of the blood.

hematoma (he-mah-**TOH**-mah) Collection of blood that has escaped from the blood vessels into surrounding tissues. Also called *bruise.*

hematuria (he-mah-**TYU**-ree-ah) Blood in the urine.

heme (**HEEM**) The iron-based component of hemoglobin that carries oxygen.

hemiparesis (**HEM**-ee-pah-**REE**-sis) Weakness of one side of the body.

hemiplegia (hem-ee-**PLEE**-jee-ah) Paralysis of one side of the body.

hemiplegic (hem-ee-**PLEE**-jik) Pertaining to or suffering from hemiplegia.

Hemoccult test (**HEEM**-o-kult **TEST**) Trade name for a fecal occult blood test.

hemodialysis (**HE**-moh-die-**AL**-ih-sis) An artificial method of filtration to remove excess waste materials and water directly from the blood.

hemodynamics (**HE**-moh-die-**NAM**-iks) The science of the flow of blood through the circulation.

hemoglobin (**HE**-moh-**GLOW**-bin) Red-pigmented protein that is the main component of red blood cells.

hemoglobinopathy (**HE**-moh-**GLOW**-bin-**OP**-ah-thee) Disease caused by the presence of an abnormal hemoglobin in the red blood cells.

hemolysis (he-**MOL**-ih-sis) Destruction of red blood cells so that hemoglobin is liberated.

hemolytic (he-moh-**LIT**-ik) Pertaining to the process of destruction of red blood cells.

hemophilia (he-moh-**FILL**-ee-ah) An inherited disease from a deficiency of clotting factor VIII.

hemoptysis (he-**MOP**-tih-sis) Bloody sputum.

hemorrhage (**HEM**-oh-raj) To bleed profusely.

hemorrhagic (**HEM**-oh-raj-ik) Pertaining to a hemorrhage.

hemorrhoid (**HEM**-oh-royd) Dilated rectal vein producing painful anal swelling. Plural *hemorrhoids.*

hemorrhoidectomy (**HEM**-oh-royd-**EK**-toh-me) Surgical removal of hemorrhoids.

hemostasis (he-moh-**STAY**-sis) Control of or stopping bleeding.

hemothorax (he-moh-**THOR**-ax) Blood in the pleural cavity.

heparin (**HEP**-ah-rin) An anticoagulant secreted particularly by liver cells.

hepatic (hep-**AT**-ik) Pertaining to the liver.

hepatitis (hep-ah-**TIE**-tis) Inflammation of the liver.

hernia (**HER**-nee-ah) Protrusion of a structure through the tissue that normally contains it.

heredity (heh-**RED**-ih-tee) Transmission of characteristics from parents to offspring through genes.

hereditary (heh-**RED**-ih-tair-ee) Transmissible from parent to offspring.

herniate (**HER**-nee-ate) To protrude.

herniation (her-nee-**AY**-shun) Protrusion of an anatomical structure from its normal location.

herniorrhaphy (**HER**-nee-**OR**-ah-fee) Repair of a hernia.

herpes simplex virus (HSV) (**HER**-peez **SIM**-pleks **VIE**-rus) Manifests with painful, watery blisters on the skin and mucous membranes.

herpes zoster (**HER**-peez **ZOS**-ter) Painful eruption of vesicles that follows a nerve root on one side of the body. Also called *shingles.*

heterograft (**HET**-er-oh-graft) A graft using tissue taken from another species. Also called *xenograft.*

hiatal (high-**AY**-tal) Pertaining to a hernia.

hiatus (high-**AY**-tus) An opening through a structure.

hilum (**HIGH**-lum) The site where the nerves and blood vessels enter and leave an organ. Plural *hila.*

histamine (**HISS**-tah-mean) Compound liberated in tissues as a result of injury or an allergic response.

histologist (his-**TOL**-oh-jist) Specialist in histology.

histology (his-**TOL**-oh-jee) Study of the structure and function of cells, tissues, and organs.

Hodgkin lymphoma (**HOJ**-kin lim-**FOH**-mah) Marked by chronic enlargement of lymph nodes spreading to other nodes in an orderly way.

holistic (ho-**LIS**-tik) Pertaining to the care of the whole person in physical, mental, emotional, and spiritual dimensions.

homeostasis (hoh-mee-oh-**STAY**-sis) Maintaining the stability of a system or the body's internal environment.

homograft (**HOH**-moh-graft) Skin graft from another person or a cadaver. Also called *allograft.*

hordeolum (hor-**DEE**-oh-lum) Abscess in an eyelash follicle. Also called *stye.*

hormonal (hor-**MOHN**-al) Pertaining to a hormone.

hormone (**HOR**-mohn) Chemical formed in one tissue or organ and carried by the blood to stimulate or inhibit a function of another tissue or organ.

Horner syndrome (**HOR**-ner **SIN**-drome) Disorder of the sympathetic nerves to the face and eye.

hospice (**HOS**-pis) Provides care to the dying and their families.

human immunodeficiency virus (HIV) (**HYU**-man **IM**-you-noh-dee-**FISH**-en-see **VIE**-rus) Etiologic agent of acquired immunodeficiency syndrome (AIDS).

human papillomavirus (HPV) (HYU-man pap-ih-**LOW**-mah **VIE**-rus) Causes warts on the skin and genitalia and can increase the risk for cervical cancer.

humerus (HYU-mer-us) Single bone of the upper arm.

humoral immunity (HYU-mor-al ihm-**YUNE**-ih-tee) Defense mechanism arising from antibodies in the blood.

Huntington disease (HUN-ting-ton diz-**EEZ**) Progressive inherited, degenerative, incurable neurologic disease. Also called *Huntington chorea.*

hyaline (**HIGH**-ah-line) Cartilage that looks like frosted glass and contains fine collagen fibers.

hyaline membrane disease (**HIGH**-ah-line **MEM**-brain diz-**EEZ**) Respiratory distress syndrome of the newborn.

hydrocele (**HIGH**-droh-seal) Collection of fluid in the space of the tunica vaginalis.

hydrocephalus (high-droh-**SEF**-ah-lus) Excess CSF in the cerebral ventricles; may cause enlarged head.

hydrochloric acid (HCl) (high-droh-**KLOR**-ik **ASS**-id) The acid of gastric juice.

hydrocortisone (high-droh-**KOR**-tih-sohn) Potent glucocorticoid with anti-inflammatory properties. Also called *cortisol.*

hydronephrosis (**HIGH**-droh-neh-**FROH**-sis) Dilation of the pelvis and calyces of a kidney.

hydronephrotic (**HIGH**-droh-neh-**FROT**-ik) Pertaining to or suffering from hydronephrosis.

hymen (**HIGH**-men) Thin membrane partly occluding the vaginal orifice.

hyperactivity (**HIGH**-per-ac-**TIV**-ih-tee) Excessive restlessness and movement.

hypercalcemia (**HIGH**-per-cal-**SEE**-me-ah) Excessive level of calcium in the blood.

hypercapnia (**HIGH**-per-**KAP**-nee-ah) Abnormal increase of carbon dioxide in the arterial bloodstream.

hyperemesis (high-per-**EM**-eh-sis) Excessive vomiting.

hyperemesis gravidarum (high-per-**EM**-eh-sis gray-vee-**DAY**-rum) Excessive nausea and vomiting during pregnancy.

hyperflexion (high-per-**FLEK**-shun) Flexion of a limb or part beyond the normal limits.

hyperglycemia (**HIGH**-per-gly-**SEE**-me-ah) High level of glucose (sugar) in blood.

hyperglycemic (**HIGH**-per-gly-**SEE**-mik) Pertaining to or having hyperglycemia.

hyperimmune globulin (**HIGH**-per-im-**YUNE GLOB**-youlin) Immunoglobulin prepared from serum of people with a high antibody titer to a specific antigen.

hyperhidrosis (**HIGH**-per-high-**DROH**-sis) Excessive production of sweat.

hyperkalemia (**HIGH**-per-kah-**LEE**-me-ah) High level of potassium in the blood.

hypernatremia (**HIGH**-per-nah-**TREE**-me-ah) High level of sodium in the blood.

hyperopia (high-per-**OH**-pee-ah) Able to see distant objects but unable to see close objects.

hyperosmolar (**HIGH**-per-os-**MOH**-lar) Marked hyperglycemia without ketoacidosis.

hyperparathyroidism (**HIGH**-per-**PAR**-ah-thigh-royd-izm) Excessive production of parathyroid hormone.

hyperplasia (**HIGH**-per-**PLAY**-zee-ah) Increase in the number of cells in a tissue or organ.

hyperpnea (high-perp-**NEE**-ah) Deeper and more rapid breathing than normal.

hyperpyrexia (**HIGH**-per-pie-**REK**-see-ah) Extremely high body temperature or fever.

hypersecretion (**HIGH**-per-seh-**KREE**-shun) Excessive secretion (of mucus or enzymes or waste products).

hypersensitivity (**HIGH**-per-sen-sih-**TIV**-ih-tee) Exaggerated abnormal reaction to an allergen.

hypersplenism (high-per-**SPLEN**-izm) Condition in which the spleen removes blood components at an excessive rate.

hypertension (**HIGH**-per-**TEN**-shun) Persistent high arterial blood pressure.

hypertensive (**HIGH**-per-**TEN**-siv) Pertaining to or suffering from high blood pressure.

hyperthyroidism (high-per-**THIGH**-royd-izm) Excessive production of thyroid hormones.

hypertrophy (high-**PER**-troh-fee) Increase in size, but not in number, of an individual tissue element.

hypochondriac (high-poh-**KON**-dree-ack) A person who exaggerates the significance of symptoms.

hypochromic (high-poh-**CROW**-mik) Pale in color, as in RBCs when hemoglobin is deficient.

hypodermic (high-poh-**DER**-mik) Pertaining to the hypodermis.

hypodermis (high-poh-**DER**-miss) Tissue layer of skin below the dermis.

hypogastric (high-poh-**GAS**-trik) Abdominal region below the stomach.

hypoglossal (high-poh-**GLOSS**-al) Twelfth (XII) cranial nerve, supplying muscles of the tongue.

hypoglycemia (**HIGH**-poh-gly-**SEE**-me-ah) Low level of glucose (sugar) in the blood.

hypoglycemic (**HIGH**-poh-gly-**SEE**-mik) Pertaining to or suffering from low blood sugar.

hypogonadism (**HIGH**-poh-**GOH**-nad-izm) Deficient gonad production of sperm or eggs or hormones.

hypokalemia (**HIGH**-poh-kah-**LEE**-me-ah) Low level of potassium in the blood.

hyponatremia (**HIGH**-poh-nah-**TREE**-me-ah) Low level of sodium in the blood.

hypoparathyroidism (**HIGH**-poh-par-ah-**THIGH**-royd-izm) Deficient production of parathyroid hormone.

hypophysis (high-**POF**-ih-sis) Another name for *pituitary gland.*

hypopituitarism (**HIGH**-poh-pih-**TYU**-ih-tah-rizm) Condition of one or more deficient pituitary hormones.

hypospadias (high-poh-**SPAY**-dee-as) Urethral opening more proximal than normal on the ventral surface of the penis.

hypotension (**HIGH**-poh-**TEN**-shun) Persistent low arterial blood pressure.

hypotensive (**HIGH**-poh-**TEN**-siv) Pertaining to or suffering from low blood pressure.

hypothalamic (high-poh-thal-**AM**-ik) Pertaining to the hypothalamus.

hypothalamus (high-poh-**THAL**-ah-muss) An area of gray matter lying below the thalamus.

hypothenar eminence (high-poh-**THAY**-nar **EM**-in-nens) The fleshy mass at the base of the little finger.

hypothermia (high-poh-**THER**-me-ah) Very low core body temperature.

hypothyroidism (high-poh-**THIGH**-royd-izm) Deficient production of thyroid hormones.

hypovolemia (**HIGH**-poh-vo-**LEE**-me-ah) Decreased blood volume in the body.

hypovolemic (**HIGH**-poh-vo-**LEE**-mik) Decreased blood volume in the body.

hypoxia (high-**POCK**-see-ah) Below-normal levels of oxygen in tissues, gases, or blood.

hypoxic (high-**POCK**-sik) Deficient in oxygen.

hysterectomy (his-ter-**EK**-toh-me) Surgical removal of the uterus.

hysterosalpingogram (**HIS**-ter-oh-sal-**PING**-oh-gram) Radiograph of the uterus and uterine tubes after injection of contrast material.

hysteroscope (**HIS**-ter-oh-skope) Endoscope to visually examine the uterine cavity.

hysteroscopy (his-ter-**OS**-koh-pee) Visual inspection of the uterine cavity using an endoscope.

I

ictal (**IK**-tal) Pertaining to, or a condition caused by, a stroke or epilepsy.

idiopathic (**ID**-ih-oh-**PATH**-ik) Pertaining to a disease of unknown etiology.

ileocecal (**ILL**-ee-oh-**SEE**-cal) Pertaining to the junction of the ileum and cecum.

ileocecal sphincter (**ILL**-ee-oh-**SEE**-cal **SFINK**-ter) A band of muscle that encircles the junction of the ileum and cecum.

ileoscopy (ill-ee-**OS**-koh-pee) Endoscopic examination of the ileum.

ileostomy (ill-ee-**OS**-toh-me) Artificial opening from the ileum to the outside of the body.

ileum (**ILL**-ee-um) Third portion of the small intestine.

ileus (**ILL**-ee-us) Dynamic or mechanical obstruction of the small intestine.

iliac (**ILL**-ee-ack) A structure related to the ilium (pelvic bone).

ilium (**ILL**-ee-um) Large wing-shaped bone at the upper and posterior part of the pelvis. Plural *ilia.*

immune (im-**YUNE**) Protected from an infectious disease.

immune serum (im-**YUNE SEER**-um) Serum taken from another human or animal that has antibodies to a disease. Also called *antiserum.*

immunity (im-**YUNE**-ih-tee) State of being protected.

immunization (**IM**-you-nih-**ZAY**-shun) Administration of an agent to provide immunity.

immunize (**IM**-you-nize) To make resistant to an infectious disease.

immunodeficiency (**IM**-you-noh-dee-**FISH**-en-see) Failure of the immune system.

immunoglobulin (**IM**-you-noh-**GLOB**-you-lin) Specific protein evoked by an antigen. All antibodies are immunoglobulins.

immunologist (im-you-**NOL**-oh-jist) Medical specialist in immunology.

immunology (im-you-**NOL**-oh-jee) The science and practice of immunity and allergy.

immunosuppression (**IM**-you-noh-suh-**PRESH**-un) Failure of the immune system caused by an outside agent.

immunotherapy (**IM**-you-noh-**THAIR**-ah-pee) Treatment to boost immune system function.

impacted (im-**PAK**-ted) Immovably wedged, as with earwax blocking the external canal.

impacted fracture (im-**PAK**-ted **FRAK**-chur) A fracture in which one bone fragment is driven into the other.

impairment (im-**PAIR**-ment) The state of being worse, weaker, or damaged.

impetigo (im-peh-**TIE**-go) Infection of the skin producing thick, yellow crusts.

implant (im-**PLANT**) To insert material into tissues; *or* the material inserted into tissues.

implantable (im-**PLAN**-tah-bul) A device that can be inserted into tissues.

implantation (im-plan-**TAY**-shun) Attachment of a fertilized egg to the endometrium.

impotence (**IM**-poh-tence) Inability to achieve an erection.

impulsive (im-**PUL**-siv) Inability to resist performing inappropriate actions.

in situ (IN **SIGH**-tyu) In the correct place.

in utero (IN **YOU**-ter-oh) Within the womb; not yet born.

in vitro fertilization (IVF) (in **VEE**-troh **FER**-til-eye-**ZAY**-shun) Process of combining sperm and egg in a laboratory dish and placing the resulting embryos inside the uterus.

inattention (**IN**-ah-**TEN**-shun) Lack of concentration and direction.

incision (in-**SIZH**-un) A cut or surgical wound.

incompatible (in-kom-**PAT**-ih-bul) Substances that interfere with each other physiologically.

incompatibility (**IN**-kom-**PAT**-ih-bil-i-tee) The quality of being incompatible.

incompetence (in-**KOM**-peh-tense) Failure of valves to close completely.

incomplete fracture (in-kom-**PLEET FRAK**-chur) A fracture that does not extend across the bone, as in a hairline fracture.

incontinence (in-**KON**-tin-ence) Inability to prevent discharge of urine or feces.

incontinent (in-**KON**-tin-ent) Denoting incontinence.

incubation (in-kyu-**BAY**-shun) Process to develp an infection.

incus (**IN**-cuss) Middle one of the three ossicles in the middle ear; shaped like an anvil.

independence (in-dee-**PEN**-dense) The state of being able to think and act for oneself.

independent (in-dee-**PEN**-dent) Pertaining to the ability to think and act for oneself.

index (**IN**-deks) A standard indicator of measurement. Plural indices.

indigestion (in-dee-**JESS**-chun) Symptoms resulting from difficulty in digesting food.

infancy (**IN**-fan-see) The first year of life.

infant (**IN**-fant) Child in the first year of life.

infantile (**IN**-fan-tile) Pertaining to an infant.

infarct (in-**FARKT**) Area of cell death resulting from blockage of its blood supply.

infarction (in-**FARKT**-shun) Sudden blockage of an artery.

infect (in-**FEKT**) To invade an organism by a microorganism.

infection (in-**FEK**-shun) Invasion of the body by disease-producing microorganisms.

infectious (in-**FEK**-shus) Capable of being transmitted to a person; *or* a disease caused by the action of a microorganism.

inferior (in-**FEER**-ee-or) Situated below.

infertility (in-fer-**TIL**-ih-tee) Failure to conceive.

infestation (in-fes-**TAY**-shun) Act of being invaded on the skin by a troublesome other species, such as a parasite.

inflammation (in-flah-**MAY**-shun) A complex of cell and chemical reactions in response to an injury or a chemical or biologic agent.

inflammatory (in-**FLAM**-ah-tor-ee) Causing or affected by inflammation.

influenza (in-flew-**EN**-zah) An acute, viral infection of upper and lower respiratory tracts.

infusion (in-**FYU**-zhun) Introduction intravenously of a substance other than blood.

ingestion (in-**JES**-chun) Intake of food, either by mouth or through a nasogastric tube.

ingredient (in-**GREE**-dee-ent) An element in a mixture.

inguinal (**ING**-gwin-ahl) Pertaining to the groin.

inhale (**IN**-hail) Breathe in.

inhibit (in-**HIB**-it-or) To curb or restrain.

inhibitor (in-**HIB**-it-or) Agent that curbs or restrains.

inotropic (**IN**-oh-**TROH**-pik) Affecting the contractility of cardiac muscle.

insanity (in-**SAN**-ih-tee) Nonmedical term for a person unable to be responsible for his or her actions.

insecticide (in-**SEK**-tih-side) Agent to destroy insects.

inseminate (in-**SEM**-ih-nate) To introduce semen into the vagina.

insemination (in-sem-ih-**NAY**-shun) The introduction of semen into the vagina.

insertion (in-**SIR**-shun) The insertion of a muscle is the attachment of a muscle to a more movable part of the skeleton, as distinct from the origin.

inspiration (in-spih-**RAY**-shun) Breathe in.

instability (in-stah-**BIL**-ih-tee) Abnormal tendency of a joint to partially or fully dislocate.

insufficiency (in-suh-**FISH**-en-see) Lack of completeness of function; for example, for a heart valve to fail to close properly.

insulin (**IN**-syu-lin) A hormone produced by the islet cells of the pancreas.

integument (in-**TEG**-you-ment) Organ system that covers the body, the skin being the main organ within the system.

integumentary (in-**TEG**-you-**MENT**-ah-ree) Pertaining to the covering of the body.

interatrial (**IN**-ter-**AY**-tree-al) Between the atria of the heart.

intercostal (**IN**-ter-**KOS**-tal) The space between two ribs.

interferon (in-ter-**FEER**-on) A small protein produced by T-cells in response to infection

interleukin (**IN**-ter-**LOO**-kin) A group of cytokines synthesized by white blood cells.

intermittent (**IN**-ter-**MIT**-ent) Alternately ceasing and beginning again.

internist (in-**TER**-nist) A physician trained in internal medicine.

interosseous (in-ter-**OSS**-ee-us) A structure between bones; for example, muscles.

interphalangeal (**IN**-ter-fah-**LAN**-jee-al) Finger or toe joint between two phalanges.

interstitial (in-ter-**STISH**-al) Pertaining to spaces between cells in a tissue or organ.

interventricular (**IN**-ter-ven-**TRIK**-you-lar) Between the ventricles of the heart.

intervertebral (**IN**-ter-**VER**-teh-bral) The space between two vertebrae.

intestinal (in-**TESS**-tin-al) Pertaining to the intestine.

intestine (in-**TESS**-tin) The digestive tube from stomach to anus.

intolerance (in-**TOL**-er-ance) Inability of the small intestine to digest and dispose of a particular dietary substance.

intracellular (in-trah-**SELL**-you-lar) Within the cell.

intracranial (in-trah-**KRAY**-nee-al) Within the cranium (skull).

intradermal (in-trah-**DER**-mal) Within the epidermis.

intramuscular (in-trah-**MUSS**-kew-lar) Within the muscle.

intraocular (in-trah-**OCK**-you-lar) Pertaining to the inside of the eye.

intrathecal (**IN**-trah-**THEE**-kal) Within the subarachnoid or subdural space.

intrauterine (**IN**-trah-**YOU**-ter-ine) Inside the uterine cavity.

intravenous (**IN**-trah-**VEE**-nus) Through a vein.

intrinsic (in-**TRIN**-sik) Any muscle located entirely within (inside) the structure under consideration; for example, muscles inside the vocal cords or the eye.

intrinsic factor (in-**TRIN**-sik **FAK**-tor) Makes the absorfption of vitamin B_{12} happen.

intubation (**IN**-tyu-**BAY**-shun) Insertion of a tube into the trachea.

intussusception (**IN**-tuss-sus-**SEP**-shun) The slipping of one part of the bowel inside another to cause obstruction.

inversion (in-**VER**-zhun) Turning inward.

invert (in-**VERT**) Turn inward.

involuntary (in-**VOL**-un-tay-ree) Not under control of the will.

involute (in-**VOH**-loot) Regressive changes in a tissue.

involution (in-voh-**LOO**-shun) Decrease in size.

iodine (**EYE**-oh-dine or **EYE**-oh-deen) Chemical element, the lack of which causes thyroid disease.

iris (**EYE**-ris) Colored portion of the eye with the pupil in its center.

irrigation (ih-rih-**GAY**-shun) Use of water to remove wax out of the external ear canal.

ischemia (is-**KEY**-me-ah) Lack of blood supply to tissue.

ischemic (is-**KEY**-mik) Pertaining to or affected by the lack of blood supply to tissue.

ischial (**IS**-key-al) Pertaining to the ischium.

ischium (**IS**-key-um) Lower and posterior part of the hip bone. Plural *ischia*.

Ishihara color system (ish-ee-**HAR**-ah) Test for color vision defects.

islet cells (**EYE**-let **SELLZ**) Hormone-secreting cells of the pancreas.

islets of Langerhans (**EYE**-lets of **LAHNG**-er-hahnz) Areas of pancreatic cells that produce insulin and glucagon. Also called *pancreatic islets*.

isotope (**EYE**-so-tope) Radioactive element used in diagnostic procedures.

isotopic (**EYE**-so-**TOP**-ick) Of identical chemical composition.

J

Jaeger reading cards (**YA**-ger) Type of different sizes for testing near vision.

jaundice (**JAWN**-dis) Yellow staining of tissues with bile pigments, including bilirubin.

jejunal (je-**JEW**-nal) Pertaining to the jejunum.

jejunum (je-**JEW**-num) Segment of small intestine between the duodenum and the ileum.

K

Kaposi sarcoma (kah-**POH**-see sar-**KOH**-mah) A skin cancer seen in AIDS patients.

keloid (**KEY**-loyd) Raised, irregular, lumpy scar due to excess collagen fiber production during healing of a wound.

karyotype (**KAIR**-ee-oh-type) Map of chromosomes of an individual cell.

Kegel exercises (**KEE**-gal **EKS**-er-size-ez) Contraction and relaxation of the pelvic floor muscles to improve urethral and rectal sphincter function

keloid (**KEY**-loyd) Raised, irregular, lumpy scar due to excess collagen fiber production during healing of a wound.

keratin (**KAIR**-ah-tin) Protein found in the skin, nails, and hair.

keratoconjunctivitis (**KAIR**-ah-toh-con-**JUNGK**-tih-**VI**-tis) Inflammation of the cornea and conjunctiva.

keratomileusis (**KAIR**-ah-toh-my-**LOO**-sis) Cuts and shapes the cornea.

keratotomy (**KAIR**-ah-**TOT**-oh-mee) Incision in the cornea.

kernicterus (kair-**NICK**-ter-us) Bilirubin staining of the basal nuclei of the brain.

ketoacidosis (**KEY**-toh-ass-ih-**DOE**-sis) Excessive production of ketones, making the blood acid.

ketone (**KEY**-tone) Chemical formed in uncontrolled diabetes or in starvation.

ketosis (key-**TOH**-sis) Excess production of ketones.

kidney (**KID**-nee) Organ of excretion.

kyphosis (kie-**FOH**-sis) A normal posterior curve of the thoracic spine that can be exaggerated in disease.

kyphotic (kie-**FOT**-ik) Pertaining to or suffering from kyphosis.

L

labium (**LAY**-bee-um) Fold of the vulva. Plural *labia.*

labor (**LAY**-bore) Process of expulsion of the fetus.

labrum (**LAY**-brum) Cartilage that forms a rim around the socket of the hip joint.

labyrinth (**LAB**-ih-rinth) The inner ear.

labyrinthitis (**LAB**-ih-rin-**THI**-tis) Inflammation of the inner ear.

laceration (lass-eh-**RAY**-shun) A tear of the skin.

lacrimal (**LAK**-rim-al) Pertaining to tears; *or* bone that forms the medial wall of the orbit.

lactase (**LAK**-tase) Enzyme that breaks down lactose (milk sugar) to glucose and galactose.

lactate (**LAK**-tate) To produce milk.

lactation (lak-**TAY**-shun) Production of milk.

lacteal (**LAK**-tee-al) A lymphatic vessel carrying chyle away from the intestine.

lactiferous (lak-**TIF**-er-us) Pertaining to or yielding milk.

lactose (**LAK**-tohs) The disaccharide found in cow's milk.

lanugo (la-**NYU**-go) Fine, soft hair on the fetal body.

laparoscope (**LAP**-ah-roh-skope) Instrument (endoscope) used for viewing the abdominal contents.

laparoscopic (**LAP**-ah-roh-**SKOP**-ik) Pertaining to laparoscopy.

laparoscopy (lap-ah-**ROS**-koh-pee) Examination of the contents of the abdomen using an endoscope.

laryngeal (lah-**RIN**-jee-al) Pertaining to the larynx.

laryngitis (lah-rin-**JEYE**-tis) Inflammation of the larynx.

laryngopharynx (lah-**RIN**-go-**FAH**-rinks) Region of the pharynx below the epiglottis that includes the larynx.

laryngoscope (lah-**RING**-oh-skope) Hollow tube with a light and camera used to visualize or operate on the larynx.

laryngotracheobronchitis (lah-**RING**-oh-**TRAY**-kee-oh-brong-**KIE**-tis) Inflammation of the larynx, trachea, and bronchi. Also called *croup.*

larynx (**LAH**-rinks) Organ of voice production.

laser surgery (**LAY**-zer **SUR**-jer-ee) Use of a concentrated, intense narrow beam of electromagnetic radiation for surgery.

lateral (**LAT**-er-al) Situated at the side of a structure.

latissimus dorsi (lah-**TISS**-ih-muss **DOOR**-sigh) The widest (broadest) muscle in the back.

leiomyoma (**LIE**-oh-my-**OH**-mah) Benign tumor derived from smooth muscle.

lens (**LENZ**) Transparent refractive structure behind the iris.

lentigo (len-**TIE**-go) Age spot; small, flat, brown-black spot in the skin of older people. Plural *lentigines.*

leptin (**LEP**-tin) Hormone secreted by adipose tissue.

lesion (**LEE**-zhun) Pathologic change or injury in a tissue.

lethargy (**LETH**-ar-jee) Abnormal drowsiness in depth, length, or time. Adj *lethargic.*

leukemia (loo-**KEE**-mee-ah) Disease when the blood is taken over by white blood cells and their precursors.

leukemic (loo-**KEE**-mik) Pertaining to or affected by leukemia.

leukocyte (**LOO**-koh-site) Another term for a white blood cell. Alternative spelling *leucocyte.*

leukocytosis (**LOO**-koh-sigh-**TOH**-sis) An excessive number of white blood cells.

leukopenia (loo-koh-**PEE**-nee-ah) A deficient number of white blood cells.

libido (lih-**BEE**-doh) Sexual desire.

life expectancy (LIFE eck-**SPEK**-tan-see) Statistical determination of the number of years an individual is expected to live.

life span (LIFE SPAN) The age that a person reaches.

ligament (**LIG**-ah-ment) Band of fibrous tissue connecting two structures.

ligature (**LIG**-ah-chur) Thread or wire tied around a tubal structure to close it.

ligate (**LIE**-gate) Tie off a structure, such as a bleeding blood vessel.

ligation (lie-**GAY**-shun) Use of a tie to close a tube.

limbic (**LIM**-bic) Array of nerve fibers surrounding the thalamus.

linear fracture (**LIN**-ee-ar **FRAK**-chur) A fracture running parallel to the length of the bone.

lipase (**LIE**-paze) Enzyme that breaks down fat.

lipectomy (lip-**ECK**-toh-me) Surgical removal of adipose tissue.

lipid (**LIP**-id) General term for all types of fatty compounds; for example, cholesterol, triglycerides, and fatty acids.

lipoprotein (**LIP**-oh-pro-teen) Bonding of molecules of fat and protein.

liposuction (**LIP**-oh-suck-shun) Surgical removal of adipose tissue using suction.

lithotripsy (**LITH**-oh-trip-see) Crushing stones by sound waves.

lithotripter (**LITH**-oh-trip-ter) Machine that generates sound waves for lithotripsy.

liver (**LIV**-er) Body's largest organ, located in the right upper quadrant of the abdomen.

lobar (**LOW**-bar) Pertaining to a lobe.

lobe (**LOBE**) Subdivision of an organ or other part.

lobectomy (low-**BECK**-toh-me) Surgical removal of a lobe.

lochia (**LOW**-kee-uh) Vaginal discharge following childbirth.

longevity (lon-**JEV**-ih-tee) Duration of life beyond the normal expectation.

Loop of Henle (**LOOP** of **HEN**-lee) Part of the renal tubule where reabsorption occurs.

lordosis (lore-**DOH**-sis) A normal forward curvature of the lumbar spine that can be exaggerated in disease.

lordotic (lore-**DOT**-ik) Pertaining to or suffering from lordosis.

louse (**LOWSE**) Parasitic insect. Plural *lice.*

lumbar (**LUM**-bar) Region in the back and sides between the ribs and pelvis.

lumen (**LOO**-men) The interior space of a tubelike structure.

lumpectomy (lump-**ECK**-toh-me) Removal of a lesion with preservation of surrounding tissue.

luteal (**LOO**-tee-al) Pertaining to a corpus luteum.

lutein (**LOO**-tee-in) Yellow pigment.

luteum (**LOO**-tee-um) Corpus luteum is the yellow (lutein) body formed after an ovarian follicle ruptures.

lymph (**LIMF**) A clear fluid collected from body tissues and transported by lymph vessels to the venous circulation.

lymphadenectomy (lim-**FAD**-eh-**NECK**-toh-me) Surgical excision of a lymph node(s).

lymphadenitis (lim-**FAD**-eh-neye-tis) Inflammation of a lymph node(s).

lymphadenopathy (lim-**FAD**-eh-**NOP**-ah-thee) Any disease process affecting a lymph node.

lymphangiogram (lim-**FAN**-jee-oh-gram) Radiographic images of lymph vessels and nodes following injection of contrast material.

lymphatic (lim-**FAT**-ic) Pertaining to lymph or the lymphatic system.

lymphedema (**LIMF**-eh-**DEE**-mah) Tissue swelling due to lymphatic obstruction.

lymphocyte (**LIM**-foh-site) Small white blood cell with a large nucleus.

lymphoid (**LIM**-foyd) Resembling lymphatic tissue.

lymphoma (lim-**FOH**-mah) Any neoplasm of lymphatic tissue.

M

macrocyte (**MACK**-roh-site) Large red blood cell.

macrocytic (mack-roh-**SIT**-ik) Pertaining to a macrocyte.

macrophage (**MACK**-roh-fayj) Large white blood cell that removes bacteria, foreign particles, and dead cells.

macula lutea (**MACK**-you-lah **LOO**-tee-ah) Yellowish spot on the back of the retina; contains the fovea centralis.

macule (**MACK**-yul) Small, flat spot or patch on the skin.

majus (**MAY**-jus) Bigger or greater; for example, labium majus. Plural *majora.*

malabsorption (mal-ab-**SORP**-shun) Inadequate gastrointestinal absorption of nutrients.

malformation (**MAL**-for-**MAY**-shun) Failure of proper or normal development.

malfunction (mal-**FUNK**-shun) Inadequate or abnormal function.

malignancy (mah-**LIG**-nan-see) State of being malignant.

malignant (mah-**LIG**-nant) Tumor that invades surrounding tissues and metastasizes to distant organs.

malleus (**MAL**-ee-us) Outer (lateral) one of the three ossicles in the middle ear; shaped like a hammer.

malnutrition (mal-nyu-**TRISH**-un) Inadequate nutrition from poor diet or inadequate absorption of nutrients.

malunion (mal-**YOU**-nee-un) The two bony ends of a fracture fail to heal together in the correct position.

mammary (**MAM**-ah-ree) Relating to the lactating breast.

mammogram (**MAM**-oh-gram) The record produced by X-ray imaging of the breast.

mammography (mah-**MOG**-rah-fee) The process of X-ray examination of the breast.

mammoplasty (**MAM**-oh-plas-tee) Surgical reshaping of the breast.

mandible (**MAN**-di-bel) Lower jawbone.

mandibular (man-**DIB**-you-lar) Pertaining to the mandible.

mania (**MAY**-nee-ah) Mood disorder with hyperactivity, irritability, and rapid speech.

manic (**MAN**-ik) Pertaining to or suffering from mania.

manic-depressive disorder (**MAN**-ik dee-**PRESS**-iv dis-**OR**-der) An outdated name for bipolar disorder.

marrow (**MAH**-roe) Fatty, blood-forming tissue in the cavities of long bones.

mastalgia (mass-**TAL**-jee-uh) Pain in the breast.

mastectomy (mass-**TECK**-toh-me) Surgical excision of the breast.

masticate (**MASS**-tih-kate) To chew.

mastication (mass-tih-**KAY**-shun) The process of chewing.

mastitis (mass-**TIE**-tis) Inflammation of the breast.

mastoid (**MASS**-toyd) Small bony protrusion immediately behind the ear.

maternal (mah-**TER**-nal) Pertaining to or derived from the mother.

matrix (**MAY**-triks) Substance that surrounds and protects cells, is manufactured by the cells, and holds them together.

maturation (mat-you-**RAY**-shun) Process to achieve full development.

mature (mah-**TYUR**) Fully developed.

maxilla (mak-**SILL**-ah) Upper jawbone, containing right and left maxillary sinuses.

maxillary (**MAK**-sih-lair-ee) Pertaining to the maxilla.

maximus (**MAKS**-ih-mus) The gluteus maximus muscle is the largest muscle in the body, covering a large part of each buttock.

meatal (me-**AY**-tal) Pertaining to a meatus.

meatus (me-**AY**-tus) The external opening of a passage.

meconium (meh-**KOH**-nee-um) The first bowel movement of the newborn.

medial (**ME**-dee-al) Nearer to the middle of the body.

mediastinal (**ME**-dee-ass-**TIE**-nal) Pertaining to the mediastinum.

mediastinoscopy (**ME**-dee-ass-tih-**NOS**-koh-pee) Examination of the mediastinum using an endoscope.

mediastinum (**ME**-dee-ass-**TIE**-num) Area between the lungs containing the heart, aorta, venae cavae, esophagus, and trachea.

medius (**ME**-dee-us) The gluteus medius muscle is partly covered by the gluteus maximus.

medulla (meh-**DULL**-ah) Central portion of a structure surrounded by cortex.

medulla oblongata (meh-**DULL**-ah ob-lon-**GAH**-tah) Most posterior subdivision of the brainstem; continuation of the spinal cord.

medullary (**MED**-ul-ah-ree) Pertaining to a medulla.

meiosis (my-**OH**-sis) Two rapid cell divisions, resulting in half the number of chromosomes.

melanin (**MEL**-ah-nin) Black pigment found in the skin, hair, and retina.

melanoma (mel-ah-**NO**-mah) Malignant neoplasm formed from cells that produce melanin.

melatonin (mel-ah-**TONE**-in) Hormone formed by the pineal gland.

melena (meh-**LEE**-nah) The passage of black, tarry stools.

membrane (**MEM**-brain) Thin layer of tissue covering a structure or cavity.

membranous (**MEM**-brah-nus) Pertaining to a membrane.

menarche (meh-**NAR**-key) First menstrual period.

Ménière disease (men-**YEAR** diz-**EEZ**) Disorder of the inner ear with acute attacks of tinnitus, vertigo, and hearing loss.

meninges (meh-**NIN**-jeez) Three-layered covering of the brain and spinal cord.

meningitis (men-in-**JIE**-tis) Inflammation of the meninges.

meningocele (meh-**NIN**-goh-seal) Protrusion of the meninges from the spinal cord or brain through a defect in the vertebral column or cranium.

meningococcal (meh-**NING**-goh-**KOK**-al) Pertaining to the *meningococcus* bacterium.

meningomyelocele (meh-nin-goh-**MY**-el-oh-seal) Protrusion of the spinal cord and meninges through a defect in the vertebral arch of one or more vertebrae.

meniscectomy (**MEN**-ih-**SEK**-toh-me) Excision (cutting out) of all or part of a meniscus.

meniscus (meh-**NISS**-kuss) Disc of cartilage between the bones of a joint; for example, in the knee joint. Plural *menisci.*

menopausal (**MEN**-oh-pawz-al) Pertaining to the menopause.

menopause (**MEN**-oh-pawz) Permanent ending of menstrual periods.

menorrhagia (men-oh-**RAY**-jee-ah) Excessive menstrual bleeding.

menses (**MEN**-seez) Monthly uterine bleeding.

menstrual (**MEN**-stru-al) Pertaining to menstruation.

menstruate (**MEN**-stru-ate) The act of menstruation.

menstruation (men-stru-**AY**-shun) Synonym of *menses.*

mesentery (**MESS**-en-ter-ree) A double layer of peritoneum enclosing the abdominal viscera.

mesothelioma (**MEZ**-oh-thee-lee-**OH**-mah) Cancer arising from the cells lining the pleura or peritoneum.

metabolic (met-ah-**BOL**-ik) Pertaining to metabolism.

metabolic acidosis (met-ah-**BOL**-ik ass-ih-**DOE**-sis) Decreased pH in the blood and body tissues as a result of an upset in metabolism.

metabolism (meh-**TAB**-oh-lizm) The constantly changing physical and chemical processes occurring in the cell that are the sum of anabolism and catabolism.

metacarpal (**MET**-ah-**KAR**-pal) The five bones between the carpus and the fingers.

metacarpophalangeal (**MET**-ah-**KAR**-poh-fah-**LAN**-jee-al) The articulations (joints) between the metacarpal bones and the phalanges.

metastasis (meh-**TAS**-tah-sis) Spread of a disease from one part of the body to another. Plural *metastases.*

metastasize (meh-**TAS**-tah-size) To spread to distant parts.

metastatic (meh-tah-**STAT**-ik) Pertaining to the character of cells that can metastasize.

metatarsal (**MET**-ah-**TAR**-sal) Pertaining to the metatarsus.

metatarsus (**MET**-ah-**TAR**-sus) The five parallel bones of the foot between the tarsus and the phalanges.

metrorrhagia (**MEE**-troh-**RAY**-jee-ah) Irregular uterine bleeding between menses.

microbe (**MY**-krohb) Short for *microorganism.*

microcephalic (**MY**-kroh-seh-**FAL**-ik) Pertaining to or suffering from a small head.

microcephaly (**MY**-kroh-**SEF**-ah-lee) An abnormally small head.

microcyte (**MY**-kroh-site) Small red blood cell.

microcytic (my-kroh-**SIT**-ik) Pertaining to a small cell.

microorganism (**MY**-kroh-**OR**-gan-izm) Any organism too small to be seen by the naked eye.

microscope (**MY**-kroh-skope) Instrument for viewing something small that cannot be seen in detail by the naked eye.

microscopic (**MY**-kroh-**SKOP**-ik) Visible only with the aid of a microscope.

microscopy (my-**CROSS**-koh-pee) Investigation of minute objects through a microscope.

microvascular decompression (**MY**-kroh-vas-kyu-lar **DEE**-kom-**PRESH**-un) Endoscopic procedure that places a sponge between the offending blood vessel and the affected nerve.

micturate (**MIK**-choo-rate) Pass urine.

micturition (mik-choo-**RISH**-un) Act of passing urine.

migraine (**MY**-grain) Paroxysmal severe headache confined to one side of the head.

mineral (**MIN**-er-al) Inorganic compound usually found in the earth's crust.

mineralocorticoid (**MIN**-er-al-oh-**KOR**-tih-koyd) Hormone of the adrenal cortex that influences sodium and potassium metabolism.

minimus (**MIN**-ih-mus) The gluteus minimus is the smallest of the gluteal muscles and lies under the gluteus medius.

minus (**MY**-nus) Smaller or lesser; for example, labium minus. Plural *minora.*

miosis (my-**OH**-sis) Constriction of the pupil.

mitochondrion (my-toh-**KON**-dree-on) Organelle that generates, stores, and releases energy for cell activities. Plural *mitochondria.*

mitosis (my-**TOH**-sis) Cell division that creates two identical cells, each with 46 chromosomes.

mitral (**MY**-tral) Shaped like the headdress of a Catholic bishop.

modify (**MOD**-ih-fie) Change the form or qualities of something.

molar (**MO**-lar) One of six teeth in each jaw that grind food.

mole (MOLE) Benign localized area of melanin-producing cells.

molecule (**MOLL**-eh-kyul) Very small particle.

molluscum contagiosum (moh-**LUS**-kum kon-**TAY**-jee-**OH**-sum) STD caused by a virus.

monoclonal (**MON**-oh-**KLOH**-nal) Derived from a protein from a single clone of cells, all molecules of which are the same.

monocyte (**MON**-oh-site) Large white blood cell with a single nucleus.

mononeuropathy (**MON**-oh-nyu-**ROP**-ah-thee) Disorder affecting a single nerve.

mononucleosis (**MON**-oh-nyu-klee-**OH**-sis) Presence of large numbers of specific, diagnostic mononuclear leukocytes.

monoplegia (**MON**-oh-**PLEE**-jee-ah) Paralysis of one limb.

monoplegic (**MON**-oh-**PLEE**-jik) Pertaining to or suffering from monoplegia.

mons pubis (**MONZ PYU**-bis) Fleshy pad with pubic hair, overlying the pubic bone.

morbidity (mor-**BID**-ih-tee) The frequency of the appearance of a disease.

morphine (**MOR**-feen) Derivative of opium used as an analgesic or sedative.

mortality (mor-**TAL**-ih-tee) Death rate.

motile (**MOH**-til) Capable of spontaneous movement.

motility (moh-**TILL**-ih-tee) The ability for spontaneous movement.

motor (**MOH**-tor) Structures of the nervous system that send impulses out to cause muscles to contract or glands to secrete.

mouth (MOWTH) External opening of a cavity or canal.

mucin (**MYU**-sin) Protein element of mucus.

mucocutaneous (**MYU**-koh-kyu-**TAY**-nee-us) Junction of skin and mucous membrane; for example, the lips.

mucolytic (**MYU**-koh-**LIT**-ik) Agent capable of dissolving or liquefying mucus.

mucosa (myu-**KOH**-sah) Lining of a tubular structure that secretes mucus. Another name for *mucous membrane.*

mucous (**MYU**-kus) Pertaining to mucus or the mucosa.

mucus (**MYU**-kus) Sticky secretion of cells in mucous membranes.

multipara (mul-**TIP**-ah-ruh) Woman who has given birth to two or more children.

murmur (**MUR**-mur) Abnormal heart sound heard with a stethoscope when a valve closes or opens abnormally.

muscle (**MUSS**-el) A tissue consisting of contractile cells.

muscular (**MUSS**-kyu-lar) Pertaining to muscle or muscles.

musculoskeletal (**MUSS**-kyu-loh-**SKEL**-eh-tal) Pertaining to the muscles and the bony skeleton.

mutation (myu-**TAY**-shun) Change in the chemistry of a gene.

mute (MYUT) Unable or unwilling to speak.

mutism (**MYU**-tizm) Absence of speech.

myasthenia gravis (my-as-**THEE**-nee-ah **GRA**-vis) Disorder of fluctuating muscle weakness.

mydriasis (mih-**DRY**-ah-sis) Dilation of the pupil.

myelin (**MY**-eh-lin) Material of the sheath around the axon of a nerve.

myelitis (**MY**-eh-**LIE**-tis) Inflammation of the spinal cord.

myelocele (**MY**-eh-low-seal) Protrusion of the spinal cord through a defect in the vertebral arch.

myelomeningocele (**MY**-eh-low-meh-**NING**-oh-seal) Protrusion of the spinal cord and meninges through a defect in the vertebral arch of one or more vertebrae.

myocardial (my-oh-**KAR**-dee-al) Pertaining to heart muscle.

myocarditis (**MY**-oh-kar-**DIE**-tis) Inflammation of the heart muscle.

myocardium (my-oh-**KAR**-dee-um) All the heart muscle.

myoma (my-**OH**-mah) Benign tumor of muscle.

myomectomy (my-oh-**MEK**-toh-me) Surgical removal of a myoma (fibroid).

myometrium (my-oh-**MEE**-tree-um) Muscle wall of the uterus.

myopathy (my-**OP**-ah-thee) Any disease of muscle.

myopia (my-**OH**-pee-ah) Able to see close objects but unable to see distant objects.

myositis (my-oh-**SIGH**-tis) Inflammation of muscle tissue.

myringotomy (mir-in-**GOT**-oh-me) Incision in the tympanic membrane.

myxedema (miks-eh-**DEE**-muh) Nonpitting, waxy edema of the skin in hypothyroidism.

N

narcissism (**NAR**-sih-sizm) A state of relating everything to oneself.

narcissistic (**NAR**-sih-**SIS**-tik) Relating everything to oneself.

narcolepsy (**NAR**-koh-lep-see) Involuntary falling asleep.

narcotic (nar-**KOT**-ik) Drug derived from opium or any drug with effects similar to those of opium derivatives.

naris (**NAH**-ris) Nostril. Plural *nares.*

nasal (**NAY**-zal) Pertaining to the nose.

nasogastric (**NAY**-zoh-**GAS**-trik) Pertaining to the nose and stomach.

nasolacrimal duct (**NAY**-zoh-**LAK**-rim-al DUKT) Passage from the lacrimal sac to the nose.

nasopharyngeal (**NAY**-zoh-fah-**RIN**-jee-al) Pertaining to the nasopharynx.

nasopharynx (**NAY**-zoh-**FAH**-rinks) Region of the pharynx at the back of the nose and above the soft palate.

natal (**NAY**-tal) Pertaining to birth.

nebulizer (**NEB**-you-liz-er) Device used to deliver liquid medicine in a fine mist.

necrosis (neh-**KROH**-sis) Pathologic death of cells or tissue.

necrotic (neh-**KROT**-ik) Pertaining to or affected by necrosis.

necrotizing fasciitis (neh-kroh-**TIZE**-ing fash-ee-**EYE**-tis) Inflammation of fascia producing death of the tissue.

neonatal (**NEE**-oh-**NAY**-tal) Pertaining to the newborn infant or the newborn period.

neonate (**NEE**-oh-nate) A newborn infant.

neonatologist (**NEE**-oh-nay-**TOL**-oh-jist) Medical specialist in disorders of the newborn.

neoplastic (**NEE**-oh-**PLAS**-tic) Pertaining to a neoplasm.

neoplasia (**NEE**-oh-**PLAY**-zee-ah) Process that results in formation of a tumor.

nephrectomy (nef-**REK**-toh-me) Surgical removal of a kidney.

nephritis (nef-**RY**-tis) Inflammation of the kidney.

nephroblastoma (**NEF**-roh-blas-**TOH**-mah) Cancerous kidney tumor of childhood. Also known as *Wilms tumor.*

nephrolithiasis (**NEF**-roe-lih-**THIGH**-ah-sis) Presence of a kidney stone.

nephrolithotomy (**NEF**-roe-lih-**THOT**-oh-me) Incision for removal of a kidney stone.

nephrologist (nef-**ROL**-oh-jist) Medical specialist in disorders of the kidney.

nephrology (nef-**ROL**-oh-jee) Medical specialty of diseases of the kidney.

nephron (**NEF**-ron) Filtration unit of the kidney; glomerulus + renal tubule.

nephropathy (nef-**ROP**-ah-thee) Any disease of the kidney.

nephroscope (**NEF**-roe-skope) Endoscope to view the inside of the kidney.

nephroscopy (nef-**ROS**-koh-pee) To examine the kidney.

nephrosis (nef-**ROH**-sis) Same as *nephrotic syndrome.*

nephrotic syndrome (nef-**ROT**-ik **SIN**-drome) Glomerular disease with marked loss of protein. Also called *nephrosis.*

nerve (NERV) A cord of nerve fibers bound together by connective tissue.

nerve conduction study (NERV kon-**DUK**-shun **STUD**-ee) Procedure for measuring the speed at which an electrical impulse travels along a nerve.

nervous (**NER**-vus) Pertaining to a nerve or the nervous system; *or* easily excited or agitated.

nervous system (**NER**-vus **SIS**-tem) The whole, integrated nerve apparatus.

neural (**NYU**-ral) Pertaining to nervous tissue.

neural tube (**NYU**-ral **TYUB**) Embryologic tubelike structure that forms the brain and spinal cord.

neuralgia (nyu-**RAL**-jee-ah) Pain in the distribution of a nerve.

neuroglia (nyu-**ROG**-lee-ah) Connective tissue holding nervous tissue together.

neurohypophysis (**NYU**-roh-high-**POF**-ih-sis) Posterior lobe of the pituitary gland.

neurologic (**NYU**-roh-**LOJ**-ik) Pertaining to the nervous sytem.

neurologist (nyu-**ROL**-oh-jist) Medical specialist in disorders of the nervous system.

neurology (nyu-**ROL**-oh-jee) Medical specialty of disorders of the nervous system.

neuroma (nyu-**ROH**-mah) Any tumor arising from cells in the nervous system.

neuromuscular (**NYU**-roh-**MUSS**-kyu-lar) A junction where a nerve supplies muscle tissue.

neuron (**NYU**-ron) Technical term for a nerve cell; consists of the cell body with its dendrites and axons.

neuropathy (nyu-**ROP**-ah-thee) Any disorder affecting the nervous system.

neurosurgeon (**NYU**-roh-**SUR**-jun) One who operates on the nervous system.

neurosurgery (**NYU**-roh-**SUR**-jer-ee) Operating on the nervous system.

neurotoxin (**NYU**-roh-tock-sin) Agent that poisons the nervous system.

neurotransmitter (**NYU**-roh-trans-**MIT**-er) Chemical agent that relays messages from one nerve cell to the next.

neutropenia (**NEW**-troh-**PEE**-nee-ah) A deficiency of neutrophils.

neutrophil (**NEW**-troh-fill) A neutrophil's granules take up (purple) stain equally, whether the stain is acid or alkaline.

neutrophilia (**NEW**-troh-**FILL**-ee-ah) An increase in neutrophils.

nevus (**NEE**-vus) Congenital lesion of the skin. Plural *nevi.*

nipple (**NIP**-el) Projection from the breast into which the lactiferous ducts open.

nitrite (**NI**-trite) Chemical formed in urine by *E. coli* and other microorganisms, indicative of UTI.

nitrogenous (ni-**TRO**-jen-us) Containing or generating nitrogen.

nocturia (nok-**TYU**-ree-ah) Excessive urination at night.

node (NOHD) A circumscribed mass of tissue.

nodule (**NOD**-yule) Small node or knotlike swelling.

nonproductive cough (**NON**-proh-**DUC**-tiv KAWF) Cough that is dry, and does not result in matter brought up from the lungs.

nonself (**NON**-self) In immunology, pertaining to foreign antigens.

normal flora (**NOR**-mal **FLOR**-uh) Microorganisms covering the exterior and interior surfaces of a healthy animal and under normal circumstances do not cause disease.

norepinephrine (**NOR**-ep-ih-**NEFF**-rin) Catecholamine hormone of the adrenal gland that is a parasympathetic neurotransmitter. Also called *noradrenaline.*

nosocomial (noh-soh-**KOH**-mee-al) Acquired while in the hospital.

nuchal cord (**NYU**-kul KORD) Loop(s) of umbilical cord around the fetal neck.

nuclear (**NYU**-klee-ar) Pertaining to a nucleus.

nucleolus (nyu-**KLEE**-oh-lus) Small mass within the nucleus.

nucleus (**NYU**-klee-us) Functional center of a cell or structure.

nutrient (**NYU**-tree-ent) A substance in food required for normal physiologic function.

nutrition (nyu-**TRISH**-un) The study of food and liquid requirements for normal function of the human body.

nystagmus (nis-**TAG**-mus) Fast uncontrollable movements of the eye in any direction.

O

obesity (oh-**BEE**-sih-tee) Excessive amount of fat in the body.

oblique fracture (ob-**LEEK FRAK**-chur) A diagonal fracture across the long axis of the bone.

obsession (ob-**SESH**-un) Persistent, recurrent, uncontrollable thoughts or impulses.

obsessive (ob-**SES**-iv) Possessing persistent, recurrent, uncontrollable thoughts or impulses.

obstetrician (ob-steh-**TRISH**-un) Medical specialist in obstetrics.

obstetrics (OB) (ob-**STET**-ricks) Medical specialty for the care of women during pregnancy and the postpartum period.

occipital (ock-**SIP**-it-al) The back of the skull.

occipital lobe (ock-**SIP**-it-al LOBE) Posterior area of the cerebral hemispheres.

occlude (oh-**KLUDE**) To close, plug, or completely obstruct.

occlusion (oh-**KLU**-zhun) A complete obstruction.

occult (oh-**KULT**) Not visible on the surface, hidden.

occult blood (oh-**KULT** BLUD) Blood that cannot be seen in the stool but is positive on a fecal occult blood test.

occupational (OCK-you-**PAY**-shun-al) A disorder resulting from exposure to an agent during performance of one's work.

ocular (OCK-you-lar) Pertaining to the eye.

olecranon (oh-**LECK**-rah-non) Prominent, proximal extremity of the ulna.

olfaction (ol-**FAK**-shun) Sense of smell.

olfactory (ol-**FAK**-toh-ree) Related to the sense of smell.

oligohydramnios (OL-ih-goh-high-**DRAM**-nee-os) Too little amniotic fluid.

oligospermia (OL-ih-go-**SPER**-me-ah) Too few sperm in the semen.

oliguria (ol-ih-**GYUR**-ee-ah) Scanty production of urine.

omentum (oh-**MEN**-tum) Membrane that encloses the bowels.

onychomycosis (oh-nih-koh-my-**KOH**-sis) Condition of a fungus infection in a nail.

oocyte (**OH**-oh-site) Female egg cell.

oogenesis (oh-oh-**JEN**-eh-sis) Development of a female egg cell.

open fracture (**OH**-pen **FRAK**-chur) The skin over the fracture is broken.

ophthalmia neonatorum (off-**THAL**-me-ah ne-oh-nay-**TOR**-um) Conjunctivitis of the newborn.

ophthalmic (off-**THAL**-mik) Pertaining to the eye.

ophthalmologist (off-thal-**MALL**-oh-jist) Medical specialist in ophthalmology.

ophthalmology (off-thal-**MALL**-oh-jee) Diagnosis and treatment of diseases of the eye.

ophthalmoscope (off-**THAL**-moh-skope) Instrument for viewing the retina.

ophthalmoscopic (**OFF**-thal-moh-**SKOP**-ik) Pertaining to the use of an ophthalmoscope.

ophthalmoscopy (**OFF**-thal-**MOS**-koh-pee) The process of viewing the retina.

opiate (**OH**-pee-ate) A drug derived from opium.

opportunistic (**OP**-or-tyu-**NIS**-tik) An organism or a disease in a host with lowered resistance.

opportunistic infection (**OP**-or-tyu-**NIS**-tik in-**FEK**-shun) An infection that causes disease when the immune system is compromised for other reasons.

optic (**OP**-tik) The eye or vision; *or* second (II) cranial nerve, which carries visual information.

optical (**OP**-tih-kal) Pertaining to the eye or vision.

optometrist (op-**TOM**-eh-trist) Someone skilled in the measurement of vision but who cannot treat eye diseases or prescribe medication.

optometry (op-**TOM**-eh-tree) The profession of the measurement of vision.

oral (**OR**-al) Pertaining to the mouth.

orbit (**OR**-bit) The bony socket that holds the eyeball.

orbital (**OR**-bit-al) Pertaining to the orbit.

orchiectomy (or-key-**ECK**-toh-me) Removal of one or both testes.

orchiopexy (**OR**-key-oh-**PEK**-see) Surgical fixation of a testis in the scrotum.

orchitis (or-**KIE**-tis) Inflammation of the testis. Also called *epididymoorchitis.*

organ (**OR**-gan) Structure with specific functions in a body system.

organelle (**OR**-gah-nell) Part of a cell having specialized function(s).

organism (**OR**-gan-izm) Any whole, living individual animal or plant.

orifice (**OR**-ih-fis) Any opening or aperture.

origin (**OR**-ih-gin) Fixed source of a muscle at its attachment to bone.

oropharyngeal (**OR**-oh-fah-**RIN**-jee-al) Pertaining to the oropharynx.

oropharynx (**OR**-oh-**FAH**-rinks) Region at the back of the mouth between the soft palate and the tip of the epiglottis.

orthopedic (or-tho-**PEE**-dik) Pertaining to the correction and cure of deformities and diseases of the musculoskeletal system; originally, most of the deformities treated were in children. Also spelled *orthopaedic.*

orthopedist (or-tho-**PEE**-dist) Specialist in orthopedics.

orthopnea (or-**THOP**-nee-ah) Difficulty in breathing when lying flat.

orthopneic (or-**THOP**-nee-ik) Pertaining to or affected by orthopnea.

orthotic (or-**THOT**-ik) Orthopedic appliance to correct an abnormality.

orthotist (or-**THOT**-ist) Maker and fitter of orthopedic appliances.

os (OSS) Opening into a canal; for example, the cervix.

osmolality (**OZ**-moh-**LAL**-ih-tee) The concentration of a solution.

osmosis (os-**MOH**-sis) The passage of a solvent across a cell membrane

osmotic (os-**MOT**-ik) Pertaining to osmosis.

ossicle (**OSS**-ih-kel) A small bone, particularly relating to the three bones in the middle ear.

osteoarthritis (**OSS**-tee-oh-ar-**THRI**-tis) Chronic inflammatory disease of the joints, with pain and loss of function.

osteoblast (**OSS**-tee-oh-blast) Bone-forming cell.

osteocyte (**OSS**-tee-oh-site) A bone-maintaining cell.

osteogenesis imperfecta (**OSS**-tee-oh-**JEN**-eh-sis im-per-**FEK**-tah) Inherited condition when bone formation is incomplete, leading to fragile, easily broken bones.

osteogenic sarcoma (**OSS**-tee-oh-**JEN**-ik sar-**KOH**-mah) Malignant tumor originating in bone-producing cells.

osteomalacia (**OSS**-tee-oh-mah-**LAY**-she-ah) Soft, flexible bones lacking in calcium (rickets).

osteomyelitis (**OSS**-tee-oh-my-eh-**LIE**-tis) Inflammation of bone tissue.

osteopath (**OSS**-tee-oh-path) Practitioner of osteopathy.

osteopathic (**OSS**-tee-oh-**PATH**-ik) Pertaining to osteopathy.

osteopathy (**OSS**-tee-**OP**-ah-thee) Medical practice based on maintaining the balance of the body.

osteopenia (**OSS**-tee-oh-**PEE**-nee-ah) Decreased calcification of bone.

osteoporosis (**OSS**-tee-oh-poh-**ROE**-sis) Condition in which the bones become more porous, brittle, and fragile and more likely to fracture.

ostomy (**OSS**-toh-me) Artificial opening into a tubular structure.

otitis externa (oh-**TIE**-tis ekz-**TER**-nah) Inflammation of the external ear.

otitis media (oh-**TIE**-tis **ME**-dee-ah) Inflammation of the middle ear.

otolith (**OH**-toh-lith) A calcium particle in the vestibule of the inner ear.

otologist (oh-**TOL**-oh-jist) Medical specialist in diseases of the ear.

otology (oh-**TOL**-oh-jee) Study of the function and diseases of the ear.

otorhinolaryngologist (oh-toh-rye-no-lah-rin-**GOL**-oh-jist) Ear, nose, and throat medical specialist.

otosclerosis (**OH**-toh-sklair-**OH**-sis) Hardening at the junction of the stapes and oval window that causes loss of hearing.

otoscope (**OH**-toh-skope) Instrument for examining the ear.

otoscopic (OH-toh-SKOP-ik) Pertaining to examination with an otoscope.

otoscopy (oh-TOS-koh-pee) Examination of the ear.

ovarian (oh-VAIR-ee-an) Pertaining to the ovary(ies).

ovary (OH-vah-ree) One of the paired female egg-producing glands. Plural *ovaries.*

ovulate (OV-you-late) Release the oocyte from a follicle.

ovulation (OV-you-LAY-shun) Release of an oocyte from a follicle.

ovum (OH-vum) Egg. Also called *oocyte.* Plural *ova.*

oxygenate (OCK-suh-jen-ate) Addition of oxygen to a molecule

oxygen (OCK-see-jen) The gas essential for life.

oxygenation (OCK-suh-juh-NAY-shun) Process of adding oxygen.

oxyhemoglobin (OCK-see-he-moh-GLOW-bin) Hemoglobin in combination with oxygen.

oxytocin (OCK-see-TOH-sin) Pituitary hormone that stimulates the uterus to contract.

P

pacemaker (PACE-may-ker) Device that regulates cardiac electrical activity.

Paget disease (PAJ-et diz-EEZ) Scaling, crusting lesion of the nipple, often associated with an underlying cancer of the breast.

palate (PAL-ate) Roof of the mouth.

palatine (PAL-ah-tine) Bone that forms the hard palate and parts of the nose and orbits.

palliative care (PAL-ee-ah-tiv KAIR) To relieve symptoms and pain without curing.

pallor (PAL-or) Paleness of the skin.

palpate (PAL-pate) To examine with the fingers and hands.

palpation (pal-PAY-shun) Examination with the fingers and hands.

palpitation (pal-pih-TAY-shun) Forcible, rapid beat of the heart felt by the patient.

palsy (PAWL-zee) Paralysis or paresis from brain damage.

pancreas (PAN-kree-as) Lobulated gland, the head of which is tucked into the curve of the duodenum.

pancreatic (PAN-kree-AT-ik) Pertaining to the pancreas.

pancreatic islets (pan-kree-AT-ik EYE-lets) Areas of pancreatic cells that produce insulin and glucagon. Also called *islets of Langerhans.*

pancreatitis (PAN-kree-ah-TIE-tis) Inflammation of the pancreas.

pancreatography (PAN-kree-ah-TOG-raff-ee) Process of recording the structure of the pancreas.

pancytopenia (PAN-site-oh-PEE-nee-ah) Deficiency of all types of blood cells.

pandemic (pan-DEM-ik) Pertaining to a disease attacking the population of whole country or the world.

panendoscopy (pan-en-DOS-koh-pee) A visual examination of the inside of the esophagus, stomach, and upper duodenum using a flexible fiber-optic endoscope.

Pap test (PAP) Examination of cells taken from the cervix.

papilla (pah-PILL-ah) Any small projection. Plural *papillae.*

papilledema (pah-pill-eh-DEE-mah) Swelling of the optic disc in the retina.

papilloma (pap-ih-LOH-mah) Benign projection of epithelial cells.

papillomavirus (pap-ih-LOH-mah-vi-rus) Virus that causes warts and is associated with cancer.

papule (PAP-yul) Small, circumscribed elevation on the skin.

paralysis (pah-RAL-ih-sis) Loss of voluntary movement.

paralytic (par-ah-LYT-ik) Suffering from paralysis.

paralyze (PAR-ah-lyze) To make incapable of movement.

paranasal (PAR-ah-NAY-zal) Adjacent to the nose.

paranoia (par-ah-NOY-ah) Presence of persecutory delusions.

paranoid (PAR-ah-noyd) Having delusions of persecution.

paraphimosis (PAR-ah-fih-MOH-sis) Condition in which a retracted prepuce cannot be pulled forward to cover the glans.

paraplegia (par-ah-PLEE-jee-ah) Paralysis of both lower extremities.

paraplegic (par-ah-PLEE-jik) Pertaining to or suffering from paraplegia.

parasite (PAR-ah-site) An organism that attaches itself to, lives on or in, and derives its nutrition from another species.

parasitic (par-ah-SIT-ik) Pertaining to a parasite.

parasympathetic (par-ah-sim-pah-THET-ik) Division of the autonomic nervous system; has opposite effects of the sympathetic division.

parathyroid (par-ah-THIGH-royd) Endocrine glands embedded in the back of the thyroid gland.

parenchyma (pah-RENG-kih-mah) Characteristic functional cells of a gland or organ that are supported by the connective tissue framework.

parenteral (pah-REN-ter-al) Giving medication by any means other than the gastrointestinal tract.

paresis (par-EE-sis) Partial paralysis (weakness).

paresthesia (par-es-THEE-ze-ah) An abnormal sensation; for example, tingling, burning, prickling. Plural *parasthesias.*

parietal (pah-RYE-eh-tal) Pertaining to the outer layer of the pericardium and the wall of any body cavity; *or* the two bones forming the sidewalls and roof of the cranium.

parietal lobe (pah-RYE-eh-tal LOBE) Area of the brain under the parietal bone.

Parkinson disease (PAR-kin-son diz-EEZ) Disease of muscular rigidity, tremors, and a masklike facial expression.

paronychia (par-oh-NICK-ee-ah) Infection alongside the nail.

parotid (pah-ROT-id) Parotid gland is the salivary gland beside the ear.

paroxysmal (par-ock-SIZ-mal) Occurring in sharp, spasmodic episodes.

passive (PASS-iv) Not active.

patella (pah-TELL-ah) Thin, circular bone in front of the knee joint and embedded in the patellar tendon. Also called *kneecap.* Plural *patellae.*

patellar (pah-TELL-ar) Pertaining to the patella.

patent (PAY-tent) Open.

patent ductus arteriosus (PAY-tent DUK-tus ar-ter-ee-OH-sus) An open, direct channel between the aorta and the pulmonary artery.

pathogen (PATH-oh-jen) A disease-causing microorganism.

pathogenic (path-oh-JEN-ik) Causing disease.

pathologic fracture (path-oh-LOJ-ik FRAK-chur) Fracture occurring at a site already weakened by a disease process, such as cancer.

pathologist (pa-THOL-oh-jist) A specialist in pathology.

pathology (pa-**THOL**-oh-jee) Medical specialty dealing with the structural and functional changes of a disease process or the cause, development, and structural changes in disease.

pectoral (**PEK**-tor-al) Pertaining to the chest.

pectoral girdle (**PEK**-tor-al **GIR**-del) Incomplete bony ring that attaches the upper limb to the axial skeleton.

pectoralis (**PEK**-tor-ah-lis) Pertaining to the chest.

pedal (**PEED**-al) Pertaining to the foot.

pediatrician (**PEE**-dee-ah-**TRISH**-an) Medical specialist in pediatrics.

pediatrics (pee-dee-**AT**-riks) Medical specialty of treating children during development from birth through adolescence.

pediculosis (peh-dick-you-**LOH**-sis) An infestation with lice.

pelvic (**PEL**-vik) Pertaining to the pelvis.

pelvis (**PEL**-viss) A basin-shaped ring of bones, ligaments, and muscles at the base of the spine; *or* a basin-shaped cavity, as in the pelvis of the kidney.

penile (**PEE**-nile) Pertaining to the penis.

penis (**PEE**-nis) Conveys urine and semen to the outside.

pepsin (**PEP**-sin) Enzyme produced by the stomach that breaks down protein.

pepsinogen (pep-**SIN**-oh-jen) Converted by HCl in stomach to pepsin.

peptic (**PEP**-tik) Relating to the stomach and duodenum.

percutaneous (**PER**-kyu-**TAY**-nee-us) Passage through the skin.

perforated (**PER**-foh-ray-ted) Punctured with one or more holes.

perforation (per-foh-**RAY**-shun) A hole through the wall of a structure.

perfusion (per-**FYU**-zhun) The act of forcing blood to flow through a lumen or a vascular bed.

perfusionist (per-**FYU**-zhun-ist) Specialist in operation of heart-lung machine.

pericardial (pair-ih-**KAR**-dee-al) Pertaining to the pericardium.

pericarditis (**PAIR**-ih-kar-**DIE**-tis) Inflammation of the pericardium, the covering of the heart.

pericardium (pair-ih-**KAR**-dee-um) A double layer of membranes surrounding the heart.

perimetrium (pair-ih-**ME**-tree-um) The covering of the uterus; part of the peritoneum.

perinatal (pair-ih-**NAY**-tal) Around the time of birth.

perineal (**PAIR**-ih-**NEE**-al) Pertaining to the perineum.

perineum (**PAIR**-ih-**NEE**-um) Area between the thighs, extending from the coccyx to the pubis.

periodontal (**PAIR**-ee-oh-**DON**-tal) Around a tooth.

periodontics (**PAIR**-ee-oh-**DON**-tiks) Branch of dentistry specializing in disorders of tissues around the teeth.

periodontist (**PAIR**-ee-oh-**DON**-tist) Specialist in periodontics.

periodontitis (**PAIR**-ee-oh-don-**TIE**-tis) Inflammation of tissues around a tooth.

periorbital (pair-ee-**OR**-bit-al) Pertaining to tissues around the orbit.

periosteal (**PAIR**-ee-**OSS**-tee-al) Pertaining to the periosteum.

periosteum (**PAIR**-ee-**OSS**-tee-um) Fibrous membrane covering a bone.

peripheral (peh-**RIF**-er-al) Pertaining to the periphery or external boundary.

peripheral vision (peh-**RIF**-er-al **VIZH**-un) Ability to see objects as they come into the outer edges of the visual field.

peristalsis (per-ih-**STAL**-sis) Waves of alternate contraction and relaxation of the muscle wall of a tube; for example, of the intestinal wall to move food along the digestive tract.

peritoneal (**PER**-ih-toh-**NEE**-al) Pertaining to the peritoneum.

peritoneum (**PER**-ih-toh-**NEE**-um) Membrane that lines the abdominal cavity.

peritonitis (**PER**-ih-toh-**NIE**-tis) Inflammation of the peritoneum.

pernicious anemia (per-**NISH**-us ah-**NEE**-me-ah) Chronic anemia due to lack of vitamin B_{12}.

pertussis (per-**TUSS**-is) Infectious disease with a spasmodic, intense cough ending on a whoop (stridor). Also called *whooping cough.*

pessary (**PES**-ah-ree) Appliance inserted into the vagina to support the uterus.

petechia (peh-**TEE**-kee-ah) Pinpoint capillary hemorrhagic spot in the skin. Plural *petechiae.*

petit mal (peh-**TEE** MAL) Old name for absence seizures.

phacoemulsification (**FACK**-oh-ee-**MUL**-sih-fih-**KAY**-shun) Breaking down and sucking out a cataract with an ultrasonic needle.

phagocyte (**FAG**-oh-site) Blood cell that ingests and destroys foreign particles and cells.

phagocytic (fag-oh-**SIT**-ik) Pertaining to a phagocyte.

phagocytosis (**FAG**-oh-sigh-**TOH**-sis) Process of ingestion and destruction.

phalanx (**FAY**-lanks) A bone of a finger or toe. Plural *phalanges.*

pharmacist (**FAR**-mah-sist) Person licensed by the state to prepare and dispense drugs.

pharmacology (far-mah-**KOLL**-oh-jee) Science of the preparation, uses, and effects of drugs.

pharmacy (**FAR**-mah-see) Facility licensed to prepare and dispense drugs.

pharyngeal (fah-**RIN**-jee-al) Pertaining to the pharynx.

pharyngitis (fah-rin-**JIE**-tis) Inflammation of the pharynx.

pharynx (**FAH**-rinks) Tube from the back of the nose to the larynx.

phenotype (**FEE**-noh-type) A visible trait.

phimosis (fih-**MOH**-sis) Prepuce cannot be retracted.

phlebitis (fleh-**BIE**-tis) Inflammation of a vein.

phlebotomist (fleh-**BOT**-oh-mist) Person skilled in taking blood from veins.

phlebotomy (fleh-**BOT**-oh-me) Taking blood from a vein.

phlegm (FLEM) Abnormal amounts of mucus expectorated from the respiratory tract.

phobia (**FOH**-bee-ah) Pathologic fear or dread.

photocoagulation (**FOH**-toh-koh-**AG**-you-**LAY**-shun) Using light (laser beam) to form a clot.

photophobia (foh-toh-**FOH**-bee-ah) Fear of the light because it hurts the eyes.

photophobic (foh-toh-**FOH**-bik) Pertaining to or suffering from photophobia.

photoreceptor (**FOH**-toh-ree-**SEP**-tor) A photoreceptor cell receives light and converts it into electrical impulses.

photosensitive (**FOH**-toh-**SEN**-sih-tiv) Abnormally sensitive to light.

photosensitivity (**FOH**-toh-sen-sih-**TIV**-ih-tee) Light produces pain in the eye.

phototherapy (foh-toh-**THAIR**-ah-pee) Treatment using light rays.

physiatrist (fizz-**I**-ah-trist) A physician who specilizes in physical medicine and rehabilitation.

physiatry (fizz-**I**-ah-tree) Physical medicine.

physical (**FIZZ**-ih-kal) Relating to the body.

physical medicine (**FIZ**-ih-cal **MED**-ih-sin) Diagnosis and treatment by means of remedial agents, such as exercises, manipulation and heat.

physical therapy (**FIZ**-ih-cal **THAIR**-ah-pee) Use of remedial processes to overcome a physical defect. Also known as *physiotherapy.*

pia mater (**PEE**-ah **MAY**-ter) Delicate inner layer of the meninges.

pica (**PIE**-kah) Eating substances not considered to be food.

pineal (**PIN**-ee-al) Pertaining to the pineal gland.

pink eye Conjunctivitis.

pinna (**PIN**-ah) Another name for *auricle.* Plural *pinnae.*

pitting edema (eh-**DEE**-mah) An indentation made by a finger in an edematous area persists for a long time.

pituitary (pih-**TYU**-ih-tar-ee) Pertaining to the pituitary gland.

placenta (plah-**SEN**-tah) Organ that allows metabolic interchange between the mother and the fetus.

placenta abruptio (plah-**SEN**-tah ab-**RUP**-she-oh) Premature detachment of the placenta.

placenta previa (plah-**SEN**-tah **PREE**-vee-ah) Placenta obstructing the fetus during delivery.

plaque (**PLAK**) Patch of abnormal tissue.

plasma (**PLAZ**-mah) Fluid, noncellular component of blood.

platelet (**PLAYT**-let) Cell fragment involved in the clotting process. Also called *thrombocyte.*

pleura (**PLUR**-ah) Membrane covering the lungs and lining the ribs in the thoracic cavity. Plural *pleurae.*

pleural (**PLUR**-al) Pertaining to the pleura.

pleural cavity (**PLUR**-al) Pertaining to the space that surrounds the lungs.

pleurisy (**PLUR**-ih-see) Inflammation of the pleura.

plexus (**PLEK**-sus) A weblike network of joined nerves. Plural *plexuses.*

pneumoconiosis (**NEW**-moh-koh-nee-**OH**-sis) Fibrotic lung disease caused by the inhalation of different dusts.

pneumonectomy (**NEW**-moh-**NECK**-toh-me) Surgical removal of a lung.

pneumonia (new-**MOH**-nee-ah) Inflammation of the lung parenchyma (tissue).

pneumonitis (new-moh-**NI**-tis) Synonym for *pneumonia.*

pneumothorax (new-moh-**THOR**-ax) Air in the pleural cavity of the chest.

podiatrist (poh-**DIE**-ah-trist) Practitioner of podiatry.

podiatry (poh-**DIE**-ah-tree) The diagnosis and treatment of disorders and injuries of the foot.

poliomyelitis (**POE**-lee-oh-**MY**-eh-lie-tis) Inflammation of the gray matter of the spinal cord, leading to paralysis of the limbs and muscles of respiration. Abbreviation *polio.*

pollutant (poh-**LOO**-tant) Substance that makes an environment unclean or impure.

pollution (poh-**LOO**-shun) Condition that is unclean, impure, and a danger to health.

polycystic (pol-ee-**SIS**-tik) Composed of many cysts.

polycythemia vera (**POL**-ee-sigh-**THEE**-me-ah **VEH**-rah) Chronic disease with bone marrow hyperplasia, increase in number of RBCs, and increase in blood volume.

polydipsia (pol-ee-**DIP**-see-ah) Excessive thirst.

polyhydramnios (**POL**-ee-high-**DRAM**-nee-os) Too much amniotic fluid.

polymenorrhea (**POL**-ee-men-oh-**REE**-ah) More than normal frequency of menses.

polymorphonuclear (**POL**-ee-more-foh-**NEW**-klee-ahr) White blood cell with a multilobed nucleus.

polymyositis (**POL**-ee-my-oh-**SIGH**-tis) Inflammation of many voluntary muscles simultaneously.

polyneuropathy (**POL**-ee-nyu-**ROP**-ah-thee) Disorder affecting many nerves.

polyp (**POL**-ip) Any mass of tissue that projects outward.

polypectomy (pol-ip-**ECK**-toh-mee) Excision or removal of a polyp.

polyphagia (pol-ee-**FAY**-jee-ah) Excessive eating.

polyposis (pol-ee-**POH**-sis) Presence of several polyps.

polysomnography (**POL**-ee-som-**NOG**-rah-fee) Test to monitor brain waves, muscle tension, eye movement, and oxygen levels in the blood as the patient sleeps.

polyuria (pol-ee-**YOU**-ree-ah) Excessive production of urine.

popliteal (pop-**LIT**-ee-al) Pertaining to the back of the knee.

popliteal fossa (pop-**LIT**-ee-al **FOSS**-ah) The hollow at the back of the knee.

portal vein (**POR**-tal) The vein that carries blood from the intestines to the liver.

postcoital (post-**KOH**-ih-tal) After sexual intercourse.

posterior (pos-**TEER**-ee-or) Pertaining to the back surface of the body; situated behind.

postictal (post-**IK**-tal) Transient neurologic deficit after a seizure.

postmature (post-mah-**TYUR**) Infant born after 42 weeks of gestation.

postmaturity (post-mah-**TYUR**-ih-tee) Condition of being postmature.

postnatal (post-**NAY**-tal) After the birth.

postpartum (post-**PAR**-tum) After childbirth.

postpolio syndrome (PPS) (post-**POE**-lee-oh **SIN**-drome) Progressive muscle weakness in a person previously affected by polio.

postprandial (post-**PRAN**-dee-al) Following a meal.

posttraumatic (post-traw-**MAT**-ik) Occurring after and caused by trauma.

potent (**POH**-tent) Possessing strength, power.

Pott fracture (**POT FRAK**-shur) Fracture of the lower end of the fibula, often with fracture of the tibial malleolus.

precancerous (pree-**KAN**-ser-us) Lesion from which cancer can develop.

precipitate labor (pree-**SIP**-ih-tate **LAY**-bore) A very rapid labor and delivery.

predictive (pree-**DIK**-tiv) The likelihood of a disease or disorder being present or occurring.

preeclampsia (pree-eh-**KLAMP**-see-uh) Hypertension, edema, and proteinuria during pregnancy.

preemie (**PREE**-me) Slang for *premature baby.*

pregnancy (**PREG**-nan-see) State of being pregnant.

pregnant (**PREG**-nant) Having conceived.

prehypertension (pree-**HIGH**-per-**TEN**-shun) Precursor to hypertension.

premature (pree-mah-**TYUR**) Occurring before the expected time; for example, an infant born before 37 weeks of gestation.

prematurity (pree-mah-**TYUR**-ih-tee) Condition of being premature.

premenstrual (pree-**MEN**-stru-al) Pertaining to the time immediately before the menses.

prenatal (pree-**NAY**-tal) Before birth.

prepatellar (pree-pah-**TELL**-ar) In front of the patella.

prepuce (**PREE**-puce) Fold of skin that covers the glans penis. Same as *foreskin*.

presbyopia (prez-bee-**OH**-pee-ah) Difficulty in nearsighted vision occurring in middle and old age.

pressor (**PRESS**-or) Producing increased blood pressure.

prevention (pree-**VEN**-shun) Process to prevent occurrence of a disease or health problem.

preterm (**PREE**-term) Baby delivered before 37 weeks of gestation. Also called *premature*.

previa (**PREE**-vee-ah) Anything blocking the fetus during its birth; for example, an abnomally situated placenta, *placenta previa*.

priapism (**PRY**-ah-pizm) Persistent erection of the penis.

primary (**PRY**-mah-ree) The first of a disease or symptom, after which others may occur as complications arise.

primigravida (pry-mih-**GRAV**-ih-dah) First pregnancy.

primipara (pry-**MIP**-ah-ruh) Woman giving birth for the first time.

prion (**PREE**-on) Small infectious protein particle.

proctoscope (**PROK**-toh-skope) Instrument to view the inside of the anus and rectum.

proctitis (prok-**TIE**-tis) Inflammation of the lining of the rectum.

proctoscopy (prok-**TOSS**-koh-pee) Examination of the inside of the anus by endoscopy.

productive cough (proh-**DUC**-tiv KAWF) Cough resulting in matter coming up from the lungs.

profile (**PRO**-file) A set of characteristics which determine the structure of a group.

progesterone (pro-**JESS**-ter-own) Hormone that prepares the uterus for pregnancy.

progestin (pro-**JESS**-tin) A synthetic form of progesterone.

prognosis (prog-**NO**-sis) Forecast of the probable future course and outcome of a disease.

prolactin (pro-**LAK**-tin) Pituitary hormone that stimulates the production of milk.

prolactinoma (proh-lak-tih-**NOH**-mah) Prolactin-producing tumor.

prolapse (pro-**LAPS**) A sinking down of an organ or tissue.

proliferate (pro-**LIF**-eh-rate) To increase in number through reproduction.

pronate (**PRO**-nate) Rotate the forearm so that the surface of the palm faces posteriorly in the anatomical position.

pronation (pro-**NAY**-shun) Process of lying face down or of turning a hand or foot with the volar (palm or sole) surface down.

prone (PRONE) Lying face down, flat on your belly.

prophylactic (pro-fih-**LAK**-tik) The act or the agent that prevents a disease.

prophylaxis (pro-fih-**LAK**-sis) Prevention of disease.

prostaglandin (**PROS**-tah-**GLAN**-din) Hormone present in many tissues but first isolated from the prostate gland.

prostate (**PROS**-tate) Organ surrounding the urethra at the base of the male urinary bladder.

prostatectomy (pros-tah-**TEK**-toh-me) Surgical removal of the prostate.

prostatic (pros-**TAT**-ik) Pertaining to the prostate.

prostatitis (pros-tah-**TIE**-tis) Inflammation of the prostate.

prosthesis (**PROS**-thee-sis) Manufactured substitute for a missing part of the body.

prosthetic (pros-**THET**-ik) Pertaining to a prosthesis.

prostrate (pros-**TRAYT**) To lay flat or to be overcome by physical weakness and exhaustion.

prostration (pros-**TRAY**-shun) To be lying flat or to be overcome by physical weakness and exhaustion.

protease (**PRO**-tee-ase) Group of enzymes that break down protein.

protein (**PRO**-teen) Class of food substances based on amino acids.

proteinuria (pro-tee-**NYU**-ree-ah) Presence of protein in urine.

prothrombin (pro-**THROM**-bin) Protein formed by the liver and converted to thrombin in the blood-clotting mechanism.

proton (**PROH**-ton) The positively charged unit of the nuclear mass.

proton pump inhibitor (**PRO**-ton PUMP in-**HIB**-ih-tor) Agent that blocks the enzyme system in the lining of the stomach that produces gastric acid.

provisional diagnosis (pro-**VIZH**-un-al die-ag-**NO**-sis) A temporary diagnosis pending further examination or testing.

proximal (**PROK**-sih-mal) Situated nearest the center of the body.

pruritic (proo-**RIT**-ik) Itchy.

pruritus (proo-**RYE**-tus) Itching.

psoriasis (so-**RYE**-ah-sis) Rash characterized by reddish, silver-scaled patches.

psychedelic (sigh-keh-**DEL**-ik) An agent that intensifies sensory perception.

psychiatric (sigh-kee-**AH**-trik) Pertaining to psychiatry.

psychiatrist (sigh-**KIGH**-ah-trist) Licensed medical specialist in psychiatry.

psychiatry (sigh-**KIGH**-ah-tree) Diagnosis and treatment of mental disorders.

psychologic (sigh-koh-**LOJ**-ik) Pertaining to psychology.

psychological (sigh-koh-**LOJ**-ik-al) Pertaining to psychology.

psychologist (sigh-**KOL**-oh-jist) One who studies and becomes a specialist in psychology.

psychology (sigh-**KOL**-oh-jee) Study of the behavior of the human mind.

psychopath (**SIGH**-koh-path) Person with antisocial personality disorder.

psychosis (sigh-**KOH**-sis) Disorder causing mental disruption and loss of contact with reality.

psychosocial (**SIGH**-koh-**SOH**-shal) Involving both the mind and various social and community aspects of life.

psychosomatic (**SIGH**-koh-soh-**MAT**-ik) Disorders of the body influenced by the mind.

psychoactive (sigh-koh-**AK**-tiv) Able to alter mood, behavior, and/or cognition.

psychotic (sigh-**KOT**-ik) Pertaining to or affected by psychosis.

ptosis (**TOH**-sis) Sinking down of the upper eyelid or an organ.

pubarche (pyu-**BAR**-key) Development of pubic and axillary hair.

puberty (**PYU**-ber-tee) Process of maturing from child to young adult.

pubic (**PYU**-bik) Pertaining to the pubis.

pubis (**PYU**-bis) Alternative name for *pubic bone.*

puerperium (pyu-er-**PEE**-reeee-um) Six-week period after birth in which the uterus involutes.

pulmonary (**PULL**-moh-**NAIR**-ee) Pertaining to the lungs.

pulmonologist (**PULL**-moh-**NOL**-oh-jist) Specialist in treating disorders of the lungs.

pulmonology (**PULL**-moh-**NOL**-oh-jee) Study of the lungs, or the medical specialty of disorders of the lungs.

pulp (**PULP**) Dental pulp is the connective tissue in the cavity in the center of the tooth.

pupil (**PYU**-pill) The opening in the center of the iris that allows light to reach the lens. Plural *pupillae.*

pupillary (**PYU**-pill-ah-ree) Pertaining to the pupil.

purge (**PURJ**) Consciously throw up or cause bowel evacuation.

purpura (**PUR**-pyu-rah) Skin hemorrhages that are red initially and then turn purple.

purulent (**PURE**-you-lent) Showing or containing a lot of pus.

pustule (**PUS**-tyul) Small protuberance on the skin that contains pus.

pyelitis (pie-eh-**LYE**-tis) Inflammation of the renal pelvis.

pyelogram (**PIE**-el-oh-gram) X-ray image of renal pelvis and ureters.

pyelonephritis (**PIE**-eh-loh-neh-**FRY**-tis) Inflammation of the kidney and renal pelvis.

pyloric (pie-**LOR**-ik) Pertaining to the pylorus.

pylorus (pie-**LOR**-us) Exit area of the stomach.

pyorrhea (pie-oh-**REE**-ah) Purulent discharge.

pyrexia (pie-**REK**-see-ah) An abnormally high body temperature or fever.

pyromania (pie-roh-**MAY**-nee-ah) Morbid impulse to set fires.

Q

quadrant (**KWAD**-rant) One-quarter of a circle; *or* one of four regions of the surface of the abdomen.

quadriceps femoris (**KWAD**-rih-seps **FEM**-or-is) An anterior thigh muscle with four heads.

quadriplegia (kwad-rih-**PLEE**-jee-ah) Paralysis of all four limbs.

quadriplegic (kwad-rih-**PLEE**-jik) Pertaining to or suffering from quadriplegia.

R

radial (**RAY**-dee-al) Pertaining to the forearm or to any of the structures (artery, vein, nerve) named after it; *or* diverging in all directions from any given center.

radiation (ray-dee-**AY**-shun) To spread out.

radiation therapy (ray-dee-**AY**-shun **THAIR**-ah-pee) Treatment using x-rays or radionuclides. *Radiotherapy* is a synonym.

radical surgery (**RAD**-ih-kal **SUR**-jeh-ree) Surgical procedure in which the affected organ is removed along with the blood and lymph supply to that organ.

radioactive iodine (**RAY**-dee-oh-**AK**-tiv **EYE**-oh-dine) Any of the various tracers that emit alpha, beta, or gamma rays.

radioallergosorbent (**RAY**-dee-oh-ah-**LUR**-go-**SOAR**-bent) A radioimmunoassay to detect IgE-bound allergens responsible for tissue hypersensitivity.

radioimmunoassay (**RAY**-dee-oh-im-you-no-**ASS**-ay) Immunoassay of a substance that has been radioactively labeled.

radiologic (**RAY**-dee-oh-**LOJ**-ik) Pertaining to radiology.

radiologist (ray-dee-**OL**-oh-jist) Medical specialist in the use of X-rays and other imaging techniques.

radiology (ray-dee-**OL**-oh-jee) Study of medical imaging.

radiotherapy (**RAY**-dee-oh-**THAIR**-ah-pee) Treatment using radiation.

radius (**RAY**-dee-us) The forearm bone on the thumb side.

rale (**RAHL**) Crackle heard through a stethoscope when air bubbles through liquid in the lungs. Plural *rales.*

rash (**RASH**) Skin eruption.

reagent (ree-**A**-jent) Any substance added to a solution of another substance to examine, produce, or measure another substance.

recombinant DNA (ree-**KOM**-bin-ant **DEE**-en-a) Deoxyribonucleic acid (DNA) altered by inserting a new sequence of DNA into the chain.

rectocele (**RECK**-toh-seal) Hernia of the rectum into the vagina.

rectal (**RECK**-tal) Pertaining to the rectum.

rectum (**RECK**-tum) Terminal part of the colon from the sigmoid to the anal canal.

reflex (**REE**-fleks) An involuntary response to a stimulus.

reflux (**REE**-fluks) Backward flow.

refract (ree-**FRAKT**) Make a change in the direction of, or bend, a ray of light.

refraction (ree-**FRAKT**-shun) The bending of light.

refractometer (ree-frak-**TAH**-meh-tur) Device that measures refractive errors of the cornea

regenerate (ree-**JEN**-eh-rate) Reconstitution of a lost part.

regeneration (ree-**JEN**-eh-**RAY**-shun) The process of reconstitution.

regurgitate (ree-**GUR**-jih-tate) To flow backward; for example, blood through a heart valve.

regurgitation (ree-gur-jih-**TAY**-shun) Expel contents of the stomach into the mouth, short of vomiting.

rehabilitation (**REE**-hah-bill-ih-**TAY**-shun) Therapeutic restoration of an ability to function as before.

remission (ree-**MISH**-un) Period when there is a lessening or absence of the symptoms of a disease.

renal (**REE**-nal) Pertaining to the kidney.

replicate (**REP**-lih-kate) To produce an exact copy.

replication (rep-lih-**KAY**-shun) Reproduction to produce an exact copy.

reproduction (ree-pro-**DUK**-shun) The process by which organisms produce offspring.

reproductive (ree-pro-**DUK**-tiv) Pertaining to reproduction.

resection (ree-**SEK**-shun) Removal of a specific part of an organ or structure.

resectoscope (ree-**SEK**-toh-skope) Endoscope for transurethral removal of lesions of the prostate.

respiration (**RES**-pih-**RAY**-shun) Process of breathing; fundamental process of life used to exchange oxygen and carbon dioxide.

respirator (**RES**-pih-**RAY**-tor) Another name for *ventilator.*

respiratory (**RES**-pih-rah-tor-ee) Pertaining to respiration.

respiratory membrane (**RES**-pih-rah-tor-ee **MEM**-brain) A thin semipermeable membrane between the alveoli and the pulmonary capillaries.

retention (ree-**TEN**-shun) Holding back in the body what should normally be discharged (e.g., urine).

retina (**RET**-ih-nah) Light-sensitive innermost layer of the eyeball.

retinal (**RET**-ih-nal) Pertaining to the retina.

retinoblastoma (**RET**-in-oh-blas-**TOH**-mah) Malignant neoplasm of primitive retinal cells.

retinoids (**RET**-ih-noydz) Keratolytic agents applied for psoriasis, acne, and photodamage.

retinopathy (ret-ih-**NOP**-ah-thee) Any disease of the retina.

retrograde (**RET**-roh-grade) Reversal of a normal flow; for example, back from the bladder into the ureters.

retroversion (reh-troh-**VER**-zhun) Tipping backward of the uterus.

retroverted (**REH**-troh-vert-ed) Tilted backward.

retrovirus (**REH**-troh-vie-rus) Virus with an RNA core.

rhesus factor (**REE**-sus **FAK**-tor) An antigen on the surface of red blood cells of Rh positive individuals. First discovered in Rhesus monkeys.

rheumatic (ru-**MA**-tik) Pertaining to or affected by rheumatism.

rheumatism (**RU**-ma-tizm) Pain in various parts of the musculoskeletal system.

rheumatoid arthritis (RA) (**RU**-mah-toyd ar-**THRI**-tis) Disease of connective tissue, with arthritis as a major manifestation.

rhinitis (rye-**NIE**-tis) Inflammation of the nasal mucosa. Also called *coryza.*

rhinoplasty (**RYE**-no-plas-tee) Surgical procedure to change size or shape of the nose.

rhonchus (**RONG**-kuss) Wheezing sound heard on auscultation of the lungs; made by air passing through a constricted lumen. Plural *rhonchi.*

ribonucleic acid (RNA) (**RYE**-boh-nyu-**KLEE**-ik **ASS**-id) Information carrier from DNA in the nucleus to an organelle to produce protein molecules.

ribosome (**RYE**-boh-sohm) Structure in the cell that assembles amino acids into protein.

rickets (**RICK**-ets) Disease due to vitamin D deficiency, producing soft, flexible bones.

rigidity (ri-**JID**-ih-tee) Increased muscle tone at rest.

Rinne test (**RIN**-eh TEST) Test for conductive hearing loss.

ritual (**RICH**-oo-al) In psychiatry or psychology, repeated set of actions to relieve or prevent anxiety.

root (ROOT) Fundamental or beginning part of a structure.

rooting reflex (**RUE**-ting) A neonatal reflex to turn toward the nipple and open the mouth when a nipple is placed on the cheek.

rosacea (roh-**ZAY**-she-ah) Persistent erythematous rash of the central face.

rotator cuff (roh-**TAY**-tor CUFF) Part of the capsule of the shoulder joint.

rumination (roo-min-**NAY**-shun) To bring back food into the mouth to chew over and over.

rupture (**RUP**-tyur) Break or tear of any organ or body part.

S

sacral (**SAY**-kral) Pertaining to or in the neighborhood of the sacrum.

sacroiliac joint (say-kroh-**ILL**-ih-ak JOINT) The joint between the sacrum and the ilium.

sacrum (**SAY**-crum) Segment of the vertebral column that forms part of the pelvis.

sagittal (**SAJ**-ih-tal) Vertical plane through the body dividing it into right and left portions.

saline (**SAY**-leen) Salt solution, usually sodium chloride.

saliva (sa-**LIE**-vah) Secretion in the mouth from salivary glands.

salivary (**SAL**-ih-var-ee) Pertaining to saliva.

salpingectomy (sal-pin-**JEK**-toh-me) Surgical excision of a uterine tube.

salpingitis (sal-pin-**JIE**-tis) Inflammation of the uterine tube.

saphenous (**SAPH**-ih-nus) Relating to the saphenous vein in the thigh.

sarcoidosis (sar-koy-**DOH**-sis) Granulomatous lesions of the lungs and other organs; cause is unknown.

sarcoma (sar-**KOH**-mah) A malignant tumor originating in connective tissue.

sarcopenia (sar-koh-**PEE**-nee-ah) Progressive loss of muscle mass and strength with aging.

scab (SKAB) Crust that forms over a wound or sore during healing.

scabies (**SKAY**-beez) Skin disease produced by mites.

scald (SKAWLD) Burn from contact with hot liquid or steam.

scapula (**SKAP**-you-lah) Shoulder blade. Plural *scapulae.*

scapular (**SKAP**-you-lar) Pertaining to the scapula.

scar (SKAR) Fibrotic seam that forms when a wound heals.

schizophrenia (skitz-oh-**FREE**-nee-ah) Disorder of perception, thought, emotion, and behavior.

sclera (**SKLAIR**-ah) Fibrous outer covering of the eyeball and the white of the eye.

scleral (**SKLAIR**-al) Pertaining to the sclera.

scleritis (sklee-**RI**-tis) Inflammation of the sclera.

scleroderma (sklair-oh-**DERM**-ah) Thickening and hardening of the skin due to new collagen formation.

sclerose (skleh-**ROSE**) To harden or thicken.

sclerosis (skleh-**ROH**-sis) Thickening or hardening of a tissue; in the nervous system, hardening of nervous tissue by fibrous and glial connective tissue.

sclerotherapy (**SKLAIR**-oh-**THAIR**-ah-pee) Injection of a solution into a vein to thrombose it.

scoliosis (skoh-lee-**OH**-sis) An abnormal lateral curvature of the vertebral column.

scoliotic (**SKOH**-lee-**OT**-ik) Pertaining to or suffering from scoliosis.

scrotal (**SKRO**-tal) Pertaining to the scrotum.

scrotum (**SKRO**-tum) Sac containing testes.

seasonal affective disorder (see-**ZON**-al af-**FEK**-tiv dis-**OR**-der) Depression that occurs at the same time every year, often in winter.

sebaceous glands (seh-**BAY**-shus GLANZ) Glands in the dermis that open into hair follicles and secrete an oily fluid called *sebum*.

seborrhea (seb-oh-**REE**-ah) Excessive amount of sebum.

seborrheic (seb-oh-**REE**-ik) Pertaining to seborrhea.

sebum (**SEE**-bum) Waxy secretion of the sebaceous glands.

secondary (**SEK**-ond-ah-ree) Diseases or symptoms following a primary disease or symptom.

secrete (seh-**KREET**) To produce a chemical substance in a cell and release it from the cell.

secretion (seh-**KREE**-shun) The production of a chemical substance in a cell and its release from the cell.

sedation (seh-**DAY**-shun) State of being calmed.

sedative (**SED**-ah-tiv) Agent that calms nervous excitement.

segment (**SEG**-ment) A section of an organ or structure.

seizure (**SEE**-zhur) Event due to excessive electrical activity in the brain.

self-examination (**SELF**-ek-zam-ih-**NAY**-shun) Conduct an examination of one's own body.

self-mutilation (self-myu-tih-**LAY**-shun) Injury or disfigurement made to one's own body.

semen (**SEE**-men) Penile ejaculate containing sperm and seminal fluid.

semilunar (sem-ee-**LOO**-nar) Appears like a half moon.

seminal vesicle (**SEM**-in-al **VES**-ih-kull) Sac of the ductus deferens that produces seminal fluid.

seminiferous (sem-ih-**NIF**-er-us) Pertaining to carrying semen.

seminiferous tubule (sem-ih-**NIF**-er-us **TU**-byul) Coiled tubes in the testes that produce sperm.

seminoma (sem-ih-**NO**-mah) Neoplasm of germ cells of a testis.

senescence (seh-**NES**-ens) The state of being old.

senescent (seh-**NES**-ent) Growing old.

senile (**SEE**-nile) Characteristic of old age.

senility (seh-**NIL**-ih-tee) Mental disorders occurring in old age.

sensation (sen-**SAY**-shun) The conscious feeling of the effects of a stimulation.

sensorineural hearing loss (**SEN**-sor-ih-**NYUR**-al) Hearing loss caused by lesions of the inner ear or the auditory nerve.

sensory (**SEN**-soh-ree) Having the function of sensation; structures of the nervous system that carry impulses to the brain.

sepsis (**SEP**-sis) Presence of pathogenic organisms or their toxins in blood or tissues.

septicemia (sep-tih-**SEE**-mee-ah) Microorganisms circulating in, and infecting, the blood (blood poisoning).

septum (**SEP**-tum) A thin wall separating two cavities or tissue masses. Plural *septa*.

serotonin (ser-oh-**TOH**-nin) A neurotransmitter in the central and peripheral nervous systems.

serous (**SEER**-us) Thicker and less transparent than water.

serum (**SEER**-um) Fluid remaining after removal of cells and fibrin clot from blood.

shock (SHOCK) Sudden physical or mental collapse or circulatory collapse.

shunt (SHUNT) A bypass or diversion of fluid; for example, blood.

sibling (**SIB**-ling) Brother or sister.

sigmoid (**SIG**-moyd) Sigmoid colon is shaped like an "S."

sigmoidoscopy (sig-moi-**DOS**-koh-pee) Endoscopic examination of the sigmoid colon.

sign (SINE) Physical evidence of a disease process.

silicosis (sil-ih-**KOH**-sis) Fibrotic lung disease from inhaling silica particles.

sinoatrial (SA) node (sigh-noh-**AY**-tree-al NODE) The center of modified cardiac muscle fibers in the wall of the right atrium that acts as the pacemaker for the heart rhythm.

sinus (**SIGH**-nus) Cavity or hollow space in a bone or other tissue.

sinus rhythm (**SIGH**-nus **RITH**-um) The normal (optimal) heart rhythm arising from the sinoatrial node.

sinusitis (sigh-nyu-**SIGH**-tis) Inflammation of the lining of a sinus.

Sjogren syndrome (**SHOR**-gren **SIN**-drome) Dryness of the mucous membranes of the eye and mouth.

skeletal (**SKEL**-eh-tal) Pertaining to the skeleton.

skeleton (**SKEL**-eh-ton) The bony framework of the body.

smegma (**SMEG**-mah) Oily material produced by the glans and prepuce.

Snellen letter chart (**SNEL**-en) Test for acuity of distance vision.

snore (SNOR) Noise produced by vibrations in the structures of the nasopharynx.

sociopath (**SOH**-see-oh-path) Person with antisocial personality disorder.

somatic (soh-**MAT**-ik) Relating to the body in general; *or* a division of the periperal nervous system serving the skeletal muscles.

somatostatin (**SOH**-mah-toh-**STAT**-in) Hormone that inhibits release of growth hormone and insulin.

somatotrophin (**SOH**-mah-toh-**TROH**-phin) Hormone of the anterior pituitary that stimulates the growth of body tissues. Also called *growth hormone*.

spasm (SPASM) Sudden involuntary contraction of a muscle group.

spasmodic (spaz-**MOD**-ik) Intermittent contractions.

spastic (**SPAS**-tik) Increased muscle tone on movement.

specific (speh-**SIF**-ik) Relating to a particular entity.

specificity (spes-ih-**FIS**-ih-tee) State of having a fixed relation to a particular entity.

speculum (**SPECK**-you-lum) An instrument inserted into a body orifice to enlarge its canal or cavity for inspection.

sperm (SPERM) Mature male sex cell. Also called *spermatozoon*.

spermatic (**SPER**-mat-ik) Pertaining to sperm.

spermatid (**SPER**-mat-id) A cell late in the development process of sperm.

spermacidal (**SPER**-mih-**SIDE**-al) Pertaining to the destruction of sperm.

spermacide (**SPER**-mih-side) Agent that destroys sperm.

spermatocele (**SPER**-mat-oh-seal) Cyst of the epididymis that contains sperm.

spermatogenesis (**SPER**-mat-oh-**JEN**-eh-sis) The process by which male germ cells differentiate into sperm.

spermatozoa (**SPER**-mat-oh-**ZOH**-ah) Sperm (plural of *spermatozoon*).

spermicidal (sper-mih-**SIGH**-dal) Pertaining to the killing of sperm; *or* destructive to sperm.

spermicide (**SPER**-mih-side) Agent that destroys sperm.

sphenoid (**SFEE**-noyd) Wedge-shaped bone at the base of the skull.

sphincter (**SFINK**-ter) Band of muscle that encircles an opening; when it contracts, the opening squeezes closed.

sphygmomanometer (**SFIG**-moh-mah-**NOM**-ih-ter) Instrument for measuring arterial blood pressure.

spina bifida (**SPY**-nah **BIH**-fih-dah) Failure of one or more vertebral arches to close during fetal development.

spina bifida cystica (**SIS**-tik-ah) Meninges and spinal cord protruding through the absent vertebral arch and having the appearance of a cyst.

spina bifida occulta (**OH**-kul-tah) The deformity of the vertebral arch is not apparent from the surface.

spinal (**SPY**-nal) Pertaining to the spine.

spinal tap (**SPY**-nal TAP) Placement of a needle through an intervertebral space into the subarachnoid space to withdraw CSF.

spine (SPINE) The vertebral column; *or* a short bony projection.

spiral fracture (**SPY**-ral **FRAK**-chur) A fracture in the shape of a coil.

spirochete (**SPY**-roh-keet) Spiral-shaped bacterium causing a sexually transmitted disease (syphilis).

spirometer (spy-**ROM**-eh-ter) An instrument used to measure respiratory volumes.

spirometry (spy-**ROM**-eh-tree) Use of a spirometer.

spleen (SPLEEN) Vascular, lymphatic organ in the left upper quadrant of the abdomen.

splenectomy (sple-**NECK**-toh-me) Surgical removal of the spleen.

splenomegaly (**SPLEE**-noh-**MEG**-ah-lee) Enlarged spleen.

spongiosum (spun-jee-**OH**-sum) Spongelike tissue.

sprain (SPRAIN) A wrench or tear in a ligament.

sputum (**SPYU**-tum) Matter coughed up and spat out by individuals with respiratory disorders.

squamous cell (**SKWAY**-mus SELL) Flat, scalelike epithelial cell.

stabilize (**STAY**-bill-ize) To make or hold firm or steady.

stable (**STAY**-bel) Steady, not varying.

stage (STAYJ) Definition of the extent and dissemination of a malignant neoplasm.

staging (**STAY**-jing) Process of determination of the extent of the distribution of a neoplasm.

stapes (**STAY**-peez) Inner (medial) one of the three ossicles of the middle ear; shaped like a stirrup.

Staphylococcus (**STAF**-ih-loh-**KOK**-us) Genus of gram-positive bacteria that divide in more than one plane to form clusters. Plural *staphylococci.*

starch (STARCH) Complex carbohydrate made of multiple units of glucose attached together.

stasis (**STAY**-sis) Stagnation in the flow of any body fluid.

statin (**STAH**-tin) A class of drugs used to lower blood cholesterol levels.

status (**STAT**-us) A state or condition.

status epilepticus (**STAT**-us ep-ih-**LEP**-tik-us) Latin phrase for being in a prolonged or recurrent seizure for longer than a specific time frame.

stem cell (STEM SELL) Undifferentiated cell found in a differentiated tissue that can divide to yield the specialized cells in that tissue.

stenosis (steh-**NOH**-sis) Narrowing of a canal or passage.

stent (STENT) Wire-mesh tube used to keep arteries open.

stereopsis (ster-ee-**OP**-sis) Three-dimensional vision.

stereotactic (**STER**-ee-oh-**TAK**-tic) A precise three-dimensional method to locate a lesion.

stereotype (**STER**-ee-oh-tipe) An image held in common by members of a group.

sterile (**STER**-il) Free from all living organisms and their spores; *or* unable to fertilize or reproduce.

sterility (steh-**RIL**-ih-tee) Inability to reproduce.

sterilization (**STER**-ih-lih-**ZAY**-shun) Process of making sterile.

sterilize (**STER**-ih-lize) To make sterile.

sternum (**STIR**-num) Long, flat bone forming the center of the anterior wall of the chest.

steroid (**STAIR**-oyd) Large family of chemical substances found in many drugs, hormones, and body components.

stethoscope (**STETH**-oh-skope) Instrument for listening to cardiac and respiratory sounds.

stimulant (**STIM**-you-lant) Agent that excites or strengthens.

stimulation (stim-you-**LAY**-shun) Arousal to increased functional activity.

stimulus (**STIM**-you-lus) Something that excites or strengthens the functional activity of an organ or part. Plural *stimuli.*

stoma (**STOW**-mah) Artificial opening.

strabismus (strah-**BIZ**-mus) Turning of an eye away from its normal position.

strain (STRAIN) Overstretch or tear in a muscle or tendon.

stratum basale (**STRAH**-tum bay-**SAL**-eh) Deepest layer of the epidermis, from which the other cells originate and migrate.

Streptococcus (strep-toh-**KOK**-us) Genus of gram-positive bacteria that grow in chains. Plural *streptococci.*

striated muscle (**STRI**-ay-ted **MUSS**-el) Another term for *skeletal muscle.*

stricture (**STRICK**-shur) Narrowing of a tube.

stridor (**STRY**-door) High-pitched noise made when there is a respiratory obstruction in the larynx or trachea.

stroke (STROHK) Acute clinical event caused by impaired cerebral circulation.

stye (STEYE) Infection of an eyelash follicle.

subarachnoid space (sub-ah-**RACK**-noyd SPACE) Space between the pia mater and the arachnoid membrane.

subclavian (sub-**CLAY**-vee-an) Underneath the clavicle.

subcutaneous (sub-kew-**TAY**-nee-us) Below the skin. Also called *hypodermic.*

subdural space (sub-**DYU**-ral SPASE) Space between the arachnoid and dura mater layers of the meninges.

sublingual (sub-**LING**-wal) Underneath the tongue.

subluxation (sub-luck-**SAY**-shun) An incomplete dislocation when some contact between the joint surfaces remains.

submandibular (sub-man-**DIB**-you-lar) Underneath the mandible.

submucosa (sub-mew-**KOH**-sa) Tissue layer underneath the mucosa.

substernal (sub-**STER**-nal) Under (behind) the sternum or breastbone.

suction (**SUK**-shun) Use of a catheter to clear the upper airway or other tubes.

sulcus (SUL-cuss) Groove on the surface of the cerebral hemispheres that separates gyri. Plural *sulci.*

superficial (soo-per-FISH-al) Situated near the surface.

superior (soo-PEER-ee-or) Situated above.

supinate (SOO-pih-nate) Rotate the forearm so that the surface of the palm faces anteriorly in the anatomical position.

supination (soo-pih-NAY-shun) Process of lying face upward or of turning a hand or foot so that the palm or sole is facing up.

supine (soo-PINE) Lying face up, flat on your spine.

suprapubic (SOO-prah-pyu-bik) Above the symphysis pubis.

surfactant (sir-FAK-tant) A protein and fat compound that creates surface tension to hold the lung alveolar walls apart.

suture (SOO-chur) Two bones are joined together by a fibrous band continuous with their periosteum, as in the skull; *or* a stitch to hold the edges of a wound together; *or* to stitch the edges of a wound together. Plural *sutures.*

swab (SWOB) Wad of cotton used to remove or apply something from/to a surface.

sympathetic (sim-pah-THET-ik) Division of the autonomic nervous system operating at an unconscious level.

sympathy (SIM-pah-thee) Appreciation and concern for another person's mental and emotional state.

symphysis (SIM-feh-sis) Two bones joined by fibrocartilage. Plural *symphyses.*

symptom (SIMP-tum) Departure from the normal experienced by a patient.

symptomatic (simp-toh-MAT-ik) Pertaining to the symptoms of a disease.

synapse (SIN-aps) Junction between two nerve cells or a nerve fiber and its target cell, where electrical impulses are transmitted between the cells.

syncope (SIN-koh-pee) Temporary loss of consciousness and posture due to diminished cerebral blood flow.

syndrome (SIN-drohm) Combination of signs and symptoms associated with a particular disease process.

synovial (si-NOH-vee-al) Pertaining to synovial fluid and the synovial membrane.

synthesis (SIN-the-sis) The process of building a compound from different elements.

synthetic (sin-THET-ik) Built up or put together from simpler compounds.

syphilis (SIF-ih-lis) Sexually transmitted disease caused by a spirochete.

syringomyelia (sih-RING-oh-my-EE-lee-ah) Abnormal longitudinal cavities in the spinal cord that cause paresthesias and muscle weakness.

systemic (sis-TEM-ik) Relating to the entire organism.

systemic lupus erythematosus (sis-TEM-ik LOO-pus er-ih-THEE-mah-toh-sus) Inflammatory connective tissue disease affecting the whole body.

systole (SIS-toh-lee) Contraction of the heart muscle.

systolic (sis-TOL-ik) Pertaining to systole.

T

tachycardia (tack-ih-KAR-dee-ah) Rapid heart rate (above 100 beats per minute).

tachypnea (tack-ip-NEE-ah) Rapid breathing.

talipes (TAL-ip-eze) Deformity of the foot involving the talus.

talus (TAY-luss) The tarsal bone that articulates with the tibia to form the ankle joint.

tampon (TAM-pon) Plug or pack in a cavity to absorb or stop bleeding.

tamponade (tam-poh-NAID) Pathologic compression of an organ, such as the heart.

tapeworm (TAPE-worm) Intestinal parasitic worm.

tarsal (TAR-sal) Pertaining to the tarsus.

tarsus (TAR-sus) The collection of seven bones in the foot that form the ankle and instep; *or* the flat fibrous plate that gives shape to the outer edges of the eyelids.

tartar (TAR-tar) Calcified deposit at the gingival margin of the teeth.

Tay-Sachs disease (TAY SAKS diz-EEZ) Congenital fatal disorder of fat metabolism.

temporal (TEM-pore-al) Bone that forms part of the base and sides of the skull.

temporal lobe (TEM-pore-al LOBE) Posterior two-thirds of the cerebral hemispheres.

temporomandibular joint (TMJ) (TEM-pore-oh-man-DIB-you-lar JOYNT) The joint between the temporal bone and the mandible.

tendinitis (ten-dih-NYE-tis) Inflammation of a tendon. Also spelled *tendonitis.*

tendon (TEN-dun) Fibrous band that connects muscle to bone.

tenosynovitis (TEN-oh-sin-oh-VIE-tis) Inflammation of a tendon and its surrounding synovial sheath.

teratogen (TER-ah-toh-jen) Agent that produces fetal deformities.

teratogenesis (TER-ah-toh-JEN-eh-sis) Process involved in producing fetal deformities.

teratogenic (TER-ah-toh-JEN-ik) Pertaining to or capable of producing fetal deformities.

teratoma (ter-ah-TOH-mah) Neoplasm of a testis or ovary containing multiple tissues from other sites in the body.

testicle (TES-tih-kul) One of the male reproductive glands. Also called *testis.*

testicular (tes-TICK-you-lar) Pertaining to the testicle.

testis (TES-tis) A synonym for *testicle.* Plural *testes.*

testosterone (tes-TOSS-ter-own) Powerful androgen produced by the testes.

tetany (TET-ah-nee) Severe muscle twitches, cramps, and spasms.

tetralogy of Fallot (TOF) (te-TRA-loh-jee ov fah-LOW) Set of four congenital heart defects occurring together.

thalamus (THAL-ah-mus) Mass of gray matter underneath the ventricle in each cerebral hemisphere.

thalassemia (thal-ah-SEE-mee-ah) Group of inherited blood disorders that produce a hemolytic anemia.

thelarche (thee-LAR-key) Onset of breast development.

thenar (THEE-nar) The thenar eminence is the fleshy mass at the base of the thumb.

therapeutic (THAIR-ah-PYU-tik) Pertaining to the treatment of a disease or disorder.

therapist (THAIR-ah-pist) Professional trained in the practice of a particular therapy.

therapy (THAIR-ah-pee) Systematic treatment of a disease, dysfunction, or disorder.

thiazide (**THIGH**-ah-zide) Abbreviated form of benzothiadiazide, a class of diuretic

thoracentesis (**THOR**-ah-sen-**TEE**-sis) Insertion of a needle into the pleural cavity to withdraw fluid or air. Also called *pleural tap*.

thoracic (**THOR**-ass-ik) Pertaining to the chest (thorax).

thoracic cavity (**THOR**-ass-ik **KAV**-ih-tee) Space within the chest containing the lungs, heart, aorta, venae cavae, esophagus, trachea, and pulmonary vessels.

thoracoscopy (thor-ah-**KOS**-koh-pee) Examination of the pleural cavity with an endoscope.

thoracotomy (thor-ah-**KOT**-oh-me) Incision through the chest wall.

thorax (**THOR**-acks) The part of the trunk between the abdomen and the neck.

thrombin (**THROM**-bin) Enzyme that forms fibrin.

thrombocyte (**THROM**-boh-site) Another name for *platelet*.

thrombocytic (**THROM**-bo-**SIT**-ik) Pertaining to a thrombocyte (platelet).

thrombocytopenia (**THROM**-boh-site-oh-**PEE**-nee-uh) Deficiency of platelets in circulating blood.

thromboembolism (**THROM**-boh-**EM**-boh-lizm) A piece of detached blood clot (embolus) blocking a distant blood vessel.

thrombolysis (throm-**BOH**-lih-sis) Dissolving of a thrombus (clot).

thrombolytic (throm-boh-**LIT**-ik) Able to dissolve a thrombus.

thrombophlebitis (**THROM**-boh-fleh-**BY**-tis) Inflammation of a vein with clot formation.

thrombosis (throm-**BOH**-sis) Formation of a thrombus.

thrombus (**THROM**-bus) A clot attached to a diseased blood vessel or heart lining. Plural *thrombi*.

thrush (**THRUSH**) Infection with *Candida albicans*.

thymectomy (thigh-**MEK**-toh-me) Surgical removal of the thymus gland.

thymoma (thigh-**MOH**-mah) Benign tumor of the thymus.

thymus (**THIGH**-mus) Lymphoid and endocrine gland located in the mediastinum.

thyroid (**THIGH**-royd) Endocrine gland in the neck; *or* a cartilage of the larynx.

thyroid hormone (**THIGH**-royd **HOR**-mohn) Collective term for the two thyroid hormones, T3 and T4.

thyroid storm (**THIGH**-royd STORM) Medical crisis and emergency due to excess thyroid hormones.

thyroidectomy (thigh-royd-**ECK**-toh-me) Surgical removal of the thyroid gland.

thyroiditis (thigh-royd-**EYE**-tis) Inflammation of the thyroid gland.

thyrotoxicosis (**THIGH**-roe-toks-ih-**KOH**-sis) Disorder produced by excessive thyroid hormone production.

thyrotropin (thigh-roe-**TROH**-pin) Hormone from the anterior pituitary gland that stimulates function of the thyroid gland.

thyroxine (thigh-**ROCK**-sin) Thyroid hormone T4, tetraiodothyronine.

tibia (**TIB**-ee-ah) The larger bone of the lower leg.

tibial (**TIB**-ee-al) Pertaining to the tibia.

tic (TIK) Sudden, involuntary, repeated contraction of muscles.

tic douloureux (tik duh-luh-**RUE**) Painful, sudden, spasmodic involuntary contractions of the facial muscles supplied by the trigeminal nerve. Also called *trigeminal neuralgia*.

tinea (**TIN**-ee-ah) General term for a group of related skin infections caused by different species of fungi.

tinea capitis (**TIN**-ee-ah **CAP**-it-us) Fungal infection of the scalp.

tinea corporis (**TIN**-ee-ah **KOR**-por-is) Fungal infection of the body.

tinea cruris (**TIN**-ee-ah **KROO**-ris) Fungal infection of the groin.

tinea pedis (**TIN**-ee-ah **PED**-is) Fungal infection of the foot.

tinea versicolor (**TIN**-ee-ah **VERSE**-ih-col-or) Fungal infection of the trunk in which the skin loses pigmentation.

tinnitus (**TIN**-ih-tus) Persistent ringing, whistling, clicking, or booming noise in the ears.

tissue (**TISH**-you) Collection of similar cells.

tolerance (**TOL**-er-ans) The capacity to become accustomed to a stimulus or drug.

tomography (to-**MOG**-rah-fee) Radiographic image of a selected slice of tissue.

tone (TONE) Tension present in resting muscles.

tongue (TUNG) Mobile muscle mass in the mouth; bears the taste buds.

tonic (**TON**-ik) State of muscular contraction.

tonic-clonic (**TON**-ik-**KLON**-ik) The body alternates between excessive muscular rigidity (tonic) and jerking muscular contractions (clonic).

tonic-clonic seizure (**TON**-ik-**KLON**-ik **SEE**-zhur) Generalized seizure due to epileptic activity in all or most of the brain.

tonometer (toh-**NOM**-eh-ter) Instrument for determining intraocular pressure.

tonometry (toh-**NOM**-eh-tree) The measurement of intraocular pressure.

tonsil (**TON**-sill) Mass of lymphoid tissue on either side of the throat at the back of the tongue.

tonsillectomy (ton-sih-**LEK**-toh-me) Surgical removal of the tonsils.

tonsillitis (ton-sih-**LIE**-tis) Inflammation of the tonsils.

topical (**TOP**-ih-kal) Medication applied to the skin to obtain a local effect.

torsion (**TOR**-shun) The act or result of twisting.

Tourette syndrome (tur-**ET SIN**-drome) Disorder of multiple motor and vocal tics.

toxic (**TOK**-sick) Pertaining to a toxin.

toxicity (tok-**SIS**-ih-tee) The state of being poisonous.

toxin (**TOK**-sin) Poisonous substance formed by a cell or organism.

trachea (**TRAY**-kee-ah) Air tube from the larynx to the bronchi.

tracheal (**TRAY**-kee-al) Pertaining to the trachea.

tracheostomy (tray-kee-**OST**-oh-me) Incision into the windpipe into which a tube can be inserted to assist breathing.

tracheotomy (tray-kee-**OT**-oh-me) Incision made into the trachea to create a tracheostomy.

tract (TRACKT) An elongated pathway.

traction (**TRAK**-shun) Pulling or dragging force.

trait (TRAYT) A discrete characteristic that has a known quality.

tranquilizer (**TRANG**-kwih-lie-zer) Agent that calms without sedating or depressing.

transdermal (tranz-**DER**-mal) Going across or through the skin.

transfusion (tranz-**FYU**-zhun) Transfer of blood or a blood component from donor to recipient.

transient (**TRAN**-see-ent) Not permanent.

transient ischemic attack (TIA) (TRAN-see-ent is-KEE-mik a-TACK) Temporary blockage of a cerebral blood vessel resulting in stroke–like symptoms lasting less than 24 hours.

transnasal (trans-NAY-zal) Through the nose.

transplant (TRANZ-plant) The tissue or organ used; *or* the act of transferring tissue from one person to another.

transplantation (TRANZ-plan-TAY-shun) The moving of tissue or an organ from one person or place to another.

transthoracic (tranz-thor-ASS-ik) Going through the chest wall.

transurethral (TRANZ-you-REE-thral) Procedure performed through the urethra.

transverse (tranz-VERS) Horizontal plane dividing the body into upper and lower portions.

transverse fracture (tranz-VERS FRAK-chur) A fracture perpendicular to the long axis of the bone.

tremor (TREM-or) Small, shaking, involuntary, repetitive movements of hands, extremities, neck, or jaw.

triceps brachii (TRY-sepz BRAY-key-eye) Muscle of the arm that has three heads or points of origin.

Trichomonas (trik-oh-MOH-nas) A parasite causing an STD.

trichomoniasis (TRIK-oh-moh-NIE-ah-sis) Infection with *Trichomonas vaginalis.*

tricuspid (try-KUSS-pid) Having three points; a tricuspid heart valve has three flaps.

trigeminal (try-GEM-in-al) The fifth (V) cranial nerve, which has three branches supplying the face.

triglyceride (try-GLISS-eh-ride) Lipid containing three fatty acids.

trimester (TRY-mes-ter) One-third of the length of a full-term pregnancy.

triplegia (try-PLEE-jee-ah) Paralysis of three limbs.

triplegic (try-PLEE-jik) Pertaining to or suffering from triplegia.

trochlear (TROHK-lee-ar) Smooth articular surface of bone on which another glides.

trochlear (TROHK-lee-ar) Pertaining to a trochlea.

tropic (TROH-pik) Tropic hormones stimulate other endocrine glands to produce hormones.

tuberculosis (too-BER-kyu-LOW-sis) Infectious disease that can infect any organ or tissue.

tumor (TOO-mor) Any abnormal swelling.

tunica (TYU-nih-kah) A covering layer in the wall of a blood vessel or other tubular structure.

tunica vaginalis (TYU-nih-kah vaj-ih-NAHL-iss) The sheath of the testis and epididymis.

tympanic (tim-PAN-ik) Pertaining to the tympanic membrane (eardrum) or tympanic cavity.

tympanostomy (tim-pan-OS-toh-me) Surgically created new opening in the tympanic membrane to allow fluid to drain from the middle ear.

U

ulcer (UL-sir) Erosion of an area of skin or mucosa.

ulceration (ul-sir-AY-shun) Formation of an ulcer or ulcers.

ulcerative (UL-sir-ah-tiv) Marked by an ulcer or ulcers.

ulna (UL-nah) The medial and larger of the bones of the forearm.

ulnar (UL-nar) Pertaining to the ulna or to any of the structures (artery, vein, nerve) named after it.

ultrasonography (UL-trah-soh-NOG-rah-fee) Delineation of deep structures using sound waves.

ultraviolet (ul-trah-VIE-oh-let) Light rays at a higher frequency than the violet end of the spectrum.

umbilical (um-BILL-ih-kal) Pertaining to the umbilicus or the center of the abdomen.

umbilicus (um-BILL-ih-kuss) Pit in the abdomen where the umbilical cord entered the fetus.

unilateral (you-nih-LAT-er-al) Pertaining to one side.

unoxygenated (un-OCK-suh-je-nay-ted) Not combined with oxygen.

urea (you-REE-ah) End product of nitrogen metabolism.

uremia (you-REE-me-ah) An accumulation of nitrogenous waste products within blood

ureter (you-REE-ter) Tube that connects a kidney to the urinary bladder.

ureteral (you-REE-ter-al) Pertaining to the ureter.

ureteroscope (you-REE-ter-oh-scope) Endoscope to view the inside of the ureter.

ureteroscopy (you-REE-ter-OS-koh-pee) To examine the ureter.

urethra (you-REE-thra) Canal leading from the bladder to the outside.

urethritis (you-ree-THRI-tis) Inflammation of the urethra.

uric acid (YUR-ik ASS-id) A chemical of white crystals poorly soluble in urine

uricosuric (YUR-ih-koh-SU-rik) Pertaining to excessive amounts of uric acid in urine

urinalysis (yur-ih-NAL-ih-sis) Examination of urine to separate it into its elements and define their kind and/or quantity.

urinary (YUR-in-ar-ee) Pertaining to urine.

urinate (YUR-in-ate) To pass urine.

urination (yur-ih-NAY-shun) The act of passing urine.

urine (YUR-in) Fluid and dissolved substances excreted by the kidney.

urological (yur-oh-LOJ-ih-kal) Pertaining to urology.

urologist (you-ROL-oh-jist) Medical specialist in disorders of the urinary system.

urology (you-ROL-oh-jee) Medical specialty of disorders of the urinary system.

urticaria (ur-tee-KARE-ee-ah) Rash of itchy wheals (hives).

uterine (YOU-ter-in) Pertaining to the uterus.

uterus (YOU-ter-us) Organ in which a fertilized egg develops into a fetus.

uvea (YOU-vee-ah) Middle coat of the eyeball—includes the iris, ciliary body, and choroid.

uveitis (you-vee-EYE-tis) Inflammation of the uvea.

uvula (YOU-vyu-lah) Fleshy projection of the soft palate.

V

vaccinate (VAK-sin-ate) To administer a vaccine.

vaccination (vak-sih-NAY-shun) Administration of a vaccine.

vaccine (VAK-seen) Preparation to generate active immunity.

vagina (vah-JIE-nah) Female genital canal extending from the uterus to the vulva.

vaginal (VAJ-ih-nal) Pertaining to the vagina.

vaginitis (vah-jih-NIE-tis) Inflammation of the vagina.

vaginosis (vah-jih-NOH-sis) A disease of the vagina.

vagus (VAY-gus) Tenth (X) cranial nerve; supplies many different organs throughout the body.

varicella (VAIR-uh-SELL-uh) An acute infectious disease caused by the varicella-zoster virus. Also called *varicella*.

varicocele (VAIR-ih-koh-seal) Varicose veins of the spermatic cord.

varicose (VAIR-ih-kos) Characterized by or affected with varices.

varicosities (vair-ih-KOS-ih-teez) Collection of varicose veins.

varix (VAIR-iks) Dilated, tortuous vein. Plural *varices*.

vasectomy (vah-SEK-toh-me) Excision of a segment of the ductus deferens.

vasoconstriction (VAY-soh-con-STRIK-shun) Reduction in the diameter of a blood vessel.

vasodilation (VAY-soh-die-LAY-shun) Increase in the diameter of a blood vessel.

vasovasostomy (VAY-soh-vay-SOS-toh-me) Reanastomosis of the ductus deferens to restore the flow of sperm. Also called *vasectomy reversal*.

vegetative (VEJ-eh-tay-tiv) Functioning unconsciously, as plant life is assumed to do.

vein (VANE) Blood vessel carrying blood toward the heart.

vena cava (VEE-nah KAY-vah) One of the two largest veins in the body. Plural *venae cavae*.

venogram (VEE-noh-gram) Radiograph of veins after injection of radiopaque contrast material.

venous (VEE-nuss) Pertaining to a vein.

ventilation (ven-tih-LAY-shun) Movement of gases into and out of the lungs.

ventilator (VEN-tih-lay-tor) Device that breathes for the patient.

ventral (VEN-tral) Pertaining to the belly or situated nearer to the surface of the belly.

ventricle (VEN-trih-kel) Chamber of the heart (pumps blood) or brain (produces cerebrospinal fluid).

venule (VEN-yule or VEEN-yule) Small vein leading from the capillary network.

vermiform (VER-mih-form) Worm shaped; used as a descriptor for the appendix.

vernix caseosa (VER-nicks kay-see-OH-sah) Cheesy substance covering the skin of the fetus.

verruca (ver-ROO-cah) Wart caused by a virus.

vertebra (VER-teh-brah) One of the bones of the spinal column. Plural *vertebrae*.

vertebral (VER-teh-bral) Pertaining to a vertebra.

vertex (VER-teks) Topmost point of the vault of the skull.

vertigo (VER-tih-go) Sensation of spinning or whirling.

vesicle (VES-ih-kull) Small sac containing liquid; for example, a blister.

vestibular (ves-TIB-you-lar) Pertaining to the vestibule.

vestibular bulb (ves-TIB-you-lar BULB) Structure on each side of the entrance to the vagina.

vestibule (VES-tih-byul) Space at the entrance to a canal.

vestibulectomy (ves-tib-you-LEK-toh-me) Surgical excision of the vulva.

villus (VILL-us) Thin, hairlike projection, particularly of a mucous membrane lining a cavity. Plural *villi*.

virus (VIE-rus) Group of infectious agents that require living cells for growth and reproduction.

viscera (VISS-er-ah) Internal organs, particularly in the abdomen.

visceral (VISS-er-al) Pertaining to the internal organs.

viscosity (viss-KOS-ih-tee) The resistance of a fluid to flow.

viscous (VISS-kus) Sticky fluid that is resistant to flow.

viscus (VISS-kus) Any single internal organ.

visual acuity (VIH-zhoo-al ah-KYU-ih-tee) Sharpness and clearness of vision.

vitamin (VYE-tah-min) Essential organic substance necessary in small amounts for normal cell function.

vitreous (VIT-ree-us) Vitreous humor is a gelatinous liquid in the posterior cavity of the eyeball with the appearance of glass.

vocal (VOH-kal) Pertaining to the voice.

vocation (voh-KAY-shun) An occupation for which a person is trained or qualified to perform.

void (VOYD) To evacuate urine or feces.

voluntary muscle (VOL-un-tare-ee MUSS-el) Muscle that is under the control of the will.

vulva (VUL-vah) Female external genitalia.

vulvar (VUL-var) Pertaining to the vulva.

vulvodynia (vul-voh-DIN-ee-uh) Chronic vulvar pain.

vulvovaginal (VUL-voh-VAJ-ih-nal) Pertaining to the vulva and vagina.

vulvovaginitis (VUL-voh-vaj-ih-NIE-tis) Inflammation of the vulva and vagina.

W

warfarin (WAR-fuh-rin) Anticoagulant; also used as rat poison; trade name *Coumadin*.

Weber test (VAY-ber, WEB-er TEST) Test for sensorineural hearing loss.

wheal (WHEEL) Small, itchy swelling of the skin. Wheals raised by an injection do not itch. Also called *hives*.

whiplash (WHIP-lash) Symptoms caused by sudden, uncontrolled extension and flexion of the neck, often in an automobile accident.

white matter (WIGHT MAT-er) Regions of the brain and spinal cord occupied by bundles of axons.

whooping cough (HOO-ping KAWF) Infectious disease with spasmodic, intense cough ending on a whoop (stridor). Also called *pertussis*.

Wilms tumor (WILMZ TOO-mor) Cancerous kidney tumor of childhood. Also known as *nephroblastoma*.

wound (WOOND) Any injury that interrupts the continuity of skin or a mucous membrane.

X

xenograft (**ZEN**-oh-graft) A graft from another species. Also called *heterograft*.

Y

yeast (YEEST) Microscopic fungus.

Z

zygoma (zye-**GO**-mah) Bone that forms the prominence of the cheek.

zygomatic (zye-go-**MAT**-ik) Pertaining to the zygoma.

zygote (**ZYE**-goat) Cell resulting from the union of the sperm and egg.

E

F

G

Lobectomy, 205, 206, 351
Lobe, of lung, 192, 194
LOC (loss of consciousness), 259
Lochia, 421–422
Long bones, 65
Longevity, 455
Loop diuretics, 374
Loop electrosurgical excision procedure (LEEP), 414
Loss of consciousness (LOC), 259
Lotion, 53
Louse, 44, 45
Low blood pressure, 12
Low-density lipoprotein (LDL), 135, 140
Lower leg, 101
Lower respiratory tract, 190–193
    disorders of, 196–199
    mechanics of respiration in, 195, 196
    trachea, lungs, and tracheobronchial tree in, 191, 192
LPN (licensed practical nurse), 409
LSD (lysergic acid diethylamide), 277
LT4 (levothyroxine), 351
L-thyroxine, 352
Lumbar puncture, 274
Lumbar region, 31, 68, 255
Lumpectomy, 437–438
Lung abscess, 198
Lung cancer, 198
Lungs, 190, 192
LUQ (left upper quadrant), 31
Luteinizing hormone (LH), 334
Lymph, 27, 152–153
Lymphadenectomy, 167–168
Lymphadenitis, 167–168
Lymphadenopathy, 167–168
Lymphangiogram, 176
Lymphatic, 27, 153
Lymphatic collecting vessels, 152
Lymphatic ducts, 153
Lymphatic network, 152
Lymphatic organs, 154
Lymphatic system, 26, 152–168
Lymphatic tissues and cells, 153
Lymphatic trunks, 153
Lymphedema, 167–168
Lymph node, 153, 172
Lymphocytes, 147, 152
Lymphoid, 153
Lymphoma, 167–168
Lysergic acid diethylamide (LSD), 277

M

Macrocyte, 5–6, 175
Macrocytic, 6, 174–175
Macrophage, 147
Macula lutea, 296, 297
Macular degeneration, 302
Macule, 42, 43
Magnesium (Mg), 219
Magnetic resonance angiography (MRA), 202, 274
Magnetic resonance imaging (MRI), 87, 110, 136, 274, 326, 349, 371
Maintenance rehabilitation, 107
Major anatomical plane, 30

Major depression, 282
Majus/majora, 398
Malabsorption, 220
Malabsorption syndromes, 230
Malaria, 171
Male infertility, 387–388
Male reproductive system, 379
    anatomy of, 378–382
    sexually transmitted diseases, 389–390
    spermatic ducts and accessory glands, 383
    testes and spermatic cord, 380–382
    testicular disorders, 386–387
Malformation, 448
Malignancy/malignant, 43
Malignant hypertension, 128
Malignant melanoma, 42
Malleus, 315, 316
Malnutrition, 230
ma/mata, 11
Mammary, 431–432
Mammary gland, 431
Mammogram, 436, 438
Mammography, 437–438
Mammoplasty, 59, 60
Mandible, 69, 70
Mandibular, 70
Maneuver, 327
Mania, 282, 283
Manic, 283
Manic-depressive disorder, 282, 283
Marijuana (THC), 277
Marrow, 65, 66
Mastalgia, 433–434
Mastectomy, 437–438
Masticate/mastication, 211
Mastitis, 433–434
Mastoid, 315, 316
Maternal, 162, 429–430, 447–448
Maternal blood, 161
Matrix, 24, 25, 38
    blood, 145
Mature, 4, 6, 443
Mature-onset diabetes of the young (MODY), 344
Maturity, 443
Maxilla, 69, 70
Maxillary bones, 69, 70
Maxillary sinuses, 187
Maximus, 101, 102
MCL (medial collateral ligament), 24
MCS (minimally conscious state), 456
MCV (mean corpuscular volume), 174
MD (Doctor of Medicine), 64, 97
MDMA (methylenedioxymethamphetamine), 277
Mean corpuscular volume (MCV), 174
Meatal, 316
Meatus, 314, 316, 363
Mechanical digestion, 210
Mechanical ventilation, 196, 198, 205
Meconium, 426–427, 443
Meconium aspiration syndrome, 426, 443
Medial, 30, 31
Medial collateral ligament (MCL), 24, 74
Medial menisci, 74
Mediastinal, 192